OPERATIVE TECHNIQUES IN COLON AND RECTAL SURGERY

Second Edition

OPERATIVE TECHNIQUES IN COLON AND RECTAL SURGERY

Second Edition

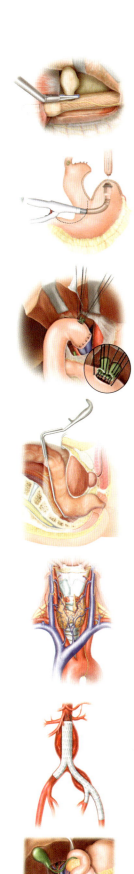

Operative Techniques in Colon and Rectal Surgery

Second Edition

Mary T. Hawn, MD, MPH
EDITOR-IN-CHIEF

Emile Holman Professor and Chair
Department of Surgery
Stanford University School of Medicine
Stanford, California

EDITOR

Daniel Albo MD, PhD, FACS
Chair, Department of Surgery
The University of Texas Rio Grande Valley (UTRGV)
  School of Medicine
Harlingen, Texas

Illustrations by: Body Scientific International, LLC

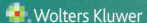 Wolters Kluwer

Philadelphia · Baltimore · New York · London
Buenos Aires · Hong Kong · Sydney · Tokyo

Senior Acquisitions Editor: Keith Donnellan
Senior Development Editor: Ashley Fischer
Development Editor: Barton Dudlick
Editorial Coordinator: Erin E. Hernandez
Marketing Manager: Kirsten Watrud
Production Project Manager: Bridgett Dougherty
Manager, Graphic Arts & Design: Stephen Druding
Manufacturing Coordinator: Beth Welsh
Prepress Vendor: TNQ Technologies

Copyright © 2024 Wolters Kluwer.

Copyright © 2015 Wolters Kluwer Health/Lippincott Williams & Wilkins. All rights reserved. This book is protected by copyright. No part of this book may be reproduced or transmitted in any form or by any means, including as photocopies or scanned-in or other electronic copies, or utilized by any information storage and retrieval system without written permission from the copyright owner, except for brief quotations embodied in critical articles and reviews. Materials appearing in this book prepared by individuals as part of their official duties as U.S. government employees are not covered by the above-mentioned copyright. To request permission, please contact Wolters Kluwer at Two Commerce Square, 2001 Market Street, Philadelphia, PA 19103, via email at permissions@lww.com, or via our website at shop.lww.com (products and services).

9 8 7 6 5 4 3 2 1

Printed in Mexico.

Library of Congress Cataloging-in-Publication Data

ISBN-13: 978-1-9751-7652-5

Cataloging in Publication data available on request from publisher.

This work is provided "as is," and the publisher disclaims any and all warranties, express or implied, including any warranties as to accuracy, comprehensiveness, or currency of the content of this work.

This work is no substitute for individual patient assessment based upon healthcare professionals' examination of each patient and consideration of, among other things, age, weight, gender, current or prior medical conditions, medication history, laboratory data and other factors unique to the patient. The publisher does not provide medical advice or guidance and this work is merely a reference tool. Healthcare professionals, and not the publisher, are solely responsible for the use of this work including all medical judgments and for any resulting diagnosis and treatments.

Given continuous, rapid advances in medical science and health information, independent professional verification of medical diagnoses, indications, appropriate pharmaceutical selections and dosages, and treatment options should be made and healthcare professionals should consult a variety of sources. When prescribing medication, healthcare professionals are advised to consult the product information sheet (the manufacturer's package insert) accompanying each drug to verify, among other things, conditions of use, warnings and side effects and identify any changes in dosage schedule or contraindications, particularly if the medication to be administered is new, infrequently used or has a narrow therapeutic range. To the maximum extent permitted under applicable law, no responsibility is assumed by the publisher for any injury and/or damage to persons or property, as a matter of products liability, negligence law or otherwise, or from any reference to or use by any person of this work.

shop.lww.com

Contributing Authors

Matthew Albert, MD, FACS, FASCRS
Medical Director, Surgical Innovation
Digestive Health and Surgical Institute
AdventHealth Orlando
Department of Colorectal Surgery
AdventHealth
Orlando, Florida

Daniel Albo, MD, PhD, FACS
Chair, Department of Surgery
Director, Cancer Center Service Line
The University of Texas Rio Grande Valley
   (UTRGV) School of Medicine
Harlingen Texas

Daniel A. Anaya, MD
Chief, Division of GI Surgery
Head, Hepatobiliary Section
Department of GI Oncology
Moffitt Cancer Center
Tampa, Florida

Avo Artinyan, MD, MS
CEO
Academic Surgical Associates
Los Angeles, California

Erik Paul Askenasy, MD
Assistant Professor of Surgery
Department of Surgery
McGovern Medical School
University of Texas Health Science Center at
   Houston
Houston, Texas

Valerie P. Bauer, MD, FACS, FASCRS
Director Colorectal Surgery
Department of Surgery
Cape Regional Medical Center
Cape May Court House, New Jersey

Jaime L. Bohl, MD
Associate Professor of Surgery
Chief, Division of Colon and Rectal
   Surgery
Department of Surgery
Virginia Commonwealth University
VCU Health
Richmond, Virginia

George J. Chang, MD, MS
Chair and Professor
Department of Colon and Rectal Surgery
The University of Texas MD Anderson
   Cancer Center
Houston, Texas

Navin Rajindra Changoor, MD
Colon and Rectal Surgeon
Department of Colon and Rectal Surgery
AdventHealth Medical Group
Orlando, Florida

William C. Chapman, Jr., MD
Department of Surgery
Washington University School of Medicine
Saint Louis, Missouri

Angel M. Charles, MD
Department of General Surgery
University of Florida College of Medicine
Gainesville, Florida

Robert R. Cima, MD, MA
Professor of Surgery
Division of Colon and Rectal Surgery
Mayo Clinic College of Medicine and Science
Rochester, Minnesota

Martin A. Croce, MD, FACS
Professor of Surgery
Department of Surgery
University of Tennessee Health Science Center
Sr. Vice President and Chief Medical Officer
Regional One Health
Memphis, Tennessee

Bidhan Das, MD
Clinical Associate Professor
Colon and Rectal Surgery
Department of Surgery
University of Texas Health Science Center at
   Houston
Houston, Texas

Vijian Dhevan, MD, MBA
Vice Chair for Clinical Affairs
Department of Surgery
The University of Texas Rio Grande Valley
   (UTRGV) School of Medicine
Harlingen, Texas

Kristen D. Donohue, MD
Assistant Professor
Department of Surgery
Rutgers New Jersey Medical School
New Brunswick, New Jersey

Antonio D'Urso, MD, PhD
Senior Consultant
IRCAD
Department of Digestive and Visceral
   Surgery
Nouvel Hospital Civil
University Hospital of Strasbourg
Strasbourg, France

Roosevelt Fajardo, MD, MBA, FACS
Associate Professor
Los Andes University School of Medicine
Department of Surgery
Director of Education
Fundación Santa Fe de Bogota University
   Hospital
Bogotá, Colombia

Barry W. Feig, MD
Professor of Surgical Oncology
Department of Surgical Oncology
The University of Texas MD Anderson
   Cancer Center
Houston, Texas

Daniel L. Feingold, MD, FACS, FASCRS
Professor of Surgery
Department of Surgery
Rutgers New Jersey Medical School
New Brunswick, New Jersey

Wayne A. I. Frederick, MD, MBA
Professor
Department of Surgery
Howard University
Washington, DC

CONTRIBUTING AUTHORS

Roger M. Galindo, MD
Assistant Professor of Surgery
Department of Surgery
The University of Texas Rio Grande Valley
(UTRGV) School of Medicine
Trauma Medical Director
Department of Surgery
Valley Baptist Medical Center Harlingen
Harlingen, Texas

Julio Garcia-Aguilar, MD, PhD
Benno C. Schmidt Chair in Surgical Oncology
Chief, Colorectal Service
Department of Surgery
Director, Colorectal Cancer Research Center
Memorial Sloan Kettering Cancer Center
Professor of Surgery
Weill Cornell Medical College
New York, New York

Kelly A. Garrett, MD
Associate Professor of Surgery
Department of General Surgery
New York Presbyterian Hospital
Weill Cornell Medicine
New York, New York

Eric Mitchell Haas, MD
Chief, Division of Colon and Rectal Surgery
Houston Methodist Hospital
Houston, Texas

Karin M. Hardiman, MD, PhD
Associate Professor
Department of Surgery
University of Alabama at Birmingham School
of Medicine
Surgeon
University of Alabama at Birmingham Health
System
Birmingham Veterans Affairs Medical System
Birmingham, Alabama

Andrew G. Hill, MBChB, MD, FRACS, FACS
Professor of Surgery
Department of Surgery
University of Auckland
Middlemore Hospital
Auckland, New Zealand

Joshua S. Hill, MD
Assistant Professor
Division of Surgical Oncology
Department of Surgery
Levine Cancer Institute
Atrium Health
Charlotte, North Carolina

Mehraneh Dorna Jafari, MD, FACS, FASCRS
Associate Professor
Department of Surgery
Weill Cornell Medicine
New York, New York

Anish Jay Jain, MD
Department of Surgery
Howard University College of Medicine
Howard University Hospital
Washington, DC

Lillian S. Kao, MD, MS
Professor
Department of Surgery
McGovern Medical School at University of
Texas
Houston, Texas

Hasan T. Kirat, MD
Associate Professor of Surgery
Department of Surgery
New York University
Colorectal Surgeon
Department of Surgery
New York University Langone Health
New York, New York

Cherry E. Koh, MBBS(Hons), MS, PhD, FRACS
Associate Professor
Department of Colorectal Surgery
Royal Prince Alfred Hospital
Director of Surgical Outcomes Research
Centre
Sydney, New South Wales, Australia

Sang W. Lee, MD
Professor and Chief, Colon and Rectal
Surgery
Department of Colon and Rectal Surgery
Keck School of Medicine of the University of
Southern California
Los Angeles, California

Edward A. Levine, MD
Professor of Surgery
Department of Surgery
Wake Forest University School of Medicine
Winston-Salem, North Carolina

Luis Jorge Lombana, MD
Colo-Rectal Surgeon
Department of Surgery
Hospital San Ignacio Universidad Javeriana
Bogotá, Columbia

Louis Jude Magnotti, MD, MS
Professor
Department of Surgery
University of Tennessee Health Science Center
Memphis, Tennessee

Lillias Holmes Maguire, MD
Assistant Professor
Department of Surgery
Perelman School of Medicine at the University
of Pennsylvania
Hospital of the University of Pennsylvania
Philadelphia, Pennsylvania

Michael R. Marco, MD
Postdoctoral Clinical Fellow
Department of Colon and Rectal Surgery
Weill Cornell Medicine
Colorectal Surgery Clinical Fellow
Department of Colon and Rectal Surgery
New York Presbyterian Hospital
New York, New York

Jacques Marescaux, MD, FACS, Hon. FRCS, Hon. FASA, Hon. FJSES, Hon. FJSS
Professor of Surgery
President and Founder of IRCAD
Research Institute against Cancers of the
Digestive System
University Hospital of Strasbourg
Strasbourg, France

John H. Marks, MD, FACS, FASCRS
Professor
Lankenau Institute for Medical Research
Chief of Colorectal Surgery
Lankenau Medical Center
Wynnewood, Pennsylvania

Craig A. Messick, MD
Associate Professor of Surgery
Department of Colon and Rectal Surgery
The University of Texas MD Anderson
Cancer Center
Houston, Texas

Stefanos G. Millas, MD
Associate Professor
Department of Surgery
McGovern Medical School at University of
Texas
LBJ General Hospital
Houston, Texas

Somala Mohammed, MD, MPH
Assistant Professor of Surgery
Harvard Medical School
Pediatric Surgeon
Department of General Surgery
Boston Children's Hospital
Boston, Massachusetts

Jayson Moloney, MBBS
Senior Lecturer
University of Queensland
Staff Surgeon
Department of Colorectal Surgery
Royal Brisbane and Women's Hospital
Brisbane, Australia

Arden M. Morris, MD, MPH
Professor
Department of Surgery
Stanford University School of Medicine
Stanford, California

CONTRIBUTING AUTHORS

Matthew G. Mutch, MD
Solan and Bettie Gershman Professor of
Surgery
Chief, Section of Colon and Rectal
Surgery
Department of Surgery
Washington University School of
Medicine
Saint Louis, Missouri

Didier Mutter, MD, PhD, FACS, FRSM
Professor of Surgery
IRCAD
Chair, Digestive and Endocrine Surgery
Department
Department of Digestive and Endocrine
Surgery
University Hospital of Strasbourg
Strasbourg, France

Govind Nandakumar, MD, FACS, FASCRS
Chief, GI Surgery
Department of Surgery
Mawipal Hospitals
Bangalore, India

Dana M. Omer, MD
Research Scholar
Department of Surgery, Colorectal Service
Memorial Sloan Kettering Cancer Center
New York, New York

Tolulope A. Oyetunji, MD, MPH, FACS
Associate Professor of Surgery
Department of Surgery
University of Missouri-Kansas City School of
Medicine
Director, Health Outcomes Research
Department of Surgery
Children's Mercy Hospital
Kansas City, Missouri

Devanshi D. Patel, MD
Department of Surgery
University of Tennessee Health Science
Center
Memphis, Tennessee

Rodrigo Pedraza, MD
Colon and Rectal Surgeon
Center for Advanced Surgery
The Oregon Clinic
Portland, Oregon

Alessio Pigazzi, MD, PhD
Chief, Colorectal Surgery
Department of Surgery
Weill Cornell Medicine
New York, New York

Harsha Polavarapu, MD, FACS, FASCRS
Attending Surgeon
Department of Surgery
Blessing Hospital
Quincy, Illinois

Dhruvesh M. Ramson, MBBS (Hons)
Adjunct Research Associate
Department of Surgery
Monash University
Melbourne, Australia
Surgical Registrar
Department of Surgery
Counties Manakau Health
Auckland, New Zealand

Scott E. Regenbogen, MD, MPH
Associate Professor
Department of Surgery
University of Michigan Medical School
Ann Arbor, Michigan

Henry A. Reinhart, MD
Assistant Professor
Department of Surgery
The University of Texas Rio Grande Valley
(UTRGV) School of Medicine
Harlingen, Texas

Feza H. Remzi, MD
Professor of Surgery
Department of Surgery
New York University
Colorectal Surgeon
Department of Surgery
New York University Langone Health
New York, New York

Saul J. Rugeles, MD
Professor of Surgery
Department of Surgery
Pontificia Universidad Javeriana
Colon and Rectal Surgeon
Department of Colon and Rectal Surgery
Hospital Universitario San Ignacio
Bogotá, Colombia

Perisa Ruhi-Williams, MD
Department of Surgery
University of California, Irvine Medical
Center
Orange, California

Tarik Sammour, BHB, MBChB, FRACS, CSSANZ, PhD
Associate Professor
Faculty of Medical and Health Sciences
University of Adelaide
Colorectal Unit
Department of Surgery
Royal Adelaide Hospital
Adelaide, Australia

William M. Sánchez, MD, FACS
Chair, Department of Surgery
Universidad Militar Nueva Granada
Hospital Militar Central
Bogotá, Colombia

Brendan F. Scully, MD
Fellow
Department of Colon and Rectal Surgery
Rutgers New Jersey Medical School
New Brunswick, New Jersey

Shiva Seetahal, MD, FACS
Medical Director, Bariatric and Weight Loss
Surgery
AdventHealth Heart of Florida
Davenport, Florida

Perry Shen, MD, FACS, FSSO
Professor of Surgery
Department of Surgery
Wake Forest University Medical Center
Winston-Salem, North Carolina

Eric J. Silberfein, MD, FACS
Associate Professor of Surgery
Associate Program Director, General Surgery
Division of Surgical Oncology
Michael E. DeBakey Department of Surgery
Baylor College of Medicine
Chief, Surgical Oncology
Chief, General Surgery
Ben Taub Hospital
Huston, Texas

Mark Soliman, MD, FACS, FASCRS
Chair, Department of Colon and Rectal
Surgery
AdventHealth Medical Group
Orlando, Florida

Michael J. Solomon, MB, BCH (Hons), BAO, MSc, DMedSc (USYD), DMed (NUI)
Professor of Surgical Research
Faculty of Medicine and Health
University of Sydney
Academic Head & VMO
Department of Colorectal Surgery
Royal Prince Alfred Hospital
Sydney Local Health District
New South Wales, Australia

Andrew RL Stevenson, MB, BS, FRACS, FASCRS (Hon)
Clinical Professor
Department of Surgery
University of Queensland
Senior Colorectal Surgeon
Department of Colorectal Surgery
Royal Brisbane and Women's Hospital
Brisbane, Australia

Zhifei Sun, MD
Assistant Professor
Section of Colorectal Surgery
Department of Surgery
Georgetown University Medical Center
Washington, DC

David Graham Taylor, MBBS, FRACS
Colorectal Surgeon
Department of Surgery
Royal Brisbane and Women's Hospital
Herston, Queensland, Australia

James P. Taylor, MBBChir, MPH
Colorectal Fellow
Department of Colon and Rectal Surgery
New York Presbyterian Hospital
Weill Cornell Medicine
New York, New York

Ryan M. Thomas, MD
Associate Professor
Department of Surgery
University of Florida College of Medicine
Section Chief, Department of General Surgery
North Florida/South Georgia Veterans Healthcare System
Gainesville, Florida

Kathrin Mayer Troppmann, MD, FACS
Professor Emeritus
Department of Surgery
University of California Davis School of Medicine
Sacramento, California

Cristian D. Valenzuela, MD
Clinical Fellow, Complex General Surgical Oncology
Department of Surgical Oncology
Wake Forest University School of Medicine
Wake Forest Baptist Atrium Health
Winston-Salem, North Carolina

Elsa B. Valsdóttir, MD
Assistant Professor
University of Iceland
Surgeon
Department of Surgery
Landspítali University Hospital
Reykjavík, Iceland

Oliver Adrian Varban, MD
Associate Professor of Surgery
Chief, Division of Minimally Invasive Surgery
Department of General Surgery
University of Michigan Medical School
Ann Arbor, Michigan

Theodoros Voloyiannis, MD, FACS, FASCRS
Chair, Colon and Rectal Surgery
US Oncology Network
Medical Director, Oncologic Surgery
HCA Houston Healthcare, Gulf Coast Division
Houston, Texas

Konstantinos I. Votanopoulos, MD, PhD, FACS
Professor of Surgery
Department of Surgery
Wake Forest University School of Medicine
Winston-Salem, North Carolina

Rebecca L. Wiatrek, MD, FACS
Surgical Oncologist
Texas Oncology Surgical Specialists
Austin, Texas

Curtis J. Wray, MD, MS
Professor
Department of Surgery
McGovern Medical School at University of Texas
Houston, Texas

Jane Yang, MD
Fellow
Colorectal Surgery
Department of Surgery
Lankenau Medical Center
Wynnewood, Pennsylvania

Y. Nancy You, MD, MHSc
Professor
Department of Colon and Rectal Surgery
The University of Texas MD Anderson Cancer Center
Houston, Texas

Jonathan Benjamin Yuval, MD
Fellow
Department of Surgery
Memorial Sloan Kettering Cancer Center
New York, New York

Series Preface

Operative interventions are complex, technically demanding, and rapidly evolving. *Operative Techniques in Surgery* seeks to provide highly visual step-by-step instructions to perform these complex tasks. The series is organized anatomically with volumes covering foregut surgery, hepato-pancreato-biliary surgery, and colorectal surgery. Breast and endocrine surgery as well as other topics related to surgical oncology are included in a separate volume. Modern approaches to vascular surgery are covered in a standalone volume. We also have a first edition standalone volume dedicated to trauma surgery. Additionally, many chapters are augmented by video clips dynamically demonstrating the critical steps of the procedure throughout the series.

The series editors are renowned surgeons with expertise in their respective fields. Each is a leader in the discipline of surgery, each recognized for superb surgical judgment and outstanding operative skill. Breast surgery, endocrine procedures, and surgical oncology topics were edited by Dr. Michael S. Sabel of the University of Michigan. Thoracic and upper gastrointestinal surgery topics were edited by Dr. Aurora D. Pryor of Donald and Barbara Zucker School of Medicine at Hofstra/Northwell, with Dr. Steven J. Hughes of the University of Florida directing the section on hepato-pancreatico-biliary surgery. Dr. Daniel Albo of University of Texas Rio Grande directed the section dedicated to colorectal surgery. Dr. Kellie R. Brown of Medical College of Wisconsin edited topics related to vascular surgery, including both open and endovascular approaches. New this year, we have added a section on Trauma and Critical Surgery, led by Dr. Amy J. Goldberg of Temple University.

In turn, the series editors recruited contributors that are world-renowned; the resulting volumes have a distinctly international flavor. Surgery is a visual discipline. *Operative Techniques in Surgery* is lavishly illustrated with a compelling combination of line art and intraoperative photography. The illustrated material provides a uniform style emphasizing clarity and strong, clean lines. Intraoperative photographs are taken from the perspective of the operating surgeon so that operations might be visualized as they would be performed.

The accompanying text is intentionally sparse, with a focus on crucial operative details and important aspects of postoperative management and potential complications. The series is designed for surgeons at all levels of practice, from surgical residents to advanced practice fellows to surgeons of wide experience.

Operative Techniques in Surgery would be possible only at Wolters Kluwer, an organization of unique vision, organization, and talent of Brian Brown, executive editor, Keith Donnellan, senior acquisition editor, and Ashley Fischer, senior development editor.

I am deeply indebted to Dr. Michael W. Mulholland, a master surgeon and leader and the editor in chief of the first series for *Operative Techniques in Surgery*. Without his leadership, this project would not have been successful. I am grateful to our new and returning series editors for their vision on how to make the second edition even more impactful. Curating and editing a major surgical techniques textbook during a worldwide pandemic has not been seamless, yet the outcome is masterful.

Mary T. Hawn, MD, MPH

Preface

Operative Techniques in Colon and Rectal Surgery, Second Edition, has been created as a comprehensive operative resource of surgeons at all levels of practice, from surgical residents to fellows and to practicing surgeons. Written by master surgeons, the chapters are presented in outline form, starting with the key elements of preoperative care, then focusing heavily on operative technique, and including essential aspects of postoperative management. The procedures are organized in a step-by-step fashion, with superb intraoperative photography and detailed artwork composed by a single artistic team. This highly visual format is particularly striking on electronic media devices, a necessary element of any modern textbook.

The authors featured in *Operative Techniques in Colon and Rectal Surgery* are a collection of international experts, selected because they are preeminent surgeon-educators in colorectal surgery, and leading innovators in the development of new surgical techniques. Special emphasis has been placed on minimally invasive approaches to the surgical treatment of colorectal disease. When multiple techniques may be used for a specific clinical problem, each approach is illustrated.

Special recognition is necessary for the editor-in-chief Mary T. Hawn, MD, MPH and the editorial and project management staff at Wolters Kluwer. Their vision and encouraging guidance are much appreciated.

Daniel Albo, MD, PhD, FACS

Contents

Contributing Authors v
Series Preface ix
Preface xi
Video Contents List xvii

Section I Surgery of the Small Intestine

1 Laparoscopic Small Bowel Resection 1
Oliver Adrian Varban

2 Strictureplasty and Small Bowel Bypass in Inflammatory Bowel Disease 9
James P. Taylor and Kelly A. Garrett

3 Surgical Management of Enterocutaneous Fistula 18
William M. Sánchez

4 End and Diverting Loop Ileostomies: Creation and Reversal 28
Kathrin Mayer Troppmann

5 Tube Jejunostomy: Open and Laparoscopic Techniques 42
Rebecca L. Wiatrek and Lillian S. Kao

Section II Surgery of the Colon, Appendix, Rectum, and Anus

6 Appendectomy: Laparoscopic Technique 48
Roosevelt Fajardo

7 Right Hemicolectomy: Open Technique 54
Somala Mohammed and Eric J. Silberfein

8 Laparoscopic Right Hemicolectomy 63
Craig A. Messick, Joshua S. Hill, and George J. Chang

9 Right Hemicolectomy: Hand-Assisted Laparoscopic Surgery (HALS) Technique 71
Matthew Albert and Harsha Polavarapu

10 Right Hemicolectomy: Single-Incision Laparoscopic Technique 78
Theodoros Voloyiannis

11 Right Hemicolectomy: Robotic-Assisted Technique 88
Michael R. Marco and Alessio Pigazzi

12 Transverse Colectomy: Open Technique 93
Y. Nancy You

13 Laparoscopic Transverse Colectomy 101
Govind Nandakumar and Sang W. Lee

14 Transverse Colectomy: Hand-Assisted Laparoscopic Surgery Technique 110
Daniel Albo

15 Left Hemicolectomy: Open Technique 118
Saul J. Rugeles and Luis Jorge Lombana

16 Left Hemicolectomy: Laparoscopic Technique 127
Erik Paul Askenasy

17 Left Hemicolectomy: Hand-Assisted Laparoscopic Technique 135
Kristen D. Donohue, Brendan F. Scully, and Daniel L. Feingold

18 Left Hemicolectomy: Robotic-Assisted Technique 143
Navin Rajindra Changoor and Mark Soliman

19 Sigmoid Colectomy: Open Technique 148
Anish Jay Jain, Shiva Seetahal, Tolulope A. Oyetunji, and Wayne A. I. Frederick

20 Sigmoid Colectomy: Laparoscopic Technique 157
Arden M. Morris

21 Sigmoid Colectomy: Hand-Assisted Laparoscopic Technique 165
Daniel A. Anaya and Daniel Albo

xiii

xiv CONTENTS

22 Sigmoid Colectomy: Single-Incision Laparoscopic Surgery Technique 176
Rodrigo Pedraza and Eric Mitchell Haas

23 Surgical Management of Complicated Diverticulitis: Perforation and Colovesical Fistula 185
Scott E. Regenbogen and Lillias Holmes Maguire

24 Total Abdominal Colectomy: Open Technique 195
Tarik Sammour and Andrew G. Hill

25 Total Abdominal Colectomy: Laparoscopic Technique 203
William C. Chapman Jr. and Matthew G. Mutch

26 Total Abdominal Colectomy: Hand-Assisted Technique 216
Daniel Albo

27 Robotic Total Abdominal Colectomy 229
Dana M. Omer, Jonathan Benjamin Yuval, and Julio Garcia-Aguilar

28 Colon and Rectal Injury: Primary Repair, Resection and Anastomosis, Colostomy 237
Louis Jude Magnotti, Devanshi D. Patel, and Martin A. Croce

Section III Rectal Resections

29 Low Anterior Resection and Total Mesorectal Excision/Coloanal Anastomosis: Open Technique 244
Konstantinos I. Votanopoulos and Jaime L. Bohl

30 Low Anterior Rectal Resection: Laparoscopic Technique 253
Antonio D'Urso, Jacques Marescaux, and Didier Mutter

31 Low Anterior Resection: Hand-Assisted Laparoscopic Surgery Technique 265
Zhifei Sun and Matthew G. Mutch

32 Low Anterior Rectal Resection: Robotic-Assisted Laparoscopic Technique 276
Perisa Ruhi-Williams, Mehraneh Dorna Jafari, and Alessio Pigazzi

33 Total Mesorectal Excision With Coloanal Anastomosis: Laparoscopic Technique 287
John H. Marks, Jane Yang, and Elsa B. Valsdottir

34 Abdominoperineal Resection: Open Technique 298
Curtis J. Wray and Stefanos G. Millas

35 Abdominoperineal Resection: Laparoscopic Technique 307
Antonio D'Urso, Jacques Marescaux, and Didier Mutter

36 Hand-Assisted Abdominoperineal Resection 322
Daniel Albo

37 Abdominoperineal Resection: Robotic-Assisted Laparoscopic Surgery Technique 335
Rodrigo Pedraza and Eric Mitchell Haas

38 Restorative Proctocolectomy: Open Technique (Ileal Pouch-Anal Anastomosis) 345
Hasan T. Kirat and Feza H. Remzi

39 Restorative Proctocolectomy: Single-Incision Laparoscopic Technique (Including Pouch Ileoanal Anastomosis) 356
Theodoros Voloyiannis

40 Restorative Proctocolectomy: Hand-Assisted Laparoscopic Surgery Ileal Pouch-Anal Anastomosis 368
Robert R. Cima

41 Pelvic Exenteration 378
Cherry E. Koh and Michael J. Solomon

42 Transanal Excision of Rectal Tumors: Open Technique 392
Angel M. Charles, Barry W. Feig, and Ryan M. Thomas

43 Transanal Minimally Invasive Surgery for Rectal Lesions 400
Avo Artinyan and Daniel Albo

44 Laparoscopic Diverting Colostomies: Formation and Reversal 409
Jayson Moloney, David Graham Taylor, and Andrew RL Stevenson

45 Surgical Management of Hemorrhoids 422
Bidhan Das

46 Surgical Management of Anal Fissures 433
Daniel Albo

47 Operative Treatment of Rectal Prolapse: Perineal Approach (Altemeier and Modified Delorme Procedures) 439
Valerie P. Bauer

48 Operative Treatment of Rectal Prolapse: Transabdominal Approach 446
Karin M. Hardiman

49 Perirectal Abscess and Perianal Fistula 455
Vijian Dhevan, Roger M. Galindo, and Henry A. Reinhart

50 Surgical Management of Pilonidal Disease 460
Vijian Dhevan and Henry A. Reinhart

51 **Surgical Management of Peritoneal Carcinomatosis** 466
Cristian D. Valenzuela, Perry Shen, Edward A. Levine, and Konstantinos I. Votanopoulos

52 **Enhanced Recovery After Surgery** 474
Dhruvesh M. Ramson and Andrew G. Hill

Index I-1

Video Contents List

Section II   **Surgery of the Colon, Appendix, Rectum, and Anus**

Chapter 23   **Surgical Management of Complicated Diverticulitis: Perforation and Colovesical Fistula**

Video 1   *Laparoscopic sigmoid colectomy for colovesical fistula*

Section III   **Rectal Resections**

Chapter 30   **Low Anterior Rectal Resection: Laparoscopic Technique**

Video 1   *Low anterior resection*

Chapter 32   **Low Anterior Rectal Resection: Robotic-Assisted Laparoscopic Technique**

Video 1   *Total mesorectal excision*

Chapter 35   **Abdominoperineal Resection: Laparoscopic Technique**

Video 1   *Abdominoperineal resection*

SECTION I: Surgery of the Small Intestine

Chapter 1 — Laparoscopic Small Bowel Resection

Oliver Adrian Varban

DEFINITION

- Laparoscopic small bowel resection involves segmental resection of the duodenum, jejunum, or ileum as well as its associated mesentery. Resection of the small bowel may be performed in the setting of necrosis, perforation, bleeding, stricture, ulceration, or malignancy.

DIFFERENTIAL DIAGNOSIS

- The following conditions represent pathology that may require a small bowel resection:
  - Polyp
  - Tumor
    - Benign: Adenoma, lipoma, hemangioma
    - Malignant: Adenocarcinoma, gastrointestinal stromal tumor, neuroendocrine tumors, lymphoma, metastatic disease
  - Crohn disease
  - Ulcer
  - Stricture (inflammatory, infectious, malignant, postsurgical)
  - Diverticula
  - Intussusception (secondary to underlying benign or malignant etiology)
  - Foreign body/bezoar
  - Small bowel injury or perforation (iatrogenic or due to trauma)
  - Prior small bowel anastomosis complicated by ulcer, stricture, or intussusception

PATIENT HISTORY AND PHYSICAL FINDINGS

- Small bowel obstruction may result in nausea, vomiting, obstipation, focal or diffuse abdominal pain, and distension with absent bowel sounds.
- Peritoneal signs, fever, and septic shock may indicate ischemia, necrosis, or perforation.
- Overt bleeding may result in hematemesis, melena, or hematochezia (depending on localization), as well as hypotension and tachycardia. Occult bleed may present with microcytic anemia and hemoccult positive stool. Abdominal pain is typically absent, unless bleeding is associated with ulcer disease, obstruction, or trauma.

IMAGING AND OTHER DIAGNOSTIC STUDIES

- Abdominal x-ray may demonstrate dilated loops of bowel indicative of a bowel obstruction. Upright views that include the chest can help identify evidence of pneumoperitoneum by demonstrating evidence of free subdiaphragmatic gas. Duodenal perforation is more commonly associated with pneumoperitoneum than jejunal or ileal perforations.
- Computed tomography (CT) with oral and intravenous (IV) contrast can assist with the location and etiology of obstruction. A transition point is noted when the proximal small bowel is dilated (with air fluid levels) and the distal small bowel is decompressed.
- Magnetic resonance imaging and magnetic resonance enteroclysis (MRE) along with CT may assist with the diagnosis of small bowel tumors.[1]
- Tagged red blood cell scan and CT angiogram may localize intraluminal bleeding in cases where bleeding rates are at least 0.1 to 1.0 mL/min.[2]
- A technetium-99m pertechnetate, or Meckel scan, can detect gastric mucosa associated with a Meckel's diverticulum.
- Small bowel enteroscopy (push enteroscopy) and capsule endoscopy may also be used to identify the location of a tumor or site of bleeding in a stable patient. If small bowel enteroscopy is performed, the location of the tumor can be tattooed to assist with intraoperative identification.
- Diagnostic laparoscopy can assist with the localization of disease and can be less morbid than performing a laparotomy.
- An elevated white blood cell count and lactate level is concerning for ischemia or necrosis.
- A decrease in hemoglobin/hematocrit is indicative of bleeding.

SURGICAL MANAGEMENT

Preoperative Planning

- The patient requires adequate IV access (ie, large bore IV in the antecubital fossa) for fluid resuscitation. Blood transfusion may be necessary if the patient is bleeding.
- A nasogastric tube assists in gastric and proximal small bowel decompression. This decreases the risk of aspiration during intubation as well as injury to the stomach or small bowel during port placement.

- A Foley catheter is placed for accurate intraoperative assessment of urine output and also to decompress the bladder for safe port placement.
- Preoperative antibiotics should cover enteric organisms in the event of spillage.

Positioning

- The patient is placed in the supine position. Arms are better tucked at the side of the patient. Tucking the arms may assist with the ergonomics of the operation by allowing both surgeon and assistant to stand on the same side of the patient comfortably. Adequate padding should be used while tucking the upper extremities to avoid potential neurovascular injuries. Additionally, IV hubs should also be padded to avoid pressure ulcers on the extremities.

ACCESS TO THE ABDOMINAL CAVITY

- Accessing the abdominal cavity can be performed in a variety of ways (ie, Hasson open cut-down technique, Veress needle insufflation, and use of an optical trocar vs radially expanding trocar) and should be guided by surgeon's preference and experience as there is insufficient evidence to recommend one technique over another.[3]
- Typical insufflation settings for laparoscopy include an intra-abdominal pressure of 15 mm Hg and a flow of 40 L/min.
    - Veress needle entry
        - With a nasogastric tube in place and the stomach decompressed, a 5-mm incision is made with a no. 11 blade scalpel through the dermis in the left upper quadrant of the abdomen, approximately 2 cm below the costal margin in the midclavicular line (ie, Palmer point) (**Figure 1**).
        - A Veress needle is placed through this incision and advanced until two distinct clicks are heard, signaling that the blunt-tip portion of the Veress needle has sprung forward. The second click is heard as the needle enters the peritoneal cavity.
        - A "drop test" can be performed by placing 10 mL of saline through the needle using a syringe without a plunger (**Figure 2**). If the saline drops into the abdominal cavity with gravity alone, then the needle may be connected to the insufflator (**Figure 3**).
        - Once the abdomen is fully insufflated to an intra-abdominal pressure of 15 mm Hg, the Veress

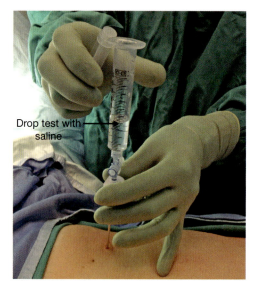

FIGURE 2 • Drop test performed with saline using a syringe without a plunger. Saline is expected to enter the abdominal cavity freely by gravity alone.

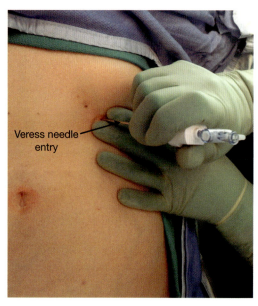

FIGURE 1 • Veress needle entry in the left upper quadrant.

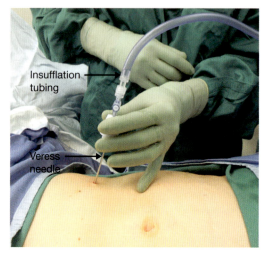

FIGURE 3 • Veress needle connected to insufflator tubing for creation of pneumoperitoneum.

- needle is removed and a 5-mm port is placed through the same incision. The port is then connected to the insufflator.
- Open cut-down technique
  - A 2-cm curvilinear incision is made with a no. 15 blade scalpel just below the umbilicus and tissue is dissected down to the level of the fascia.
  - S-shaped or L-shaped retractors are placed to assist with exposure of the anterior fascia and linea alba.
  - The umbilical stalk is then grasped with a Kocher clamp and elevated, thus pulling the fascia away from the underlying bowel.
  - A 2-cm longitudinal incision is made in the fascia with a no. 15 blade scalpel, and the edges are grasped and retracted using Kocher clamps. The peritoneum is identified below, grasped with DeBakey forceps in two separate locations, and then incised with Metzenbaum scissors under direct vision.
  - A Hasson port is placed into the abdominal cavity and then connected to the insufflator, first at low flow (10 L/min) to reduce the risk of bradycardia and hypotension. Once target pressure has been achieved (15 mm Hg) and hemodynamics have not been compromised, insufflation can be increased to high flow (40 L/min).
- Optical trocar entrance technique
  - A small incision is placed on the skin with a 11-blade scalpel in either the right or left upper quadrant of the abdomen.
  - Using a 0° scope, a 5-mm trocar is advanced under direct visualization through all layers of the abdominal wall (in sequence: fat, Scarpa fascia, fat, anterior fascia, three muscle layers, posterior fascia, preperitoneal fat, peritoneum, until the omentum/bowel is visualized) using a twisting motion. Care must be taken to avoid overpenetration into the abdominal cavity.
  - The trocar is then connected to the insufflator, first at low flow (10 L/min) to reduce the risk of bradycardia and hypotension. Once target pressure has been achieved (15 mm Hg) and hemodynamics have not been compromised, insufflation can be increased to high flow (40 L/min).
  - At this point, you may switch to a 30° scope if desirable.

PORT PLACEMENT

- After the first port is placed, a 5-mm 30° angled laparoscope is introduced into the abdominal cavity and used to examine the bowel and organs just below the site of port entry to ensure no inadvertent injury occurred during insufflation/entry of the abdominal cavity.
- The remaining ports are placed under laparoscopic visualization, which assists in avoiding injury to intra-abdominal organs and the inferior epigastric vessels.
- The 5-mm ports accommodate most laparoscopic grasping and dissecting instruments (**Figure 4**). Atraumatic graspers are preferred to avoid injuring the small bowel.
- The 12-mm ports accommodate laparoscopic stapling devices and autosuturing devices.
- Port placement for optimal exposure and manipulation of the proximal small bowel is demonstrated in **Figure 5**.
- Port placement for optimal exposure and manipulation of the distal small bowel is demonstrated in **Figure 6**.

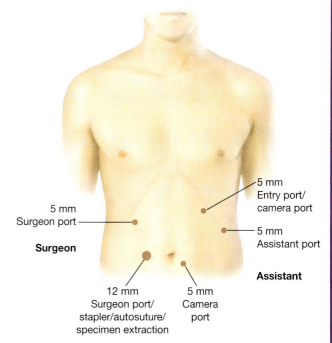

FIGURE 5 • Optimal port placement for exposure of the proximal small bowel.

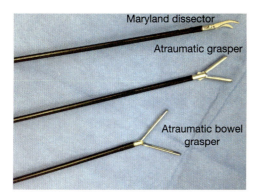

FIGURE 4 • Laparoscopic atraumatic graspers and dissectors that can be used through a 5-mm port.

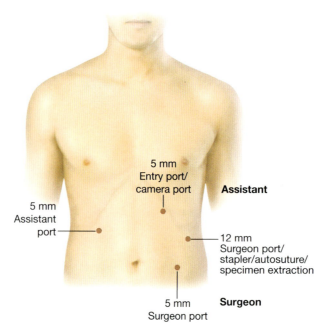

FIGURE 6 • Optimal port placement for exposure of the distal small bowel.

IDENTIFICATION OF DISEASE

- The small bowel is run from the ligament of Treitz to the terminal ileum using atraumatic nonlocking graspers.
- To identify the ligament of Treitz, the greater omentum is reflected cephalad. Next, the assistant grasps the epiploicae of the transverse colon or the mesentery of the transverse colon to retract it cephalad and expose the base of the transverse mesocolon. The surgeon then grasps the small bowel located to the patient left of midline and follows it back hand over hand in the proximal direction toward the base of its mesentery until they feel resistance and can see that the proximal jejunum emanates from the retroperitoneum (**Figure 7**).
- With the proximal small bowel identified, the small bowel can be run, hand over hand to the terminal ileum until the diseased portion can be identified.

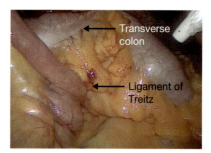

FIGURE 7 • Identification of the ligament of Treitz requires elevation of the transverse colon and exposure of the transverse mesocolon. The small bowel is grasped and followed hand over hand proximally until it can be seen emanating from the retroperitoneum.

SMALL BOWEL RESECTION

- The surgeon grasps the proximal small bowel and the assistant grasps the distal small bowel.
- Creation of a mesenteric window is performed using a Maryland dissector (**Figure 8**) at a location both proximal and distal to the diseased portion of small bowel.
- A laparoscopic dividing stapler (gastrointestinal anastomosis [GIA] type) is then placed through this window and the bowel is divided at proximal and distal points of resection. Staple height varies from 2.5 to 4.5 mm and choice of application depends on tissue thickness (**Figure 9**).[4]

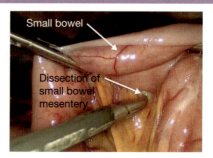

FIGURE 8 • Creation of mesenteric window, allowing for the placement of the laparoscopic dividing stapler.

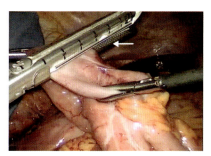

FIGURE 9 • Placement of the laparoscopic dividing stapler through the mesenteric window. Arrow represents laparoscopic stapler.

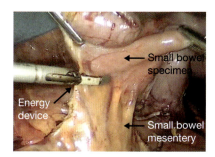

FIGURE 10 • Mesenteric division using an energy device (ie, ultrasonic scalpel or bipolar cautery).

- The mesentery is divided using an energy device, such as an ultrasonic scalpel or bipolar device (**Figure 10**).

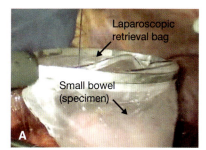

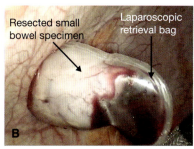

FIGURE 11 • Placement of specimen in a laparoscopic retrieval bag **(A)** and removal from 12-mm port site **(B)**.

- The segment of resected bowel is then placed into a laparoscopic specimen retrieval bag (**Figure 11A**) and removed through the 12-mm port site (**Figure 11B**). This can be performed either before or after the creation of anastomosis.

SMALL BOWEL ANASTOMOSIS

- The two divided ends of small bowel are placed side to side and a seromuscular traction suture is placed using 2-0 absorbable suture, approximately 8 to 10 cm from the ends along the antimesenteric surface of the bowel. A freehand suture may be performed or may be placed using an autosuture device. The tails of the suture are cut approximately 5 cm long so that they may be grasped and used for retraction.

- With the assistant holding the traction suture, the surgeon creates an enterotomy in each segment of the bowel, approximately 1 cm from the stapled ends. Enterotomies may be created with an L-hook monopolar cautery or with an ultrasonic scalpel. The enteric contents are suctioned in order to contain spillage.
- Each limb of a laparoscopic linear stapler (2.5-mm staples, 60 mm in length) is placed separately into each enterotomy and aligned along the antimesenteric border (**Figure 12**). The stapler is closed and fired to create a

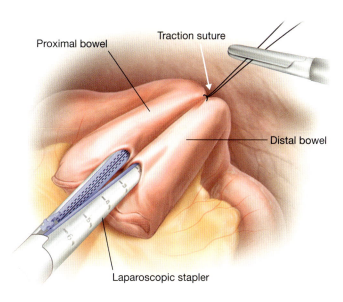

FIGURE 12 • Placement of a laparoscopic linear stapler in separate enterotomies made on each limb of bowel for creation of anastomosis. A traction suture placed 8 to 10 cm from the ends is held by the assistant.

SECTION I SURGERY OF THE SMALL INTESTINE

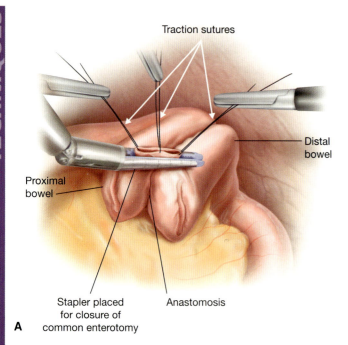

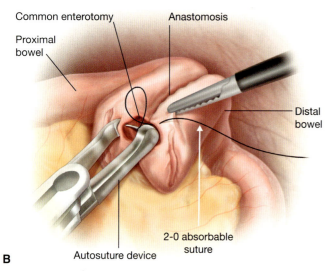

FIGURE 13 • **A,** Stapled closure of the common enterotomy is performed by placing traction sutures at either end of the enterotomy and one in the middle. The tails of the sutures are left long so they may be grasped and assist with placement of the stapler. The enterotomy is closed transversely so as to avoid narrowing the anastomosis. **B,** Suture closure of the common enterotomy is performed using an autosuture device. It may be performed with freehand suturing as well. The first row is performed with a 2-0 absorbable suture in a running fashion, closing the enterotomy transversely. The second layer consists of interrupted seromuscular imbricating sutures using a 2-0 nonabsorbable suture.

common channel between each segment of the bowel. Once the stapler is removed, the inside of the staple line is examined for hemostasis.

- The common enterotomy can be closed using a running suture or in a stapled fashion.
- When closing the common enterotomy with a stapler, three traction sutures are placed (one at each end and one in the middle) to approximate the enterotomy and elevate the edges. The tails of each suture are left long (approximately 5 cm) to allow for easy manipulation. A laparoscopic stapler (2.5-mm staples, 60 mm in length) is positioned beneath the cut edges and fired. Care is used to avoid including excessive amount of tissue in the stapler as it can narrow the anastomosis (**Figure 13A**).
- When closing the common enterotomy with suture, a running 2-0 absorbable suture may be placed for the inner layer and interrupted 2-0 permanent sutures may be placed in the seromuscular layer for the outer layer. Sutures may be placed freehand or with an autosuture device (**Figure 13B**).
- The mesenteric defect (**Figure 14A**) is closed with either a running or an interrupted series of 2-0 permanent sutures to prevent an internal hernia. Sutures are placed superficially in order to avoid injuring the blood supply (**Figure 14B**).

Chapter 1 LAPAROSCOPIC SMALL BOWEL RESECTION   7

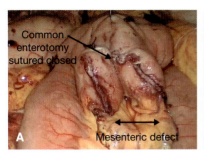
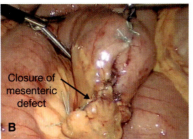

FIGURE 14 • The mesenteric defect (A) is approximated with a running permanent suture (B).

REMOVAL OF SPECIMEN

- Once the specimen is placed in a laparoscopic retrieval bag, it may be removed by expanding the size of one of the port sites. Alternatively, the specimen may be removed from a separate incision and with the use of a wound protection device.

CLOSURE

- It is recommended to close the fascia for all port sites greater than 10 mm to prevent port site herniation. (Owens, 2011 #7 This may be performed using a single absorbable or permanent 0-suture and a Carter-Thomason suture-passer device (Figure 15A-C).
- The site of specimen extraction may be closed in a similar fashion; however, larger defects do not maintain pneumoperitoneum and are more difficult to close laparoscopically. As such, these may be closed by placing interrupted sutures in an open fashion using a suture on a UR-6 needle.
- The skin is closed with interrupted absorbable subcuticular sutures.
- Drains are not required.

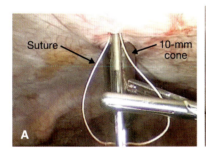
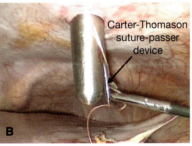
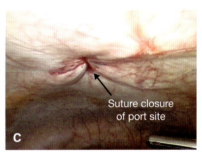

FIGURE 15 • A, A Carter-Thomason suture-passer device is used to pass a free suture through the port site defect using a cone to direct the passage of the suture through one side of fascial defect. B, The Carter-Thomason is then passed without the suture on the opposite site of the defect in order to grasp the suture. C, The end of the suture is then pulled up through the fascia and tied.

PEARLS AND PITFALLS

Port placement	■ Decompression of the stomach with a nasogastric tube allows for safer placement of a Veress needle at Palmer point. ■ Ports should be placed at least 10 cm apart and allow for triangulation of camera and instruments. ■ Placement of additional ports can enhance operative exposure and use of laparoscopic instruments in an ergonomic fashion. ■ Always begin the operation with 5-mm ports and upsize to a 12-mm port only after it has been decided whether a proximal or distal bowel resection will be performed.
Identification of disease	■ The surgeon may begin the case on the right side of the patient to evaluate the proximal bowel and then move to the left side of the patient to evaluate the distal bowel. ■ Localization of intraluminal tumors can be facilitated with MRE or preoperative double-balloon enteroscopy and tattooing. ■ If unsure, areas of suspected disease can be marked with a suture laparoscopically and then a hand-port or minilaparotomy incision can be used for a tactile evaluation.

Small bowel resection	▪ Creation of a mesenteric window allows for optimal placement of a laparoscopic GIA stapler, ensuring that the entire bowel is within the stapler load. ▪ Staple height of 2.5 mm is adequate for normal small bowel. However, edematous or thicker bowel may require 3.5- or 4.5-mm stapler cartridge.
Small bowel anastomosis	▪ Traction sutures placed along the common enterotomy assist in accurate placement of a laparoscopic GIA stapler during closure of the common enterotomy. If the anastomosis appears narrowed with placement of the stapler, a sutured closure is preferred. ▪ Ensure that the bowel undergoing anastomosis is well vascularized and not under tension. Edematous bowel is best approximated by a hand-sewn anastomosis. This may also be performed as an extracorporeal anastomosis through a small incision.
Removal of specimen	▪ Use of a laparoscopic catch bag or wound protector can reduce the risk of wound infection.
Closure	▪ Remove ports under laparoscopic visualization and inspect for bleeding prior to closure.

POSTOPERATIVE CARE

- After a laparoscopic small bowel resection, patients are admitted to the hospital for observation. If an extensive adhesiolysis is performed, a nasogastric tube may be placed at the end of the operation as the risk of ileus is higher. Return of bowel function is signaled by production of flatus or formed bowel movements.
- A clear liquid diet may be started on postoperative day 1 after an uncomplicated laparoscopic small bowel resection. A solid diet may be started after return of bowel function.
- The patient may ambulate immediately after laparoscopic surgery and does not require prolonged bladder catheterization.

OUTCOMES

- When compared to open surgery, laparoscopic small bowel resection results in shorter hospital length of stay, less wound complications and pain, better cosmesis, and also lower risk of adhesive disease when compared to an open approach.[5,6]
- Conversion from laparoscopic to open surgery is more likely in the setting of small bowel obstruction as dilated loops of small bowel can decrease operative exposure during laparoscopy. Additional factors include prior radiotherapy, history of previous intestinal obstruction or bowel resection, and significant bleeding.[7,8]
- Advanced operative skills such as laparoscopic suturing are necessary in order to perform a safe laparoscopic small bowel resection and anastomosis.[9]
- Complete recovery is expected after small bowel resection. However, outcomes can depend on preoperative comorbidities, severity of disease, and the length of bowel removed. A minimum of 50 to 70 cm of small bowel is necessary to achieve nutritional autonomy if there is a portion of the colon present and 110 to 150 cm is necessary if there is no colon in continuity.[10]

COMPLICATIONS

- Postoperative ileus
- Superficial site infection
- Port site hernia
- Intra-abdominal abscess
- Anastomotic leak
- Anastomotic stricture
- Adhesive small bowel disease
- Short bowel syndrome

REFERENCES

1. Williams EA, Bowman AW. Multimodality imaging of small bowel neoplasms. *Abdom Radiol (NY)*. 2019;44(6):2089-2103.
2. Parekh PJ, Buerlein RC, Shams R, Vingan H, Johnson DA. Evaluation of gastrointestinal bleeding: update of current radiologic strategies. *World J Gastrointest Pharmacol Ther*. 2014;5(4):200-208.
3. Ahmad G, Baker J, Finnerty J, Phillips K, Watson A. Laparoscopic entry techniques. *Cochrane Database Syst Rev*. 2019;1:CD006583.
4. Chekan E, Whelan RL. Surgical stapling device-tissue interactions: what surgeons need to know to improve patient outcomes. *Med Devices (Auckl)*. 2014;7:305-318.
5. Krielen P, Stommel MWJ, Pargmae P, et al. Adhesion-related readmissions after open and laparoscopic surgery: a retrospective cohort study (SCAR update). *Lancet*. 2020;395(10217):33-41.
6. Nordin A, Freedman J. Laparoscopic versus open surgical management of small bowel obstruction: an analysis of clinical outcomes. *Surg Endosc*. 2016;30(10):4454-4463.
7. Nakamura T, Sato T, Naito M, et al. Laparoscopic surgery is useful for preventing recurrence of small bowel obstruction after surgery for postoperative small bowel obstruction. *Surg Laparosc Endosc Percutan Tech*. 2016;26(1):e1-e4.
8. Nakamura T, Ishii Y, Tsutsui A, Kaneda M, Sato T, Watanabe M. Safety and indications of laparoscopic surgery for postoperative small-bowel obstruction: a single-center study of 121 patients. *Surg Laparosc Endosc Percutan Tech*. 2017;27(4):301-305.
9. Lim S, Ghosh S, Niklewski P, Roy S. Laparoscopic suturing as a barrier to broader adoption of laparoscopic surgery. *J Soc Laparoendosc Surg*. 2017;21(3).
10. Wilmore DW, Lacey JM, Soultanakis RP, Bosch RL, Byrne TA. Factors predicting a successful outcome after pharmacologic bowel compensation. *Ann Surg*. 1997;226(3):288-292; discussion 292-283.

Chapter 2

Strictureplasty and Small Bowel Bypass in Inflammatory Bowel Disease

James P. Taylor and Kelly A. Garrett

DEFINITION

- Strictureplasty and small bowel bypass are methods used to avoid bowel resection in patients with Crohn disease.
- The technique of strictureplasty was initially described in the treatment of tuberculous strictures as an alternative to resection. This procedure is mainly used in patients with jejunoileal Crohn disease, but it may also be used in select patients with duodenal disease. There are different techniques described, but all involve division of the strictured area either transversely or longitudinally with a distinctive closure that serves to widen the lumen of the small bowel.
- Small bowel bypass involves bypass of an affected segment of small intestine that is deemed unsuitable for resection or strictureplasty. Resection of the diseased segment is usually preferred. Bypass may be used in gastroduodenal Crohn disease, complex small bowel disease, or ileocolic disease when a patient's comorbidities preclude resection.

DIFFERENTIAL DIAGNOSIS

- At initial presentation, imaging findings may be nonspecific, and the differential diagnosis of diseases causing similar findings can be broad, including infectious processes and bowel ischemia.
- There are several disease processes that may present with some of the imaging features that are typical of Crohn disease, including skip lesions, mural thickening, luminal stenosis, or strictures.[1]
- The differential includes:
  - NSAID enteropathy
  - Cryptogenic multifocal ulcerous stenosis enteritis
  - Tuberculosis
  - Behcet disease
  - Henoch–Schonlein purpura
  - Endometriosis

PATIENT HISTORY AND PHYSICAL FINDINGS

- A thorough history and physical examination should be performed. History should include duration of symptoms and distribution of disease as well as current or prior medical therapy.
- Crohn disease may manifest in one of three disease patterns: (1) nonstricturing, nonpenetrating; (2) stricturing, and (3) penetrating. Sticturing disease is the most common and typically presents with a progressive course in which stricturing of the small bowel leads to obstructive symptoms.[2]
- Pattern of disease distribution should be determined prior to operative intervention. Anatomic location of disease can be classified as terminal ileal, colonic, ileocolonic, and upper gastrointestinal (GI). Over time, 15% of patients experience a change in anatomic location and 46% of patients demonstrate an alteration in disease behavior.[3]

- Past surgical history is of particular importance because many patients with Crohn disease have had prior abdominal surgery, and this may affect operative planning. A detailed surgical history also allows for an estimation of the length of remaining small bowel.
- A detailed description of the patient's medical management should be obtained. The disease can be managed with anti-inflammatory medications such as derivatives of 5-aminosalicylic acid; with immunosuppressors such as corticosteroids, azathioprine, 6-mercaptopurine, and methotrexate; and/or with immunomodulators such as antibodies targeting tumor necrosis factor-α. These medications can influence perioperative morbidity.
- A detailed history should also be obtained to distinguish Crohn disease from ulcerative colitis. The two inflammatory bowel diseases can have similar patterns of presentation, although they have different principles of surgical management.

IMAGING AND OTHER DIAGNOSTIC STUDIES

- The distribution of active disease needs to be mapped out preoperatively. Thought should be given to the risk of exposure to ionizing radiation as many patients with Crohn disease can have flares over the course of many decades and hence require repeat imaging studies.
- Conventional radiologic techniques for imaging the small bowel include small bowel enteroclysis and small bowel follow-through. Strictures may appear as narrowed areas with delayed passage of contrast. Dynamic images may reveal impaired peristalsis in strictured areas. Computed tomography (CT) and magnetic resonance (MR) enterography have almost completely replaced the use of these studies at most academic centers.
- CT performed with intravenous and oral contrast is helpful in identifying abscesses and other inflammatory processes outside the bowel lumen. Recent developments have also improved the ability of CT to identify strictures, fistulas, and areas of active inflammation. CT enterography uses low-density oral contrast in place of barium or iodine-based oral contrast used in standard scans. This in combination with intravenous iodinated contrast allows for better definition of the mucosa and thickness of the bowel wall.
- MR enterography is being increasingly used to evaluate extent of active disease.[1] MR enterography can also be performed using low-density oral contrast and offers the additional benefit of sparing patients' exposure to radiation; thus, it should be used where possible instead of CT.
- Ultrasound, although not as widely used, may be able to identify areas of bowel wall thickening, strictures, and decreased peristalsis. It is also useful for identifying abscesses and fistulas. Although ultrasound spares patients' exposure

to ionizing radiation, it is operator dependent and may not be able to distinguish inflammatory vs fibrotic strictures.
- Leukocyte scintigraphy is an additional imaging modality that is well tolerated and noninvasive and can allow for assessment of the presence, extent, and activity of inflammation. However, there is associated radiation exposure and limited sensitivity.
- All the previously described imaging studies may help determine whether an area of stricture has an active inflammatory component that may respond to medical therapy, aid in determining the extent of disease prior to surgery, and facilitate operative planning.

SURGICAL MANAGEMENT

Preoperative Planning

- Indications for surgery in patients with Crohn disease include the following[4]:
  - Failure of medical or endoscopic therapy
  - Perforation
  - Enterovesicular fistula resulting in recurrent infections
  - Intestinal obstruction
  - Worsening inflammation
  - Hemorrhage
  - Neoplasia
  - Growth retardation
  - Extraintestinal manifestations
- When preoperative imaging reveals stricturing small bowel disease with minimal area of inflammation in patients with obstructive symptoms, additional medical therapy is unlikely to resolve the symptoms and the patient should be considered for surgery. Patients with suspected active inflammation who have failed medical therapy should also be considered for surgery.
- Strictureplasty should not be performed in every patient with stricturing Crohn disease. In most patients, simple resection and reanastomosis is sufficient. Indications for strictureplasty are the following[5]:
  - Diffuse jejunoileitis causing obstructive symptoms unresponsive to medical therapy
  - Recurrent stricturing disease in patients with multiple prior intestinal resections (high risk for short bowel syndrome)
  - Recurrence of strictures within 12 months of prior resection
  - Isolated ileocolonic anastomotic strictures
  - Selected duodenal strictures such as proximal lesions near the pylorus[6]
- Contraindications to strictureplasty are the following[5]:
  - Diffuse peritonitis
  - Free intra-abdominal perforation of the affected bowel segment
  - Phlegmon or abscess of affected bowel segment
  - Fistulous disease with significant inflammation of affected bowel segment
  - Multiple areas of stricture, within a short distance of each other, more amenable to single resection and anastomosis

- Suspicion for neoplasia
- Hypoalbuminemia
- In some cases, bypass of affected segments of the GI tract are indicated. These include the following:
  - Gastroduodenal Crohn disease—The duodenum is involved in 0.5% to 4% of patients with Crohn disease and can cause obstruction or hemorrhage.[7] In this scenario, resection is excessively morbid, so strictureplasty and bypass play a larger role.
    - With obstruction of the first or second portions of the duodenum, a gastrojejunostomy should be performed. Although vagotomy is traditionally performed to prevent marginal ulceration, current use of effective acid-suppressing medications have rendered vagotomy unnecessary.[7,8] Furthermore, vagotomy may increase morbidity in patients already predisposed to diarrhea from extensive or poorly controlled Crohn disease or short-gut syndrome.
    - In patients with obstruction of the third or fourth portions of the duodenum, a duodenojejunal bypass should be performed.[9]
  - Active inflammation of the duodenum and small bowel can lead to duodenoenteric fistula formation, commonly involving recurrence at a previous ileocolic anastomosis. Resection of diseased areas may require partial resection of involved duodenum as well. In these cases, bypass with a gastrojejunostomy may be required.
  - In complex small bowel or ileocolonic Crohn disease,[10] bypass should be considered when resection would be unsafe as in the presence of an ileocecal phlegmon that is adherent to the retroperitoneum or iliac vessels.
- Bypass of small bowel disease should be avoided if resection is possible. An excluded segment should eventually be resected in order to avoid development of perforation, recurrent disease, carcinoma, or blind loop syndrome.[10]

Preparation

- A mechanical bowel preparation is not necessary for patients who are undergoing small bowel or ileocolic resection and should be avoided in patients with stricturing disease.
- If there is a chance that a stoma will be created, the patient should be evaluated by an enterostomal nurse to help avoid the development of pouching problems postoperatively.
- Appropriate antibiotic and venous thromboembolism prophylaxis are administered prior to incision, and normothermia is maintained throughout the case.

Positioning

- Supine position is useful for patients who have uncomplicated ileocolic disease or gastroduodenal disease.
- Modified lithotomy position is preferred if patients have distal disease that may require intervention. This allows for intraoperative colonoscopy to be performed for diagnostic purposes or to interrogate an anastomosis or repair if necessary. This position is also advantageous if the procedure will be done laparoscopically as it allows the surgeon to stand between the patient's legs, which can assist with running the small bowel or with mobilization of the flexures if needed.

APPROACH

Placement of Incision

- The procedure can be performed via a laparoscopic or open approach.
- Laparoscopy for ileocolic Crohn disease has been shown to result in earlier return of bowel function, shorter length of stay, and decreased postoperative pain.[11] This approach may not be feasible for all patients, however, as many will have had extensive previous abdominal surgery.
- For open surgery, particularly in those with multiple prior surgeries, a standard midline laparotomy incision is usually performed. This can be limited to the upper midline if minimally active disease is suspected.
- In patients with multiple abdominal operations, entering the abdomen in an area that has not previously been opened is recommended to avoid inadvertent bowel injury.

Evaluation of the Bowel

- Adhesiolysis may be necessary to allow for complete evaluation of the small bowel. Strictured areas are often identified by fibrotic, narrowed bowel with proximal dilation. Other external indications of stricture are fat wrapping, thickened mesentery, and serosal corkscrew vessels.[5] Areas of suspected stricture are marked with a stitch on the antimesenteric bowel surface.
- In patients with multiple previous abdominal operations and obliterative scar tissue, the use of injectable saline can be useful to help delineate bowel loops.
- After the most obvious area of stricture is identified, the lumen is opened longitudinally along the antimesenteric border in preparation for strictureplasty or resection. A Foley catheter is placed into the bowel lumen and filled with varying amounts of water. The catheter is then advanced or withdrawn through the bowel in both directions to identify the area of stricture that may not be externally evident.
- Patients may have multiple areas of disease that require a combination of resection and strictureplasty. Resections should be performed first.
- Once the decision is made to perform a strictureplasty, the length of affected small bowel must be determined as this dictates the type of strictureplasty performed.
    - Less than 8 to 10 cm: Heineke–Mikulicz strictureplasty
    - 10 to 25 cm: Finney strictureplasty
    - Extensive, long-segment disease: side-to-side isoperistaltic strictureplasty

HEINEKE–MIKULICZ STRICTUREPLASTY

- The stricture is isolated proximally and distally using umbilical tape or bowel clamps. The stricture is opened longitudinally on the antimesenteric border, beginning in normal bowel approximately 2 to 3 cm from the stricture. A clamp is placed into the bowel lumen, and the incision is carried across the stricture using electrocautery and ending 2 to 3 cm into normal bowel.
- Two 3-0 polyglactin stay sutures are placed on opposite sides of the incision in the center of the stricture. These are used to create tension perpendicular to the incision, thereby opening the incised area of bowel and allowing the bowel to be closed transversely.
- Interrupted seromuscular 3-0 polyglactin sutures are then placed to close the incision transversely[12] (**FIGURE 1**).

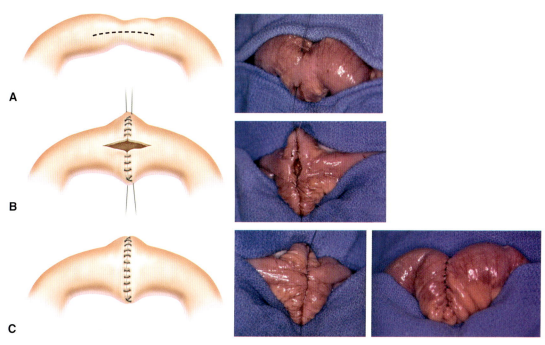

FIGURE 1 • Heineke–Mikulicz strictureplasty. The bowel is opened longitudinally across the stricture **(A)** and then closed transversely **(B)** to increase the bowel lumen **(C)**.

FINNEY STRICTUREPLASTY

- For strictures 10 to 25 cm in length, a Heineke–Mikulicz strictureplasty creates excessive tension, so the Finney strictureplasty is preferred. A Finney strictureplasty should not be performed in a strictured segment that is longer than 25 cm, however, because this may risk a blind loop syndrome.
- The strictured area of bowel is isolated as previously described and the bowel is placed in a U shape with the midpoint of the stricture as the apex to simulate the finished strictureplasty and guide the bowel incision.
- The bowel is incised on the antimesenteric border beginning in normal bowel 2 to 3 cm from the stricture. This incision is then carried through the stricture using electrocautery. As the incision reaches the apex of the U shape, it should take a gradual course toward the mesenteric border as this allows for better tissue apposition. The incision finishes in 2 to 3 cm of normal bowel after having been brought back to the antimesenteric border.
- Interrupted, full-thickness 3-0 polyglactin sutures are used as marking sutures to approximate normal bowel edges at the base of the strictureplasty and are also used to fix the diseased bowel at the apex. Continuous 3-0 polyglactin suture is then used to close the posterior wall followed by the anterior wall of the strictureplasty. Interrupted sutures may also be used to reinforce and imbricate the continuous suture at various points and maintain tissue apposition[5] (**FIGURE 2**).

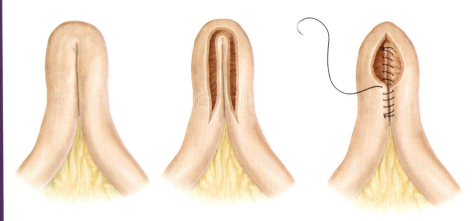

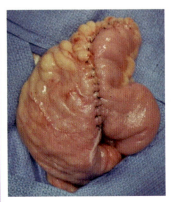

FIGURE 2 • Finney strictureplasty. The bowel opening is made longitudinally across the stricture along "an omega loop" and is then closed side to side (posterior and anterior rows).

SIDE-TO-SIDE ISOPERISTALTIC STRICTUREPLASTY

- For extensive stricturing Crohn disease not amenable to strictureplasty of isolated segments, the side-to-side isoperistaltic strictureplasty can be performed.
- The affected bowel is first transected at the midpoint. The proximal bowel is then brought to overlie the distal segment in an isoperistaltic fashion (**FIGURE 3**). An enterotomy is performed on the antimesenteric border and extended 2 to 3 cm into normal mucosa (**FIGURE 4**).
- The transected ends of bowel are spatulated to avoid creation of blind stumps.
- Similar to the Finney strictureplasty, tissues are brought together at both ends of the treated segment with interrupted 3-0 polyglactin sutures. The posterior layer is closed with a running 3-0 polyglactin suture followed by closure of the anterior layer (**FIGURE 5**).

Chapter 2 STRICTUREPLASTY AND SMALL BOWEL BYPASS IN INFLAMMATORY BOWEL DISEASE

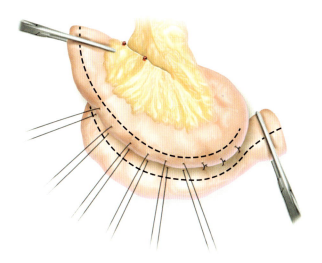

FIGURE 3 • Side-to-side isoperistaltic strictureplasty. The affected bowel is first transected at the midpoint. The proximal bowel is then brought to overlie the distal segment in an isoperistaltic fashion.

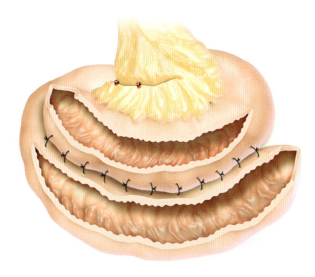

FIGURE 4 • Side-to-side isoperistaltic strictureplasty. An enterotomy is performed on the antimesenteric border and extended 2 to 3 cm into normal mucosa.

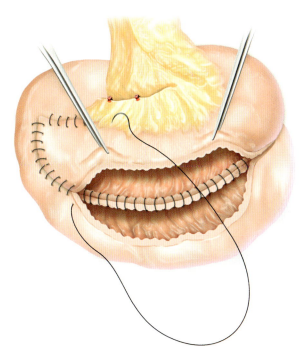

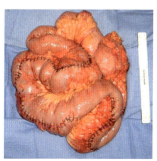

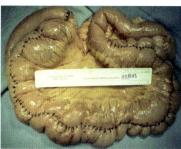

FIGURE 5 • Side-to-side isoperistaltic strictureplasty. Similar to the Finney strictureplasty, tissues are brought together at both ends of the treated segment with 3-0 polyglactin sutures.

SMALL BOWEL BYPASS

Gastrojejunal Bypass

- Gastrojejunostomy is performed by bringing the most proximal loop of jejunum that easily reaches the greater curvature of the stomach. The anastomosis can be done using either a hand-sewn (FIGURE 6) or stapled technique (FIGURE 7).

It can also be done antecolic or retrocolic. The antecolic approach avoids dissection through the transverse colon mesentery and also keeps the anastomosis away from the retroperitoneum.

Duodenojejunal Bypass

- A longitudinal enterotomy in the proximal jejunum is made in an area that is free of disease. A Foley catheter

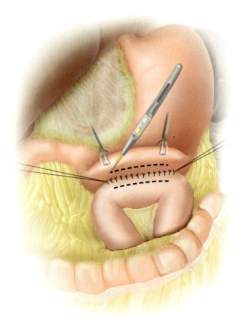
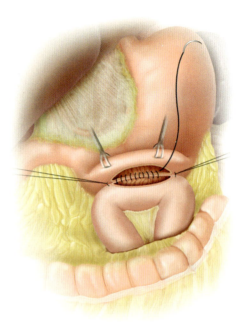

FIGURE 6 • Gastrojejunal bypass: hand-sewn technique.

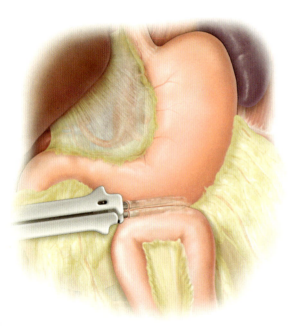

FIGURE 7 • Gastrojejunal bypass: stapled technique.

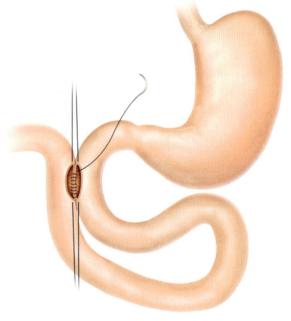

FIGURE 8 • Duodenojejunal bypass: A posterior layer of interrupted 3-0 silk sutures is placed to approximate the duodenal and jejunal segments.

is inserted and passed proximally through the duodenal sweep and filled with varying amounts of water to assess for duodenal stricture. If there is a stricture isolated to the third and fourth portions of the duodenum and it is determined that there is healthy, patent bowel in the first and second portions, then a bypass may be performed. A longitudinal duodenotomy is performed in the healthy portion of the duodenum. 3-0 Polyglactin sutures are placed to approximate the jejunal enterotomy to the duodenotomy.

- A posterior layer of interrupted 3-0 silk sutures is placed to approximate the duodenal and jejunal segments (**FIGURE 8**). This is followed by a continuous inner suture layer of 3-0 polyglactin suture. A layer of interrupted 3-0 silk is then placed on the anterior surface to complete the anastomosis (**FIGURE 9**). The use of a stapler is not recommended.[10]

Chapter 2 STRICTUREPLASTY AND SMALL BOWEL BYPASS IN INFLAMMATORY BOWEL DISEASE   15

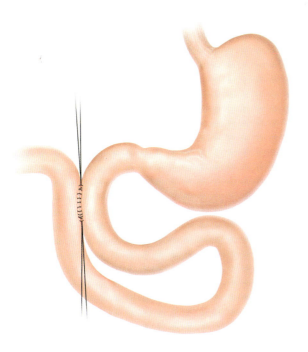

FIGURE 9 • Duodenojejunal bypass: A continuous inner suture layer of 3-0 polyglactin suture and a layer of interrupted 3-0 silk are then placed on the anterior surface to complete the anastomosis.

ILEOTRANSVERSE BYPASS

- When ileocolic disease is severe and resection is deemed unsafe, an ileotransverse bypass may be performed.
- The small bowel is transected proximal to the involved ileum.
- A hand-sewn anastomosis is performed in an end-to-side fashion with the end of the transected ileum anastomosed to the side of a segment of transverse colon (**FIGURE 10**). This is done in a similar fashion as described for the duodenojejunal bypass. Alternatively, the anastomosis can be performed in a side-to-side fashion using a gastrointestinal anastomosis stapler[10] (**FIGURE 11**).

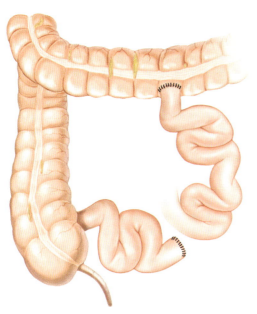

FIGURE 10 • Ileotransverse bypass: hand-sewn technique.

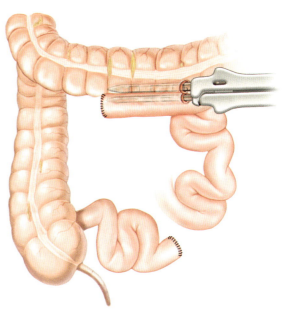

FIGURE 11 • Ileotransverse bypass: stapled technique.

16 SECTION I **SURGERY OF THE SMALL INTESTINE**

OTHER CONSIDERATIONS

- Duodenal strictures
  - Patients with nonperforated, nonphlegmonous strictures of the duodenum can undergo Heineke–Mikulicz strictureplasty.
  - Patients with refractory obstruction, pain, or extensive duodenal stricturing may require bypass with gastrojejunostomy or duodenojejunostomy. The role of vagotomy in this setting has been debated; however, as stated previously it can most often be omitted.
    - Duodenal resection is not indicated for Crohn disease due to its excessive morbidity.
- Colonic strictures that cannot be evaluated by colonoscopy biopsy or cytology should be resected as approximately 7% of these may contain occult malignancy.[13] Biopsy of the strictured bowel wall should be considered to evaluate for possible occult malignancy.[14]

PEARLS AND PITFALLS

Imaging	- Preoperative imaging studies should be used to determine the extent of disease and to facilitate surgical planning, with MRI the preferred modality. - Extent of active inflammation should be estimated preoperatively as this is potentially responsive to medical therapy.
Choice of procedure	- Resection with simple reanastomosis should be performed for most patients with small bowel and ileocolic disease. - Strictureplasty should be performed in patients with previous resections who are at risk for short bowel syndrome or patients with diffuse or recurrent stricturing disease. - Bypass of affected segments is most useful for gastroduodenal Crohn disease and should only be employed in small bowel or ileocolonic Crohn disease if resection is deemed too unsafe. - When a strictured area is identified, a longitudinal incision is made and the proximal and distal bowel is evaluated with a Foley catheter to determine extent of disease. - Metallic clips should be placed on the mesentery at the strictureplasty sites for future identification during imaging or surgery. - The length of remaining small bowel should be measured and recorded, especially in patients who are having reoperations. This will help in planning during possible future operations.

POSTOPERATIVE CARE

- Patients undergoing resection, strictureplasty, or bypass for Crohn disease often have proximally dilated small bowel. Chronically dilated intestine should be expected to have dysfunctional peristalsis, and as such, recovery of full bowel function may take up to 1 week or more. For severe obstruction, nasogastric tube decompression may be indicated. Total parenteral nutrition may also be useful in the postoperative period to optimize patients and allow adequate healing at anastomosis or strictureplasty sites.

OUTCOMES

- Resection: Recurrence of stricturing disease requiring surgery occurs in 25% and 50% of patients at 5 and 10 years, respectively.[2] Recurrence is unaffected by the presence of active microscopic inflammation at the resection margin and as such, only macroscopically involved segments of bowel should be resected.[12]
- Strictureplasty: Recurrence following strictureplasty occurs in 28% and 34% of patients at 3.5 and 7.5 years, respectively. Younger patients are at higher risk for recurrence following strictureplasty.[2] Overall recurrence rates are comparable with those following resection.

- Duodenal Crohn disease: Bypass or strictureplasty of the duodenum are relatively uncommon procedures but have been performed with good results. Major morbidity of these procedures may be as high as 27%. It is thought that use of laparoscopy to perform gastrojejunostomy may decrease complication rates.[7] Recurrence and reoperation rates are variable and data are limited.

COMPLICATIONS

- Surgical site infection
- Intra-abdominal infection
- Anastomotic leak
- Anastomotic hemorrhage
- Ileus
- Small bowel obstruction
- Short bowel syndrome
- Recurrence

REFERENCES

1. Guimaraes L, Greer M, Dillman J, et al. Magnetic resonance in Crohn's disease: diagnosis, disease burden and classification. *Magn Reson Imaging Clin N Am.* 2020;28(1):31-44.
2. Dietz DW, Laureti S, Strong SA, et al. Safety and longterm efficacy of strictureplasty in 314 patients with obstructing small bowel

Crohn's disease. *J Am Coll Surg.* 2001;192(3):330-337; discussion 337-338.

3. Louis E, Collard A, Oger AF, et al. Behaviour of Crohn's disease according to the Vienna classification: changing pattern over the course of the disease. *Gut.* 2001;49(6):777-782.

4. Meima-van Praag EM, Buskens CJ, Hompes, et al. Surgical management of Crohn's disease: a state of the art review. *Int J Colorectal Dis.* 2021;36(6):1133-1145.

5. Milsom JW. Strictureplasty and mechanical dilation in strictured Crohn's disease. In: Michelassi F, Milsom JW, eds. *Operative Strategies in Inflammatory Bowel Disease.* Springer; 1999:259-267.

6. Lu KC, Hunt SR. Surgical management of Crohn's disease. *Surg Clin North Am.* 2013;93(1):167-185.

7. Shapiro M, Greenstein AJ, Byrn J, et al. Surgical management and outcomes of patients with duodenal Crohn's disease. *J Am Coll Surg.* 2008;207(1):36-42.

8. Worsey MJ, Hull T, Ryland L, et al. Strictureplasty is an effective option in the operative management of duodenal Crohn's disease. *Dis Colon Rectum.* 1999;42(5):596-600.

9. Lightner A. Duodenal Crohn's disease. *Inflamm Bowel Dis.* 2018;24(3):546-551.

10. Wolff BG, Nyam D. Bypass procedures. In: Michelassi F, Milsom JW, eds. *Operative Strategies in Inflammatory Bowel Disease.* Springer; 1999:268-278.

11. Tan JJ, Tjandra JJ. Laparoscopic surgery for Crohn's disease: a meta-analysis. *Dis Colon Rectum.* 2007;50(5):576-585.

12. Fazio VW, Marchetti F, Church M, et al. Effect of resection margins on the recurrence of Crohn's disease in the small bowel. A randomized controlled trial. *Ann Surg.* 1996;224(4):563-571; discussion 571-573.

13. Strong SA, Koltun WA, Hyman NH, et al. Practice parameters for the surgical management of Crohn's disease. *Dis Colon Rectum.* 2007;50(11):1735-1746.

14. Strong SA. Surgical treatment of inflammatory bowel disease. *Curr Opin Gastroenterol.* 2002;18(4):441-446.

Chapter 3: Surgical Management of Enterocutaneous Fistula

William M. Sánchez

- Intestinal fistulas are a major public health problem. They are the source of significant morbidity and mortality risk to the individuals affected and of a major economic impact to society.
- Brooks et al utilized the US National Inpatient Sample database to investigate the impact of enteric fistulas on the US healthcare system between 2004 and 2014.
- They found that enteric fistulas require a median of 8 days of hospital stay per admission at a median cost of approximately US$16,000 per admission.
- Overall, there are 28,000 hospital admissions resulting in a total of 230,000 hospital days per year at an estimated cost of US$1.5 billion annually.[1]
- In this way, the reported cost of hospital admission associated with enteric fistulas is similar to the average annual cost of diabetes management per patient in the United States in 2017.[2]

DEFINITION

- A fistula is the abnormal communication between two epithelialized surfaces. An enterocutaneous fistula (ECF) is the abnormal communication between the bowel lumen and the skin. An enteroatmospheric fistula (EAF) is the communication between the bowel and the environment, with absence of skin continuity (open abdomen fistula) (**FIGURE 1**).
- In our hospital, anastomotic leaks occurring during the first postoperative week are considered anastomotic line failures and not fistulas (no epithelialized tract has formed during that short period of time). They are usually detected because of drainage of intestinal material or the pooling of secretions in the peritoneal cavity leading to the formation of an abscess or diffuse peritonitis. In those cases, patients are taken to surgery immediately in order to repair the leak, if possible, or to perform proximal diversion ostomies so as to ensure patient recovery.

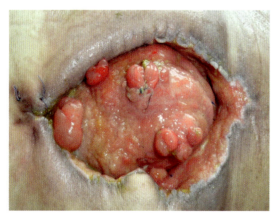

FIGURE 1 • Patient with open abdomen and multiple enteroatmospheric fistulas.

CLASSIFICATION AND PROGNOSTIC FACTORS

Multiple fistula classifications have been described, based on the fistula anatomy, etiology, and/or physiology of the fistula.

- Anatomic: fistulas are described based on the affected segment:
  - Gastrocutaneous, duodenocutaneous, enterocutaneous, and colocutaneous
- Etiology: multiple causes are described, including the following[3-5]:
  - Infectious and inflammatory (Crohn disease, ulcerative colitis, tuberculosis, mycosis, diverticulitis, Salmonellosis, amebic abscess)
  - Iatrogenic (postoperative, open abdomen, postradiation)
  - Traumatic
  - Cancer
  - Foreign bodies
- Fistula output:
  - High output: greater than 500 mL/d. These fistulas are associated with severe electrolyte and nutritional abnormalities.
  - Intermediate output: 200 to 500 mL/d
  - Low output: less than 200 mL/d

Prognostic Factors

- Deep EAFs drain the intestinal content into the abdominal cavity, giving rise to peritonitis. Mortality associated with this condition is higher than that of the superficial fistula that drains its content to the outside, creating an abdominal granulation wound with no diffuse contamination of the abdominal cavity.[6-8]
- In surgical patients with secondary fistula, we characterize the most important adverse prognostic factors associated with the course of treatment, which are analyzed following the initial resuscitation and stabilization stage (initial 48-72 hours). These factors include the following:
  - Open abdomen
  - Diameter >5 mm
  - Output >500 mL/d
  - Presence of abscess and/or diffuse peritonitis
  - Need for mechanical ventilation
  - Generalized sepsis
  - Inability to provide enteral feeding
  - Presence of multiple fistulae (**FIGURE 1**)
  - Severe comorbidities (cancer, immunosuppression, radiation therapy, etc).
- The probability of a spontaneous fistula closure is related to different factors summarized in **TABLE 1**. Three risk groups are then established in order to arrive at an objective determination of the degree of complexity of the fistula, the goals of the proposed treatment, and the predicted clinical course (**TABLE 2**).

Table 1: Probability of Spontaneous Fistula Closure

Spontaneous closure	No spontaneous closure
Esophageal, duodenal stump, jejunal	Gastric, Treitz, ileal
Enteric wall defects <1 cm	Enteric wall defects >1 cm
Fistula tracts <2 cm	Fistula tracts >2 cm
No abdominal wall defect	Open abdomen
Albumin level >25 g/L	Albumin level <25 g/L
No FRIEND factors	FRIEND factors
Output >500 mL/d	Output <200 mL/d
Conservative treatment	Surgical treatment

Nonhealing enterocutaneous fistulas are associated with FRIEND factors: a foreign body, radiation, inflammation/infection/inflammatory bowel disease, epithelization of the fistula tract, neoplasms, and distal obstructions.

Table 2: Fistula Treatment Outcomes: Prognostic Risk Groups

Prognostic group	I	II	III
Degree of complexity of the fistula	Low	Intermediate	High
Goals of the proposed treatment	Spontaneous closure	Early surgical closure	Late surgical closure
Predicted clinical course (mortality)	Very low mortality	Mortality 10%-25%	Mortality >25%

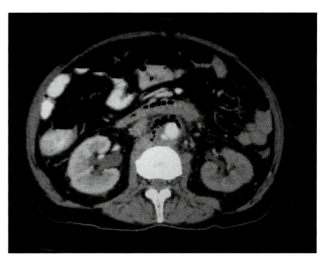

FIGURE 2 • Computed tomography scan showing aortoenteric fistula with gas around the aorta.

- Risk group I: good prognosis: This group includes patients with no debilitating disease who are in good general condition and have no systemic inflammatory response syndrome (SIRS), with fistulae that have a good probability of closing spontaneously (diameter <5 mm, output <200 mL/d, single). Treatment is limited to support, and surgical closure is not considered initially.
- Risk group II: intermediate prognosis: This group includes patients in acceptable general condition with no SIRS but with fistulas that have a small probability of closing spontaneously (diameter >5 mm, output >500 mL/d, multiple). The treatment strategy is to initially stabilize the patient and subsequently perform early surgical closure.
- Risk group III: poor prognosis: This group includes patients in poor condition who are malnourished, with severe comorbidities, who exhibit SIRS and who have fistulas with small probability of closing spontaneously. The initial goal of the treatment is to reduce output, achieve granulation and ostomization of the fistula, and care for the open abdomen. The surgical closure is performed at a later stage (6-12 months) once the patient has recovered and both objective and subjective signs of recovery are satisfactory.[8]

IMAGING AND OTHER DIAGNOSTIC STUDIES

- The role of imaging is to define the anatomy, evaluate associated processes, and provide therapeutic alternatives for treatment.
- Fistulograms, the first choice in the evaluation of ECF, are the most direct method of linking a cutaneous opening with the gastrointestinal (GI) tract. In the absence of sepsis, fistulograms may be the only imaging study needed. Two classes of contrast media are commonly used to evaluate the fistula tract, each with particular risks and benefits. Barium is a non–water-soluble media with high radiographic density, isotonic osmolarity, and an inert nature. Barium provides high-quality mucosal images, demonstrating areas of inflammation and the presence of fistula tracts with good accuracy. Unfortunately, if extravasated, barium causes significant peritoneal inflammation, including foreign body granulomas and peritoneal adhesions. Aqueous contrast agents, such as Gastrografin, are hyperosmolar and water-soluble. Water-soluble agents provide less mucosal detail; areas of inflammation, mucosal projections, and fistula tracts themselves may be missed. Gastrografin is rapidly absorbed within the peritoneal cavity if extravasated with minimal inflammation. To minimize risk and maximize benefits, water-soluble contrast material is often injected initially, followed by barium if no extravasation is seen and additional information is required.[4,7,9]
- Small bowel follow-through (SBFT) studies provide a more global view of the intestinal tract. Multiple views are typically taken to optimize visualization. Ideally, barium is used for contrast as Gastrografin can be diluted as it moves distally through the GI tract. Fistulas with narrow lumen and distal fistulas may not be detected in SBFT studies. Previously opacified loops of bowel may complicate visualization of the fistula.
- Ultrasound: Limitations of ultrasound include operator dependency, obesity, and difficulty of evaluating certain portions of the small bowel including the duodenum and jejunum. Injection of hydrogen peroxide through the fistula orifice has been reported to increase the diagnostic accuracy of ultrasound from 29% to 88% in ECF complicating Crohn disease.[10]
- Computed tomography (CT) allows for the identification of extraluminal pathology, downstream disease, and inflammation (**FIGURE 2**).
- Computed tomography enterography uses "negative" contrast, which appears dark, allowing for distention of the bowel. With the concomitant administration of intravenous contrast that will delineate mucosa, negative contrast provides additional information concerning the mucosa surrounding a fistula tract.[9]

- Magnetic resonance imaging is a promising adjunct to primary imaging modalities. Its use in ECF evaluation is beginning to be understood.
- Early diagnosis of a fistula after the initial surgery, before generalized peritonitis develops, is key in improving survival of GI anastomotic leaks. Unfortunately, there is no imaging study that is 100% sensitive and specific to diagnose this operative complication at an early stage. A proposal has been used for early diagnosis of this complication based on analysis of the peritoneal fluid collected through the drainage and measuring various proinflammatory molecular mediators including cytokines and metalloproteinases (IL-1B, IL-6, IL-10, TNF-α, MMP-2, MMP-9) which are necessary in the early phase of healing. The C-index of the nomogram was 0.93, suggesting that anastomotic leakage can be diagnosed early using this nomogram.[11]

SURGICAL MANAGEMENT

Preoperative Planning

- The fundamental pillars for fistula management, initially described by Chapman,[8] can be summarized by the **SOWATS** acronym: management of the *septic* condition, *optimization* of the nutritional status, surgical *wound* care, fistula *anatomy*, right *timing* for surgery, and *surgical* strategy.[1] By adopting this strategy, they reduced ECF mortality from 40% down to 15%.[2,8,9]
- **Sepsis:** Associated infection is the primary cause of death in fistula patients. The initial management of a patient with an ECF, with or without associated infection, is fluid resuscitation to address dehydration and prevent renal failure. Blood transfusion must be considered if required. There are two stages associated with the management of infection:
  - Early stage: When a fistula is suspected or diagnosed, the goal is to prevent or control the generalized contamination of the abdominal cavity and subsequent peritonitis. Treatment at this stage is surgical or percutaneous invasive therapy together with the use of antibiotics.
  - Late stage: After the fistula tract has been established, the goal is to prevent or treat any secondary focus of infection, usually nosocomial (catheter-related sepsis, pneumonia, residual abscesses, etc). Treatment at this stage is systemic or preventive.
- **Optimization of the nutritional status:** Effective nutritional support is a priority. Although parenteral nutrition may be needed in some cases, recent publications favor enteral nutrition as a protective factor against associated infections. The enteral route must be considered when it is suspected that the fistula will not close spontaneously, when it is a low-output fistula, or when it is localized in the terminal ileum or the colon. The use of somatostatin and octreotide, which lower endocrine and exocrine secretion, reduces fistula output. The use of antiperistaltic agents such as loperamide and codeine is also helpful. The basic nutritional requirements consist of carbohydrates and fats 20 kcal/kg/d and proteins 0.8 g/kg/d. Caloric and protein requirements may increase to 30 kcal/kg/d and 1.5 to 2.5 g/kg/d, respectively, in patients with high-output fistulas.[4,7,12,13]
- Glucagon-like peptic-2 (GLP-2) therapy has recently been introduced to restore intestinal functionality in short bowel syndrome. The therapeutic action makes it possible to inhibit the apoptosis of intestinal villus cells, favoring the proliferation of intestinal crypt epithelial cells. From a pharmacological and functional point of view, GLP-2 should be evaluated in the near future not only in the treatment of short bowel syndrome but also in the early treatment of complex intestinal fistulas.[14]
- In enteroatmospheric fistula when the distal limb of the fistula is accessible, chime reinfusion, a technique that restores artificially digestive continuity, can be instituted until definitive surgical repair. This management is recommended by ESPEN and ASPEN when possible. This therapy has been associated with weaning off intravenous fluids in 89% of the patients, and with an improved nutritional status, as determined by weight gain and albumin, absorption of nitrogen, and citrulline increases.[15]
- In these challenging clinical situations, it is sometimes necessary to use unorthodox treatments or surgical techniques. We temporarily reconstitute the intestinal tract using low-density silicone-coated Dacron prosthesis bridge joining the intestinal fistulas and thus the patient can start oral intake improving the nutritional status to finally plan the reparative surgery.
- **Surgical wound care:** The goal of treatment is to avoid maceration and excoriation of the skin surrounding the ECF, one of the main causes of chronic pain in these patients. Multidisciplinary treatment is recommended preferably in a specialized wound clinic.
- **Fistula anatomy:** It is crucial to identify the origin and tract of the fistula to plan proper treatment. Diagnostic imaging studies with water-soluble contrast through the fistula tract or through the GI route provide accurate information about the problem. CT scans are useful to assess the entire abdominal cavity and to identify other associated problems requiring treatment (abscesses, free fluid collections, obstructions, etc). In some cases, endoscopic evaluation is useful, given the possibility of performing therapeutic maneuvers to obliterate the fistulous tract (stent, clips, glue sealant).[16-19]
- **Right timing for surgery:** The ideal timing for ECF closure is still somewhat controversial. The decision on the right timing for the surgical closure of an ECF must be made after analyzing all prognostic variables for each individual patient. A period of 6 weeks is considered the minimum time between the development of the fistula and the surgical repair procedure because it is the time required for the patient to recover from the inflammatory response and to achieve a good nutritional status that will help avoid a new, possibly fatal, complication. Preoperative albumin level of less than 2.5 g/L is a strong adverse prognostic factor associated with mortality; this result has been replicated in other series.[2] In open abdomens, the time required for regression of the inflammatory state, the nutritional recovery, and the best course of potential abdominal adhesions is between 6 and 12 months. Patients are eligible for surgery when septic foci have been treated adequately and the subjective criteria for a good clinical and nutritional condition are satisfactory. These criteria include a patient who can walk, feels well, interacts actively, and is impatiently waiting for the restorative surgery. The absence of signs of sepsis is determined by the increase in albumin and hemoglobin levels, together with lower leukocyte, reactive protein C, and thrombocytosis values.[4,6,7]

- **Surgical strategy:** There are multiple surgical techniques and strategies for the treatment of ECFs. There is no single technique, and the combination of several different strategies is usually required. Generally, the surgical goals include the following:
  - Fistula resection.
  - Restore continuity of bowel transit.
  - Address the factors that promote fistula formation (obstruction, foreign body, tumors, diverticular disease, inflammations).
  - Abdominal wall closure
  - Perform as few anastomoses as possible, all of which need to be covered by healthy tissue and separated from other anastomosis lines.
  - Avoid the use of nonabsorbable mesh for closure of the abdominal wall.
  - Avoid leaving skin defects that might promote the formation of a new fistula.
  - Ensure adequate nutrition.

Surgical Tips

- In established fistulas with a defect larger than 5 mm in diameter and an output greater than 500 mL/d, attempting a primary closure with sutures is often ineffective and may increase the size of the damage to the intestinal wall. In order to attempt the primary closure of the fistula, all granulation tissue at the edges must be removed, the closure must be done under no tension, and the defect must be covered.
- No balloon catheters (Foley) must be introduced or inflated inside the fistula tract or the gut lumen because this will increase the size of the fistula. When the fistula is close to the ligament of Treitz, a feeding tube may be introduced distally for enteral nutrition.
- In fistulas with an open abdomen, the use of the Bogota bag is not very effective because it does not allow for the control of ongoing contamination of the abdominal cavity and there is persistence of skin erosion. These problems are solved with the use of the wound vacuum-assisted closure (VAC) system (the right foam must be selected in accordance with the clinical situation). In some cases, VAC therapy together with other strategies results in primary closure of the fistula. If primary closure is not achieved, VAC therapy promotes granulation and wound healing, maturation of the fistula into a controlled stoma, and patient recovery so that surgical closure and abdominal wall reconstruction may follow (**FIGURES 3-5**).[20-22]

- Patients with ECF difficult to reach and/or control (ie, ECF in frozen open abdomen, duodenal fistulas, aortoenteric fistula, etc) can develop ongoing peritonitis leading to persistent sepsis. Attempting extensive surgery (pancreatoduodenectomy, diverticulization, etc) or multiple diversions in this setting usually results in a poor outcome and extremely high mortality rates. In these critical situations, we pass a self-expandable coated stent or an impermeable corrugated prosthetic tube through the fistula defect and into the intestinal lumen to seal off the fistula, to restore intestinal transit, and to prevent ongoing soilage of the peritoneal cavity. The use of the wound VAC therapy in this setting collects any spillage of bowel fluid leaks that may occur and promotes granulation and healing of the abdominal cavity. We also use fibrin and thrombin sealants and hemostatic matrix patches in combination with local cell growth factors. Surgery must be performed at an early stage before the patient goes into multiple organ failure and is beyond rescue. After the patient recovers (weeks or months later), and if the fistula has closed, an attempt is made to recover the prosthesis through enteroscopy or surgery. If the fistula has not closed, the relevant repair surgery is planned. The introduction of this concept is controversial, but its use may be acceptable in extreme situations, based on the wide clinical experience with the use of stents or shunts in other GI, vascular, and colonic diseases (**FIGURE 6**).[23-25]

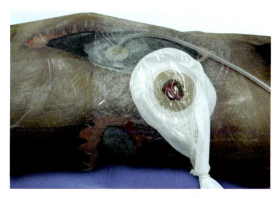

FIGURE 4 • Wound VAC therapy is very effective to allow control of fistula fluids or of contamination of the abdominal cavity.

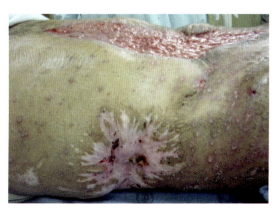

FIGURE 5 • Wound VAC therapy promotes granulation, wound healing, and control of the fistula. This allows the patient to recover in preparation for surgical closure and abdominal wall reconstruction.

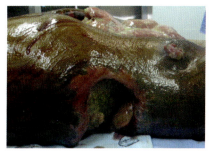

FIGURE 3 • Soldier wounded in combat with multiple intra-abdominal injuries and complex enterocutaneous fistula.

- The use of a self-expandable impermeable corrugated prosthetic stent (illustrated in **FIGURE 6**) used as a bridge to restore intestinal continuity and transit allows for oral feeding and enhanced nutritional status. This technique is particularly useful in the management of complex enteric fistulas (**FIGURE 7**) using a self-expandable impermeable corrugated prosthetic stent (**FIGURE 7B**). After several weeks of enteral support, the patient's nutritional status improved, and the wound has almost completed healed (**FIGURE 7C**) as well as for the management of complex duodenal fistulas (**FIGURE 8**) using a self-expandable impermeable corrugated prosthetic stent to control abdominal soilage by duodenal/pancreatic fluid (**FIGURE 8B**). After several weeks of duodenal stent bridge VAC therapy and enteral support, the patient's nutritional status improved, and the wound is granulating well (**FIGURE 8C**). Once the wound granulates in completely (**FIGURE 8D**), the wounds are ready for a skin graft closure (**FIGURE 8E**).

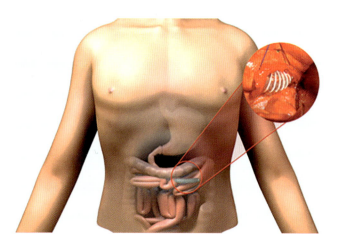

FIGURE 6 • Fistula in the fourth portion on duodenum, stent, or corrugated prosthetic tube with intestinal bypass.

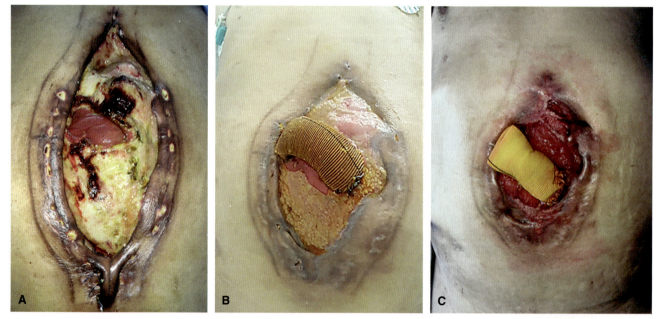

FIGURE 7 • Temporizing treatment of a complex enterocutaneous fistula **(A)** using a self-expandable impermeable corrugated prosthetic stent **(B)**. After several weeks of enteral support, the patient's nutritional status improved, and the wound has almost completed healed **(C)** as well as for the management of complex duodenal fistulas.

Chapter 3 SURGICAL MANAGEMENT OF ENTEROCUTANEOUS FISTULA   23

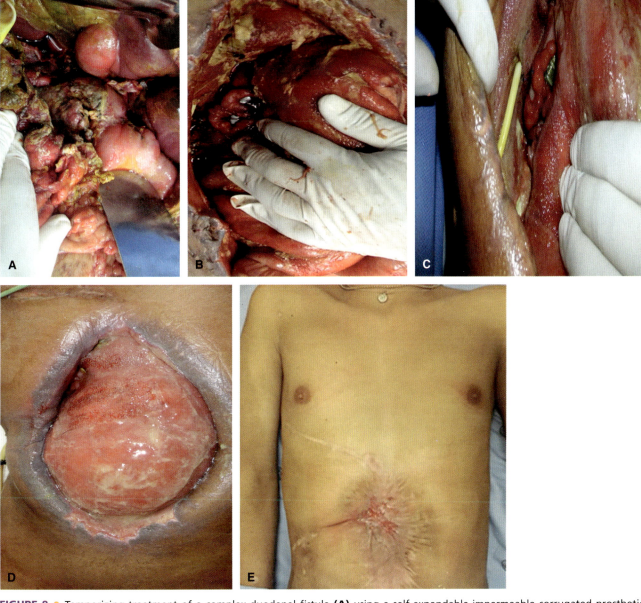

FIGURE 8 • Temporizing treatment of a complex duodenal fistula **(A)** using a self-expandable impermeable corrugated prosthetic stent to control abdominal soilage by duodenal/pancreatic fluid **(B)**. After several weeks of duodenal stent bridge VAC therapy and enteral support, the patient's nutritional status improved, and the wound is granulating well **(C)**. Once the wound granulates in completely **(D)**, the wounds are ready for a skin graft closure **(E)**.

SURGICAL CLOSURE OF COMPLEX ENTEROATMOSPHERIC FISTULA

Step 1: Peritoneal Contamination Control

- Remove the Bogota bag **(FIGURE 9)**, wash and clean the abdominal cavity, and then place a tube for enteral feeding, covering the open abdomen partially with a wound VAC system **(FIGURE 10)**.

Step 2: Granulation of the Abdominal Wound and Conversion of the Fistula into a Stoma

- Continue with wound VAC therapy until the peritoneal contamination is under control, promoting granulation of the abdominal wound **(FIGURE 11)**. The end point of this step is to achieve conversion of the fistula into a functional stoma **(FIGURE 12)**.

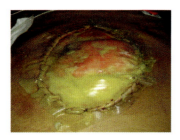

FIGURE 9 • Temporary abdominal closure with a Bogota bag.

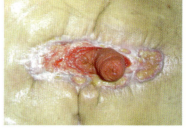

FIGURE 12 • The end point of therapy prior to surgical excision of the enterocutaneous fistula is when the fistula has been transformed into a stable stoma.

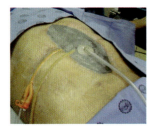

FIGURE 10 • Placement of a feeding tube and a wound VAC system.

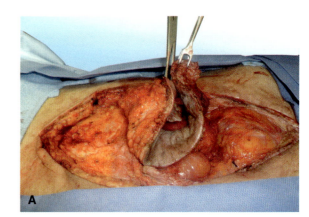

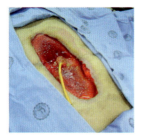

FIGURE 11 • This strategy allowed for excellent granulation tissue to form around the enterocutaneous fistula in the open abdominal wound.

FIGURE 13 • **A** and **B**, En bloc dissection of enterocutaneous fistula and granulation tissue bed.

Step 3: En Bloc Resection of the Fistula and Abdominal Wound

- En bloc dissection is performed on the entire abdominal scar component and the fistula, working inward from the surface (**FIGURE 13A** and **B**).

Step 4: Reconstruction of the Intestinal Transit and the Abdominal Wall

- The ECF is then resected (**FIGURE 14**), and the intestinal tract is reconstructed with a hand-sewn (**FIGURE 15**) or stapled technique (**FIGURE 16**). The abdominal wall is reconstructed using partially absorbable mesh with carboxymethyl cellulose coating or, preferably, with a biologic coating (**FIGURE 17**).

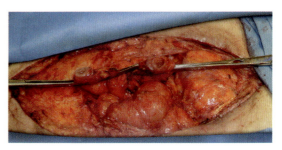

FIGURE 14 • Resection of the enterocutaneous fistula.

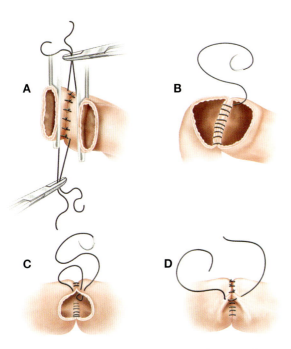

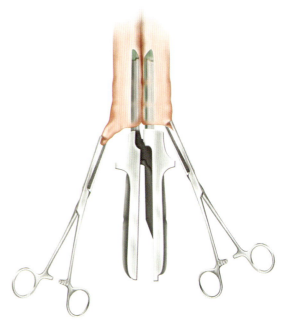

FIGURE 15 • Reestablishment of intestinal continuity. End-to-end hand-sewn anastomosis technique. **A,** The two ends are approximated with interrupted Lambert 3-0 silk sutures. **B,** The posterior row of the anastomosis is performed with running 4-0 PDS sutures. **C,** The anterior row of the anastomosis is completed with running 4-0 PDS sutures. **D,** The anastomosis is reinforced with interrupted 3-0 silk Lambert sutures.

FIGURE 16 • Reestablishment of intestinal continuity. Side-to-side stapled anastomosis technique.

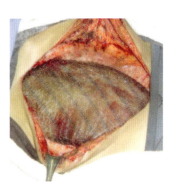

FIGURE 17 • The abdominal wall is reconstructed using partially absorbable mesh with carboxymethyl cellulose coating.

NONSURGICAL CLOSURE OF A COMPLEX ENTEROATMOSPHERIC FISTULA

- A newborn, 31 weeks of gestation with necrotizing enterocolitis, develops EAF after right hemicolectomy (**FIGURE 18**). In patients such as this one, with otherwise no significant comorbidities, a nonsurgical approach to ECF closure may be attempted.

Step 1: Peritoneal Contamination Control

- Start with general resuscitation measures and use of the SOWATS protocol. Control contamination and intestinal fluid leaks using wound VAC therapy (**FIGURE 19**).

Step 2: Granulation of the Abdominal Wound and Fistula Control

- Continue the wound VAC therapy until the peritoneal contamination is under control, promoting granulation of the abdominal wound, and channel the fistula to reduce output gradually (**FIGURE 20**).

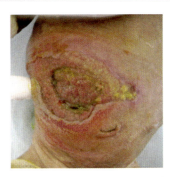

FIGURE 18 • Newborn with enterocutaneous fistula secondary to necrotizing enterocolitis.

Step 3: Closure of the Fistulous Tract Using Fibrin Glue

- Once the fistula output is down to a minimum, fibrin glue is applied through the fistula tract (**FIGURE 21**). Continue with general measures and wound VAC therapy until healing of the fistula and closure of the abdominal wall are achieved (**FIGURE 22**).

SECTION I SURGERY OF THE SMALL INTESTINE

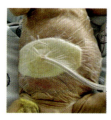

FIGURE 19 • A wound VAC has been placed to control the fistula, protect the skin, and promote granulation tissue formation.

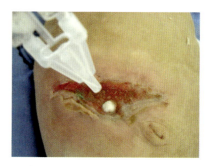

FIGURE 21 • Fibrin glue application into the fistula tract to accelerate enterocutaneous fistula closure.

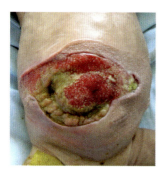

FIGURE 20 • Excellent granulation tissue has been achieved.

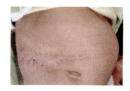

FIGURE 22 • Full healing of enterocutaneous fistula (ECF) after nonoperative management of ECF fistula.

PEARLS AND PITFALLS—PROPHYLACTIC

Burn injury	A fistula may originate from a bowel lesion created inadvertently by diathermia (**FIGURE 23**) during open or laparoscopic surgery.

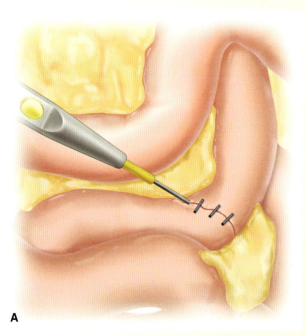
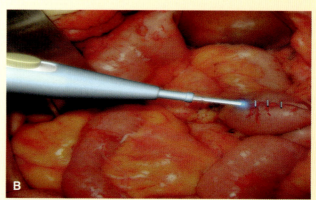

FIGURE 23 • A fistula may originate from a bowel lesion created inadvertently by diathermia secondary to technical defects or the inadequate use of surgical resources. **A,** Schematic. **B,** operative image.

Suture line protection	Anastomosis lines should not be in contact with other suture lines or prostheses.
	A vascularized omental patch is a good option to protect the anastomosis. Although the use of fibrin glue sealant has also been advocated for this purpose, there is inconclusive evidence in the literature about their benefit.
	The use of nonabsorbable mesh in direct contact with the bowels should be avoided. A good option is the use of biologic mesh or nonadherent synthetic mesh coated with carboxymethyl cellulose.
Fistulae secondary to adhesions	The prophylactic use of antiadhesive substances, such as carboxymethyl cellulose and hyaluronic acid, has been shown to reduce the presence and degree of complexity of the adhesions and, consequently, lower the possibility of fistula formation secondary to surgical injuries.[26]
Open abdomen-related fistulae (25% incidence)	The fistula forms as a result of direct injury, desiccation, or erosion due to foreign bodies that become incorporated into the gut wall (ie, Packing, Wittmann Patch, etc). Partial coverage of the abdominal cavity using the VAC system is a good option for lowering the probability of fistula formation.[20-22,25]

COMPLICATIONS

- **Local:** abscess, diffuse peritonitis, other fistulas, bleeding from erosion of adjacent structures, skin lesions.
- **Systemic:** fluid and electrolyte imbalances, malnutrition, abscess of distant solid viscera (liver, lung, brain), sepsis, SIRS.

CONCLUSION

- Currently the main cause of ECFs are those associated to the complications of surgery. Review and practice of prophylactic surgical tips can reduce its incidence.
- The treatment of fistulas must be multidisciplinary and adherence to a driving guide as SOWATS allows a sequential ordered therapeutic strategy with a chance of better clinical outcomes.
- Patients with intestinal fistulas should be categorized into risk groups in order to predict its prognosis and to define the management strategy necessary. There is no one single standard treatment; the selection of the treatment depends on the individual condition of each patient and the characteristics of the fistula itself.

REFERENCES

1. Brooks NE, Idress JJ, Steinhagen E, Giglia M, Stein SL. The impact of enteric fistulas on US hospital systems. *Am J Surg.* 2021;221(1):26-29.
2. Hu KY, Peterson CY. Enteric fistula: an overlooked but significant healthcare burden. *Am J Surg.* 2021;221(1):25.
3. Henry Edmunds L Jr, Williams GM, Welch CE. External fistulas arising from the gastro-intestinal tract. *Ann Surg.* 1960;152(3):445-469.
4. Schecter WP, Hirsberg A, Chang DS, et al. Enteric fistulas: principles of management. *J Am Coll Surg.* 2009;209(4):484-491.
5. Berry SM, Fischer JE. Classification and pathophysiology of enterocutaneous fistulas. *Surg Clin North Am.* 1996;76:1009-1018.
6. Martinez JL, Luque-de-leon E, Mier J, et al. Systematic management of postoperative enterocutaneous fistula: factors related to outcomes. *World J Surg.* 2008;32:436-443;discussion 444.
7. Lee SH. Surgical management of enterocutaneous fistula. *Korean J Radiol.* 2012;13(suppl 1):S17-S20.
8. Chapman R, Foran R. Management of intestinal fistulas. *Am J Surg.* 1964;108:157-164.
9. Lee JK, Stein SL. Radiographic and endoscopic diagnosis and treatment of enterocutaneous fistulas. *Clin Colon Rectal Surg.* 2010;23(3):149-160.
10. Maconi G, Parente F, Porro G. Hydrogen peroxide enhanced ultrasound fistulography in the assessment of enterocutaneous fistulas complicating Crohn's disease. *Gut.* 1999;45(6):874-878.
11. Shi J, Wu Z, Wu X, Shan F, Zhang Y, Ying X, Li Z, Ji J. Early diagnosis of anastomotic leakage after gastric cancer surgery via analysis

of inflammatory factors in abdominal drainage. *Ann Surg Oncol.* 2022;29(2):1230-1241. doi:10.1245/s10434-021-10763-y
12. Visschers RG, Olde Damink SW, Winkens BJ, et al. Treatment strategies in 135 consecutive patients with enterocutaneous fistulas. *World J Surg.* 2008;32(3):445-453.
13. Dudrick SJ, Wilmore DW, Vars HM, Rhoads JE. Can intravenous feeding as the sleep means of nutrition support growth in the child and restore weight loss in an adult? An affirmative answer. *Ann Surg.* 1969;169:974-984.
14. Jeppesen PB, Gabe SM, Seidner DL, Lee HM, Oliver C. Factors associated with response to teduglutide in patiens with short—bowell syndrome and intestinal failure. *Gastroenterology.* 2018;154(4):874-885.
15. Picot D, Layec S, Seynhaeve E, Dussaulx L, Trivin F, Carsin-Mahe M. Chyme reinfusion in intestinal failure related to temporary double enterostomies and enteroatmospheric fistulas. *Nutrients.* 2020;1376:2-15.
16. Groitl H, Scheele J. Initial experience with the endoscopic application of fibrin tissue adhesive in the upper gastrointestinal tract. *Surg Endosc.* 1987;1:93-97.
17. Nakagawa K, Momono S, Sasaki Y, Furusawa A, Ujiie K. Endoscopic examination for fistula. *Endoscopy.* 1990;22:208-210.
18. Lange V, Meyer G, Wenk H, Schildberg FW. Fistuloscopy—an adjuvant technique for sealing gastrointestinal fistulae. *Surg Endosc.* 1990;4:212-216.
19. Avalos-Gonzales J, Portilla-deBuen E, Leal-Cortes C. Reduction of the closure time of postoperative enterocutaneous fistulas with fibrin sealant. *World J Gastroenterol.* 2010;16(22):2793-2800.
20. Cro C, George KJ, Donnelly J, et al. Vacuum assisted closure system in the management of enterocutaneous fistulae. *Postgrad Med J.* 2002;78:364-365.
21. Sánchez MW. VAC ® Una Opción Terapéutica para el Abdomen abierto. *Investigaciones Médicas.* 2005;24(131):6-8.
22. D'Hondt M, Devriendt D, Van Rooy F. Treatment of small-bowel fistulae in the open abdomen with topical negative-pressure therapy. *Am J Surg.* 2011;202(2):20-24.
23. Puli SR, Spofford IS, Thompson CC. Use of self-expandable stents in the treatment of bariatric surgery leaks: a systematic review and meta-analysis. *Gastrointest Endosc.* 2012;75(2):287-293.
24. Van Boeckel PG, Sijbring A, Vleggaar FP, Siersema PD. Systematic review: temporary stent placement for benign rupture or anastomotic leak of the oesophagus. *Aliment Pharmacol Ther.* 2011;33(12):1292-1301.
25. Sanchez MW, Rodriguez GE, Rojas D, Asensio J. Results of the medical strategy for military trauma in Colombia. In: Asensio J, Trunkey D. eds. *Current Therapy of Trauma and Surgical Critical Care.* 2nd ed. Elsevier; 2016:7-12.
26. Kumar S, Wong PF, Leaper DJ. Intraperitoneal prophylactic agents for preventing adhesions and adhesive intestinal obstructions after non gynecological abdominal surgery. *Cochrane Database Syst Rev.* 2009;2009(1):CD005080.

Chapter 4

End and Diverting Loop Ileostomies: Creation and Reversal

Kathrin Mayer Troppmann

END AND DIVERTING LOOP ILEOSTOMIES: CREATION

DEFINITION

- An ileostomy is an artificially created opening of the distal ileum that is externalized on the abdominal wall. It can be temporary or permanent. Furthermore, it can be constructed as end ileostomy or as diverting loop ileostomy.

PATIENT HISTORY AND PHYSICAL FINDINGS

- A thorough review of the patient's history, including a review of all past operative notes and diagnostic studies, and a physical examination are necessary to carefully select patients who are appropriate candidates for an ileostomy and to determine the most appropriate type of ileostomy to be created.
- The history and the physical examination should be obtained with the functional and anatomic implications, treatment plan, and prognosis of the underlying disease in mind.
- Additionally, the patient's comorbidities, ability to perform activities of daily living and self-care, mobility limitations, and body contour must be thoroughly assessed.

IMAGING AND OTHER DIAGNOSTIC STUDIES

- Appropriate imaging studies must be obtained according to the patient's underlying disease and diagnosis. Any abnormal findings should be thoroughly worked up to ensure that the correct operation and diversion techniques are chosen. These tests may include the following:
  - Colonoscopy with biopsy if malignancy or inflammatory bowel disease is suspected
  - Computed tomography scan, upper gastrointestinal contrast study, and fistulogram to rule out intestinal obstruction or leak and to assess underlying disease severity
  - Anal manometry and endorectal ultrasound to evaluate the anal sphincter
  - Colonic motility study (eg, SITZMARKS test) to identify the region of intestinal dysmotility and to tailor the procedure and type of stoma to the patient's needs
  - Prior to ileostomy formation, the nutritional status must be assessed (including albumin and prealbumin levels) and the patient's comorbidities must be addressed (eg, coronary artery disease, diabetes [HbA_{1c}]) to minimize perioperative risk

SURGICAL MANAGEMENT

General Considerations

- If possible, a stoma should be avoided, as the morbidity of ileostomy creation and reversal can be significant.
- An ileostomy can be constructed as an end ileostomy (Brooke ileostomy) or as a diverting loop ileostomy. Alternatives to the more commonly used end and loop ileostomy techniques include the divided (or separated) loop ileostomy for maximizing fecal diversion and the end-loop (or loop-end) ileostomy for patients with a contracted mesentery and a short vascular pedicle.
- An end ileostomy is the preferred configuration for a permanent ileostomy because it allows for a symmetric and protruding spout that is more easily constructed and managed.
- Permanent end ileostomies are usually created when the distal intestine is not suitable for restoration of intestinal continuity due to underlying disease or poor intestinal function. Typical scenarios include:
  - Following total proctocolectomy for inflammatory bowel disease or familial adenomatous polyposis
  - Following subtotal colectomy for slow-transit constipation with concomitant severe pelvic floor dyssynergia
  - Fecal incontinence
  - Congenital anomalies
- Temporary end ileostomies are typically created under the following circumstances:
  - Following subtotal colectomy for acute diverticular bleeding or ulcerative colitis–related toxic megacolon
- Temporary or permanent diverting loop ileostomies are created when diversion of the fecal stream and decompression of the distal bowel are necessary:
  - Following distal ileal or colonic anastomoses at high risk for disruption due to:
    - Malnutrition or immunocompromised status
    - Anastomotic location within an irradiated, inflamed, or contaminated field
    - Low pelvic anastomotic location following sphincter-preserving procedures (eg, ileal pouch–anal anastomoses, coloanal or low colorectal anastomoses)
  - Disruption of a previously created distal anastomosis
  - Distal bowel perforation
  - Pelvic sepsis
  - Rectal trauma
  - Complicated diverticulitis
  - Following anal sphincter reconstruction
  - Following rectovaginal fistula repair
  - Fecal incontinence
  - Severe radiation proctitis
  - Obstructing or nearly obstructing colorectal cancer, carcinomatosis, and Crohn disease
  - Sacral decubitus ulcer
  - Necrotizing perineal and gluteal soft-tissue infections

Preoperative Planning

- The ideal stoma has no necrosis, prolapse, or retraction. Daily output ranges from 500 to 1000 mL, the appliance does not leak, and the skin is healthy. The importance of appropriate planning to ensure an optimal ileostomy location and to maximize the opportunity for creation of a viable,

tension-free, and well-functioning ileostomy cannot be overemphasized. Attention to these principles will decrease the time required for stoma management and minimize patient frustration.
- A comprehensive discussion with the patient about the proposed ileostomy procedure, alternatives, and postoperative lifestyle is imperative.
- The majority of stoma patients are elderly, and many have their stoma care performed by a spouse, offspring, or caretaker; it is thus critical to involve these providers in the stoma education process.
- Ideally, patients must be mentally and physically ready for a stoma and must therefore be informed as early as possible in their course of disease regarding the potential need for a stoma. For many patients, though, an ileostomy is created in an acute setting at the end of a long, often life-saving procedure.

Stoma Education

- A comprehensive perioperative educational program decreases readmissions and complications related to dehydration and appliance problems and optimizes postoperative patient satisfaction and participation in activities of daily life.
  - Wound ostomy continence nurse or enterostomal therapy nurse
    - Optimal stoma management begins with preoperative patient education regarding diet, activities, clothing, and sexuality. The nurse can provide emotional and physical support. The patient must be informed that self-care may be awkward initially, but that it can be learned and mastered.
  - Patient support groups, United Ostomy Association visitor
    - Patients should be introduced to other individuals with ileostomies who have similar socioeconomic and disease backgrounds. These encounters and relationships can help to improve morale and can reassure patients that they can have a satisfactory quality of life. Meetings should occur pre- and postoperatively (particularly during the first 3 to 6 months).
  - Stoma preparedness literature
    - The American College of Surgeons has created a comprehensive stoma preparedness kit including an educational DVD and manual, a stoma model, and stoma appliance samples.

Stoma Site Marking

- The stoma location must be carefully planned to minimize complications and to prevent leakage.
- The patient may wear the stoma appliance faceplate prior to the operation. The optimal location of the stoma should be assessed with the patient standing, sitting, and bending. Where does the patient wear the waist of the pants? Range of motion and physical limitations must be evaluated to determine if the patient can visualize the stoma and can manipulate the appliance (eg, the site may be placed higher on the abdomen for a wheelchair-bound patient). Care must be taken to avoid stoma placement beneath an abdominal pannus so that the stoma remains visible and easy to access for the patient or caretaker.
- In general, the ileostomy should be placed through the rectus muscle (to minimize parastomal herniation), at the summit of the right paramedian infraumbilical fat pad. The umbilicus, bone, scars, skin folds, and abdominal panni should be avoided (**FIGURE 1**). The skin site can be identified with a permanent marker or a scratch can be made with a small needle.

Intraoperative Positioning

- Supine or lithotomy position may be used based on the need for an adjunctive procedure for assessment of the colon, rectum, or perineum prior to ileostomy creation (eg, colonoscopy).

Antibiotic Prophylaxis

- Intravenous antibiotics covering enteric flora must be given prior to the incision.

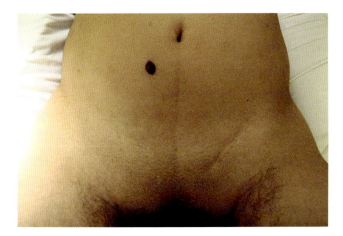

FIGURE 1 • Preoperative marking of the ileostomy site. The ileostomy is placed in the right lower quadrant of the abdomen in a right paramedian, infraumbilical position.

CREATION OF AN END ILEOSTOMY

- Meticulous construction of an end ileostomy is paramount because the ileal contents are liquid, bilious, and voluminous. An everted, spout-shaped end ileostomy (Brooke ileostomy) is best suited to address these challenges.

Abdominal Wall Skin Incision for Exploratory Laparotomy and/or Bowel Resection

- If an abdominal incision for bowel resection is necessary, a left paramedian skin incision (slightly to the left of midline) can be made and angled toward the midline. The abdomen can then be entered through the linea alba between the rectus muscles. This approach maximizes the distance and amount of skin between the ileostomy and the skin incision.

Ileal Mobilization

- The ileum is prepared by releasing the lateral attachments along the pelvic brim and by fully mobilizing the embryonic root of the terminal ileal mesentery to the level of the duodenum.

Stoma Site Skin Incision

- Following the intestinal resection, the skin opening is created in the right lower quadrant at the premarked site. The skin is grasped with a Kocher clamp and a circular skin incision of 2 cm in diameter (**FIGURE 2A**) is made tangentially beneath the Kocher clamp with a No. 10 blade. The excised skin disc is removed.

Abdominal Wall Aperture Creation for the Stoma

- Bovie electrocautery is used to perpendicularly divide the subcutaneous fat in the right paramedian plane at the ileostomy site. Handheld retractors can be gently used. The subcutaneous fat should be preserved as much as possible.
- The anterior rectus sheath is identified and incised in a cruciate fashion for approximately 1 cm in both directions. (The horizontal limb should not be placed too close to the midline.)
- Mayo clamps are used to split the rectus muscle bluntly to expose the posterior rectus sheath and peritoneum. The rectus muscle fibers are not divided (**FIGURE 2B**).
- The surgeon places one hand into the abdominal cavity behind the intended stoma site to protect the abdominal contents.
- The abdominal cavity is entered through the stoma incision with a thin-point clamp (eg, Schnidt or tonsil clamp).
- The defect in the posterior rectus sheath and peritoneum is widened to allow for passage of the ileum without compromising its mesenteric blood supply. The appropriate defect size is obtained by digitally dilating the stoma site with the tips of two digits to create an approximately 2-cm aperture (**FIGURE 2C**).

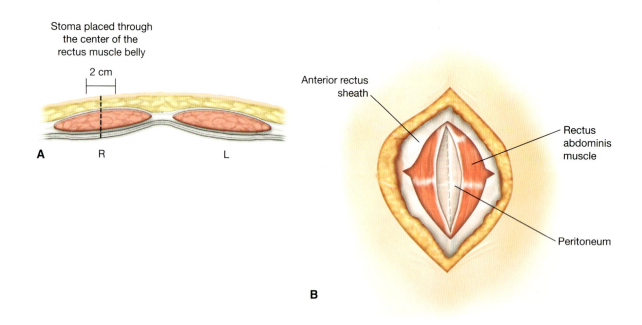

FIGURE 2 • Creation of an end ileostomy. **A,** A circular skin incision for the ileostomy is made over the center of the rectus muscle belly and carried through the subcutaneous fat. **B,** A cruciate incision is made in the anterior rectus sheath to expose the underlying rectus muscle. The rectus muscle is split bluntly along the direction of its fibers to expose the posterior sheath and peritoneum. **C,** The peritoneum is incised longitudinally, and the incision is widened by stretching it with two digits to obtain the desired aperture. **D,** The vascular end arcade and the mesentery are preserved on the ileal segment that is to be used for the end ileostomy *(dotted arrow)*. **E,** The ileum is advanced through the abdominal wall stoma aperture so that it protrudes for about 4 cm beyond the skin level. Following removal of the staple line, three-point sutures are placed through the end of the ileum (full thickness), the seromuscular layer at the base of the stoma 4 cm from the end of the ileum, and the dermis, respectively. No epidermis should be included in stitch. **F,** The sutures are placed circumferentially. They are only tied after all of them have been placed, everting the ileum to create a 2-cm-high ileostomy.

Chapter 4 END AND DIVERTING LOOP ILEOSTOMIES: CREATION AND REVERSAL 31

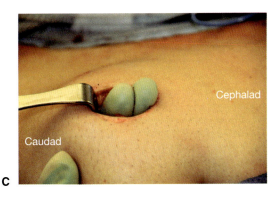

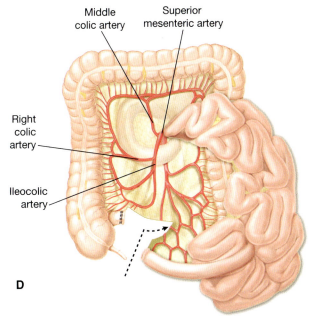

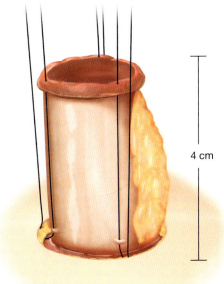

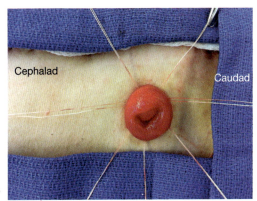

FIGURE 2 • (continued)

Ileal Limb Preparation and Placement

- At least 6 cm of viable distal or terminal ileum with the adjacent marginal artery should be preserved to maintain an optimal blood supply. The mesentery should not be stripped (**FIGURE 2D**). The ileal limb preparation should be performed as early as possible during the operation to allow for sufficient time to observe and assess the ileum's viability. The mesentery must be handled gently to avoid hematomas and mesenteric vascular injury.
- The ileum is advanced (gently "pushed" from the abdominal side, rather than "pulled" through the skin opening) through the split muscle and the abdominal wall to about 4 cm beyond the skin level (using a Babcock clamp to grasp the ileum only if necessary). If the ileum and adjacent tissues are too bulky to pass easily through the aperture, the epiploic fat can be excised.

- To facilitate a future ileostomy reversal procedure, an adhesion barrier (eg, Seprafilm) can be used at the time of ileostomy creation. The adhesion barrier is wrapped around the ileal limb used for the ileostomy, extending along the intra-abdominal ileal segment for approximately 5 cm.
- The ileal mesentery may be secured to the peritoneum over a length of 3 to 4 cm if a permanent stoma is planned. (This step may prevent torsion, retraction, and prolapse of the ileum.)
- Both edges of the rectal stump (or other potentially remaining distal bowel segment) are tagged with polypropylene suture to facilitate identification of the distal intestinal segment for potential ileostomy reversal.
- To prevent wound contamination, the surgical abdominal incision is closed next and then covered with a protective wound dressing prior to maturing the stoma.

Stoma Maturation

- The staple line is removed from the ileum.
- The 3-0 absorbable (eg, Vicryl) interrupted stitches are placed (but not immediately tied), with the stitches running through the following three points (**FIGURE 2E**):
  - End of the ileum (full thickness)
  - Skin-level base of the stoma (4 cm from the end of the ileum) (seromuscular layer)
  - Dermis (large bites of the subcuticular layer should be avoided to prevent "buttonholing" and mucosal islands)
- One stitch is placed in each quadrant followed by one stitch between each quadrant stitch for a total of seven to eight stitches. Ensure that one stitch is on each side of, and adjacent to, the mesentery (but not through the mesentery).
- To allow for more precise placement, each stitch should be individually tagged and tied only when all stitches have been placed. The subcutaneous and mesenteric fat can be tucked in as each suture is tied. The goal is to create a stoma with a spout that protrudes about 2 cm beyond the skin level when completed (**FIGURE 2F**).
- The ileostomy appliance is placed over the stoma. Waterproof, nonallergenic tape can be used to further secure the edge of the appliance to the skin.

CREATION OF A LOOP ILEOSTOMY

Stoma Site Skin Incision and Abdominal Wall Aperture Creation

- The skin incision for a loop ileostomy is like the incision for an end ileostomy, except that it is made slightly longer and oblong. In obese patients, some of the subcutaneous tissues may have to be excised down to the fascia in the shape of a cone (apex at skin level) to not constrict the afferent and efferent limbs of the loop ileostomy.

Ileal Limb Preparation and Placement

- An ileal segment 20 to 30 cm proximal to the ileocecal valve is identified. The segment is selected to maximize mesenteric pedicle length and to avoid compromising the ileocecal valve. The segment's mesentery and vasculature are preserved (**FIGURE 3A**).
- Two different orienting sutures are placed on the antimesenteric side of the ileum to mark the afferent and efferent aspects of the ileal segment (eg, by using sutures of different colors, or sutures with one knot for the afferent segment and two knots for the efferent segment) (**FIGURE 3B**).
- An umbilical tape is passed behind the ileum at the ilealmesenteric interface. The ileal loop is advanced through the abdominal wall using the umbilical tape as a guide, taking care to maintain proper orientation and to avoid torsion.
- The afferent (productive) limb of the loop ileostomy is placed inferiorly so that its spout will be located on the caudal aspect of the stoma. Alternatively, the afferent limb can be placed on the medial side of a transversely oriented loop ileostomy, depending on surgeon preference and amount of tension on the ileostomy.
- Optionally, sutures may be placed between the ileal mesentery and peritoneum to maintain the appropriate rotation, especially in obese patients.
- The umbilical tape is removed and may optionally be replaced with a supporting rod or a 6-cm segment of red rubber catheter (which may be looped and sutured to itself above the loop ileostomy or secured to the skin).
- To prevent contamination of the laparotomy incision, the surgical abdominal incision (midline or left paramedian) is closed next, and a protective wound dressing is placed prior to stoma maturation.

Stoma Maturation

- It is important to create an adequate spout on the afferent bowel limb.
- First, the efferent (distal) limb of the ileum is transversely incised 1 cm above the skin surface for approximately 75% of the circumference of the ileum to allow for appropriate stoma eversion (**FIGURE 3C**). This allows for a large "hood" and for the os on the afferent productive limb to be larger (encompassing 80%-90% of the ileostomy) than the os of the efferent limb.
- The stoma is created and matured with 3-0 absorbable suture (eg, Vicryl). First, the efferent stoma is sewn relatively flush with the dermis by using a two-point suturing technique, with each stitch taking a full-thickness bite through the cut edge of ileum and then through the dermis. Next, the afferent stoma is matured with a three-point suturing technique as already described in principle for the end ileostomy (**FIGURE 3D**). However, the seromuscular stitches of the afferent limb are taken 3 to 4 cm from the mucosal edges. The main difference in appearance between the loop ileostomy and end ileostomy is that the loop ileostomy will not protrude as far from the skin surface compared with an end ileostomy. Also, ileal eversion sutures cannot be placed on the posterior bridge of ileum that joins the afferent and efferent limbs.
- Optionally, as the sutures are tied, the spout can be formed over a supporting rod (or catheter), which is left in place for 3 to 5 days postoperatively. The edge of the aperture in the ileostomy faceplate is placed beneath the rod or catheter.

Chapter 4 **END AND DIVERTING LOOP ILEOSTOMIES: CREATION AND REVERSAL** 33

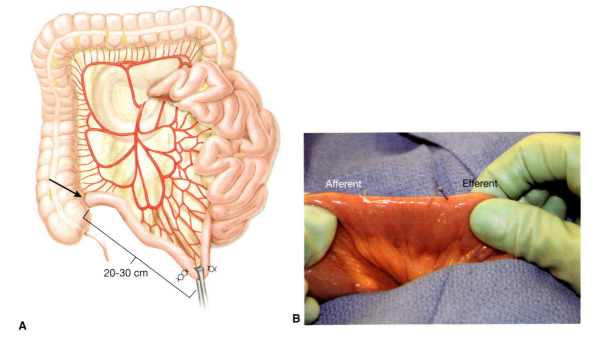

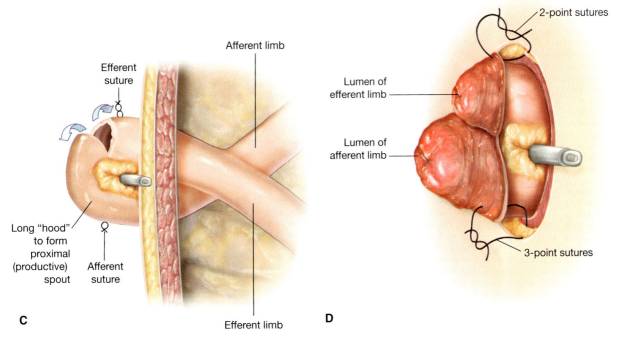

FIGURE 3 • Creation of a loop ileostomy. **A,** An ileal segment that is 20 to 30 cm proximal to the ileocecal junction *(arrow)* is identified. The segment's mesentery and vasculature are preserved. **B,** Marking sutures (eg, sutures of different colors or with differing numbers of knots) are placed on the afferent and efferent limbs. The ileum is advanced through the abdominal wall stoma aperture so that it protrudes for about 3 to 4 cm beyond the skin level. **C,** The ileum is incised 1 cm above the skin level on the efferent limb side for 75% of the circumference to create a large afferent spout. **D,** The loop ileostomy is matured by placing two-point sutures (full thickness through the end of the ileum and the dermis) on the efferent limb and three-point sutures (full thickness through the end of ileum, the seromuscular layer at the base of stoma, and the dermis) on the afferent limb to evert the ileum.

CREATION OF A DIVIDED LOOP ILEOSTOMY

- A divided (or separated) loop ileostomy is an alternative technique for creating a protecting loop ileostomy; it may result in a more complete fecal diversion.

Stoma Site Skin Incision and Abdominal Wall Aperture Creation

- The skin incision and abdominal wall aperture are created as for a loop ileostomy.

Ileal Limb Preparation and Placement

- The ileum is divided with a linear cutting stapler 20 to 30 cm proximal to the ileocecal valve. The mesentery and vasculature are only minimally divided (**FIGURE 4A**).
- The stapled afferent limb is advanced through the abdominal wall aperture so that it protrudes 4 cm beyond the skin and the staple line is removed. Only the antimesenteric corner of the efferent limb is externalized, thus minimizing the need for division of the mesentery. Alternatively, the efferent limb can remain stapled closed if complete fecal diversion is desired and only if there is no risk of distal obstruction (**FIGURE 4B**).

Stoma Maturation

- Afferent limb—The stoma is constructed in the same manner as described for an end ileostomy, using a three-stitch technique (**FIGURE 4C**).
- Efferent limb—The antimesenteric corner is excised to decompress the distal bowel if desired. A two-stitch technique is then used, placing sutures that encompass the full-thickness edge of the ileum and the dermis.

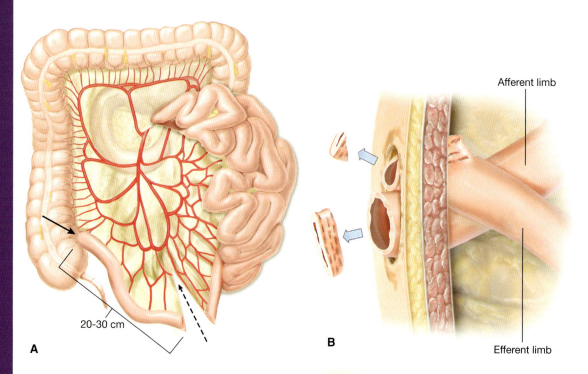

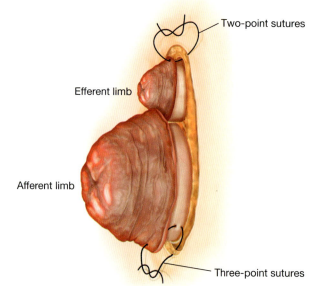

FIGURE 4 • Creation of a divided loop ileostomy. **A,** The ileum is divided using a linear cutting stapler, 20 to 30 cm proximal to the ileocecal valve (solid arrow). The mesentery and vasculature are only minimally divided (dotted arrow). **B,** The stapled afferent limb is advanced through the abdominal wall aperture so that it protrudes for about 4 cm beyond the skin level, and the entire staple line is then cut off. Optionally, if distal decompression is desired for the efferent limb, only the antimesenteric corner is externalized, excised, and matured. The staple line may also be left intact on the efferent limb for total diversion, yet only if there is no risk of distal obstruction. **C,** The afferent limb of the ileostomy is matured with three-point sutures. If distal decompression is desired, the efferent limb can be matured with two-point sutures.

CREATION OF AN END-LOOP ILEOSTOMY

- An end-loop (or loop-end) ileostomy is functionally not different from an end ileostomy, but the stoma maturation is like the technique for a loop ileostomy. An end-loop ileostomy allows for preservation of an adequate mesenteric blood supply when the mesentery would otherwise be too short for adequate advancement through the abdominal wall (eg, in case of a shortened mesentery or a thickened abdominal wall). This technique is more likely to be used in obese patients and those with prior operations.

Stoma Site Skin Incision and Abdominal Wall Aperture Creation

- The skin and stoma site are prepared as described for a loop ileostomy.

Ileal Limb Preparation and Placement

- The mesentery and vasculature are divided to obtain as much length as possible (**FIGURE 5A**).
- Following the distal intestinal resection or division, the staple line at the end of the ileum is oversewn.
- The segment of ileum to be used for the stoma creation is typically located about 10 cm proximal to the oversewn ileal staple line. The segment must have adequate mobility to reach the proposed stoma site without tension. Within the abdominal cavity, the afferent limb is oriented inferiorly and the efferent limb superiorly. The segment of ileum to be used for the stoma is then advanced through the abdominal wall as for a loop ileostomy (**FIGURE 5B**).
- Optionally, a supporting rod or catheter can be passed behind the ileum at the ileal-mesenteric interface.
- Optionally, the intra-abdominal ileal mesentery may be sutured to the peritoneum.

Stoma Maturation

- The end-loop ileostomy is matured as described for a loop ileostomy (**FIGURE 3C** and **D**).

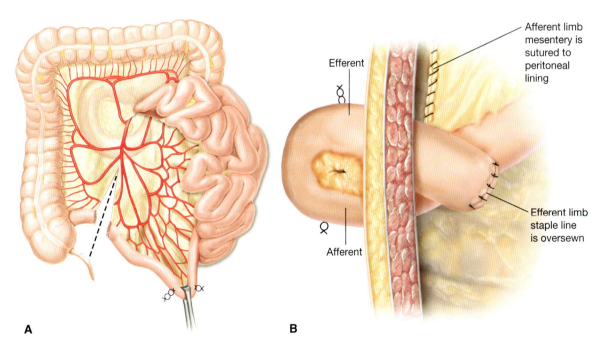

FIGURE 5 • Creation of an end-loop ileostomy. **A,** The mesentery and vasculature are divided proximally to obtain as much length as possible. **B,** Marking sutures are placed on the afferent and efferent limbs. The staple line closing off the ileum is oversewn with Lembert sutures and remains in the abdomen. A more proximal segment of ileum to be used for the ileostomy, approximately 10 cm proximal to the oversewn ileal staple line, is externalized so that the afferent limb is in the inferior position on the abdominal wall. The mesentery may be affixed to the abdominal wall to prevent stoma prolapse, torsion, or an internal hernia.

LAPAROSCOPIC CREATION OF AN ILEOSTOMY

- The laparoscopic approach can be used for temporary and permanent end ileostomies, loop ileostomies, divided loop ileostomies, and end-loop ileostomies.
- The entire abdominal cavity can be visualized and inspected, which can be beneficial as it allows for assessment of the underlying disease and the extent of adhesions. Additionally, laparoscopy allows for precise identification of the ileal segment to be used for the stoma and can help to ensure its proper orientation.
- The laparoscopic approach may not be feasible if the patient has extensive adhesions from prior operations or an insufficient intra-abdominal domain due to intestinal dilatation.

- Laparoscopic ileostomy creation may result in shorter total incision length, shorter operative time, decreased pain, fewer wound complications, more rapid return of bowel function, and shorter hospital stay.

Stoma Site Skin Incision and Port Placement

- The 2 cm skin incision for the stoma site can be made prior to insufflation at the time of port site creation *or* after diagnostic laparoscopy and selection of the ileal segment to be externalized (see "Abdominal Wall Aperture Creation for the Stoma").
- A 5-mm or 10-mm port is placed through the upper midline for the camera.
- A 10-mm port is placed through the intended ileostomy site.
- A 5-mm port is placed in the left lower quadrant for bowel manipulation and adhesiolysis as necessary.
- An additional 5-mm port may be placed in the left suprapubic region if needed.

Ileal Limb Preparation and Placement

- The most distal segment of ileum that can reach the intended stoma site without tension is identified laparoscopically.
- For loop ileostomies, sutures or clips are placed to mark the afferent and efferent ileum prior to externalization.
- A laparoscopic bowel clamp is placed through the 10-mm port at the stoma site to grasp the ileum.
- The pneumoperitoneum is released.
- To facilitate the passage of the loop of ileum, the anterior rectus sheath can be further stretched or incised with a cruciate incision.
- The ileum, bowel clamp, and 10-mm port are pulled out of the abdomen.

Laparoscopic Confirmation of Proper Stoma Orientation

- Adequate stoma loop orientation and hemostasis are confirmed after reestablishing pneumoperitoneum.
- All ports are removed and the skin incisions are closed with absorbable suture.

Stoma Maturation

- The stoma is matured as described for the open technique.

PLACEMENT OF THE ILEOSTOMY APPLIANCE

- Most appliances are disposable and available as one-piece or two-piece products. A basic appliance consists of an adhesive faceplate with a central opening and a collection bag. When cutting out the definitive stoma aperture in the appliance faceplate, the stoma aperture is cut offset (ie, medially in relation to the precut stoma aperture) in order to shift the entire appliance laterally on the patient. As a result, the portion of the appliance directly over any midline incision can be minimized. The edges of the cutout area of the appliance should be 1 to 2 mm away from the edges of the ileostomy to avoid unnecessary skin exposure to the bowel contents (which would excoriate the exposed skin) and also to avoid appliance trauma to, and leakage from, the ileostomy (**FIGURE 6**).

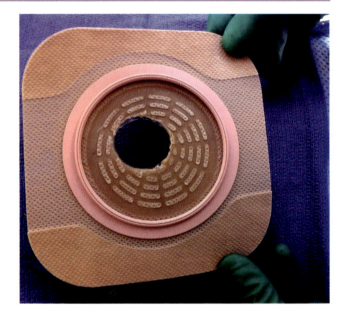

FIGURE 6 • Ileostomy appliance. The faceplate stoma aperture is cut off-center in a medial direction to minimize the portion of the faceplate that lays directly over a midline incision (allows for a shift laterally off the midline if an incision if present).

END AND DIVERTING LOOP ILEOSTOMIES: REVERSAL

DEFINITION

- Ileostomy reversal (synonyms: ileostomy takedown or closure) is a procedure that reestablishes intestinal continuity in a patient with an ileostomy.

PATIENT HISTORY AND PHYSICAL FINDINGS

- Reversal of a temporary ileostomy has traditionally been performed at 3 months after index procedure to allow for optimal healing of the area from which the enteric contents were diverted (eg, distal anastomosis, bowel repair) or to allow for the distal inflammation to subside.
- Ileostomy reversal earlier than 3 months after index procedure may be performed in carefully selected patients.
  - Reversal may be necessary at an earlier date for selected patients in the presence of an ileostomy complication such as prolapse or recurrent serious fluid and electrolyte abnormalities.
  - Reversal may be acceptable at an earlier date in relatively healthy patients under certain circumstances (eg, an end ileostomy following subtotal colectomy may be reversed if the rectal and anal complexes are healthy and without disease or malfunction).

- Modifiable risk factors (eg, malnutrition) must be optimized and any chemotherapy and radiation should be completed.
- Ileostomy reversal can be associated with considerable morbidity.
- Up to 30% of patients with potentially reversible ileostomies never have their ileostomies reversed due to underlying health issues, underlying disease prognosis, or patient preference.

IMAGING AND OTHER DIAGNOSTIC STUDIES

- The indications for preoperative imaging and diagnostic (eg, functional) studies must be individualized for each patient.
- The routine use of contrast studies prior to ileostomy takedown to assess the distal bowel or anastomosis for stricture, obstruction, leak, recurrence of disease, or pouch anatomy is controversial. If a study is performed, the contrast can be instilled through the efferent limb of a loop ileostomy or per anum, depending on the location of the area to be studied.
- An examination under anesthesia and an endoscopic assessment may be performed to ascertain if a J-pouch is intact, to confirm that a distal anastomosis or repair has healed, and to ensure that a malignancy has not recurred.
- If the anal sphincter was involved in the disease or repair, an anal manometry or endoscopic ultrasonography may be helpful to evaluate the sphincter.

SURGICAL MANAGEMENT

Preoperative Planning

- Ileostomy reversal is not a minor operation and sometimes requires a full laparotomy.
- A loop ileostomy often facilitates subsequent ileostomy reversal by potentially obviating the need for a full laparotomy.
- The groundwork for successful ileostomy reversal is laid at the time of the construction of the ileostomy. To facilitate the ileostomy takedown procedure, an adhesion barrier should be placed at the time of ileostomy creation.
- Bowel preparation for the proximal intestine consists of 24 hours of clear liquids.
- Bowel preparation distal to the ileostomy is optional but is strongly recommended if no formal bowel preparation was performed prior to creation of ileostomy (eg, in case of an emergency operation). Bowel preparation can be achieved under those circumstances as follows:
  - Patients with an end ileostomy and a rectal stump: transanal enema.
  - Patients with a loop ileostomy: irrigation through the efferent limb or transanal retrograde enema, depending on the location of disease, repair, or anastomosis.
  - The radiologist can be asked to irrigate the diverted segment (efferent limb or colon) with saline solution at the completion of a contrast study.
  - Preoperative (day of surgery) ureteral stents should be strongly considered if the patient has had significant pelvic inflammation.

Positioning

- The patient is placed in lithotomy position if an endoscopic assessment or examination under anesthesia is required, if the rectal vault requires irrigation and evacuation of inspissated mucus secretions, or if an ileorectal or ileoanal anastomosis is to be created.
- Supine position is adequate if no access to the anus or rectum is required.

REVERSAL OF END ILEOSTOMY

Stoma Closure

- The stoma is closed with a running 0 silk suture.

Mobilization and Resection of Ileostomy

- A circumferential skin incision is made sharply around the closed ileostomy just peripheral to the mucocutaneous junction.
- Sharp dissection is used next to the bowel wall, with judicious use of electrocautery, to release the stoma from the subcutaneous fat, rectus muscle, and rectus sheath (**FIGURE 7**). Caution is used to avoid an injury to the bowel wall or mesentery. Eastman or Army-Navy retractors can facilitate exposure and visualization.
- Any internal adhesions of the ileostomy to the abdominal peritoneum are lysed circumferentially to clear the peritoneal surface for safe subsequent approximation and closure of the abdominal wall defect.
- A wound protector may be placed to minimize wound contamination.
- The ileostomy is excised with its adjacent fibrofatty tissue.
- A viable segment of ileum with intact serosa and adequate blood supply is prepared for the anastomosis. If a stapled anastomosis is planned, the anvil from the circular stapler is placed and secured into the lumen of the ileum.

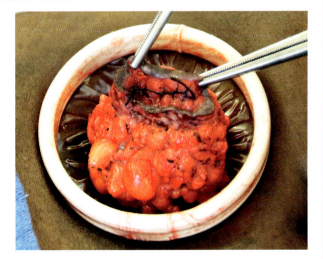

FIGURE 7 • Skin incision and stoma mobilization for reversal of an end or loop ileostomy. A circumferential skin incision is made directly adjacent to the closed ileostomy. The incision is deepened across all abdominal wall layers down to the level of the abdominal cavity. The ileostomy and adherent fibrofatty tissues are resected.

Preparation of the Distal Bowel Segment

- Utilizing the open or laparoscopic technique, the distal bowel segment to which the ileum is to be anastomosed (often the rectum) is carefully mobilized and prepared for anastomosis. The intestinal segment must be viable and of adequate length.

Anastomosis after Takedown of the End Ileostomy

- A standard ileorectal (or ileoanal or ileocolic) anastomosis can be created with a stapler (eg, by using a circular end-to-end anastomosis [EEA] stapler) or a handsewn technique (**FIGURE 8**).
- A leak test is performed. Water is poured into the pelvis until the anastomosis is submerged. The bowel is occluded proximal to the anastomosis. Air is insufflated per anum with a proctoscope.
  - Small leaks can be oversewn and the leak test is repeated. If the leak test remains positive, the anastomosis can be redone with a low threshold for the placement of a proximal diverting loop ileostomy and a pelvic drain.
  - Small leaks low in the pelvis or large leaks should be repaired or the anastomosis should be redone. Creation of a proximal diverting loop ileostomy and insertion of a pelvic drain should be strongly considered under those circumstances. The omentum should be wrapped around the anastomosis.
- Alternatively, the anastomosis can be visualized endoscopically (with or without injection of intravenous fluorescein to assess the intestinal blood supply).

Fascial Closure

- The abdominal wall stoma defect is closed without tension in two layers with running or interrupted 1-polydioxanone suture. Omentum is placed between the anastomosis and the fascial closure, if available.
- Biologic or prosthetic mesh can be used for reinforcement at the stoma site to decrease risk of incisional hernia.

Stoma Site Skin Closure

- The skin can be closed with numerous different techniques, but in principle, the closure should not be watertight. Options include the following:
  - Primary skin closure
    - Loose skin closure with interrupted 2-0 nylon sutures or staples. Wound fluid drainage should be facilitated, for instance, by application of wicks made of Kendall Telfa dressing pads (the wicks should be removed on postoperative day 2 or 3).

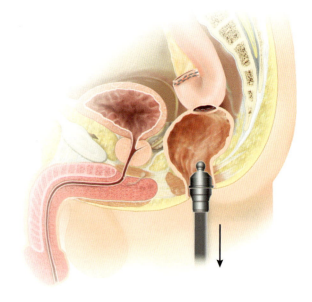

FIGURE 8 • Reversal of an end ileostomy. Intestinal continuity is restored with a circular cutting stapler (eg, by creating an ileorectal anastomosis).

  - Delayed primary closure (performed on postoperative day 2 or 3).
  - Purse-string closure. Loose circular (purse-string) skin closure with 2-0 running, subcuticular polypropylene. The approximately 1 to 1.5 cm central opening resulting from the purse-string closure is packed with moist gauze that is first removed on postoperative day 2 and then exchanged daily. The suture is removed on postoperative day 21. The purse-string closure is associated with a lower surgical site infection rate than a primary closure.
  - Wound healing by secondary intention. The wound is left open and wet-to-dry dressing changes are initiated. Alternatively, a wound VAC can be applied to the wound if a large pannus is present to accelerate wound healing.

REVERSAL LOOP ILEOSTOMY

- The loop ileostomy closure can usually be performed through the ileostomy site, without requiring a complete laparotomy.
- The steps leading up to the anastomosis are the same as for the reversal of the end ileostomy discussed earlier.
- A wound protector is placed to minimize wound contamination.

Anastomosis after Takedown of Loop Ileostomy

- The anastomosis between the proximal (afferent) and distal (efferent) ileal limbs can be either handsewn or stapled.
- The stoma and fibrofatty tissues are resected with a linear cutting stapler to a level where there are two distinct ileal limbs (**FIGURE 9A**).
  - For a stapled side-to-side anastomosis, the antimesenteric corner of each ileal end is cut and removed.
- A side-to-side, functional EEA is created with a linear cutting stapler (**FIGURE 9B**). The enteric defect is closed with a linear stapler or a handsewn technique.
- The anastomosis can also be constructed with a circular stapler or handsewn.
- Alternatively, a direct transverse closure of the enteric defect at the stoma site can be performed. With this technique, the stoma and fibrofatty tissues are resected sparingly so that the connecting bridge of intestinal wall on the posterior (mesenteric) aspect of the loop stoma remains intact (**FIGURE 10A**).
  - The antimesenteric defect can then be closed either by a handsewn technique (double layer technique consisting of 3-0 absorbable full-thickness sutures [eg, Vicryl], followed by 3-0 nonabsorbable Lembert seromuscular sutures [eg, silk]) (**FIGURE 10B**) or stapled technique (with a linear stapler) with optional oversewing of the staple line (**FIGURE 10C**).

Chapter 4 **END AND DIVERTING LOOP ILEOSTOMIES: CREATION AND REVERSAL** 39

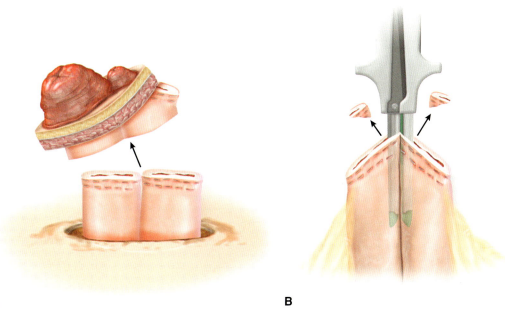

FIGURE 9 • Reversal of a loop ileostomy: option 1 (results in larger anastomotic cross section). **A,** The ileum is mobilized from the abdominal wall. The stoma itself (including the staples in case of a divided loop ileostomy) and adjacent fibrofatty tissues are resected with a linear cutting stapler to a level where both limbs are completely separated. **B,** A side-to-side (functional end-to-end) stapled anastomosis is created with a linear cutting stapler inserted into the antimesenteric aspect of each ileal limb. The remaining ileal opening is closed off with a linear stapler application or by using a handsewn technique.

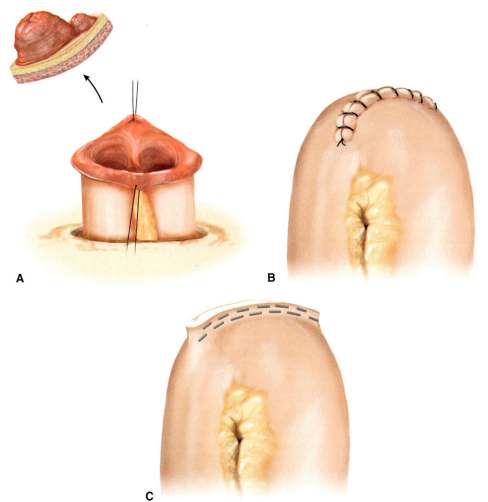

FIGURE 10 • Reversal of a loop ileostomy: option 2. **A,** The ileum is mobilized from the abdominal wall. The stoma itself and adjacent fibrofatty tissues are resected sparingly so that the connecting bridge of ileum on the posterior/mesenteric aspect of the loop ileostomy is left intact. **B,** The ileal defect is closed with a transverse two-layer handsewn technique or **(C)** with a linear stapler.

40 SECTION I **SURGERY OF THE SMALL INTESTINE**

PEARLS AND PITFALLS

Ileostomy Creation	
Indications	■ A diverting ileostomy may prevent morbidity by preventing a distal anastomotic disruption in high-risk patients.
Preoperative education	■ Stoma education is crucial to familiarize the patient with the impending stoma and to minimize potential complications.
Stoma placement	■ Preoperative ileostomy site determination and marking is critical. The stoma must be placed away from bony prominences, panni, and scars to create a viable, tension-free ileostomy with a reliable appliance seal.
Orientation of loop ileostomy	■ Orienting, marking sutures are advised on afferent and efferent limbs. Avoid torsion and mesenteric vascular compromise during stoma creation.
Stoma maturation	■ Creation of a 2-cm Brooke ileostomy (end or diverting loop) minimizes the morbidity that stems from the ileostomy effluent.
Follow-up	■ Close follow-up and the use of ileostomy care pathways are critical to recognize and address stoma-site problems and to minimize readmissions for dehydration and electrolyte abnormalities.
Ileostomy Reversal	
History and physical examination	■ Ileostomy reversal is usually an elective procedure. Ideally, the patient should attain an optimal health status before reversal is performed.
Diagnostic tests	■ Diagnostic studies should be considered to assess the distal bowel or anastomosis prior to closure. These studies may prevent morbidity and improve outcome.
Preparation of the ileum for takedown	■ The ileum should be prepared using viable ileum with adequate blood supply of sufficient length. Tension on the anastomosis is to be avoided.
Skin closure	■ "Purse-string" skin closure is increasingly used as a skin closure option with lower risk of stoma site surgical infection.
Follow-up	■ Patients undergoing ileostomy reversal are at risk for major morbidity and mortality and must be followed up closely postoperatively.

POSTOPERATIVE CARE

For Ileostomy Creation Patients

■ Creation of an ileostomy results in the loss of the function of the ileocecal valve and of the colonic water reabsorption, leading to dehydration and electrolyte abnormalities. Postoperatively, the newly created ileostomy begins to function within 72 hours, often with high output (>1 L) per day. Within weeks, the proximal small bowel adapts (at least partially) as water absorption increases and the effluent thickens. Ideal daily effluent volume after adaptation is 500 to 1000 mL.

■ Appropriate hydration and electrolyte levels (sodium, potassium, magnesium, and calcium) must be maintained using electrolyte solutions (eg, Pedialyte) or oral/intravenous sodium chloride. After discharge, the patient must contact their medical provider if the ileostomy output is greater than 1 L/d for 2 consecutive days.

■ Psyllium (eg, Metamucil) can be used to thicken the enteric contents.

■ Anticholinergic agents, opioid receptor agonists (eg, loperamide), bile acid binders (eg, cholestyramine), and narcotic agents (eg, tincture of opium) can be used to decrease ileostomy output.

■ Vitamin B_{12} is administered as indicated for patients who have had ileal resection.

■ Support belts may be helpful for securing poorly fitting appliances, especially in obese patients.

■ Maintaining healthy skin around the stoma is paramount. Allergic reactions to the appliance can occur and may be managed by changing appliance type or manufacturer.

■ Pooling of ileal effluent must be avoided by frequent appliance changes or bag emptying. The appliance should be changed immediately postoperatively if the patient experiences leakage or peristomal skin problems.

For Ileostomy Reversal Patients

■ The patients must be followed closely postoperatively to identify problems and complications after ileostomy takedown. This is especially important in high-risk patients.

■ Dehydration and electrolyte abnormalities may persist after ileostomy takedown.

OUTCOMES

■ Readmission with dehydration following ileostomy formation is a serious problem with several risk factors. Eight variables with significant association with dehydration-related readmission include age ≥65 years, body mass index ≥30 kg/

m², diabetes mellitus, hypertension, renal comorbidity, regular diuretic use, ileal pouch–anal anastomosis procedure, and length of stay after index admission.[1]

- An "ileostomy care pathway," including a standardized set of perioperative patient education tools, direct patient engagement with stoma care, strict monitoring of stoma output postdischarge, and visiting nurse involvement, may all positively impact overall readmission rates (eg, 35% prepathway implementation vs 21% postpathway implementation) and may decrease or even eliminate readmissions for dehydration (eg, 15.5% prepathway implementation vs 0% postpathway implementation).[2]
- The use of a sodium hyaluronate and carboxymethylcellulose-based bioabsorbable membrane can significantly decrease adhesion formation around a loop ileostomy as identified at the time of ileostomy reversal (eg, no Seprafilm vs Seprafilm around stoma, 30.6% vs 14.1%).[3]
- In patients requiring a diverting loop ileostomy, a bridge (rod) does not significantly impact retraction or leakages.[4]
- Laparoscopic creation of an ileostomy is safe and effective and should be considered for patients.[5]
- Over 10% of patients require ileostomy-related reoperations. Obesity is an independent risk factor for ileostomy complications and, along with smoking history, is associated with a lower likelihood of subsequent ileostomy reversal.[6]
- Reversal of a temporary ileostomy has traditionally been performed at 3 months after ileostomy creation. Yet, in highly selected patients without clinical or radiological signs of anastomotic leakage or other complications, it is safe to close a temporary ileostomy earlier than 3 months after ileostomy creation.[7]
- Handsewn vs stapled ileo-ileostomy anastomoses for ileostomy closure have similar major complications such as bowel obstruction (in about 15% of cases) and anastomotic leak (in about 2% of cases), with stapled anastomoses resulting in shorter operation times.[8]
- Despite longer operative times, prophylactic mesh reinforcement at the site of stoma closure is effective with lower incidence of stoma site incisional hernia and need for reoperation, and with similar short-term outcomes compared with standard stoma site closure technique. A significant superiority of a specific mesh type (biologic, polypropylene, or biosynthetic) was not identified.[9]
- Purse-string skin closure after stoma reversal has a lower risk of stoma site surgical site infection than conventional primary closure (purse-string vs conventional primary closure, 2% vs 15%, $P = .01$).[10]

COMPLICATIONS

Ileostomy Creation Patients

- Over 80% of patients experience one or more stoma-related complications. Common problems include skin irritation (in up to 60%), fixation problems (in up to 50%), and peristomal leakage (in up to 40%). Superficial necrosis, bleeding, and retraction can occur in up to 20%, 15%, and 10% of

patients, respectively. Stoma-related complications are even more common for stomas in suboptimal locations.

- Parastomal hernia
- Parastomal fistula
- High-output ileostomies may result in dehydration, electrolyte abnormalities, and fat/fat-soluble vitamin malabsorption. Severe dehydration may lead to acute renal failure and, potentially, chronic renal failure.

Ileostomy Reversal Patients

- An analysis of the National Surgical Quality Improvement Program demonstrated that following elective ileostomy closure, 9.3% of patients had major complications (eg, mortality, sepsis, return to the operating room, renal failure, major cardiac, neurologic, or respiratory episode) and 8.4% had minor complications (eg, wound infection or urinary tract infection) within 30 days. Mortality was 0.6%. Independent predictors of major complications were American Society of Anesthesiologists physical status classification system score, functional status, history of chronic obstructive pulmonary disease, dialysis, disseminated cancer, and prolonged operative time.
- Handsewn ileo-ileostomy and stapled ileo-ileostomy anastomoses for ileostomy closure have similar major complications.
- Wound infections following ileostomy reversal are significantly lower in patients undergoing delayed primary closure or purse-string closure vs primary closure, with similar cosmetic outcomes.

REFERENCES

1. Liu C, Bhat S, Sharma P, et al. Risk factors for readmission with dehydration after ileostomy formation: a systematic review and meta-analysis. *Colorectal Dis.* 2021;23:1071-1082.
2. Nagle D, Pare T, Keenan E, et al. Ileostomy pathway virtually eliminates readmissions for dehydration in new ostomates. *Dis Colon Rectum.* 2012;55(12):1266-1272.
3. Salum M, Wexner SD, Nogueras J, et al. Does sodium hyaluronate- and carboxy cellulose-based bioresorbable membrane (Seprafilm) decrease operative time for loop ileostomy closure? *Tech Coloproct.* 2006;10(3):187-190.
4. Speirs M, Leung E, Hughes D, et al. Ileostomy rod—is it a bridge too far? *Colorectal Dis.* 2006;8(6):484-487.
5. Oliveira L, Reissman P, Nogueras J, et al. Laparoscopic creation of stomas. *Surg Endosc.* 1997;11(1):19-23.
6. Chun L, Haigh P, Tam M, et al. Defunctioning loop ileostomy for pelvic anastomoses: predictor of morbidity and nonclosure. *Dis Colon Rectum.* 2012;55(2):167-174.
7. Danielsen A, Park J, Jansen J, et al. Early closure of a temporary ileostomy in patients with rectal cancer: a multicenter randomized controlled trial. *Ann Surg.* 2017;265(2):284-290.
8. Löffler T, Rossion I, Bruckner T, et al. Hand suture versus stapling for closure of loop ileostomy (HASTA trial): results of a multicenter randomized trial. *Ann Surg.* 2012;256(5):828-835.
9. Peltrini R, Imperatore N, Altieri G, et al. Prevention of incisional hernia at the site of stoma closure with different reinforcing mesh types: a systematic review and meta-analysis. *Hernia.* 2021;25(3):639-648.
10. Lee J, Marquez T, Clerc D, et al. Pursestring closure of the stoma site leads to fewer wound infections: results from a multicenter randomized controlled trial. *Dis Colon Rectum.* 2014;57(11):1282-1289.

Chapter 5

Tube Jejunostomy: Open and Laparoscopic Techniques

Rebecca L. Wiatrek and Lillian S. Kao

DEFINITION

- A jejunostomy feeding tube is a tube placed into the proximal jejunum and brought out through the skin to allow for feeding distal to the stomach. Jejunostomy tubes are indicated in patients who are unable to maintain adequate nutrition orally and who are unable to be fed via the stomach. Examples of conditions that may require a jejunostomy tube include, but are not limited to, gastric outlet obstruction, esophageal perforation, gastroparesis, or recurrent aspiration. Jejunostomy tubes may be placed via a nasojejunal or percutaneous route; the latter can be approached via interventional radiology, via laparoscopic or open surgery, or via endoscopy, as an extension through a percutaneous gastrostomy tube.

PATIENT HISTORY AND PHYSICAL FINDINGS

- A complete surgical history should be elicited, focusing on prior abdominal operations.
- A complete abdominal examination should be performed, noting prior incisions and hernias.
- Because malnutrition may be an indication for placement of a jejunostomy tube, a complete nutritional history should be obtained including recent weight loss.
- Physical examination should be focused on signs of severe malnutrition such as loss of subcutaneous fat, muscle wasting, and/or presence of edema and ascites.
- The Subjective Global Assessment Score combines the history and physical examination to provide a rating from A (*well nourished*) to C (*severely malnourished*).

IMAGING AND OTHER DIAGNOSTIC STUDIES

- A nutritional assessment should be performed. Severe malnutrition may be a reason for placement of a jejunostomy tube, such as prior to major elective surgery. Indicators of preoperative malnutrition include weight loss greater than 10% to 15% over the previous 6 months, body mass index less than 18.5 kg/m², Subjective Global Assessment Grade C, and/or serum albumin less than 3 g/dL.[1]
- Electrolytes should be checked and replaced prior to surgery. An electrocardiogram should also be checked in order to rule out cardiac abnormalities and arrhythmias.
- Additional studies and radiologic imaging should be based on the primary diagnosis. In patients with underlying malignancy, staging studies should be recent enough to ensure that there are no changes in the cancer status that may affect the operative plan.

SURGICAL MANAGEMENT

Preoperative Planning

- Although enteral feeding is preferred to the parenteral route, the surgeon should ensure that there are no contraindications to enteral nutrition such as distal obstruction, ileus, high-output enterocutaneous fistula, or shock.
- Alternatives to jejunostomy tubes include temporary nasally inserted feeding tubes and gastrostomy tubes. Temporary feeding access can be achieved using a nasogastric or a nasojejunal feeding tube; the latter can be placed with the assistance of fluoroscopy or endoscopy. Smaller-diameter feeding tubes may be more comfortable for the patient but also may be more prone to clogging. Gastrostomy tubes for longer-term feeding access can be placed endoscopically, radiologically, or surgically.
- If enteral access is not the primary indication for surgery, then the complete operative plan should be considered. The anticipated duration of inability to take in oral nutrition or of inadequate nutrition (<60% of caloric requirement) should be taken in consideration when deciding whether or not to place a feeding jejunostomy tube as well as in deciding the route of placement (nasojejunal vs surgical).[1] In patients with cancer, whether the goal of surgery is curative or palliative should be considered. A temporary feeding jejunostomy tube may be indicated after resection of cancer of the esophagus, stomach, or pancreas to allow continued distal enteral nutrition in the event of an anastomotic leak.
- Palliative care may include placement of a surgical jejunostomy tube. Patients with cancer who are not candidates for curative treatment should be assessed for their preferences, quality of life, and resources. The risks of surgical intervention should be weighed against the potential benefits of enteral nutrition. A candid discussion should be held with the patient regarding advanced directives and end-of-life care.
- When enteral access is the primary indication for surgery, the surgeon should discuss the planned operative approach with the patient. When a laparoscopic jejunostomy tube is planned, the surgeon should discuss the possibility of conversion to open. If the jejunostomy tube is palliative, the surgeon should discuss the possibility of aborting the procedure when the risks outweigh the benefits (ie, in the setting of carcinomatosis and inability to safely dissect the proximal jejunum).
- Although no randomized trials exist regarding antibiotic prophylaxis prior to jejunostomy tube placement, there is high-quality evidence that antibiotic prophylaxis reduces surgical site infections across procedures and baseline risks.[2] In addition, a meta-analysis of randomized controlled trials of antibiotic prophylaxis to prevent peristomal infection after percutaneous endoscopic gastrostomy demonstrated a significant risk reduction with cephalosporin and penicillin-based prophylaxis.[3]

Positioning

- The patient should be positioned in the supine position. This is required for both laparoscopic and open techniques. For the laparoscopic approach, it is important to secure the patient to the bed with straps or tapes to allow for safe manipulation of the operating table.

OPEN JEJUNOSTOMY FEEDING TUBE PLACEMENT

First Step—Placement of Skin Incision

- A limited midline incision, approximately 5 cm in length, is made above the umbilicus. This allows for identification of the ligament of Treitz. A larger incision may be needed if the patient has had multiple prior operations requiring adhesiolysis.
- Once the abdomen is entered, the omentum can be followed to the transverse colon, which is retracted cephalad. The ligament of Treitz is located at the base of the transverse mesocolon to the left of the fourth portion of the duodenum (**FIGURE 1**) and is identified by visualization and palpation. A segment of jejunum distal to the ligament of Treitz is identified. A distance of 15 to 20 cm from the ligament of Treitz will allow the jejunum to reach the abdominal wall without tension, while also providing for enough length for a proximal revision of the jejunal segment, should one be necessary in the future.
- An exit site is identified in the skin of the left upper quadrant, several centimeters lateral from the midline. A stab incision is made at this level, and tonsil clamps are used to deliver the jejunostomy tube into the abdominal cavity.

Second Step—Choice of Tubes

- The type of jejunostomy tube used can be as simple as a 10- or 12-Fr red rubber catheter or a silicone jejunostomy tube similar to those used in laparoscopic cases. Silicone tubes may have more longevity.[4] Avoid using balloon-tipped catheters (ie, Foley catheters) or, alternatively, ensure that the ability to inflate the balloon has been disabled to prevent future attempts at insufflating the balloon that could lead to subsequent bowel obstruction.
- If using a red rubber catheter, the tip may be cut off, which allows for exchange over a wire should the tube become clogged. Additional side holes may also be cut at the distal end of the tube in order to improve flow through the catheter.

Third Step—Suturing Tube Into the Bowel

- The previously chosen site of proximal jejunum is delivered into the wound. The site of entry of the tube should be on the antimesenteric side of the jejunum. Once this is identified, a 3-0 silk is used to create a diamond-shaped purse-string suture. A small opening is made inside the purse-string suture with cautery, only large enough to allow for the tube to be inserted into the bowel.
- The tube is placed into the bowel and advanced into the distal portion of the jejunum. The length of advancement into the jejunum should be long enough to prevent backflow of feeds into the proximal small intestine.
- The purse-string suture is secured, and the tube is placed along the proximal bowel wall. The Witzel technique is then used to prevent extravasations of enteric feeds at the jejunostomy tube entrance site. In this technique, 3-0 silk seromuscular sutures are placed perpendicularly on the antimesenteric border of the bowel on both sides of the feeding tube (Lembert sutures) in order to imbricate the bowel wall over the feeding tube, creating a serosal tunnel (**FIGURE 2**). This should be approximately 2 to 3 cm in length and care should be taken to not narrow the

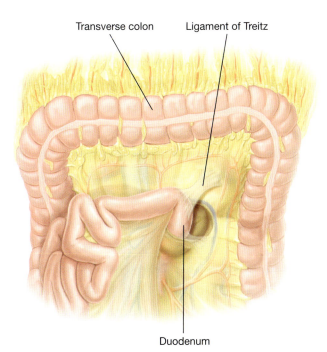

FIGURE 1 • Identification of the ligament of Treitz. With the transverse colon retracted superiorly, the ligament of Treitz can be easily identified at the base of the transverse mesocolon and to the left of the fourth portion of the duodenum.

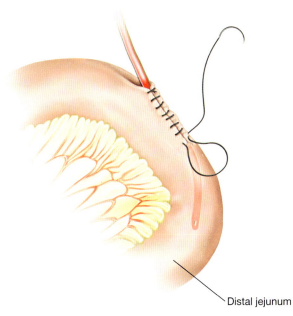

FIGURE 2 • The open Witzel technique. 3-0 Silk seromuscular sutures are placed perpendicularly on the antimesenteric border of the bowel on both sides of the feeding tube (Lembert sutures) in order to imbricate the bowel wall over the feeding tube, creating a serosal tunnel.

lumen of the bowel or tube with these sutures. Care should also be taken to avoid perforating the feeding tube during the placement of these sutures, as this could lead to extravasation of the enteric feeds into the abdominal cavity.

Fourth Step—Suturing the Tube to the Abdominal Wall

- The tube should then be secured with 3-0 silk seromuscular sutures to the abdominal wall parietal peritoneum in four quadrants around the exit point of the tube just proximal to the last Witzel suture. Care should be taken to avoid perforating the feeding tube during the placement of these sutures, as this could lead to extravasation of the enteric feeds into the abdominal cavity. One additional suture can be used to tack the jejunum to the abdominal wall distal to the tube entrance site to prevent kinking or volvulus of the jejunum around the tube site.

LAPAROSCOPIC JEJUNOSTOMY FEEDING TUBE PLACEMENT

First Step—Laparoscopic Port Placement

- The abdomen may be entered either by a cut-down technique, by use of an insufflation needle followed by entry with an optical access trocar, or with an optical access trocar alone. One 5-mm port should be placed periumbilically and two additional 5-mm ports should be placed in a triangulated fashion to allow for manipulation of the jejunum; these should be placed under direct visualization to prevent bowel injury. These are traditionally placed in the right upper and left lower quadrants.

Second Step—Identification of the Ligament of Treitz

- The patient is placed in a Trendelenburg position and is rotated to the right side in order to facilitate identification of the ligament of Treitz.
- The transverse colon is elevated with an atraumatic grasper to identify the ligament of Treitz, located at the base of the transverse mesocolon and to the left of the fourth portion of the duodenum (**FIGURE 1**). A segment of jejunum approximately 15 to 20 cm distal from the ligament that will easily allow the jejunum to reach the abdominal wall without tension is identified.

Third Step—Placing the Tube in the Jejunum

- A purse-string suture of 3-0 silk can be placed with a laparoscopic needle driver or with an endoscopic sewing device in a circular manner, in the same fashion as performed in open cases (**FIGURE 3**). Using electrocautery, make an opening in the small bowel and deliver the feeding tube through the opening and into the distal jejunum. The purse-string suture is tied intracorporeally.
- Lembert sutures are placed to create a Witzel serosal tunnel around the feeding tube. The jejunostomy tube is then tacked to the anterior abdominal wall with a four-quadrant suture placed intracorporeally proximally to the Witzel tunnel.
- If using a laparoscopic jejunostomy tube kit that provides T-fasteners, the jejunum is grasped with two atraumatic graspers and the percutaneous T-fastener is placed through the skin and into the bowel just proximal to where the tube will enter the jejunum. Care should be taken not to place the needle through and through the bowel (back-wall perforation), which would lead to leakage of tube feeds and enteric contents into the abdominal cavity postoperatively. Once the needle is inside the bowel, the T-fastener is released by pushing in the stylet (**FIGURE 4**). The needle is then removed, and a hemostat is used to pull up on the suture in order to pull the jejunum up flushed to the abdominal wall. Additional T-fasteners are placed in a diamond shape around the planned insertion site.
- The jejunum is then accessed with a needle, and a guidewire is threaded into the bowel (**FIGURE 5**). The wire is followed laparoscopically to ensure it is going down the distal jejunal limb. A skin incision is made at the guidewire exit site, and the dilator is placed over the wire and into the jejunum. The dilator is exchanged for the peel-away sheath. The wire is removed and the tube is placed through the peel-away sheath. The sheath is then peeled away from the catheter (**FIGURE 6**).
- Confirmation that the tube is in the bowel lumen can be achieved by injecting air into the tube and observing the bowel distend.

Fourth Step—Securing the Jejunum to the Abdominal Wall

- The bowel can be fastened to the abdominal wall in four corners with 3-0 silks using laparoscopic needle drivers

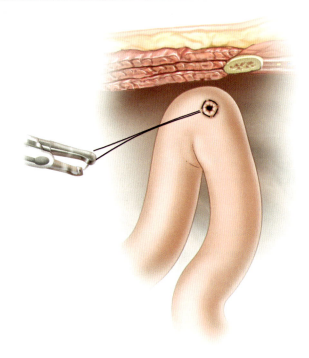

FIGURE 3 • A purse-string suture of 3-0 silk is placed with an endoscopic sewing device in a circular manner at the site where the feeding tube will be inserted.

Chapter 5 **TUBE JEJUNOSTOMY: OPEN AND LAPAROSCOPIC TECHNIQUES** 45

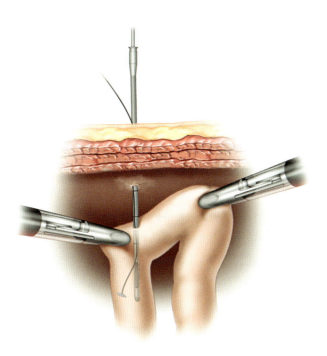

FIGURE 4 • Laparoscopic jejunostomy kit technique. Once the needle is inserted inside the bowel, pushing in the stylet deploys the T-fastener.

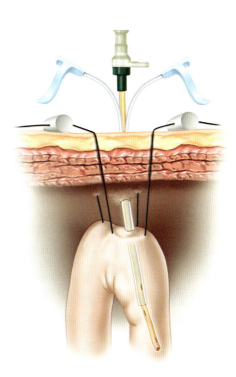

FIGURE 6 • Laparoscopic jejunostomy kit technique. The jejunostomy tube is placed through the peel-away sheath and into the distal jejunal limb.

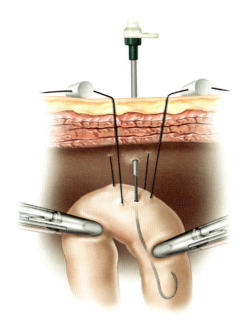

FIGURE 5 • Laparoscopic jejunostomy kit technique. The jejunum is then accessed with a needle, and a guidewire is threaded into the bowel.

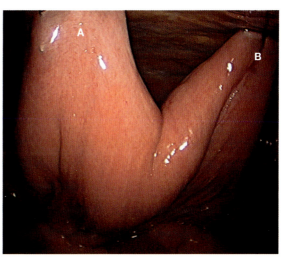

FIGURE 7 • Laparoscopic jejunostomy kit technique. *A*, The T-fasteners have been secured by crimping the metal fasteners above the bolsters, thus approximating the jejunum to the abdominal wall at the jejunostomy site. *B*, An additional T-fastener was placed to tack the jejunum to the abdominal wall distal to the tube insertion site to prevent volvulus.

(**FIGURE 3**). An alternative method is to place sutures on all four quadrants around the purse-string site and deliver them through the abdominal wall with a suture passer.
- If T-fasteners are used, they are then secured by crimping the metal fasteners above the bolsters with a straight hemostat,

thus approximating the jejunum to the abdominal wall. An additional T-fastener can be used to tack the jejunum to the abdominal wall distal to the tube insertion site to prevent volvulus (**FIGURE 7**).
- Inject a small amount of saline or air into the tube after it has been secured to the abdominal wall to ensure there is no leak and that the tube is patent.

PEARLS AND PITFALLS

Technique	
Open jejunostomy tube placement	
Creating the serosal tunnel	▪ When creating the Witzel tunnel, it is possible to cause narrowing of the proximal bowel. The sutures should be carefully placed close to the feeding tube to avoid this problem.
Laparoscopic jejunostomy tube placement	
Using T-fasteners	▪ Care should be taken not to place the needle through and through the bowel (avoid back-wall perforation of the bowel). ▪ When crimping the T-fasteners, ensure that the jejunum is flush to the abdominal wall. However, do not indent the skin significantly, which can cause necrosis of the skin and cause the patient significant pain. ▪ Fasteners should be carefully planned as kits only carry five fasteners and once through the skin and fascia, the fastener is not reusable.
Wire placement	▪ Ensure that the wire is traveling distally when placed. ▪ Ensure that the wire is freely mobile in the bowel and has not dissected into the layers of the intestinal wall.
Confirmation of tube placement	▪ Ensure that the dilator and tube are visualized laparoscopically while entering into the distal aspect of the jejunum. ▪ Inject a small amount of saline or air into the tube after it has been secured to the abdominal wall to ensure there is no leak and that the tube is patent.

POSTOPERATIVE CARE

- Postoperatively, the patient's jejunostomy tube can be used immediately.
- The jejunostomy tube should be flushed daily, before and after administration of medications and after stopping tube feeds to prevent clogging and to ensure patency.
- If a laparoscopic jejunostomy kit was used, the T-fasteners can be cut at the skin level 2 weeks after tube placement.
- Nutritional consultation should be considered in order to determine the patient's caloric needs. Nutritionists may also assist in the choice of enteral formula. There are data from meta-analyses of randomized trials suggesting a benefit to using immunonutrition in perioperative head/neck and gastrointestinal cancer patients.[5,6]
- In malnourished patients who are at high risk for refeeding syndrome, nutritional support should be started slowly.[7] Fluid and electrolyte imbalances should be corrected. In addition, high-risk patients should be monitored closely in terms of their vital signs, electrolytes, weight, and neurologic signs and symptoms. Patients should be monitored for hypophosphatemia, hypokalemia, hypomagnesemia, hyperglycemia, and hyponatremia upon initiation of feeds. Because of the risk of arrhythmias, telemetry may be indicated in severe cases.
- Diarrhea is a common side effect of enteral nutrition. High-quality data on preventive interventions are lacking.[8] Persistent diarrhea (>72 hours) should trigger evaluation for *Clostridium difficile* infection, rectal examination to rule out fecal impaction, cessation of laxatives, and restoration of fluid and electrolyte balance. Addition of soluble fiber or modification of the composition of the enteral formula may reduce diarrhea.[8]

- Nonocclusive bowel necrosis is a rare but devastating complication of enteral feeding. Tube feed tolerance should be monitored closely, particularly among patients with preexisting impaired gastrointestinal function. Signs of intolerance may be nonspecific such as nausea, diarrhea, bloating, and abdominal pain. Mechanisms that may contribute to nonocclusive bowel necrosis include mesenteric hypoperfusion, bacterial contamination, and hyperosmolarity of the tube feeds. Unfortunately, due to the rarity of nonocclusive bowel necrosis, specific risk factors cannot be identified.[9] Therefore, a low threshold for diagnosis should be maintained and early reexploration performed when suspected.

OUTCOMES

- Outcomes after jejunostomy tube placement are dependent on the primary diagnosis.
- In patients with cancer undergoing curative treatment, enteral nutrition improves the tolerance and response to therapy.[10,11] In patients with cancer undergoing palliative treatment, enteral nutrition may improve symptoms and quality of life while reducing loss of autonomy.[10]

COMPLICATIONS

- Diarrhea
- Dermatitis
- Infection
- Tube leakage (peristomal or intraperitoneal)
- Small bowel perforation
- Displacement of the jejunostomy tube
- Enterocutaneous fistula

- Refeeding syndrome
- Mechanical small bowel obstruction at the jejunostomy tube site
- Volvulus around the jejunostomy tube site
- Nonocclusive bowel necrosis

REFERENCES

1. Weimann A, Braga M, Harsanyi L, et al. ESPEN guidelines on enteral nutrition: surgery including organ transplantation. *Clin Nutr*. 2006;25:224-244.
2. Bowater RJ, Stirling SA, Lilford RJ. Is antibiotic prophylaxis in surgery a generally effective intervention? Testing a generic hypothesis over a set of meta-analyses. *Ann Surg*. 2009;249:551-556.
3. Jafri NS, Mahid SS, Minor KS, et al. Meta-analysis: antibiotic prophylaxis to prevent peristomal infection following percutaneous endoscopic gastrostomy. *Aliment Pharmacol Ther*. 2007;25:647-656.
4. Boullata JI, Nieman Carney L, Guenter P, et al. *A.S.P.E.N. Enteral Nutrition Handbook*. American Society for Parenteral and Enteral Nutrition; 2010.
5. Zhang Y, Gu Y, Guo T, et al. Perioperative immunonutrition for gastrointestinal cancer: a systematic review of randomized controlled trials. *Surg Oncol*. 2012;21:e87-e95.
6. Osland E, Hossain MB, Khan S, et al. Effect of timing of pharmaco-nutrition (immunonutrition) administration on outcomes of elective surgery for gastrointestinal malignancies: a systematic review and meta-analysis. *J Parenter Enteral Nutr*. 2014;38(1):53-69.
7. Khan LU, Ahmed J, Khan S, et al. Refeeding syndrome: a literature review. *Gastroenterol Res Pract*. 2011;2011:410971.
8. Whelan K, Schneider SM. Mechanisms, prevention, and management of diarrhea in enteral nutrition. *Curr Opin Gastroenterol*. 2011;27:152-159.
9. Melis M, Fichera A, Ferguson MK. Bowel necrosis associated with early jejunal tube feeding: a complication of postoperative enteral nutrition. *Arch Surg*. 2006;141:701-704.
10. Marin Caro MM, Laviano A, Pichard C. Nutritional intervention and quality of life in adult oncology patients. *Clin Nutr*. 2007;26:289-301.
11. Paccagnella A, Morassutti I, Rosti G. Nutritional intervention for improving treatment tolerance in cancer patients. *Curr Opin Oncol*. 2011;23:322-330.

SECTION II: Surgery of the Colon, Appendix, Rectum, and Anus

Chapter 6: Appendectomy: Laparoscopic Technique

Roosevelt Fajardo

DEFINITION
- Acute appendicitis is the most frequent cause of acute surgical abdominal pain seen in the emergency services around the world. Close to 7% of the total world population will suffer from appendicitis at some point in their lives. Although it may occur at any age, its incidence is higher in childhood, with a peak incidence between 10 and 30 years of age. It is more frequent in men, with a male-to-female ratio of 1.4:1. Advances in laparoscopic surgery around the world have made laparoscopic appendectomy a safe and simple procedure.

DIFFERENTIAL DIAGNOSIS
- Urinary tract infection
- Intestinal obstruction
- Acute cholecystitis
- Mesenteric adenitis
- Meckel diverticulitis
- Colonic diverticulitis
- Right ureteric colic
- Ectopic pregnancy
- Salpingitis, pelvic inflammatory disease
- Ruptured ovarian follicle
- Ovarian torsion
- Gastroenteritis
- Terminal ileitis

PATIENT HISTORY AND PHYSICAL FINDINGS
- Despite advances in diagnostic imaging, diagnosis of acute appendicitis continues to be predominantly clinical. A good clinical history and a thorough physical examination should provide the surgeon with a high degree of suspicion. The characteristic clinical picture is one of abdominal pain that exacerbates with movement, starting in the periumbilical region and then migrating to the right lower quadrant. Fever, anorexia, nausea, and vomiting are frequent.
- There are several score systems for the diagnosis of acute appendicitis. The Alvarado score, AIR score, and RIPASA score are probably the ones that are most frequently used.
- The Alvarado score, a clinical scoring system used in the diagnosis of acute appendicitis, assigns points to six clinical items and two laboratory measurements with a maximum possible total of 10 points. With scores greater than 5, the probability of acute appendicitis increases.
- A popular mnemonic used to remember the Alvarado score factors is **MANTRELS**: **M**igration to the right iliac fossa, **A**norexia, **N**ausea/Vomiting, **T**enderness in the right iliac fossa, **R**ebound pain, **E**levated temperature (fever), **L**eukocytosis, and **S**hift of leukocytes to the left. Owing to the popularity of this mnemonic, the Alvarado score is sometimes referred to as the MANTRELS score.
- The Appendicitis Inflammatory Response (AIR) score: AIR also contributes to the diagnosis of acute appendicitis. The AIR score associates clinical criteria and two simple laboratory tests. The probability of acute appendicitis based on the AIR score is: 0 to 4 = low probability, 5 to 8 = mild probability, 9 to 12 = high probability.
- RIPASA (Raja Isteri Pengiran Anak Saleha Appendicitis) score: The RIPASA score was developed in the Department of Surgery at Raja Isteri Pengiran Anak Saleha Hospital, Brunei Darussalam, in 2008. It includes 14 clinical parameters that are easily obtained from a good clinical history and examination.
- The location of the appendix may change the clinical presentation. With the appendix in a retrocecal location, patients may present with right flank pain. With an appendix in a pelvic location, patients typically present with urinary symptoms and diarrhea.

IMAGING AND OTHER DIAGNOSTIC STUDIES
- The hemogram typically shows a leukocytosis, with a left-sided shift.
- Female patients in fertile age should have a pregnancy test prior to surgery.
- Ultrasound (**FIGURE 1**) has been shown to have 86% sensitivity and 81% specificity for the diagnosis of acute appendicitis and has the benefit of not being invasive, but it is operator-dependent.

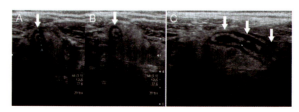

FIGURE 1 • Ultrasound imaging in appendicitis. *Arrows* show a distended appendix with a thickened wall. **A** and **B** show transverse views of the appendix. **C** shows a longitudinal view of the appendix.

Chapter 6 APPENDECTOMY: LAPAROSCOPIC TECHNIQUE   49

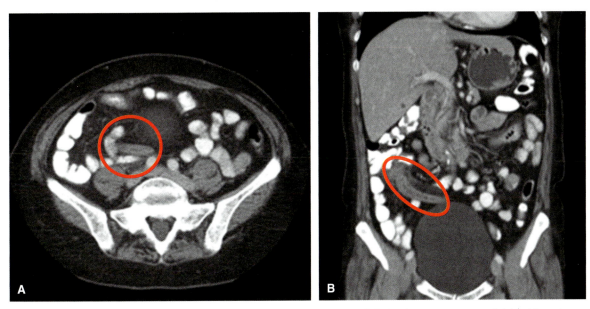

FIGURE 2 • CAT scan imaging in appendicitis. **A,** Axial view. **B,** Coronal view. Red circles show acute appendicitis with periappendiceal inflammation.

- Computed axial tomography (CAT; **FIGURE 2**) scan, with a 94% sensitivity and a 95% specificity, has been shown to be the most accurate imaging study for the diagnosis of acute appendicitis but is expensive and may delay surgical intervention.
- Magnetic resonance imaging (MRI) is reserved for patients who cannot be exposed to radiation, such as pregnant women suspected of having appendicitis.

SURGICAL MANAGEMENT
Indications
- Operative indications are the same as that for open appendectomy.
- Any patient with diagnosis of appendicitis who can tolerate pneumoperitoneum and general anesthesia, provided that trained staff and the necessary equipment for a safe procedure are available.

Preoperative Planning
- Appropriate prophylactic antibiotic should be administered within 30 minutes of surgery.
- Decompression of the bladder by voiding before surgery or by using a Foley catheter may avoid injury of the bladder during trocar placement.

Patient and Team Positioning
- The patient is secured to the table with the arms padded and tucked to the side.

- The surgeon and the camera operator stand on the patient's left side (**FIGURE 3**).
- The monitor is placed in front of the surgeon (at eye level) on the patient's right side.

Port Placement
- A traditional laparoscopic appendectomy is performed using a three-port system (**FIGURES 3** and **4**). The surgeon should be able to work two-handed.
- The ports are triangulated to enhance maneuverability and exposure.

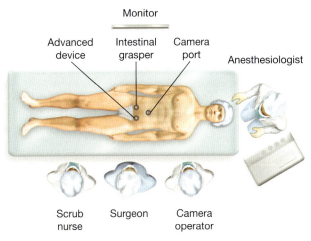

FIGURE 3 • Patient, port, team, and operating room setup.

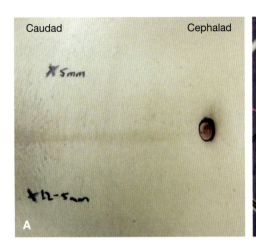 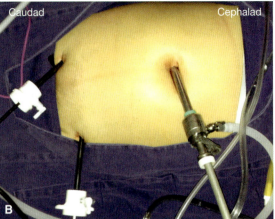

FIGURE 4 • **A** and **B**, Port placement. The three ports are triangulated to enhance maneuverability and visualization.

- A 10-mm Hasson trocar is inserted in the umbilicus. This trocar will be used for CO_2 insufflation and as a camera port.
- A 12-mm trocar is inserted in the left lower quadrant. In addition to being the main dissection port, this port will be used for the stapler and as an extraction site. If a good quality 5-mm camera is available, then a 5-mm port can be inserted in this location; in this alternative setup, the specimen would be retrieved through the umbilical port site.
- A 5-mm trocar is inserted in the right lower quadrant. This trocar will be used to help retract and expose. Placement of a urinary catheter may be required before introducing the lower abdominal trocars in order to reduce the risk of bladder perforation during this step of the procedure.

STEP 1. EXPOSURE OF THE APPENDIX AND IDENTIFICATION OF THE APPENDICEAL BASE

- The patient is placed in a Trendelenburg position and rotated with the right side up to help mobilize the small bowel out of the field of view and to enhance operative exposure.
- The fold of Treves (an antimesenteric fat fold also known as the sail sign) allows for identification of the terminal ileum (**FIGURE 5**). Following the terminal ileum distally to the ileocecal junction facilitates identification of the cecum. The appendix can usually be seen at the base of the cecum.
- In retrocecal appendicitis cases, the cecum may have to be mobilized medially by transecting its lateral peritoneal attachments in order to expose the appendix.
- The base of the inflamed appendix is localized by identifying the convergence of the three teniae coli at the base of the cecum (**FIGURE 5**).

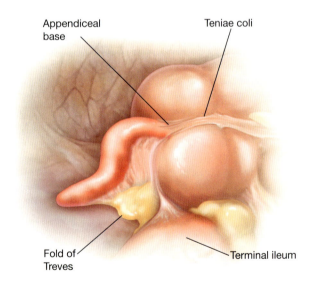

FIGURE 5 • The appendiceal base can be identified by the convergence of the teniae coli at the base of the cecum. Identifying the ileocecal junction, with the fold of Treves in the antimesenteric aspect of the terminal ileum, facilitates identification of the cecum and the appendix in patients with severe inflammation.

STEP 2. DIVISION OF THE MESOAPPENDIX

- Once identified, the tip of the appendix is pulled up with a grasper introduced through the right lower quadrant port site. This allows for the exposure of the triangular-shaped space between the appendix, the cecum, and terminal ileum, where the mesoappendix can be readily identified (**FIGURE 6**).
- The mesoappendix can then be sequentially transected with an advance energy device (LigaSure or a Harmonic) (**FIGURE 7**) very close to the appendix. Transection of the mesoappendix is carried down to the base of the appendix (**FIGURE 8**). Alternatively, the mesoappendix may be transected with a linear vascular load stapler.

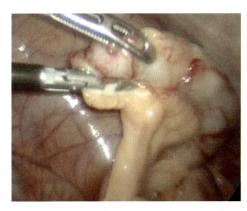

FIGURE 7 • Transection of the mesoappendix with an energy device.

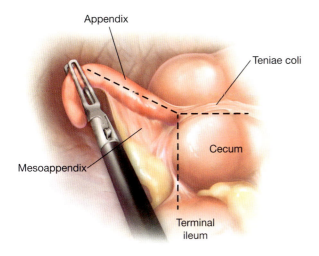

FIGURE 6 • Exposure of the mesoappendix. Pulling up on the tip of the appendix exposes the triangular space between the appendix, the cecum, and terminal ileum, where the mesoappendix can be readily identified.

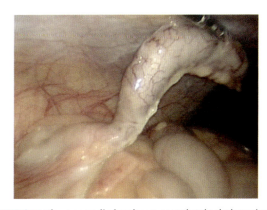

FIGURE 8 • The appendix has been completely skeletonized by transecting the mesoappendix down to the level of the appendiceal base. The appendix is now ready for transection.

STEP 3. TRANSECTION OF THE APPENDIX

- The appendix is transected at its base, flush to the cecal wall.
- This is critical to avoid potentially leaving a fecalith impacted in a retained, long appendiceal stump. In this situation, a dead space will be left between the stapled transected end of the appendix and the persistent luminal obstruction produced by the fecalith at the base of the appendix. Progressive fluid and gas accumulation in this dead space could lead to a "blown" appendiceal stump and the development of severe peritonitis postoperatively.
- If the base of the appendix is sufficiently narrow, it may be ligated with 8- to 10-mm Hem-o-Lok clips (**FIGURE 9**) or with

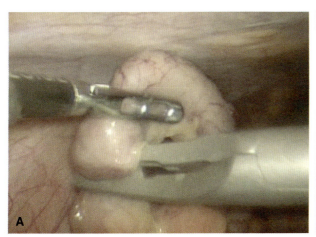
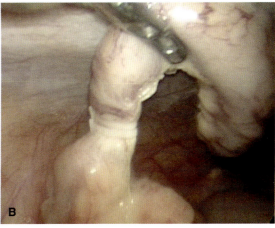

FIGURE 9 • A and B, Ligation of the appendiceal base with Hem-O-Lock clips. This is only possible when the appendiceal base is sufficiently narrow.

a pretied Roeder endoloop. In cases where the appendix is thicker and inflamed, a linear 30- or 45-mm stapling device (introduced through the right lower quadrant port site) may be used to transect the appendix at its base (**FIGURE 10**).

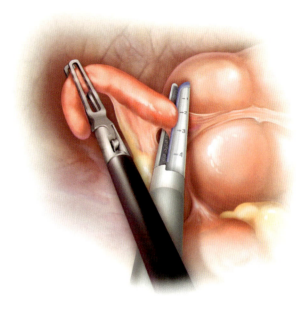

FIGURE 10 • In cases with a thick appendix with severe inflammation, the appendix is transected at its base with a linear stapler device.

STEP 4. RETRIEVAL OF THE SPECIMEN

- With the appendix transected, the appendiceal stump staple line is checked for integrity and hemostasis (**FIGURE 11**).

- The appendix may then be retrieved through the 12-mm trocar site using an endoretrieval bag (**FIGURE 12**).

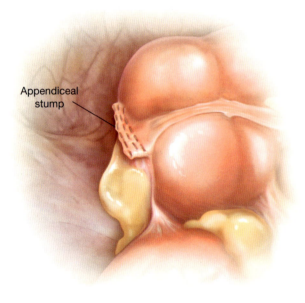

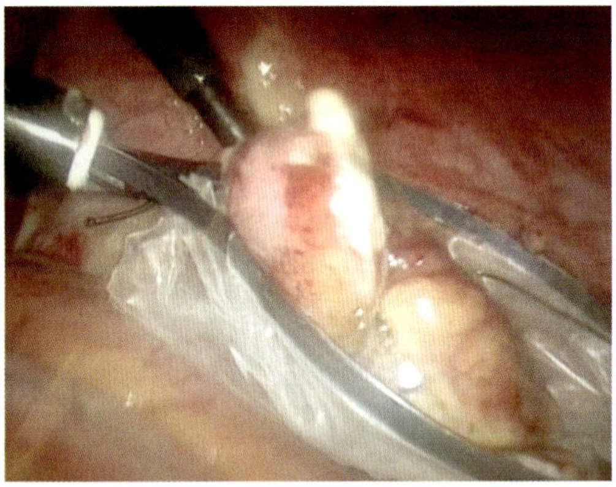

FIGURE 12 • The appendix may be then retrieved through the 12-mm trocar site using an endoretrieval bag.

FIGURE 11 • With the appendix transected, the appendiceal stump staple line is checked for integrity and hemostasis.

STEP 5. CLOSURE

- The operative site is irrigated with sterile normal saline solution.
- A drain is placed by the appendiceal stump only in cases of perforated appendicitis.
- The pneumoperitoneum is evacuated.
- All ports are removed.
- The skin incisions are closed with reabsorbable subcuticular sutures.

PEARLS AND PITFALLS

Localization on the appendix	▪ By identifying the cecum and following the teniae coli distally or using the terminal ileum as a guide to reach the ileocecal valve.
Transection of the mesoappendix	▪ Stay close to the appendix; this will minimize cumbersome bleeding and will facilitate the extraction of the specimen from the abdominal cavity.
Transection of the base of the appendix	▪ It is imperative to transect the base of the appendix to prevent a potential blown appendiceal stump syndrome. ▪ If the base of the appendix is too thick, use a linear stapling device.
Extraction from the abdominal cavity	▪ Use an endoretrieval bag to protect the wound. You may need to expand the 12-mm trocar site if the appendix is bulky.
Use of drainage	▪ Only leave a closed drainage in cases of perforation of the appendix.

POSTOPERATIVE CARE

- This procedure, done through laparoscopy, is less painful, and it may be done as an outpatient procedure in most cases of uncomplicated appendicitis.
- The patient can resume oral feeding within a few hours of the surgery and go back to routine activities sooner than with traditional open surgery.
- Patients with perforated or complicated appendicitis are generally admitted for intravenous (IV) antibiotics until they are afebrile with a normal white blood cell count. Antibiotics are usually targeted toward gram-negative and anaerobic organisms.
- Discharge criteria include ability to tolerate oral intake and appropriate pain control.
- If patients continue to have abdominal pain, develop leukocytosis, or become febrile after undergoing appendectomy for perforated or complicated appendicitis, their symptoms may be signs of an intra-abdominal abscess. Image-guided percutaneous drainage may be needed for resolution.

OUTCOMES

- Laparoscopic appendectomy has been shown to have multiple advantages over the open procedure, including a lower rate of wound site infection, although there are reports in the literature of an increased rate of residual abscesses when compared with open appendectomy.

COMPLICATIONS

- Complications of acute appendectomy are relatively rare, and they are more frequently associated with the disease status or the presence of perforation
- In nonperforated appendicitis, reported mortality is 0.8 per 1000, and it increases to 5.1 per 1000 in cases of perforation
- Wound infection may vary from 5% to 50% in cases of perforated appendicitis

- Surgical site infection is directly related to the status of the disease, and it increases by up to 20% in cases of perforated appendicitis. With the advent of laparoscopic appendectomy, this rate of infection has dropped dramatically
- Hematoma
- Appendiceal stump leak/blowout
- Port site hernia

SUGGESTED READINGS

1. Addiss D, Shaffer N, Fowler B, et al. The epidemiology of appendicitis and appendectomy in the United States. *Am J Epidemiol.* 1990;132(5):910-925.
2. Andersson RE. Meta-analysis of the clinical and laboratory diagnosis of appendicitis. Review. *Br J Surg.* January 2004;91(1):28-37.
3. Chong CF, Thien A, Mackie AJ, et al. Evaluation of the RIPASA score: a new scoring system for the diagnosis of acute appendicitis. *Brunei Int Med J.* 2010;6:17-26.
4. Fajardo R. *Guia para el manejo de apendicitis aguda en adultos.* Ministerio de la Proteccion Social; 2005.
5. Grunewald B, Keating J. Should the 'normal' appendix be removed at operation for appendicitis?. *J R Coll Surg Edinb.* 1993;38:158-160.
6. Humes DJ, Simpson J. Acute appendicitis. *BMJ.* 2006;333:530-534.
7. Katkhouda N, Mason RJ, Towfigh S, et al. Laparoscopic versus open appendectomy: a prospective randomized double-blind study. *Ann Surg.* 2005;242:439-449.
8. Patiño JF. Apendicitis aguda. In: Patiño JF, ed. *Lecciones de Cirugía.* Editorial Médica Panamericana; 2001.
9. Rathod S, Ali I, Bawa AP, Singh G, Mishra S, Nongmaithem M. Evaluation of Raja Isteri Pengiran Anak Saleha appendicitis score: a new appendicitis scoring system. *Med J DY Patil Univ.* 2015;8:744-749.
10. SAGES guidelines for laparoscopic appendectomy. *SAGES Society of American Gastrointestinal and Endoscopic Surgeons Website*; 2009. Accessed January 2012http://www.sages.org/publications/guidelines/guidelines-for-laparoscopic-appendectomy/. .
11. Temple CL, Huchcroft SA. The natural history of appendicitis in adults: a prospective study. *Ann Surg.* 1995;221:278-281.
12. Vargas Domínguez A, Ortega León LH, Miranda Fraga P. Sensibilidad, especificidad y valores predictivos de la cuenta leucocitaria en apendicitis. *Ciruj General (México).* 1994;16:1-7.

Chapter 7: Right Hemicolectomy: Open Technique

Somala Mohammed and Eric J. Silberfein

DEFINITION
- Right hemicolectomy refers to the removal of the cecum, the appendix, the ascending colon, the hepatic flexure, the proximal portion of the transverse colon, and part of the terminal ileum (**FIGURE 1**). It is the standard surgical treatment for malignant neoplasms of the right colon and involves ligation of the ileocolic, right colic, and right branch of the middle colic vessels.

DIFFERENTIAL DIAGNOSIS
- Various benign and malignant conditions require right hemicolectomy. The most common indication is a mass in the right colon. Other indications include neoplasms of the cecum or appendix. Benign conditions for which right hemicolectomy is performed include adenomatous polyps that cannot be removed endoscopically, cecal volvulus, inflammatory bowel disease, and right-sided diverticulitis, among others.

PATIENT HISTORY AND PHYSICAL FINDINGS
- A thorough history and physical examination is mandatory.
- Findings such as ascites or diffuse adenopathy may result in additional diagnostic workup to rule out metastatic disease and this may alter the overall care plan for the patient.
- A baseline nutritional and functional status should also be ascertained in the preoperative setting.
- Previous abdominal surgeries should be noted.
- A thorough family history, including history of colonic polyps and cancers, should be obtained.

IMAGING AND OTHER DIAGNOSTIC STUDIES
- A full colonoscopy should be obtained to examine the remainder of the colon, which has up to a 5% chance of synchronous disease. Colonoscopy can also allow for India ink tattooing of the lesion to facilitate accurate intraoperative localization (**FIGURE 2**).
- Preoperative imaging also includes high-quality dual phase computed tomography (CT) imaging of the abdomen and pelvis to not only assess for metastatic disease but also to evaluate the primary tumor's relationship to nearby structures such as the kidney, ureter, duodenum, and nearby vessels such as the vena cava, superior mesenteric vessels, and middle colic vessels. Tumors that involve adjacent organs require additional preoperative planning and consultation with ancillary services may be necessary. Attempts at en bloc resection should be made in cases where the tumor involves adjacent organs or structures.
- Additional workup includes a CT of the chest, complete blood cell count, and comprehensive metabolic panel. A baseline carcinoembryonic antigen level should be obtained to assist with postoperative surveillance for recurrence in cancer patients. Positron emission tomography-CT is not routinely indicated.

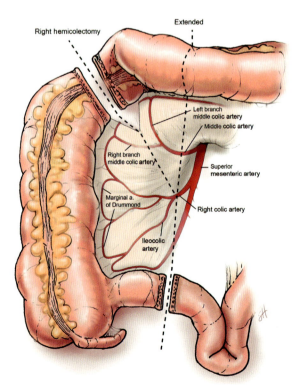

FIGURE 1 • Vascular anatomy of a right hemicolectomy. (Illustration by Scott Holmes, CMI, copyright Baylor College of Medicine.)

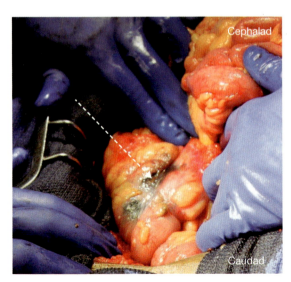

FIGURE 2 • Tattooed lesion in the cecum.

SURGICAL MANAGEMENT

Preoperative Planning

- Preoperative mechanical bowel preparation is not mandatory but it may make manipulation of the colon more manageable. If intraoperative colonoscopy is required, a prepped colon would also be preferred.
- Preoperative antibiotic prophylaxis for skin and bowel flora is recommended. Intravenous broad-spectrum antibiotics that contain second- or third-generation cephalosporins (such as cefoxitin or ceftriaxone) or fluoroquinolones (such as ciprofloxacin) along with metronidazole will adequately cover gram-negative and anaerobic pathogens. Alternatively, ertapenem, a carbapenem with activity against gram-positive, gram-negative, and anaerobic flora, can be used. Prophylactic antibiotics should be at therapeutic bloodstream levels at the time of incision. Redosing the antibiotic should be considered when taking into account the length of the operation, the estimated blood loss, and the half-life of the antibiotic.
- Venous thromboembolic prophylaxis for patients undergoing right hemicolectomy includes both mechanical interventions, such as pneumatic compression devices, and pharmacologic interventions, such as low molecular weight heparin or unfractionated heparin. These agents should be delivered prior to induction of anesthesia as the dramatically decreased level of vascular tone associated with anesthesia results in venous stasis and risks thrombosis. Patients on preoperative warfarin should be transitioned to either low molecular weight or unfractionated heparin prior to surgery.
- Preoperative thoracic epidural placement for postoperative pain control should be offered to patients without contraindications to this form of analgesia. Epidural pain control reduces narcotic requirements postoperatively and decreases risk of postoperative ileus and pulmonary complications. Alternatively, bilateral transversus abdominis plane block with long-acting local anesthetic can be used. The use of multimodal analgesia, as part of an enhanced recovery after surgery program, is strongly recommended as it has been proven to reduce pain, reduce narcotic use, accelerate recovery, reduce postoperative complications, reduce length of stay, and decrease cost of care after open colon surgery. Otherwise, patient-controlled analgesia is preferred. Intravenous nonsteroidal anti-inflammatory drugs should also be considered in the perioperative period to decrease the use and side effects of narcotic analgesia.
- Ancillary surgical services may be required to assist in the patient's care for procedures such as preoperative placement of ureteral stents or assistance in resection or reconstruction of involved adjacent organs, such as the kidneys, ureters, or the duodenum.

ANESTHESIA AND PATIENT POSITIONING

- General endotracheal anesthesia is preferred for right hemicolectomy. However, spinal anesthesia alone is feasible if necessary.
- The patient is placed in a supine position with or without the arms tucked.
- After induction of anesthesia, the bladder is catheterized and an orogastric tube is placed.
- The entire abdomen is prepped and draped.
- The surgeon stands on the patient's left and the first assistant on the right.

INCISION

- A midline laparotomy is made.
- Upon entering the abdominal cavity, inspect for evidence of metastatic disease. The liver should be palpated for masses and biopsied as needed, and the small bowel is eviscerated and inspected from the ligament of Treitz to the ileocecal valve. The colon and rectum should be inspected and palpated. The omentum and peritoneum should be evaluated for tumor implants or carcinomatosis. In women, the ovaries should also be inspected for abnormalities.

RIGHT COLON MOBILIZATION

- Placement of self-retaining retractors, such as a Balfour or Bookwalter retractor, may be used to improve exposure. Otherwise, the abdominal wall is retracted with handheld instruments.
- The cecum and ascending colon are freed from the peritoneal reflection by incising along the white line of Toldt (**FIGURE 3**). The terminal ileum is also freed from the retroperitoneum and mobilized by incising the peritoneum along the root of the mesentery.
- As the colon and terminal ileum are reflected anteriorly and medially, the right gonadal vessels and right ureter should be identified in the retroperitoneum and not mobilized anteriorly to avoid injuring them.
- The lateral dissection is carried sharply up and around the hepatic flexure in the avascular, embryologic plane between the mesocolon and the duodenum. The second and third portions of the duodenum are identified near the hepatic flexure and injury to this structure must be avoided.
- The hepatocolic ligament is transected (**FIGURE 4**).
- The gastrocolic ligament, extending from the greater curvature of the stomach to the transverse colon, is divided from left to right to complete the mobilization of the hepatic flexure (**FIGURE 5**).

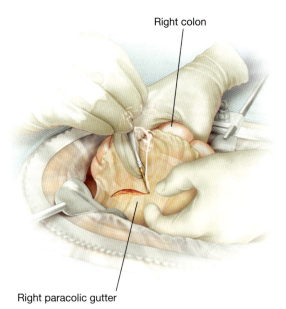

FIGURE 3 • Ascending colon mobilization. The surgeon retracts the ascending colon medially. Dissection proceeds along the right paracolic gutter by transecting the white line of Toldt.

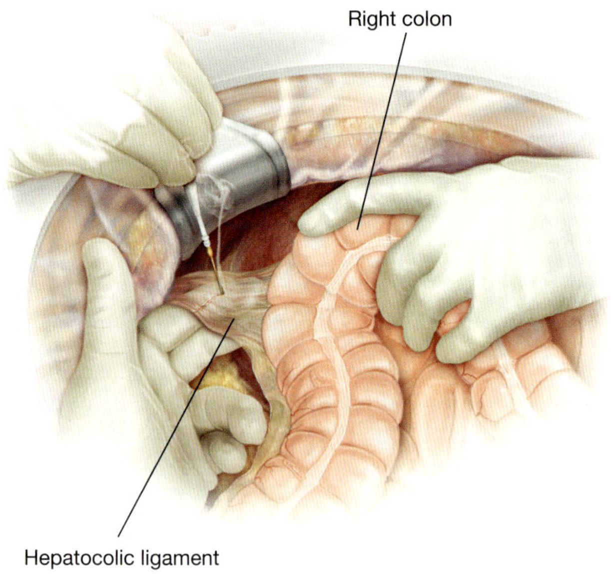

FIGURE 4 • Hepatic flexure mobilization. Gentle traction on the hepatic flexure of the colon exposes the hepatocolic ligament, which is then transected with electrocautery.

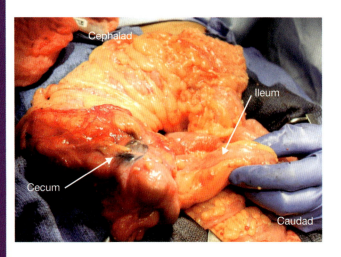

FIGURE 5 • Fully mobilized terminal ileum and right colon. The tattooed area can be seen on the surface of the cecum.

VASCULAR PEDICLE TRANSECTION

- For a right hemicolectomy, the lymphovascular pedicles of interest include the ileocolic, the right colic, and the right branch of the middle colic pedicles.
- An avascular window between the right branch of the middle colic and the right or ileocolic vessel arcade is made (FIGURE 6).
- The right branch of the middle colic is doubly clamped, divided, and tied while the left branch is spared.
- The right colic arcade, if present, is also taken at its origin to ensure adequate resection of lymphatics. This arcade, however, rarely branches directly off the superior mesenteric vessels. It is most often a branch of the ileocolic arcade.
- The ileocolic arcade is therefore ligated at its origin off the superior mesenteric vessels in the majority of circumstances (FIGURE 7).

- The lymphatic drainage pattern mirrors that of the vascular system. There are two possible paths of lymphatic spread: paraintestinal (along the intestine) and central (along the vessels). To reduce the risk of recurrence, an adequate lymph node harvest should be attempted by ligating the required mesenteric vessels at their origin. A minimum of 12 resected nodes is required for American Joint Committee on Cancer for adequate staging of colorectal cancer. Intramural spreading of cancer beyond 2 cm is rare, but an oncologic resection should aim for proximal and distal mucosal margins of at least 5 to 7 cm to ensure adequate harvest of paraintestinal and mesenteric nodes.
- An extended right hemicolectomy may be performed for lesions located at the hepatic flexure or transverse colon. This procedure involves transection of the middle colic vessels at their origin and an anastomosis of the distal ileum

Chapter 7 RIGHT HEMICOLECTOMY: OPEN TECHNIQUE

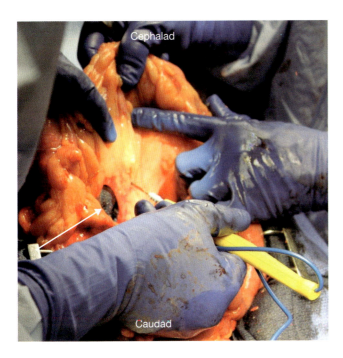

with the distal transverse colon, relying on the margin artery of Drummond for blood supply. If the integrity of this blood vessel is questionable, the resection must be extended to include the splenic flexure and the distal ileum is anastomosed to the descending colon.

- For an extended right hemicolectomy, mobilization of the splenic flexure is required. In order to mobilize the splenic flexure, the splenocolic, phrenocolic, and gastrocolic ligaments must be divided (**FIGURE 8**). The splenic flexure is then carefully dissected off the tail of the pancreas. Care must be taken to avoid injury to the spleen and the ascending branch of the left colic artery.

FIGURE 6 • Avascular window adjacent to right branch of the middle colic vessels (arrow).

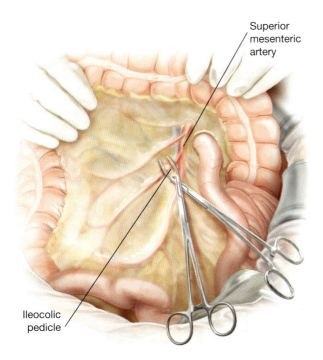

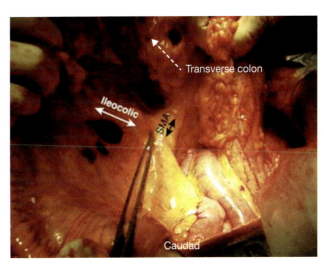

FIGURE 7 • Transection of the ileocolic pedicle. The ileocolic vessels are transected at their origin of the superior mesenteric vessels. *SMA*, superior mesenteric artery.

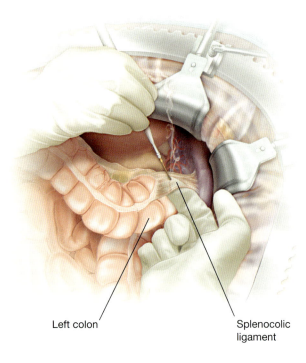

Left colon | Splenocolic ligament

FIGURE 8 • Splenic flexure mobilization (for extended right hemicolectomies). After medial and lateral mobilization of the splenic flexure attachments, the surgeon hooks their right index finger under the splenocolic ligament, providing good exposure and allowing for a safe transection of this ligament.

BOWEL TRANSECTION

- The colon is cleared of epiploic fat at the proposed site of anastomosis to allow the bowel wall to be visualized, thereby facilitating precise placement of staplers. The transverse colon is then transected to the right of the middle colic vessels with a linear 75-mm blue load stapler (**FIGURE 9**).
- The distal ileum is divided approximately 10 cm proximal to the ileocecal valve with a linear 75-mm blue load stapler (**FIGURE 10**).

- If adjacent organs are involved (T4 lesions), every attempt at a complete en bloc resection must be made. The specimen should be assessed with the pathologist to ensure that the diseased segment is acquired and that adequate margins have been obtained. If there is any doubt about margin status, an intraoperative frozen section evaluation should be conducted.

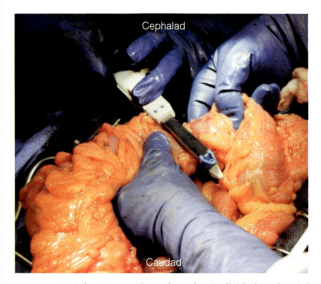

FIGURE 9 • Colon transection. The colon is divided to the right side of the middle colic vessels with a linear stapler.

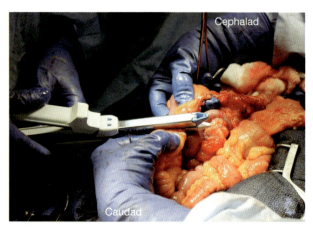

FIGURE 10 • Ileal transection. The terminal ileum is divided with a linear stapler.

ILEOCOLONIC ANASTOMOSIS

- After resection, reconstruction proceeds with an anastomosis between the ileum and the transverse colon.
- A primary ileocolic anastomosis is almost always possible. Either a hand-sewn or a stapled anastomosis can be performed in an end-to-end, end-to-side, side-to-side, or side-to-end fashion. The viability of the proximal and distal segments of bowel should be assessed and further resection to well-perfused bowel should be performed if there is any question regarding the viability of the bowel.
- Atraumatic bowel clamps should be placed proximal and distal to the anastomotic site to prevent spillage of bowel contents. Gauze pads should also be placed in the abdomen to protect surrounding structures and the skin from contamination during the process of transection of the colon and creation of the anastomosis.
- The ileal and transverse colon segments should be brought into apposition to allow a tension-free anastomosis.
- For the stapled technique, the antimesenteric borders of the bowel segments are approximated with interrupted 3-0 silk sutures. A small enterotomy is made on the antimesenteric border of both the ileum and the transverse colon (**FIGURE 11**) to allow insertion of a stapling device (**FIGURE 12**). The stapler is allowed to gently close, bringing together the ileum and transverse colon (**FIGURE 13**). Once it is assured that the mesentery is clear and the stapler is in good position, the stapling device is fired and then slowly removed.
- This fuses the two previous enterotomies into a single enterotomy. The anterior common channel of this newly constructed anastomosis can be then closed either with a stapler, placed at a right angle to the previous staple line (**FIGURE 14**), or with sutures, in one or two layers (**FIGURES 15** and **16**).
- The completed anastomosis is visually inspected to ensure that it is well perfused and is palpated to check for patency (**FIGURE 17**).
- Alternatively, a hand-sewn anastomosis can be performed in either one or two layers. The type of suture (monofilament, braided, absorbable), type of stitch (interrupted, continuous, Lembert), or configuration used is probably not as important as are the principles of approximating well-perfused bowel without tension. The authors prefer a two-layer, side-to-side anastomosis using an outer layer of interrupted Lembert silk sutures and an inner continuous running layer of monofilament absorbable suture.
- Closure of the mesenteric defect is optional and is based on surgeon preference. Oftentimes, the omentum can be placed around the anastomosis.

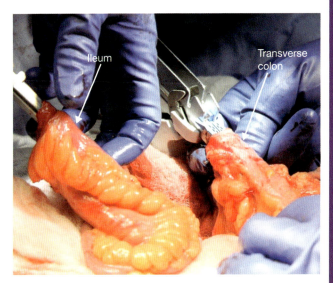

FIGURE 12 • Stapled ileocolonic anastomosis: inserting the stapling device into the enterotomy.

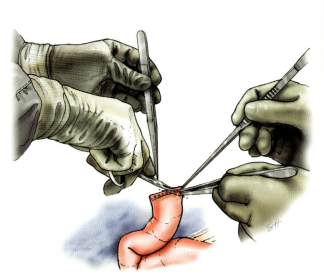

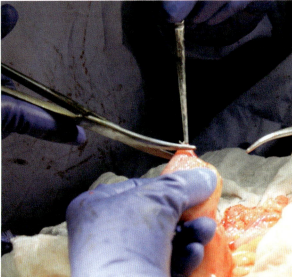

FIGURE 11 • Stapled ileocolonic anastomosis. Scissors are used to make a small enterotomy on the antimesenteric border of the bowel. (Illustration by Scott Holmes, CMI, copyright Baylor College of Medicine.)

60 SECTION II SURGERY OF THE COLON, APPENDIX, RECTUM, AND ANUS

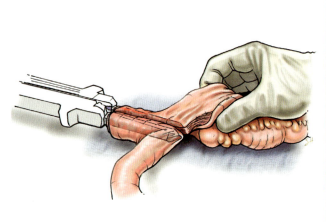
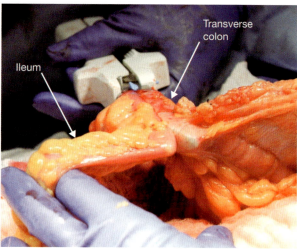

FIGURE 13 • Stapled ileocolonic anastomosis. The stapler is inserted in the ileum and transverse colon and is then closed. (Illustration by Scott Holmes, CMI, copyright Baylor College of Medicine.)

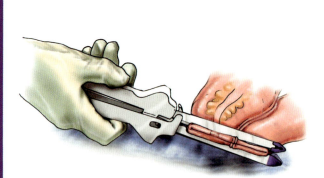

FIGURE 14 • Stapled ileocolonic anastomosis: closing the common enterotomy with a stapler. (Illustration by Scott Holmes, CMI, copyright Baylor College of Medicine.)

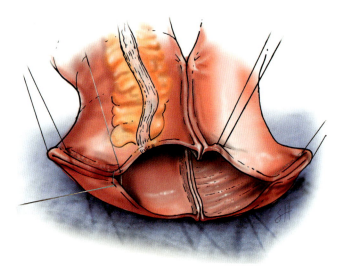

FIGURE 15 • Stapled ileocolonic anastomosis: closing the inner layer of the common enterotomy with an absorbable running suture. (Illustration by Scott Holmes, CMI, copyright Baylor College of Medicine.)

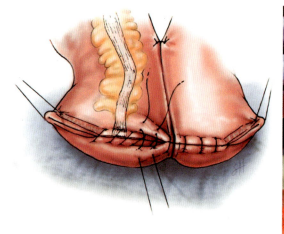
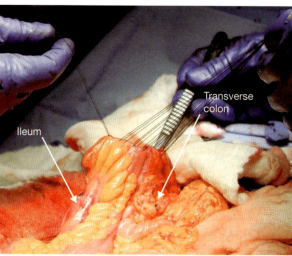

FIGURE 16 • Stapled ileocolonic anastomosis: closing the outer layer of the common enterotomy with interrupted Lembert sutures. (Illustration by Scott Holmes, CMI, copyright Baylor College of Medicine.)

Chapter 7 RIGHT HEMICOLECTOMY: OPEN TECHNIQUE   61

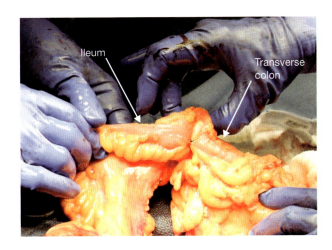

FIGURE 17 • The completed ileotransverse colon side-by-side stapled anastomosis. Palpation of the anastomosis between the thumb and index finger shows that the anastomosis is patent. Notice that both the ileal and colonic segment are well perfused. Closure of the mesenteric defect is optional and is based on surgeon preference.

CLOSURE

- Once hemostasis is ensured and the abdomen is irrigated, the abdominal fascia and skin are closed in standard fashion. Drains are not routinely required, although in cases of infection or abscess, a drain may be placed.

PEARLS AND PITFALLS

Colon mobilization	■ The plane between the mesocolon and the retroperitoneum is an avascular embryologic plane that can be dissected sharply. Excess blood loss during this dissection alerts the surgeon that the incorrect plane was entered.
Vascular dissection	■ During dissection of the middle colic vessels, avulsion of the large collateral branch that connects the inferior pancreaticoduodenal vein with the middle colic vein and superior mesenteric vein can result in bleeding that is difficult to control because the vein retracts and cannot be isolated easily. ■ In order to avoid this, avoid excess upward and medial traction of the right colon while mobilizing the hepatic flexure. ■ Transillumination of the mesocolon and the mesentery of the terminal ileum can help to identify vascular arcades to minimize iatrogenic injury in patients with thick mesentery and can assure good blood supply to the anastomosis.
Anastomosis	■ A well-vascularized, tension-free anastomosis minimizes the risk of anastomotic breakdown. ■ If there is any doubt regarding the integrity of the anastomosis, the bowel segments should be further resected to healthy, vascularized bowel. ■ Blood supply to the anastomosis can also be further assessed with Doppler ultrasound if necessary.

POSTOPERATIVE CARE

- In the absence of intra-abdominal infection, antibiotic therapy does not need to be continued postoperatively.
- A nasogastric tube is not routinely placed.
- The patient should begin ambulating on postoperative day 1.
- The Foley catheter can usually be removed on postoperative day 1 or 2 unless an epidural remains in place.
- The patient can be started on a liquid diet. The diet can be advanced based on clinical progress.
- Deep venous thrombosis prophylaxis should be continued until the time of discharge and can be considered as an outpatient in certain subsets of patients.
- The patient should be counseled about the initial changes in bowel habits including more frequent, loose stools and the possible appearance of blood clots in the first few bowel movements.

COMPLICATIONS

- Intraoperative complications include injury to the right ureter, duodenum, nearby bowel or colon segments, nearby blood vessels such as the inferior pancreaticoduodenal vessels or the superior mesenteric vessels, or an anastomosis that is poorly vascularized or under tension.
- Early postoperative complications include wound infection, anastomotic leak, or intra-abdominal abscess formation.
- Late postoperative complications include development of colocutaneous fistulas, recurrence of cancer, anastomotic stricture, incisional or internal hernia, or ureteral stricture from ureteral devascularization.
- An extended right hemicolectomy adds the potential complication of splenic injury, as the splenic flexure must be mobilized to achieve a tension-free anastomosis. Because most of the proximal colon absorbs fecal water, an extended right hemicolectomy also predisposes to postoperative diarrhea.

SUGGESTED READINGS

1. Larson DW. Right colectomy: open and laparoscopic. In: Evans SRT, ed. *Surgical Pitfalls*. Elsevier; 2009:257-264.
2. Morris A Colorectal cancer. In: Mulholland MW, Lillemoe KD, Doherty GM, et al, eds. *Greenfield's Surgery: Scientific Principles and Practice*. 5th ed. Lippincott Williams & Wilkins; 2010:1090-1119.
3. Rosenberg BL, Morris AM. Colectomy. In: Minter RM, Doherty GM, eds. *Current Procedures: Surgery*. McGraw-Hill; 2010:180-191.
4. Silberfein EJ, Chang GJ, You YN, et al. Cancer of the colon, rectum, and anus. In: Feig BW, Ching CD, eds. *The MD Anderson Surgical Oncology Handbook*. 5th ed. Lippincott Williams & Wilkins; 2012:347-415.
5. Sonoda T, Milsom JW. Segmental colon resection. In: Ashley SW, Cancer WG, Jerkovich GJ, et al, eds. *ACS Surgery: Principles and Practice*. Decker Publishing Inc; 2012:921-932.
6. Wolff BG, Wang JY. Right hemicolectomy for treatment of cancer: open technique. In: Fischer JE, ed. *Fischer's Mastery of Surgery*. 6th ed. Lippincott Williams & Wilkins; 2012:1698-1703.

Chapter 8

Laparoscopic Right Hemicolectomy

Craig A. Messick, Joshua S. Hill, and George J. Chang

DEFINITION

- Right hemicolectomy is defined as the resection of a portion of the terminal ileum, cecum, ascending colon, and portion of the transverse colon. When performed for neoplastic disease, it includes resection of lymphovascular pedicles including the ileocolic, right colic (when present), and sometimes right branches of the middle colic vessels. An extended right hemicolectomy is one in which the middle colic vessels are incorporated in the resection.
- Laparoscopic right hemicolectomy has been shown to be a preferred alternative technique to open surgery in the resection of benign and malignant diseases of the colon. In experienced hands, it has been shown to have equivalent oncologic outcomes with improvements in speed of recovery and other short term outcome advantages when compared with open resection.[1-3]

INDICATIONS

- Right hemicolectomy may be performed for either benign or malignant indications, but the same underlying principles of surgical resection apply to both open and laparoscopic approaches.
- A thorough preoperative workup to define the underlying disease plays a critical role in determining the nature of the operative intervention and optimizing the surgical treatment.
- Benign pathology (common etiologies)
  - Crohn disease: most frequently occurs in the terminal ileum and may include the ascending colon with an associated inflammatory phlegmon or fistula. Right hemicolectomy for Crohn disease is performed when the disease is refractory to medical therapy or when there are penetrating or fibrostenotic complications.
  - Right-sided diverticulitis: occurs uncommonly in the US population, and it is felt to arise as a congenital lesion occurring more commonly in Asian patients. It is commonly misdiagnosed as acute appendicitis.
  - Ischemic colitis: uncommonly affects the right colon in isolation owing to its collateral blood supply. It may present with abdominal pain, bloating due to stricture, or hematochezia.
  - Cecal volvulus: caused by a twist (typically clockwise) of the terminal ileum and colonic mesentery around fixed retroperitoneal attachments, presents with acute abdominal pain and obstructive symptoms.
- Neoplastic pathology
  - Endoscopically unresectable polyps should be treated with colectomy. As they have potential to harbor malignant foci not detected on biopsy, they should be managed according to oncologic principles. Right-sided polyps include high-risk adenomas with high-grade dysplasia or villous components, large hyperplastic polyps, or sessile serrated adenoma/polyps.
  - Malignancy is the most common indication for laparoscopic right hemicolectomy. Equivalent outcomes to open resection have been demonstrated in large multicenter randomized controlled trials.[2-6] A bulky cancer or one that has invaded into adjacent organs should be resected en bloc with associated tissues and may be considered for open resection.
  - Adenocarcinoma: The location with respect to the anatomy of the blood supply determines the extent of bowel resection.
  - Carcinoid: Right colectomy is indicated for carcinoid tumors of the terminal ileum or appendix when 2 cm or greater. Colectomy is also indicated for adverse features such as goblet cell carcinoid histology or presence of lymphovascular or perineural invasion.

PATIENT HISTORY AND PHYSICAL FINDINGS

- Patients with adenocarcinoma are commonly asymptomatic but can present with anemia, melena, altered stool patterns (diarrhea or constipation), abdominal pain, and weight loss.
- A thorough history and physical examination is essential for identifying candidates for laparoscopic surgery. Several patient factors that can affect the feasibility of laparoscopic resection are shown in **TABLE 1**. Patient characteristics or underlying disease issue may preclude safety of the laparoscopic approach or greatly increase the operative difficulty and time, and these factors should be considered when making the decision to proceed with laparoscopy and during operative planning.
- Obesity poses unique challenges during laparoscopic right hemicolectomy. The ease of finding the correct plane and the identification of the central vascular anatomy is greatly diminished in obese patients. Patient positioning may also be impacted by obesity as obese patients may not tolerate extreme Trendelenburg, reverse Trendelenburg, or side to side positioning. In addition, obesity has been associated with a higher risk for conversion to open surgery. Despite these challenges, patients who are obese have increased risk for morbidity such as wound infection when compared with nonobese patients and thus may derive significant benefit from laparoscopic surgery.

Table 1: Patient Factors That Can Affect the Feasibility of Laparoscopic Resection

Obesity
Prior abdominal surgery
Cardiac dysfunction
Pulmonary dysfunction
Large tumor burden
Potential local involvement of adjacent vital organs
Abnormal intra-abdominal anatomy

- Patients with decreased cardiac output may not tolerate increased intra-abdominal pressures resulting in decreased venous return secondary to pneumoperitoneum.
- Intra-abdominal adhesions caused by prior surgery may preclude laparoscopy. Laparoscopic lysis of adhesions may be performed, although surgeon experience and the extent of adhesions should be considered.
- Patients with nutritional deficiencies and impaired healing, such as those on high-dose steroids, recent immunomodulators, or systemic chemotherapy, are at higher risk for anastomotic failure. In those patients with ongoing life-threatening illnesses, ileocolonic anastomosis should be deferred in favor of end ileostomy. An ileocolostomy anastomosis should not be performed in patients with hemodynamic instability.

DIAGNOSTIC STUDIES

- Colonoscopy: All tumors should be localized, biopsied, and tattooed prior to embarking on laparoscopic surgery. Tattooing allows for intraoperative localization of the tumor, although it may be faint when localized to the mesenteric border (FIGURE 1). The tattoo can also be on the retroperitoneal surface and not seen (FIGURE 2). Synchronous tumors (present in 3%-5% of patients with colon cancer) and unresected polyps should be noted and considered in the treatment plan.[7] Colonoscopy may not be possible in patients with a complete obstruction. In these patients, intraoperative palpation of the entire colon should be performed to assess for secondary lesions. After recovery from surgery, a short interval completion colonoscopy should be performed.
- Computed tomography (CT) colonography/enterography: Can be useful in patients not amenable to colonoscopy. Use of CT enterography provides additional information of the small intestines in patients with Crohn disease that may alter surgical strategy.
- CT scan of the abdomen and pelvis: In patients with inflammatory bowel disease, CT scan provides information pertaining to the extent of colitis, presence of a fistula, and/or abscess. In patients with malignancy, CT scans of the chest, abdomen, and pelvis should be performed to assess for pulmonary, hepatic, and lymphatic metastasis as well as infiltration of the primary tumor into adjacent structures.[8]

SURGICAL MANAGEMENT

Preoperative Planning

- Appropriate preoperative antibiotic coverage before incision has been shown to decrease the risk of surgical-site infections, but courses of antibiotics greater than 24 hours are actually associated with worse outcomes.[9]
- The need for a preoperative mechanical bowel preparation in patients undergoing right hemicolectomy is controversial.[10,11] We use mechanical bowel preparation because it lightens the colon, thus facilitating laparoscopic handling of the colon.

Patient Positioning

- The patient is positioned on a supine position and is secured with Trendelenburg straps on the ankles (FIGURE 3). If an extended right hemicolectomy will be performed, the patient may be placed in a lithotomy position to facilitate the mobilization of the splenic flexure, if necessary.
- Gravity is the single greatest facilitator of exposure during laparoscopic colectomy. During the course of the case, the patient may be placed in steep Trendelenburg, reverse Trendelenburg and rotated right side up. For this reason, the patient must be secured to the operating table. A variety of devices have been used to secure the patient. We prefer to use ankle and chest straps, but commercially available foam pads placed under the patient to prevent slippage may also be used. We avoid using pads of beanbags placed above the shoulder that can cause brachial plexus injuries.
- Both arms should be padded and tucked at the patient's side. If the patient is too wide for the table, the right arm may be left out so that the operative team standing together on the patient's left side still has sufficient working space. The patient's hands should be turned such that their palms face medially with the thumbs up and the in a neutral position.
- Ensure that intravenous (IV) lines are working after positioning and prior to the start of the case. A second IV is recommended because the patient's arms will be inaccessible during the operation, thus making the establishment of another IV difficult.

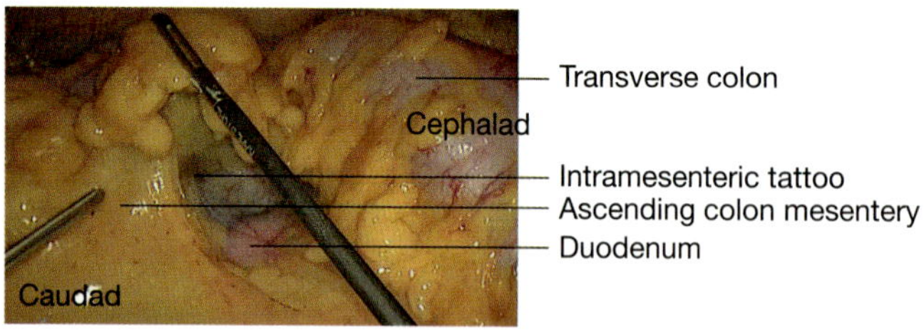

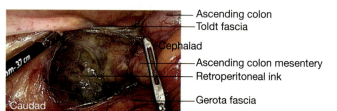

FIGURE 1 • Tattooing the target. Tattoos placed within the colonic mesentery may not be visible upon initial inspection. As shown in this operative photograph, the distal ascending colon at the hepatic flexure has been anteriorly reflected to reveal the location of a previously placed intramesenteric tattoo.

FIGURE 2 • Tattooing the target. In some instances, a tattoo placed within the mesentery is not visible until dissection into the retroperitoneum. Here, the dissection of Toldt fascia (anterior) has been performed and the retroperitoneum exposed, revealing the location of the tattoo within the retroperitoneum of the ascending colon.

Chapter 8 LAPAROSCOPIC RIGHT HEMICOLECTOMY 65

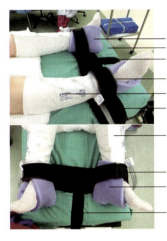

FIGURE 3 • Securing the patient to the table. Velcro straps are secured to the patient's ankles, then attached to the operating room table to protect the patient's legs from sliding laterally off the table's sides with extreme left-right positioning and to assist in keeping the patient from slipping toward the head of the table when placed in steep Trendelenburg position.

PORT PLACEMENT

- A variety of methods may be employed for the entry into the abdomen during laparoscopic surgery. Two commonly used options are the use of a Veress needle or the authors' preferred technique of a direct fascial cutdown (Hassan technique). Pneumoperitoneum is established with carbon dioxide to 15 mm Hg as tolerated.
- Standard port placement includes a 10- to 12-mm umbilical port (camera port), 5-mm working ports in the left upper quadrant, and either a 5-mm or 10- to 12-mm port in the left lower quadrant. A fourth port is used in either the suprapubic or right lower quadrant positions. An optional 5-mm port is placed in the patient's right upper quadrant to assist with the distal transverse colon or splenic flexure mobilization as needed for an extended right hemicolectomy (FIGURE 4).

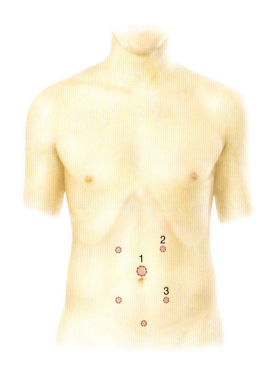

FIGURE 4 • Port placement. This diagram shows the standard and additional laparoscopic port sites for a laparoscopic right hemicolectomy. Standard placement includes a 10- to 12-mm umbilical port (1), 5-mm left upper quadrant port (2), and either a 5-mm or 10- to12-mm left lower quadrant port. A fourth port is used in the optional locations (o), either suprapubic or right lower quadrant positions. An optional 5-mm port is placed in the patient's right upper quadrant to assist with the distal transverse colon or splenic flexure as needed for an extended right hemicolectomy.

VASCULAR TRANSECTION AND MEDIAL TO LATERAL MOBILIZATION OF THE ILEOCOLIC MESENTERY

- The abdomen should be thoroughly inspected to rule out metastatic sites or synchronous pathology with evaluation of the peritoneum, liver, retroperitoneum, and adnexal structures in women.
- The patient is positioned with the left side down and in slight Trendelenburg.
- The omentum is retracted cephalad over the transverse colon into the upper abdomen. In an obese patient with a bulky omentum, an assistant can hold retraction of the omentum through the left upper quadrant port.
- The small intestine is swept to the left lower quadrant, allowing for complete visualization of the mesenteric attachments

to the right colon and the superior mesenteric artery (SMA). The ileocolic vessels (ICVs) can be identified as they cross over the third portion of the duodenum. The fold of Treves is grasped and retracted laterally to demonstrate the course of the ICVs and to identify their origin from the SMA and the confluence of the ileocolic vein into the superior mesenteric vein (SMV) (**FIGURE 5**).

- The peritoneal surface is scored on the dorsal surface of the ICV near their origin off the SMA/SMV (**FIGURE 6**). While ensuring that the lymph node–bearing tissue is dissected into the ileocolic mesentery (specimen side), the retroperitoneal attachments to the colonic mesentery are divided.
- The correct, avascular plane can be developed with a combination of sharp and blunt dissection. The small retroperitoneal vessels can act as a guide and should be dissected downward, away from the colonic mesentery. If these are bluntly torn, minimal, yet bothersome bleeding can ensue. This careful medial-to-lateral dissection of the ileocolic mesentery is carried cephalad to the origin of the ICV, with care taken not to inadvertently injure the duodenum, and laterally releasing the colonic mesentery from retroperitoneal attachments without injury to the ureter or gonadal vessels. The dissection plane should be anterior to the duodenum and pancreatic head, taking care to avoid inadvertent duodenal mobilization or dissection between the duodenum and pancreas (**FIGURE 7**).
- The ICV can then be divided at the origin from the SMA/SMV with either an endoscopic GIA stapler with a vascular load (our preference; see **FIGURE 8**), with an energy device, or between endoclips. Node-bearing tissue should be kept with the specimen.
- Next, the dissection is taken up along the SMA to identify the right colic artery and vein (when present) (**FIGURE 9**) as well as the middle colic vessels (MCVs) and their bifurcation (**FIGURE 10**). This step is facilitated by anterior and cephalad traction on the transverse colon to tent the mesentery.
- By following the SMA from the point of ICV ligation, the variably present right colic artery is identified to arise from the SMA between the ICV and the MCV where it should be divided at its origin with an energy-sealing device.
- The venous drainage of the right colon is also highly variable, and the right colic vein is missing in up to 50% of patients. It can be found joining the right gastroepiploic and superior pancreaticoduodenal veins at the gastrocolic trunk of Henle.
- In cases of more distal ascending colon or hepatic flexure tumors, transaction of either the right branch or the entire

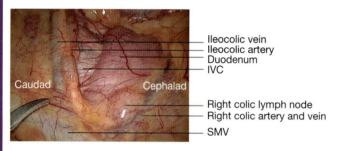

FIGURE 5 • Exposure of the ileocolic pedicle. After the small bowel has been placed in the patient's left hemiabdomen exposing the right colon mesentery, the ileocolic pedicle is often seen pulsating within its mesentery. The duodenum is often seen through a thin layer of colon mesentery; the ICVs can be identified as they cross the third portion of the duodenum. In this image, the SMV, inferior vena cava, and right colic artery and vein are seen. IVC, inferior vena cava; SMV, superior mesenteric vein.

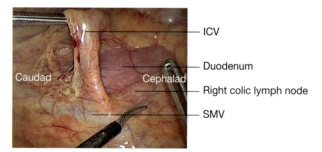

FIGURE 6 • Dissection of the ICV. Scoring of the peritoneum along the inferior sulcus of the ICV allows for a posterior dissection to the ICV. Gentle lifting of the pedicle will allow for dissection of the tissue to the origin of the ICV at the SMA and SMV. ICV, ileocolic vessels; SMV, superior mesenteric vein.

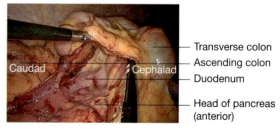

FIGURE 7 • Medial-to-lateral dissection. The medial-to-lateral dissection of the ileocolic mesentery is *continued* both laterally and superiorly anterior to the duodenum and head of pancreas along the course of the SMA and SMV to the origin on the middle colic vessels.

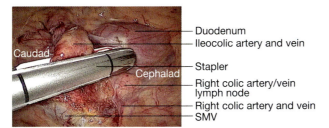

FIGURE 8 • Transection of the ICV. Once the ileocolic artery and vein have been cleared of their surrounding fat and lymphatic tissue, they can be transected at their origins off the SMA and SMV. This can be performed with a 30-mm stapler (as shown) or with an energy device as appropriate. The vessels can be separated and ligated either separately or together, as per surgeon preference.

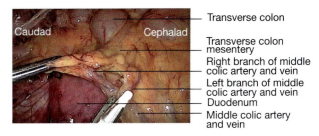

FIGURE 10 • Exposure of the middle colic vessels. The colon mesentery is incised along the border of the superior mesenteric vessels to the bifurcation of the right and left branches of the middle colic artery and vein as shown here, ensuring that all lymphatic tissue within the distribution of the right and proximal transverse colon is removed with the specimen. This dissection is performed anteriorly to the duodenum and head of pancreas. The right branch of the middle colic artery and vein are typically small enough to transect with a sealing energy device.

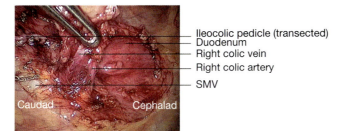

FIGURE 9 • Transection of the right colic vessels. A right colic artery and vein are shown originating from the superior mesenteric artery and vein. This is often discovered only after transection of the ileocolic artery and vein has been completed. These vessels are typically smaller than the ileocolic artery and vein and may be ligated with staples, endoclips, or an energy device. SMV, superior mesenteric vein.

trunk of the MCVs should be performed after exposing the origin of these vessels from the SMA/SMV. Tearing the vein at this level will result in rapid bleeding; therefore, it is important to identify the vascular anatomy of the right colon carefully and completely prior to dividing the mesentery.

LATERAL COLON MOBILIZATION

- Placing the patient in Trendelenburg position and retracting the small bowel out of the pelvis into the upper abdomen facilitates this step.
- The ascending colon is mobilized in an inferior to superior fashion by lifting the cecum away from the retroperitoneum and scoring the base of the cecal and terminal ileal mesenteries until the medial-to-lateral dissection is met (**FIGURE 11**). Care should be taken to avoid inadvertent dissection and injury of the ureter and gonadal vein.
- The lateral attachments along Toldt fascia are then incised up to the level of the hepatic flexure. We prefer an inferior to superior approach as this minimizes the risk for kidney mobilization or duodenal Kocherization during bowel mobilization (**FIGURE 12**).
- After the ascending colon has been mobilized, the mobilization of the transverse colon and hepatic flexure is performed. With the patient in reverse Trendelenburg position, the lesser sac is opened by releasing the omentum from the transverse colon. At this level the omentum is frequently fused to the transverse mesocolon, so care should be taken to avoid inadvertent mesenteric vascular injury.
- The proximal transverse colonic attachments along the hepatocolic ligament can then be divided with an energy device

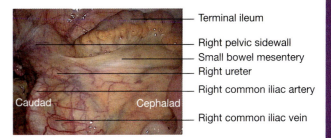

FIGURE 11 • Exposure of the right pelvic inlet. With the patient positioned in steep Trendelenburg and the small intestine removed from the pelvis, the proximal lateral pelvic and abdominal attachments of the terminal ileum and cecum are identified. Important anatomy is appreciated in this photo: right common iliac artery and vein and the right ureter. These peritoneal attachments must be incised and freed to allow complete mobility of the small intestine.

to meet the plane over the duodenum previously established during the medial-to-lateral dissection (**FIGURE 13**). The previous exposure of the duodenum minimizes the risk of inadvertent Kocherization and/or injury to the duodenum at this stage.

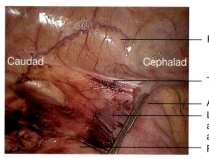

FIGURE 12 • Lateral mobilization of the ascending colon. Once the lateral pelvic and initial abdominal attachments are incised, gentle traction on the cecum and ascending colon toward the patient's left upper quadrant will assist in the dissection of Toldt fascia. The dark purple–appearing tissue toward the bottom of this operative photo reveals the retroperitoneum previously dissected during the initial medial-to-lateral dissection. The ureter maintains a close approximation to the dissection planes.

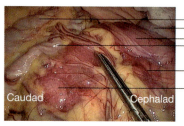

FIGURE 13 • Mobilization of the hepatic flexure. With the patient in reverse Trendelenburg position and the transverse colon with its omentum reflected inferiorly, the superior portion of the previous medial-to-lateral dissection is easily visualized and is seen here in the middle of the photo. Incision into this thin tissue connects with the previous dissection plane, and the dissection continues laterally to incise and release the hepatocolic ligaments completing the mobilization of the right colon. After this has been completed, the right colon should be able to be medialized across the midline of the abdomen.

ENTEROCOLONIC ANASTOMOSIS

- Ileocolonic anastomosis may be performed either intracorporeally or extracorporeally.
- We prefer an extracorporeal anastomosis through a periumbilical extraction site, incorporating the supraumbilical port site. An advantage of this approach is that the anastomosis may be performed according to standard open technique.
- In patients with cancer, the extraction site must be sufficiently large to allow for the passage of the tumor-bearing segment. A wound protector is placed into the incision to reduce infection.
- If the terminal ileal or colon mesenteries have not been completely mobilized, or the mesenteries have not been properly ligated, bowel exteriorization may be difficult and associated with a risk for avulsion injury to the mesenteric vessels.
- During bowel exteriorization, it is helpful to initially maintain the reverse Trendelenburg position with the table slightly rotated left side down to keep the small bowel from falling over the colon and entrapping it.

EXTRACORPOREAL TRANSECTION AND ENTEROCOLONIC ANASTOMOSIS

- Once the right colon and terminal ileum have been delivered through the wound protector, attention is turned to the bowel resection. Investigation of the vascular supply to the planned resection sites prior to division and anastomosis is paramount.
- The mesentery should be carefully inspected, and the terminal vessels should be visually assessed for pulsations or pulsatile blood flow should be confirmed by Doppler interrogation. If no pulsations are present, then another site for resection and anastomosis is chosen.
- The terminal ileum and the transverse colon (typically to the right side of the MCV) are transected with a linear stapler. The intervening mesentery is transected with an energy device.
- There are multiple methods to create an anastomosis. We suggest that surgeons use the method with which they are most comfortable. Our preferred approach is to perform a side-to-side, antimesenteric, functional end-to-end, stapled anastomosis in continuity to avoid potential for twisting of the bowel.
- This is done with a colotomy and an enterotomy on the antimesenteric side of the specimen about 1 or 2 cm away proximal to the planned transection sites. A linear stapler is placed into the enterotomy and colotomy and approximated at their antimesenteric sides. After ensuring that the ileal and colonic mesenteries are free from the closed stapler, it is fired creating the side-to-side enterocolostomy anastomosis (**FIGURE 14**).
- The common enterocolostomy is closed by using an 85- to 100-mm linear stapler (reload), avoiding narrowing the anastomosis (**FIGURE 15**).
- The anastomosis is inspected for gross defects or bleeding, both of which can be oversewn. The corners and intersections of the staple lines may be imbricated or reinforced with Lembert sutures.
- An alternative technique includes bowel division and intracorporeal anastomosis with a variety of options for specimen extraction. One advantage of this approach is the ability to avoid a periumbilical incision with its associated risk for hernia in favor of a Pfannenstiel incision.

Chapter 8 LAPAROSCOPIC RIGHT HEMICOLECTOMY   69

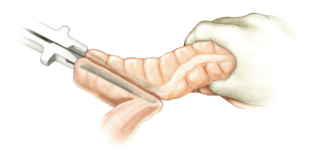

FIGURE 14 • Creation of an extracorporeal side-to-side stapled ileocolonic anastomosis with a linear stapler.

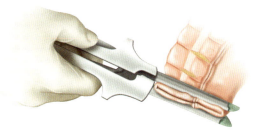

FIGURE 15 • Closure of the common enterocolostomy anastomosis opening with a linear stapler.

CLOSURE

- The abdomen should be inspected for hemostasis and to ensure that there has been no inadvertent avulsion injury to the mesentery or twisting of the mesentery. The mesenteric defect will be large after colectomy with proximal vascular ligation; therefore, neither there is the need to close the mesentery nor is it generally possible to do so.
- Any 12-mm port sites are closed, and the extraction site can be closed with interrupted suture or according to the surgeon's preference.

PEARLS AND PITFALLS

Patient selection	■ Patients who meet criteria for hereditary nonpolyposis colorectal cancer (HNPCC) or Lynch syndrome should be considered for a subtotal colectomy. ■ Patient should be assessed to ensure they will tolerate pneumoperitoneum and changes in positioning during surgery.
Preoperative planning	■ Ensure a complete colonoscopy was performed. As many as 1 in 20 patients will have synchronous primary cancers. ■ Localize the tumor with CT imaging for larger lesions and colonoscopic tattoo or metallic clip for smaller ones. ■ Careful review of preoperative CT imaging identifies locally advanced disease, distant metastases, or aberrant vascular anatomy.
Patient positioning and port placement	■ Securing the patient to the bed with chest and leg straps is key and allows for extremes in patient positioning. ■ Placing ports in either the midline or contralateral to the target facilitates orientation and maximizes instrument range of motion.
Procedure	■ Completing the medial-to-lateral dissection from the right branch of the middle colic artery down to the cecum is key to the dissection, allowing easier dissection of the lateral ascending colon off of Toldt fascia. ■ Careful attention to the duodenum and pancreatic head should be maintained while freeing the transverse mesocolon. The duodenum also serves as a landmark for proximal ligation of the ICV. ■ Anticipate variations in the vascular anatomy of the hepatic flexure. The course of the right colic vein in particular is highly variable, and it is therefore at risk for avulsion injury especially at the trunk of Henle. ■ Mobilization along the base of the terminal ileal mesentery over the inferior vena cava and toward the ligament of Treitz ensures adequate mobilization for bowel exteriorization and tension-free anastomosis. ■ Sweeping the ascending colon and terminal ileum to the left side of the patient's abdomen is a good test to ensure complete mobilization of the entire right and transverse colon. ■ Ensure an appropriate oncologic resection is performed during all steps of the procedure not leaving behind ileocolic and middle colic lymph nodes.
Orientation	■ Prior to closure, inspect the orientation of the small bowel and its mesentery to ensure that no twists in the bowel were introduced. ■ Closure of the mesenteric defect to prevent internal hernias is not necessary if the defect is large.

POSTOPERATIVE CARE

- Following the procedure, principles of early mobilization and oral intake are observed.
- Early ambulation is encouraged to assist in return of bowel function, and any invasive lines or catheters are also removed within 48 hours.
- Diet is initiated with clear liquids on the day of surgery and advanced as tolerated.
- Discharge criteria include (1) ability to maintain oral hydration, (2) adequate pain control without the need for IV narcotics, (3) signs of bowel function (flatus), and (4) afebrile for at least 24 hours. A narcotic minimizing regimen improves recovery.

OUTCOMES

- Laparoscopic procedures, when compared with traditional open surgery, have been shown to have quicker return of bowel function, less requirement of IV narcotics, earlier patient ambulation, fewer surgical-site infections, and earlier discharge from the hospital.
- Most importantly, randomized control trials comparing laparoscopic and open colectomies, when performed adequately, provide equivalent oncologic outcomes with no differences in tumor recurrence and patient survival.

COMPLICATIONS

- Surgical-site infection (superficial, deep, and organ space)
- Wound dehiscence
- Hemorrhage
- Anastomotic leak/breakdown
- Bowel obstruction

REFERENCES

1. Kuhry E, Bonjer HJ, Haglind E, et al. Impact of hospital case volume on short-term outcome after laparoscopic operation for colonic cancer. *Surg Endosc.* 2005;19(5):687-692.
2. Clinical Outcomes of Surgical Therapy Study Group. A comparison of laparoscopically assisted and open colectomy for colon cancer. *N Engl J Med.* 2004;350(2):2050-2059.
3. Jayne DG, Guillou PJ, Thorpe H, et al. Randomized trial of laparoscopic-assisted resection of colorectal carcinoma: 3-year results of the UK MRC CLASICC Trial Group. *J Clin Oncol.* 2007;25(21):3061-3068.
4. Bohm B, Milsom JW, Fazio VW. Postoperative intestinal motility following conventional and laparoscopic intestinal surgery. *Arch Surg.* 1995;130(4):415-419.
5. Fleshman JW, Fry RD, Birnnaum EH, et al. Laparoscopic-assisted and minilaparotomy approaches to colorectal diseases are similar in early outcome. *Dis Colon Rectum.* 1996;39(1):15-22.
6. Weeks JC, Nelson H, Gelber S, et al. Short-term quality-of-life outcomes following laparoscopic-assisted colectomy vs open colectomy for colon cancer: a randomized trial. *JAMA.* 2002;287(3):321-328.
7. Latournerie M, Jooste V, Cottet V, et al. Epidemiology and prognosis of synchronous colorectal cancers. *Br J Surg.* 2008;95(12):1528-1533.
8. Pihl E, Hughes ES, McDermott FT, et al. Lung recurrence after curative surgery for colorectal cancer. *Dis Colon Rectum.* 1987;30(6):417-419.
9. Mahid SS, Polk HC Jr, Lewis JN, et al. Opportunities for improved performance in surgical specialty practice. *Ann Surg.* 2008;247(2):380-388.
10. Pineda CE, Shelton AA, Hernandez-Boussard T, et al. Mechanical bowel preparation in intestinal surgery: a meta-analysis and review of the literature. *J Gastrointest Surg.* 2008;12(11):2037-2044.
11. Englesbe MJ, Brooks L, Kubus J, et al. A statewide assessment of surgical site infection following colectomy: the role of oral antibiotics. *Ann Surg.* 2010;252(3):514-519; discussion 519-520.

Chapter 9

Right Hemicolectomy: Hand-Assisted Laparoscopic Surgery (HALS) Technique

Matthew Albert and Harsha Polavarapu

DEFINITION

- Hand-assisted laparoscopic surgery (HALS) is a hybrid technique, which allows the surgeon to insert their hand into the abdominal cavity through a relatively small incision while preserving the ability to work under pneumoperitoneum. This approach aids in tactile feedback, retraction, and dissection by hand assistance in turn eliminating the technical challenges of conventional laparoscopy while maintaining nearly all of its benefits.[1,2]

INDICATIONS

- Colon cancer
- Colon polyps not amenable to colonoscopic removal
- Inflammatory bowel disease
- Angiodysplasia
- Recurrent right colonic diverticulitis

PATIENT HISTORY AND PHYSICAL FINDINGS

- A thorough history should be taken, including a detailed past medical history, past surgical history, present medications and allergies, and a personal and family history of colon and rectal cancer.
- A detailed family history to assess the risk of hereditary polyposis syndromes is critical in selecting the optimal procedure for the patient. Suspected patients should be offered genetic counseling and testing.
- A detailed physical examination of the patient should be performed to identify any prior surgical incisions and palpable masses to plan for the operation.
- The location, histopathology, and the clinical stage of the lesion are crucial prior to any planned procedure.

IMAGING AND OTHER DIAGNOSTIC STUDIES

- Colonoscopy remains the investigation of choice for localizing the target lesion, for obtaining tissue for histopathology, and for tattooing for intraoperative localization. This is also helpful in identifying synchronous lesions in the remaining colon.
- Computed tomography (CT) scan of the chest/abdomen/pelvis with IV and oral contrast is recommended as the primary staging tool to assess for local organ invasion and for distant metastasis.[3]

- Serum carcinoembryonic antigen (CEA) level is a valuable marker for postoperative surveillance.
- Bone scan and brain imaging should be reserved for symptomatic patients only.

SURGICAL MANAGEMENT

- The goal of surgery is an en bloc resection of the involved segment of bowel and to perform a high ligation of the vascular pedicle permitting adequate removal of associated lymphatics and lymph nodes.
- At least 12 lymph nodes must be harvested to adequately stage the patient and to avoid risk of understaging.[3]

Preoperative Planning

- Routine use of mechanical bowel preparation is not recommended.[4]
- Deep vein thrombosis prophylaxis with sequential compression devices and subcutaneous heparin dosing before induction of anesthesia is administered.
- A Foley catheter is placed prior to the operation.
- Nasogastric/orogastric tube is placed prior to the operation.
- Preoperative antibiotics covering skin and bowel flora are administered prior to induction of anesthesia.

Positioning

- Patient is positioned in a supine position. In order to prevent the patient from sliding during the case, the arms are tucked to the sides, the feet are placed against a padded footboard, and a strap is placed over the thighs (**FIGURE 1**).
- Alternatively, the patient can be placed in the low lithotomy position to avoid instrument conflict with the lower extremities. The knees should be slightly flexed and the feet firmly planted on the stirrups to prevent undue pressure on the calves and on the lateral peroneal nerves.
- Depending on the location of pathology and body habitus, a 5- to 7-cm incision is made for the hand port in an epigastric, periumbilical, or Pfannenstiel location (**FIGURE 2**).
- Location of the trocars can be variable based on surgeon's preference. In general, it is best to triangulate all ports to enhance visualization and to prevent instrument conflict inside the abdomen.
- A traditional port placement includes (**FIGURE 2**):
  - A GelPort hand port through a 6-cm epigastric incision
  - A 5-mm infraumbilical camera port
  - A 5-mm left lower quadrant instrument port
  - A 5-mm left upper quadrant/left anterior flank

72 SECTION II SURGERY OF THE COLON, APPENDIX, RECTUM, AND ANUS

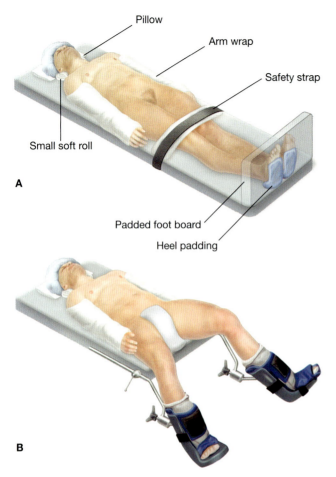

FIGURE 1 • The patient is positioned in the supine position with the arms tucked, a foot board, and a strap over the legs to prevent patient sliding during table movement **(A)**. Alternatively, the patient can be placed in the low lithotomy position to facilitate a surgeon or assistant standing between the legs **(B)**.

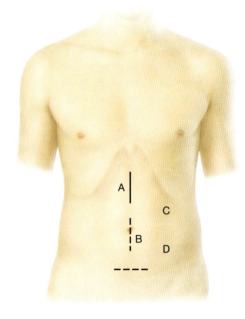

FIGURE 2 • Port placement. The hand access port is placed through a 5- to 7-cm epigastric incision (*A*). Alternatively, it can be placed through a Pfannenstiel or periumbilical incision *(dotted lines)*. A 5-mm camera port is placed infraumbilically (*B*). Two 5-mm working ports are placed in the left upper (*C*) and left lower (*D*) quadrants.

TECHNIQUES

EXPOSURE

- After placement of the hand port, the abdomen is explored to locate the lesion, to assess the extent of spread, and to palpate the liver and peritoneal cavity for distant metastatic spread.
- In female patients, the ovaries should be examined for metastatic spread or primary neoplasms.
- Pneumoperitoneum is created with carbon dioxide (CO_2) and additional trocars are inserted.
- Patient is placed in a left lateral tilt and slight Trendelenburg position. The small bowel is fanned out along its mesentery to aid in the exposure of the right colon.
- The greater omentum along with the transverse colon is retracted cephalad.
- The cecum is grasped with the hand and retracted toward the anterior abdominal wall using gentle traction to identify the ileocolic vessels.

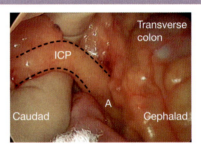

FIGURE 3 • The ileocolic pedicle (ICP), identified at its origin off the inferior mesenteric vessels at the root of the mesentery (*A*), is grasped and retracted toward the anterior abdominal wall.

- The ileocolic pedicle is grasped and retracted toward the anterior abdominal wall (**FIGURE 3**).

DIVISION OF ILEOCOLIC PEDICLE

- With the ileocolic pedicle on stretch, a parallel incision is made on the peritoneal layer underneath the pedicle (**FIGURE 4**) extending to the root of the mesentery and the superior mesenteric vein, using monopolar electrocautery.
- A window is created under the ileocolic pedicle in the avascular plane that separates the pedicle from the retroperitoneum (**FIGURE 5**).
- The ileocolic pedicle is isolated and divided close to its origin off the superior mesenteric vessels using an energy device, a linear vascular stapler, or surgical clips based on surgeon's preference (**FIGURE 6**).

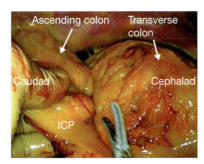

FIGURE 4 • With the ileocolic pedicle (ICP) on stretch, a parallel incision has been made on the peritoneal layer underneath the ICP extending to the root of the mesentery. The surgeon, with the left hand now holding the ICP anteriorly, is now ready to open a window through the mesocolon lateral to the ICP.

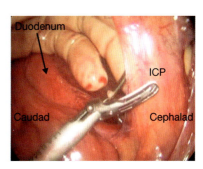

FIGURE 5 • The ileocolic pedicle (ICP) has now been completely encircled and is now ready for transection. Notice that the pedicle has been completely separated from the duodenum and other retroperitoneal structures.

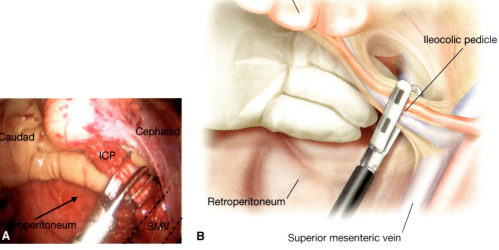

FIGURE 6 • **A,** The ileocolic pedicle (ICP) is isolated and divided in between vascular clips with a 5-mm energy device close to its origin off the superior mesenteric vessels (SMV). **B,** Illustration of this step.

MOBILIZATION OF RIGHT MESOCOLON

- Using blunt dissection with a 5-mm energy device, the ascending mesocolon is mobilized off the retroperitoneum (duodenum and Gerota's fascia) using a medial to lateral dissection approach.
- To facilitate exposure, the surgeon's left hand should be pronated and placed underneath the mesocolon, giving upward traction for the retroperitoneal dissection (**FIGURE 7**).
- Mobilization of the right mesocolon is carried out laterally to the abdominal wall (**FIGURE 8A**), superiorly to the hepatorenal recess (**FIGURE 8B**), and medially exposing the third portion of the duodenum (**FIGURE 8C**).
- At this point, critical structures including the right ureter, the right gonadal vein, and the duodenum are identified and preserved intact in the retroperitoneum (**FIGURE 9**).

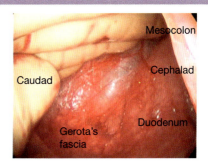

FIGURE 7 • The ascending mesocolon is mobilized off the retroperitoneum (duodenum and Gerota's fascia), using a medial to lateral dissection approach. To facilitate exposure, the surgeon's left hand should be pronated and placed underneath the mesocolon, giving upward traction for the retroperitoneal dissection.

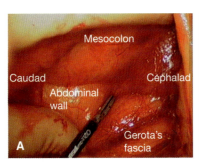
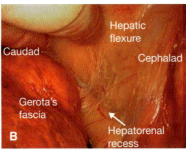
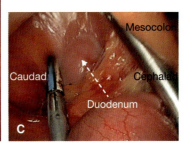

FIGURE 8 • **A,** The medial to lateral dissection, performed bluntly with a 5-mm energy device, separates the ascending mesocolon from the retroperitoneal structures (Gerota's fascia and duodenum) until reaching the lateral abdominal wall. **B,** The dissection is carried superiorly until the hepatorenal recess. **C,** The third portion of the duodenum is exposed medially.

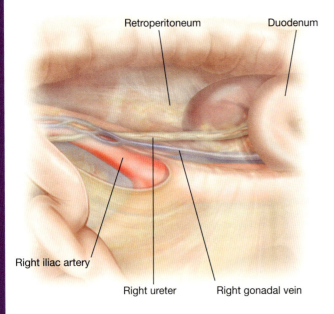

FIGURE 9 • After completion of the medial to lateral mobilization of the ascending mesocolon, critical structures including the right ureter, the right gonadal vein, and the duodenum are identified and preserved intact in the retroperitoneum.

LATERAL MOBILIZATION OF THE ASCENDING COLON

- With the patient in a steep Trendelenburg position, the small bowel is retracted out of pelvis, and the base of cecum is grasped and retracted anteriorly toward the abdominal wall.
- With the ileum on stretch, a peritoneal incision is created from the cecum medially along the root of the ileal mesentery (**FIGURE 10**) to communicate with the retrocolic space previously created by the medial to lateral mobilization of the ascending mesocolon.
- The right ureter and the right gonadal vein are most easily identified at this phase of the operation coursing over the right iliac vessels and into the pelvis (**FIGURE 11**). Lateral and anterior to the psoas muscle, the lateral femoral cutaneous nerve is also frequently identified.
- The white line of Toldt is incised (**FIGURE 12**), dividing the only remaining attachments of the ascending colon if the medial to lateral dissection was carried out adequately during the previous step.

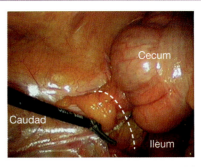

FIGURE 10 • With the patient in a steep Trendelenburg position, the small bowel is retracted out of pelvis, and the base of cecum is grasped and retracted anteriorly toward the abdominal wall. With the ileum on stretch, a peritoneal incision is created from the cecum medially along the root of the terminal ileal mesentery.

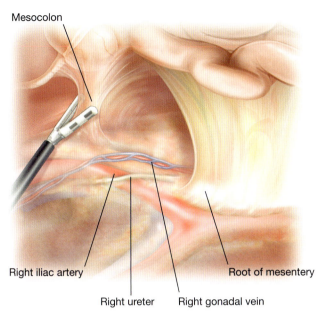

FIGURE 11 • After mobilization of the cecum and terminal ileum, the right gonadal vein and the right ureter are seen in the retroperitoneum crossing over the right iliac artery and into the pelvis.

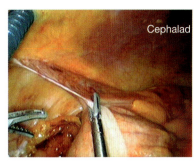

FIGURE 12 • With the surgeon retracting the colon medially, the lateral attachments of the ascending colon (white line of Toldt) are transected with an energy device in a cephalad direction.

MOBILIZATION OF THE HEPATIC FLEXURE AND THE PROXIMAL TRANSVERSE COLON

- The patient is positioned in reverse Trendelenburg position and the hepatic flexure can easily be exposed by grasping the colon in your palm and pulling it downward and medially, as one would do during open surgery.
- The hepatocolic ligament is transected with a 5-mm energy device. The surgeon can facilitate this step by hooking their index finger under the hepatocolic ligament (**FIGURE 13**).
- By pulling the transverse colon now downward, the gastrocolic ligament is readily exposed.
- The gastrocolic ligament is transected up to the midtransverse colon with a 5-mm energy device, and the lesser sac entered.
- The extent of mobilization is dictated by the location of the pathology, body habitus, and extraction site.

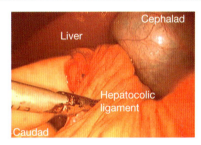

FIGURE 13 • Transection of the hepatocolic ligament. The hepatocolic ligament is transected with a 5-mm energy device. The surgeon can facilitate this step by hooking their index finger under the hepatocolic ligament as shown.

- With the hepatic flexure and the ascending colon now fully mobilized, we are now ready for the extracorporeal mobilization of the specimen.

BOWEL RESECTION AND ANASTOMOSIS

- Once the colon is completely mobilized, the pneumoperitoneum is desufflated, and the right colon and terminal ileum are exteriorized through the hand port site with the wound protector in place to prevent oncologic and infectious contamination of the wound (**FIGURE 14**).
- The extracorporeal mobilization of the right colon and terminal ileum should be feasible without any tension. Should there be any tension during the extracorporeal delivery of the specimen, reintroduce it into the abdomen, reinsufflate the pneumoperitoneum, and mobilize the right colon further to avoid potentially troublesome mesenteric tears that could lead to significant bleeding.
- The remaining mesentery of the small bowel and the large bowel is divided followed by the division of the terminal ileum and midtransverse colon with a linear stapler device (**FIGURE 15**).
- The resected right colon is opened on a side table to confirm complete resection of the target lesion and the specimen is sent for final pathology.
- A side-to-side ileocolic anastomosis is performed (**FIGURE 16A**). The completed anastomosis is introduced back into the abdominal cavity (**FIGURE 16B**). Surgeons may choose from either a stapled or a hand-sewn technique for ileocolic anastomosis.
- The abdomen is reinsufflated to assure that there is good hemostasis as well as a correct bowel orientation.

SECTION II SURGERY OF THE COLON, APPENDIX, RECTUM, AND ANUS

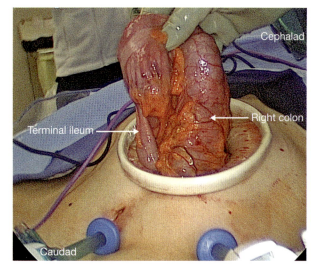

FIGURE 14 • Extracorporeal mobilization. The right colon and the terminal ileum are exteriorized through the hand port site with the wound protector in place.

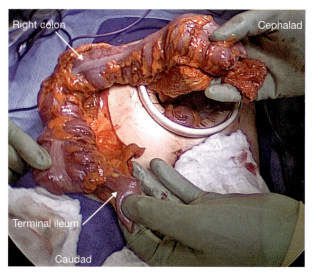

FIGURE 15 • Extracorporeal transection. The terminal ileum and the transverse colon have been transected with a linear stapler.

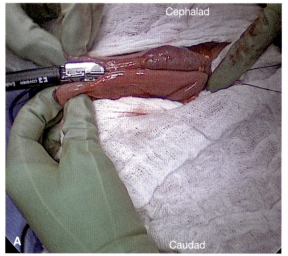
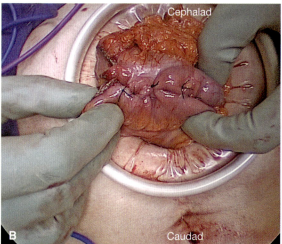

FIGURE 16 • Extracorporeal anastomosis. **A,** A stapled side-to-side ileotransverse colon anastomosis technique is shown. **B,** The completed anastomosis will be introduced back into the abdomen.

CLOSURE

- The ports, the hand-assisted device, and the wound protector are removed under direct vision.
- Surgical gloves are changed to minimize the chance of a wound infection.
- The hand-port fascial incision is closed with a running absorbable monofilament suture (no. 1 polydioxanone [PDS]).
- All wounds are irrigated and closed with subcuticular 4-0 PDS sutures.

PEARLS AND PITFALLS

Preoperative localization	▪ Preoperative localization of the lesion with a tattoo is crucial, especially for polyps, as these can be difficult to identify even with tactile feedback.
Identification of the ileocolic pedicle	▪ The ileocecal junction should be elevated to identify the ileocolic vessels, as the superior mesenteric vessels can easily be mistaken for the ileocolic vessels.
Avoid the superior mesenteric vein	▪ When dissecting high on the ileocolic vessels, care should be taken to avoid the superior mesenteric vein.
Identifying the right ureter	▪ The right ureter should be identified and preserved as it can be easily injured if you are in the wrong plane. Stay in the loose areolar plane located between the ascending mesocolon anteriorly and the retroperitoneum posteriorly.
Small bowel orientation	▪ Before performing an ileocolic anastomosis, the orientation of the small bowel should be checked, as the small bowel can easily get twisted on itself during the extracorporeal mobilization.

POSTOPERATIVE CARE

- Patients are monitored on a surgical floor bed.
- Start a clear liquid diet on postoperative day 1 and advance diet as tolerated.
- Foley catheter is removed on postoperative day 1.
- Most of the patients are discharged home on postoperative days 2 and 3.

OUTCOMES

- Hand-assisted colectomy has been shown to decrease the total operative time and conversion rate compared to conventional laparoscopy.[2,5]
- The long-term survival of patients with colon cancer correlates with the American Joint Committee on Cancer (AJCC) stage published guidelines.

COMPLICATIONS

- Surgical site infection
- Anastomotic leak
- Postoperative bleeding
- Postoperative ileus
- Intra-abdominal infection
- Incisional hernia

REFERENCES

1. Naitoh T, Gagner M, Garcia-Ruiz A, et al. Hand-assisted laparoscopic digestive surgery provides safety and tactile sensation for malignancy or obesity. *Surg Endosc.* 1999;13(2):157-160.
2. Marcello PW, Fleshman JW, Milsom JW, et al. Hand-assisted laparoscopic vs. laparoscopic colorectal surgery: a multicenter, prospective, randomized trial. *Dis Colon Rectum.* 2008;51(6):818-826.
3. *NCCN clinical practice guidelines in oncology: colon cancer (Version 3.2014).* Accessed January 7, 2014. http://www.nccn.org/professionals/physician;usgls/f;usguidelines.asp#site
4. Mutch M, Cellini C. Surgical management of colon cancer. In: Beck DE, Roberts PL, Saclarides TJ, et al, eds. *The ASCRS Textbook of Colon and Rectal Surgery.* 2nd ed. Springer; 2011:711-720.
5. Aalbers AG, Biere SS, van Berge Henegouwen MI, et al. Hand-assisted or laparoscopic-assisted approach in colorectal surgery: a systematic review and meta-analysis. *Surg Endosc.* 2008;22(8):1769-1780.

Chapter 10

Right Hemicolectomy: Single-Incision Laparoscopic Technique

Theodoros Voloyiannis

DEFINITION

- Single-incision laparoscopic right hemicolectomy represents the most advanced technique of conventional laparoscopy where a single multichannel laparoscopic port with a wound protector is used via a 2.5- to 5-cm total incision length.
- The procedure offers comparable outcomes to hand-assisted or multiport laparoscopic technique and it follows the same steps and oncologic principles.
- It can be accomplished without difficulty with an extracorporeal anastomosis allowing for a much faster completion of the procedure. An intracorporeal anastomosis can be performed as well; however, it requires advanced laparoscopic skills and the addition of laparoscopic Endo GIA staplers.

DIFFERENTIAL DIAGNOSIS

- The procedure can be performed for benign or neoplastic diseases or conditions, including the following:
  - Appendectomy
  - Laparoscopic-assisted colonoscopic polypectomy
  - Ileocecectomy
  - Formal right colectomy
  - Extended right colectomy
  - Ileocolonic anastomotic resection with new anastomosis or creation of ileostomy
  - Synchronous other laparoscopic single-incision surgery such as left colectomy, small bowel resection, hysterectomy, etc

PATIENT HISTORY AND PHYSICAL FINDINGS

- A detailed history and physical exam is essential preoperatively to determine if the patient is suitable for laparoscopic single-incision right hemicolectomy. Potential contraindications to laparoscopic single-incision right hemicolectomy are summarized in **TABLE 1**.
- Virtual visit with the patient such as telemedicine preoperatively maybe sufficient in several cases of planned right colectomy; however, an immediate preoperative physical exam is always required.

Table 1: Absolute Contraindications to Single-Incision Laparoscopic Right Colectomy

- Complex terminal ileal or right colonic inflammatory bowel disease with abscess or fistula
- Extensive peritoneal adhesions
- Extensive abscess, feculent peritonitis
- Colon tumor size of more than 10 cm
- Colonic obstruction with proximal massive intestinal dilation
- Preoperative decision for complex en bloc resection
- Midline incisional hernia longer than the maximum single incision of 7 cm

---

- In case of underlying neoplasia, the size of the tumor determines if it can be extracted without tension via the single-port wound protector. In general, tumors up to 10 cm can be extracted via a 7-cm maximum length single incision. The procedure can still be performed with elongation of the incision for extraction of larger tumors. In that case, the benefit of the single port is compromised, with the exception of the avoidance of use of multiple laparoscopic ports.
- A large palpable tumor preoperatively with fixation to the abdominal wall or other organs such as the duodenum, liver, gallbladder or invasion into the perinephric fascia and kidney may challenge the single-incision laparoscopic approach, although excision en bloc with soft tissue abdominal wall or synchronous cholecystectomy or liver wedge resection is still possible via a single incision in most cases.
- Signs and symptoms of obstructing neoplastic lesion with massive proximal distended right colon with or without competent ileocecal valve and small intestinal dilation may also suggest contraindication to laparoscopic approach due to difficulty establishing a safe working space with pneumoperitoneum. Anastomosis may be contraindicated in this case.
- It is important to define the underlying pathology—benign vs malignant disease and the location of the lesion preoperatively. Ileocecectomy or right hemicolectomy for neoplasia may require formal lymphadenectomy with high ligation of the ileocolic vascular pedicle. Hepatic flexure or proximal transverse colon lesions may require additional resection of the right colic vein or right branch or the middle colic artery and vein and further mobilization of the proximal transverse colon.
- Involvement of other organs or structures, such as right ovary, small intestine, abdominal wall, right ureter, right kidney, duodenum, small intestine, omentum, liver, and gallbladder, may require extension of the incision and conversion to a hand-assisted laparoscopy or open laparotomy. Intraoperative consultation prior to the planned procedure to subspecialist surgeons who are experienced with single-incision laparoscopy may be required in these cases.
- Failure to identify the tumor extent and involvement to adjacent organs or structures preoperatively may lead to longer operative time if a single-port technique is used. Conversion to hand-assisted or open approach is prudent in these cases.
- Diagnosing an umbilical or other ventral hernia does not preclude a single-incision approach; however, it may require lengthier operative time, extension of the incision, and possibly removal of an old mesh and placement of a xenograft.
- Previous abdominal surgeries with extensive abdominal or pelvic adhesions may increase the operative time. A single incision may actually facilitate a faster abdominal adhesiolysis, as it can partially be performed under direct visualization via the single port's wound protector.

Chapter 10 **RIGHT HEMICOLECTOMY: SINGLE-INCISION LAPAROSCOPIC TECHNIQUE** **79**

- Crohn's terminal ileitis or right colitis with a large phlegmon or perforation with complex fistulae or abscess may preclude a single-incision laparoscopic approach.
- Previous appendectomy, ileocecectomy with ileocolonic anastomosis, pelvic gynecologic surgery such as salpingo-oophorectomy, surgery for endometriosis or hysterectomy with adhesions of the cecum and terminal ileum in the pelvis is not a contraindication to single-incision approach, as adhesions may be the only intraoperative finding with minimal to moderate increase to operative time.

IMAGING AND OTHER DIAGNOSTIC STUDIES

- Preoperative colonoscopy with India ink tattoo injection is of paramount importance for smaller nonpalpable benign or malignant lesions or polyps, which are not resectable endoscopically. The surgeon must clearly identify the site of the tattoo distal to the lesion preoperatively in the absence of other anatomic landmarks, such as the ileocecal valve or the appendiceal orifice and the cecum itself.
- India ink tattoo by different gastroenterologists has been reported to be placed proximally or around the lesion, distal to the lesion, or both proximal and distal to the lesion, leading occasionally to a false distal colonic resection margin; therefore, personal review of the colonoscopy report and the pictures by the surgeon is necessary.
- Inadvertent extracolonic India ink injection may lead to inflammatory—diverticulitis type—reaction of the surrounding mesentery and omentum, thus making the single-incision laparoscopic colonic mobilization challenging.
- Absence of preoperative tattoo for smaller or nonpalpable lesions distal to the ileocecal valve may lead to failure to localize the lesion intraoperatively, lengthy procedure and possible need for intraoperative colonoscopy, and conversion to laparotomy. This may lead to significant air insufflation of the colon and small intestine unless a carbon dioxide (CO_2) colonoscopic insufflation is available. Compressing the terminal ileum with a laparoscopic grasper during the intraoperative colonoscopy may prevent small intestinal distension. A repeat colonoscopy by the surgeon or the gastroenterologist for proper tattoo identification of the lesion maybe required preoperatively. In this case, a repeat colonoscopy with tattoo localization can be performed the day prior to surgery after formal bowel preparation and the patient may stay on clear liquids for the remainder of the day in order to avoid another bowel preparation.
- Computed tomography of the chest, abdomen, and pelvis with oral and intravenous (IV) contrast helps determine the feasibility and planning of a single-incision laparoscopic approach and identifies the exact location of larger right colonic neoplastic lesions, involvement of adjacent organs or structures, mesenteric adenopathy and possible metastatic lesions, hernia, and other abdominal nonrelated pathology. Inflammatory disease of the terminal ileum or right colon is suspected by the presence of phlegmon, abscess, fistula, or obstruction.
- CT colonography is another diagnostic modality for screening; however, findings of a lesion, mass, or polyp will require a colonoscopy preoperatively.
- Magnetic resonance imaging (MRI) of the abdomen may assist with the identification of indeterminate liver lesions and the assessment of metastatic lesions preoperatively.

- Positron emission tomography (PET) computed tomography is not generally needed preoperatively.
- Preoperative barium enema or small bowel follow-through contrast study has generally been replaced by colonoscopy.
- Ultrasound (US) of the abdomen has limited usefulness for the identification of colonic pathology.
- A carcinoembryonic antigen is obtained as baseline tumor marker for surveillance.
- Circulating Tumor DNA (ct-DNA) is a new assay for molecular residual disease (MRD) and recurrence monitoring, and it may have better application for immediate post-right colectomy assessment of MRD and stratify stage 2 patients for adjuvant therapy.
- Positive FIT-DNA test requires further diagnostic evaluation with colonoscopy as above.

SURGICAL MANAGEMENT

Preoperative Planning

- The administration of the enhanced surgery recovery protocol is proven to expedite the recovery of the patients by allowing early oral feedings, ambulation, avoidance or elimination of use of opioid analgesics, decrease of cost of hospitalization, leading to earlier discharge from the hospital. Most hospitals, institutions, and surgical practices already apply the protocol in different but similar formats and names and in many the application of the protocol is mandatory for elective colon surgery.
- Full bowel preparation is administered the day prior to surgery with the addition of oral antibiotics neomycin and metronidazole at 2, 3, and 10 PM the day prior to surgery. New bowel prep products have essentially replaced the one-gallon PGE bowel prep and much tolerable by the majority of the patients. Right colectomy without bowel preparation can still be performed in certain cases, such as in underlying partial bowel obstruction, but it may increase the weight and volume of the right colon and impair the laparoscopic handling of the colon. Furthermore, extraction of the specimen via a small 3.5-cm single incision may become challenging. Contraindications to the bowel preparation such as complete bowel obstruction or underlying medical conditions remain in place.
- Preoperative medical, renal, or pulmonary and cardiac clearance as necessary.
- Correction of preoperative anemia as needed.
- IV antibiotics for surgical site infection prophylaxis, venous thromboembolism (VTE) prophylaxis, μ-receptor antagonist (alvimopan, others) immediately preoperatively, and correction of electrolyte abnormalities.

Instrumentation

- A bariatric length, 10-mm 30° camera is used. A right-angle adaptor for fiberoptic attachment to the camera is used, if needed, to avoid conflict of the fiberoptic cord with other laparoscopic instruments. Use a preheated camera or other devices for camera lens cleansing. Repeated camera cleansing requires frequent removal via the single port, which adds time to the procedure. High definition 4K camera and monitors is the latest technology for enhanced laparoscopic visualization.
- One bariatric length 5 mm laparoscopic bowel grasper.
- One bariatric length laparoscopic energy device, preferably a 43-cm LigaSure L-hook, or LigaSure impact with

5 mm with monopolar tip, Enseal, or ultrasound powered energy devices or similar is used. Energy devices that produce excessive moisture/plume may impair the visibility as most single-incision laparoscopic ports have a side port for smoke evacuation at the same level with the channel for air insufflation.
- AIRSEAL-CONMED 8-mm laparoscopic insufflation port via the gel of the single port provides an excellent solution for maintaining the pneumoperitoneum during suctioning of blood or peritoneal fluids while the device itself eliminates smoke and plum from the abdomen. In addition, the suctioning system is connected to a ULPA filter that successfully captures viral particles of 0.05μ or larger such as HPV or COVID-19. The AIRSEAL allows for performing the procedure in lower pressure setting without compromising the visualization, such as 8 to 10 mm Hg compared to conventional laparoscopy at 15 mm Hg, thus potentially reducing postoperative pain and enhancing patient recovery.
- Indocyanine green (ICG) and camera for monitoring the vascular supply of the resection margins and the anastomosis.
- Bariatric length laparoscopic 5-mm suction-irrigation. Suction is connected preferably to powered device with UPLA filter such as the Neptune device.
- Laparoscopic smoke evacuator channel with other devices such as STRYKER when AIRSEAL insufflation port is not used.
- Electrocautery attached to powered suctioning system connected to ULPA filter (Ethicon, CONMED, others) is preferable.
- Laparoscopic scissors (optional).
- Laparoscopic 5-mm or 10-mm clip applier (optional).
- Laparoscopic Endoloop polydioxanone (PDS) for the ileocolic vascular pedicle.
- Staplers: linear gastrointestinal anastomosis (GIA) 75-mm, triple line, blue staple cartridges.
- Second set of instruments and drapes, gowns, and gloves for the extracorporeal anastomosis (Duke protocol).
- Hemostatic agents such as Vistaseal for application via laparoscopic spray at the surgical bed as needed or over the staple anastomotic lines for hemostasis.
- Eliminate the set of open instruments used to the necessary only for the procedure. It decreases cost and allows for faster turn over between surgeries.

Patient, Team, and Operating Room Setup

- The patient is placed over a foam pad on supine position with the arms and legs tucked to the side and secured to the table with a Velcro safety strap or broad tape across the chest and belts over the lower extremities (**FIGURE 1**).
- Sequential compression devices (SCDs) are applied to the lower extremities.
- A laparoscopic operating room (OR) table with steep tilting is used. Test maximum tilting prior to draping to assess patients' secure positioning on the table.
- A Foley catheter is inserted and taped over the right thigh in order to avoid urethral trauma during patient positioning changes throughout the operation.
- A bear hugger or other thermal device is applied to the chest and legs.
- Protecting foam pad is placed over the head to avoid injury to the patient's face from laparoscopic instruments and laying equipment on the surgical field.

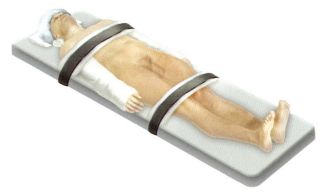

FIGURE 1 • Patient positioning. The patient is placed over a foam pad on supine position with the arms and legs tucked to the side and secured to the table with a Velcro safety strap or broad tape across the chest and lower extremities.

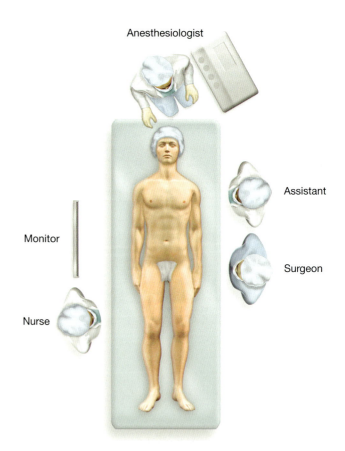

FIGURE 2 • Team positioning. The surgeon stands to the patient's left side with the assistant standing to the surgeon's right side. The scrub nurse stands by the patient's right leg. One or two high-definition monitors are placed to the patient's right side at eye level, in front of the surgeon.

- The laparoscopic tower and other energy devices are placed to the right of the patient's head.
- After the single port is inserted and pneumoperitoneum is established the surgeon stands to the patient's left side with the assistant standing to the surgeon's right side (**FIGURE 2**). The scrub nurse stands by the patient's right leg. One or two high-definition monitors are placed to the patient's right side at eye level in front of the surgeon and the first assistant.

DIAGNOSTIC LAPAROSCOPY—SINGLE MULTICHANNEL PORT TECHNIQUE

- After positioning and securing the patient, the abdominal field is prepped preferably with chlorhexidine-based antiseptic and draped. We recommend laparoscopic draping with side plastic bags/pockets to allow for bariatric instrument placement and ioban strips attached to the edges of the drape to the skin to avoid detachment from the weight of the laparoscopic equipment placed in the side bags. All laparoscopic cords are brought via the patient's upper chest side and secured with the drape's Velcro.
- A 3-7 cm vertical midline incision is performed with a no. 11 scalpel through the umbilicus (**FIGURE 3A** and **B**).
- Insert the three 10-mm ports and the single 12-mm port as well as the 8-mm CONMED AIRSEAL port if used via the gel of the APPLIED MEDICAL Gel Point Port on the back table to avoid losing parts outside the sterile field. Insert the wound protector with the "fan" over it and then cap the assembled laparoscopic multichannel single port and secure it (**FIGURE 4A** and **B**). Insufflate CO_2 pneumoperitoneum to 15 mm Hg or if AIRSEAL is used to 8 to 10 mm Hg.
- Perform a diagnostic laparoscopy. The surgical assistant/camera holder and the surgeon stand by the patient's left side, with the assistant to the surgeon's right side. Tilt the OR table to a minus 5° to 10° Trendelenburg position and airplane it to the left maximum degrees (usually 15°-19°) for better exposure of the ileocolic pedicle and the medial mobilization of the small intestine. There is no need for placement of sponges or Ray-Tecs in the abdomen for retraction.
- Minimize excursion/cluster effect around hands and camera between the surgical assistant and the operating surgeon. Adhere to the principle that the surgeon should position the assisting (nondominant hand) instrument's distal tip (for grasping, retracting, or suctioning) as close as possible to the dominant operating instrument's tip (ie, energy device at the dissecting surgical plane). This distance should be about 3 to 4 cm between the two instruments' tips. For example, hold the ileocolic vascular pedicle just above the site of the division site rather than holding the cecum itself, which is far more

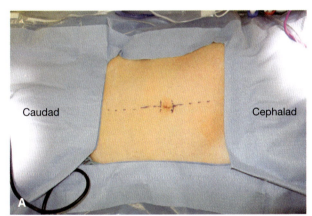 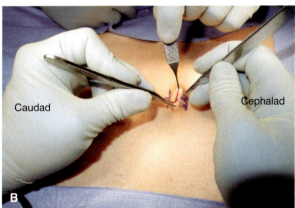

FIGURE 3 • Single-incision laparoscopic surgery (SILS) port placement. **A**, Skin markings. **B**, Skin incision.

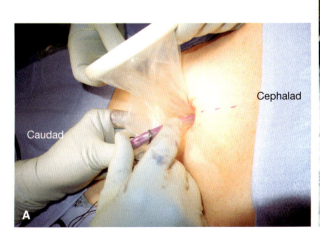 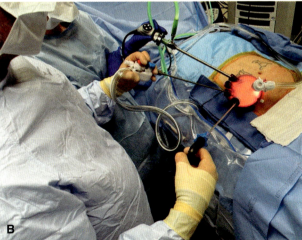

FIGURE 4 • Single-incision laparoscopic surgery (SILS) port placement and configuration. **A**, A wound protector is used. **B**, A multiport channel with three working ports and insufflation port and a smoke evacuator port is used. The port is assembled on a side table prior to insertion in the patient.

distant from the pedicle. This technique allows achieving a wide angle between the two instruments outside the abdomen as they exit and cross via the single port, thus leading to no instrument cluster effect between the surgeon's hands.
- The assistant camera holder will avoid clustering with the surgeon's instruments outside the abdomen if they abduct the camera as far as possible from the surgeon's hands and use the camera's 30° angulation for side view as well as the zoom-in option.
- Minimize the need for frequent instrument exchange via the single port, such as for camera lens cleaning or exchange of graspers with monopolar laparoscopic scissors. Instead, consider avoiding using laparoscopic scissors or elongated cautery and replace with energy devices that provide both dissection and sealing-cutting effect, thus allowing constant progress in the operating field and significant time saving.
- The surgeon and the assistant can either switch sides (caudal and cephalad to the patient's left side) during the various steps of the procedure or just rotate the single port clockwise or counterclockwise while the instruments stay in the abdomen under direct visualization with the camera, thus achieving different angles with the camera, better exposure, and visualization.
- If the surgeon's hands are crossing, then rotating the port or switching positions with the assistant (caudal–cephalad) will improve exposure.
- The OR table is also tilted accordingly during the various steps of the procedure to increase exposure and prevent instrument clustering. Sometimes, the table is placed on reverse Trendelenburg position depending on the anatomic location of the colon and the identified lesion in relation to adjacent organs or structures.

DIVISION OF THE ILEOCOLIC VASCULAR PEDICLE AND MEDIAL TO LATERAL MOBILIZATION OF THE ASCENDING MESOCOLON

- The patient is positioned in a minus 5° to 10° Trendelenburg position with the table tilted maximally toward the patient's left side. The surgeon stands on the patient's lower left side, using a grasper in the nondominant hand and an energy device on the dominant hand. The assistant stands up the surgeon's right side holding the camera.
- If the omentum is adherent medially to the right colon, we start the procedure with the dissection of the omentum off the colon or perform an omentectomy to allow for maximum exposure of the ileocolic pedicle and the ascending colon mesentery.
- Dissect the terminal ileal retroperitoneal attachments and mobilize it medially toward the midline.
- Identify the ileocolic vessels as they cross over the third portion of the duodenum (**FIGURE 5**).
- Perform a medial to lateral mobilization of the ascending mesocolon (**FIGURE 6**). Dissect under (dorsal) the ileocolic vessels, entering the plane between the ascending mesocolon and the retroperitoneal structures (duodenum and Gerota's fascia). The transition between the fat planes of the ascending mesocolon and Gerota's fascia can be easily identified and aids to stay in the proper dissection plane.
- Using an energy device, we divide the ileocolic vascular pedicle at the origin as it crosses the third portion of the duodenum (**FIGURE 7**) while holding the vessel stump with a grasper to avoid retraction or post division bleeding.

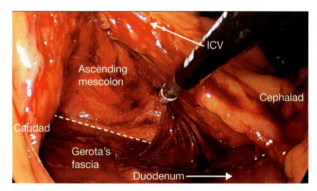

FIGURE 6 • Medial to lateral dissection of the ascending mesocolon. Dissect under (dorsal) the ileocolic vessels, entering the plane between the ascending mesocolon and the retroperitoneal structures (duodenum and Gerota's fascia). The transition between the two fat planes (mesocolon and Gerota's fascia) can be easily visualized *(dotted line)*.

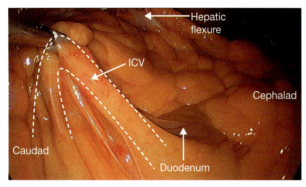

FIGURE 5 • Identification the ileocolic vessels (ICV) as they cross over the third portion of the duodenum.

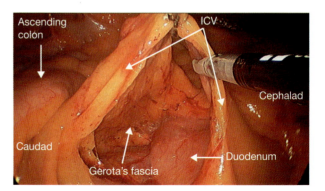

FIGURE 7 • Transection of the ileocolic vessels (ICVs). Using an energy device, we divide the ileocolic vascular pedicle at its origin as it crosses the third portion of the duodenum.

- Place hemostatic clips or Endoloop PDS at the divided stump to secure hemostasis.
- There is no need for laparoscopic stapled pedicle division unless severe atherosclerosis or vessels larger than 7 to 10 mm in size are present. In that case, usage of a laparoscopic energy device for vessel sealing is not recommended by most manufactures and it is the surgeon's choice and decision to proceed. In that case, we may use an Endo GIA stapler with a vascular load.
- Complete the medial to lateral dissection of the ascending colon mesentery, off the retroperitoneal avascular attachments without entering the Gerota's fascia, identifying and protecting the right gonadal vessels and the right ureter.
- Placement of a right ureteral stent for localization by a urologist is rarely required during right colectomy. Examples are severe inflammatory bowel disease and neoplasia with possible involvement of the right ureter.
- Continue the medial to lateral dissection of the ascending colon mesentery in a cephalad direction, separating it from the second and third portion of the duodenum and the head of the pancreas in an atraumatic fashion. This will allow for an easier mobilization of the hepatic flexure later during the case.

MOBILIZATION OF TERMINAL ILEUM, ASCENDING COLON, HEPATIC FLEXURE, AND PROXIMAL TRANSVERSE COLON

- Divide the terminal ileal mesentery with energy device flush to the ileocolic vascular pedicle up to the mesenteric border of the terminal ileum at the selected site of proximal intestinal division. A high ligation of the pedicle is preferred even in absence of neoplasia, as it allows for complete mobilization of the entire mesocolon via the avascular planes without bleeding (**FIGURE 8**).
- In addition, the terminal ileum is mobilized off the retroperitoneal attachments toward the midline. This will allow for a tension-free extraction via the single port site for the extracorporeal division without tension or risk for avulsing the mesentery. Morbidly obese patients require generous terminal ileum medial mobilization to allow for a tension-free specimen extraction via the single port. Previous pelvic surgery may lead to significant adhesions of the terminal ileum into the inner pelvis requiring additional time for adhesiolysis.
- Mobilize the ascending colon medially by transecting its lateral peritoneal attachments (the white line of Toldt) (**FIGURE 9**).
- Place the patient on a reverse Trendelenburg position by 5° to 10° and keep the OR table tilted to the left. The surgeon is positioned now cephalad, and the assistant/camera holder is positioned to their left side.
- Enter the lesser sac via the antimesenteric border of the proximal transverse colon (**FIGURE 10**) and perform a formal hepatic flexure mobilization using the energy device.

- Elect the point of distal division of the right colon and divide the corresponding mesentery up to the site of the distal resection margin and to the right of the middle colic vessels (**FIGURE 11**).
- A more generous distal mobilization of the colon is required compared to hand-assisted laparoscopy, by approximately another 5 cm, to allow for a tension-free extraction of the specimen and to avoid mesenteric avulsion during specimen extraction and the extracorporeal anastomosis.
- Infuse 3 mL IV of ICG and flush with 10 mL of normal saline and at the same time use the laparoscopic ICG camera (Stryker or Karl Storz 5 mm non bariatric). Evaluate the proximal and the distal resection division intestinal sites for vascular supply. Bright green, fluorescent color of the intestine

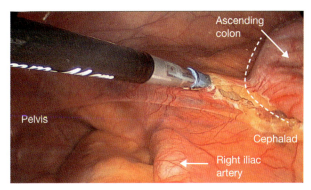

FIGURE 9 • Lateral mobilization of the ascending mesocolon. Transect the white line of Toldt (*dotted line*) with the energy device.

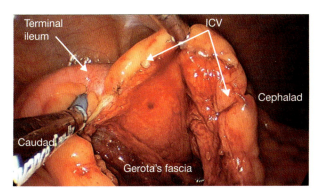

FIGURE 8 • Division of terminal ileum mesentery. Transect the terminal ileum mesentery down to the bowel wall with the energy device, keeping the ileocolic vessels (ICVs) in the specimen side.

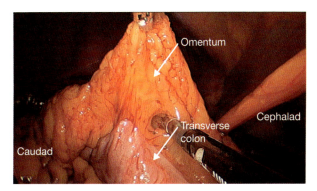

FIGURE 10 • Entrance to the lesser sac. Enter the lesser sac via the antimesenteric border of the proximal transverse colon and perform a formal hepatic flexure mobilization using the energy device.

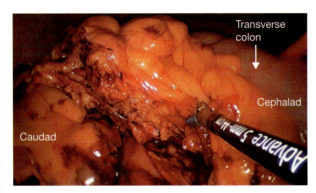

FIGURE 11 • Division of the midtransverse colon mesentery. Elect the point of distal division of the right colon and divide the corresponding mesentery up to the site of the distal resection margin and to the right of the middle colic vessels.

suggests excellent vascular supply and black color adjacent to that suggests nonviable intestinal segment, which was devascularized. Mark the transition site at the proximal and distal resection margins with the energy sealing device and take pictures. This confirmatory test prevents to a great degree anastomotic leak from ischemic intestinal segments that

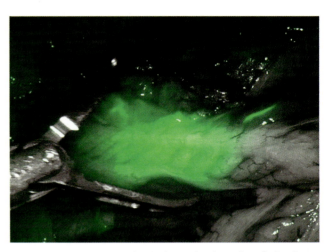

FIGURE 12 • Intraoperative Indocyanine bowel perfusion imaging showing a clear demarcation between viable (green) and non viable (not green) colon.

appear viable macroscopically. In case of ischemia, an additional intestinal segment may be resected prior to formation of the anastomosis (**FIGURE 12**).

EXTRACORPOREAL MOBILIZATION AND TRANSECTION OF THE SPECIMEN

- Grasp the terminal ileum at the proximal resection site securely before evacuating the pneumoperitoneum.
- Place wet lap sponges around the wound protector and use a second towel for the instruments used for creation of the anastomosis in order to avoid fecal contamination to the laparoscopic surgical drapes.
- Extract the terminal ileum first and divide it with a GIA linear 75-mm, triple, blue staple load (**FIGURE 13**). Use a grasper to hold into the terminal ileum stapled stump line and reintroduce temporarily into the abdomen.
- Extract the right colon and divide it at the distal resection marked site with another GIA linear 75-mm, triple, blue staple load (**FIGURE 14**).
- If the colon with the attached mesentery is too thick or in case of neoplasia, the tumor is larger than the incision, then elongate the incision superiorly using an army navy retractor to "hook" under the midline fascia and protect the wound protector from perforation. Use a no. 11 scalpel in a sawing motion or electrocautery to elongate the incision as necessary and extract the specimen.
- Pass the specimen to pathology or open the specimen at the back table to photograph, confirm adequate margins and place marking sutures in case of neoplasia.

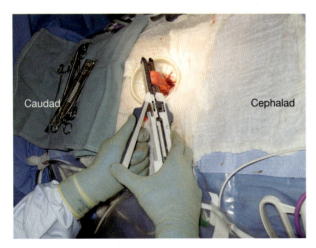

FIGURE 13 • Extracorporeal transection of the terminal ileum. Extract the terminal ileum first and divide it with a GIA linear 75-mm double or triple blue staple load.

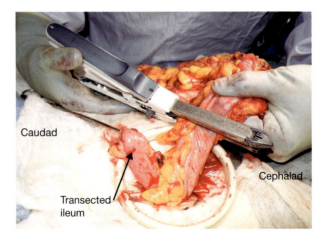

FIGURE 14 • Extracorporeal transection of the midtransverse colon. Extract the right colon and divide it at the distal site with a GIA linear 75-mm, double or triple, blue staple load.

EXTRACORPOREAL ANASTOMOSIS

- Perform an extracorporeal side-to-side, functional end-to-end ileotransverse anastomosis with a GIA linear 75-mm, triple, blue staple load (**FIGURE 15A** and **B**).
- Inspect the ileal and colonic segments to rule out torsion or tension prior to firing the stapler. The surgeon can palpate with a finger along the mesenteric margin of the terminal ileum mesentery and the distal colon mesentery toward the base at the retroperitoneum and ensure that there is no intestinal torsion.
- Inspect for bleeding from the anastomotic line inside and outside the bowel.
- Approximate the anastomotic stump defect with another GIA linear 75-mm, triple, blue staple load. Most times a second load of the same staple line is required. Triple line blue load stapler is superior to the two lines one in preventing anastomotic leaks.
- Introduce the anastomosis into the abdomen; inspect for bleeding and fecal spillage. Cover the anastomosis with the rest of the omentum or small intestine and ensure there is no torsion of the anastomosis. When in doubt, proceed again with laparoscopic inspection. Coating the anastomotic staple lines with a hemostatic agent such as Vistaseal is optional for prevention-control of bleeding.

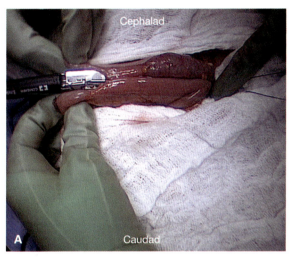 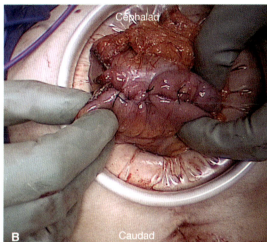

FIGURE 15 • Extracorporeal anastomosis. **A,** An anatomic side-to-side, functional end-to-end stapled ileocolonic anastomosis is constructed. **B,** The anastomosis is tension-free and has excellent blood supply.

WOUND CLOSURE

- It is advised to place an antiadhesive sheet such as Seprafilm posterior to the midline fascia edges while avoiding contact with the anastomotic staple lines. Finally, remove the wound protector and close the fascial incision with no. 1 PDS suture in running fashion. New braided sutures for fascia closure and with antimicrobial capabilities (such as Strattafix) have become available lately but there are no long-term data yet and their usage is currently on the surgeon's discretion.
- Irrigate the wound copiously with normal saline; obtain wound hemostasis.
- Approximate the skin edges with staples while leaving the umbilical skin edges opened and tucked with a Vaseline gauze with a cotton ball. Alternatively, approximate the dermis with inverted interrupted 3-0 PDS sutures and avoid the usage of staples.
- The procedure is a clean contaminated one and leaving the umbilicus skin edges slightly open may prevent a superficial wound infection.

PEARLS AND PITFALLS

Preoperative workup	■ Correct identification of the underlying pathology and extent of the tumor in relation to other organs and structures allows for careful selection of the laparoscopic single-incision technique. New enhanced recovery protocol allows for shorter and safer hospitalization.
Lesion localization	■ India ink tattoo placement when indicated for preoperative localization of the lesion and the distal resection margin is of paramount importance.
Patient positioning, laparoscopic instruments	■ Securing the patient's position, use of OR table tilting, single port rotation, and usage of bariatric length instruments and camera are necessary for laparoscopic single-incision surgery.

New technology	■ ICG infusion and camera for evaluation of the vascular perfusion, high-definition 4K laparoscopic tower, AIRSEAL laparoscopic lower pressure insufflation and smoke evacuation solution, new energy sealing and dissecting devices, and hemostatic agents provide significant assistance for a successful single-incision procedure.
Surgeon and assistant position	■ The surgeon should change their position in relation to the assistant several times during the procedure in order to achieve adequate exposure and visualization.
Laparoscopic instrument and tissue handling	■ The tip of the assisting and dominant laparoscopic instruments are positioned as close as possible to each other in the surgical field in order to avoid hand clustering outside the abdomen.

POSTOPERATIVE CARE

■ A Enhanced Recovery postoperative course is initiated.
■ The orogastric tube is discontinued in the OR upon completion of the procedure.
■ IV or PO acetaminophen, alvimopan, intraoperative decadron, gabapeptine, IV/IM ketorolac or other NSAIDs such as Celebrex are some of the options of the Enhanced Recovery protocol widely used.
■ Avoid opioid patient-controlled anesthesia (PCA).
■ Abdominal wall nerve block- "tap block" is used as per surgeon's preference the day of surgery; however, secondary to the minor single incision, it may not offer significant advantage for pain control.
■ Ice chips/water sips in PACU and clear liquid diet is introduced the day of surgery with the goal to advance to regular diet within 18 to 24 hours. Chewing gum may benefit postoperatively for early GI function.
■ The Foley catheter is discontinued within 24 hours.
■ Perioperative antibiotics, VTE protocol—mechanical and pharmacologic—as well as early ambulation is initiated within 24 hours of surgery.
■ Incentive spirometer is initiated as per standard hospital policy.
■ Wound care need is minimal: Remove the umbilical dressing 1 to 2 days postoperatively.
■ The patient usually can be safely discharged home within 36 to 72 hours when passage of flatus is documented and regular diet is tolerated by at least two consecutive meals, pain is controlled, patient ambulates, and there are no other adverse postoperative findings such as abnormal labs or signs of infection.
■ There is no need to wait until the patient has a bowel movement prior to discharge.
■ No weightlifting more than 20 lb is recommended for 4 to 6 weeks postoperatively in order to avoid incisional hernia.

OUTCOMES

■ Single-port laparoscopic hemicolectomy is an equally safe and possibly more cost-effective approach with better cosmesis, faster operative time with the extracorporeal anastomosis, less postoperative pain and faster return to full activities, short hospital stay, and comparable oncologic outcomes when performed for neoplastic diseases to conventional hand-assisted or multiport laparoscopic approach.
■ It is achieved with equipment that the hospital already has available, including the widely available single port and requires no additional training for the operative room personnel while it is reproducible by surgeons who perform advanced laparoscopy.
■ It requires a first assistant to the surgeon who has advanced laparoscopic skills for cameral maneuvering and laparoscopic suctioning.
■ The single-incision laparoscopic approach with the addition of the Enhanced Recovery protocol may transform the right colectomy to a one midnight hospital stay surgery in the future.

COMPLICATIONS

■ The procedure has similar morbidity and mortality rates and comparable rates for conversion to laparotomy when compared to conventional laparoscopy.
■ Anastomotic leak rate is less than 1% especially with the introduction of the ICG and new triple line stapling devices.
■ The single-incision laparoscopic technique for right hemicolectomy has the option for conversion to multiport or hand-assisted laparoscopy.
■ Because a larger sized laparoscopic port is used, there is a slight increase in the incidence of incisional hernia (1% or more) compared to multiport laparoscopy. However, the incisional hernia rates are similar to the ones in hand-assisted laparoscopy. Newer braided sutures for fascia closure may improve the hernia rates in the future.
■ Single-incision laparoscopy may require a longer operative time during the early learning curve. This can complicate an already challenging operation especially for hepatic flexure or proximal transverse colon neoplastic lesions.
■ It is intrinsically a one-operating surgeon technique with less involvement of the assistant surgeon and with a potential negative impact on resident of fellows' education during the learning curve period.

SUGGESTED READING

1. Ceppa EP, Park CW, Portenier DD, et al. Single-incision laparoscopic right colectomy: an efficient technique. *Surg Laparosc Endosc Percutaneous Tech*. 2012;22(2):88-94.
2. Dong B, Luo Z, Lu J, et al. Single-incision laparoscopic versus conventional laparoscopic right colectomy: a systematic review and meta-analysis. *Int J Surg*. 2018;55:31-38.
3. Gustafsson UO, Scott MJ, Hubner M, et al. Guidelines for perioperative care in elective colorectal surgery – enhanced recovery after surgery (ERAS®) Society Recommendations: 2018. *World J Surg*. 2019;43(3):659-695.

4. Lin J, Zheng B, Lin S et al. The efficacy of intraoperative ICG fluorescence angiography on anastomotic leak after resection for colorectal cancer: a meta-analysis. *Int J Colorectal Dis.* 2021;36(1):27-39.

5. Mufty H, Hillewaere S, Appeltans B, et al. Single-incision right hemicolectomy for malignancy: a feasible technique with standard laparoscopic instrumentation [Review]. *Colorectal Dis.* 2012;14(11): e764-e770.

6. Obaro AE, Burling DN, Plumb AA. Colon cancer screening with CT colonography: logistics, cost effectiveness, efficiency and progress. *Br J Radiol.* 2018;91(1090):20180307.

7. Toh JWT, Phan K, Hitos K. Association of mechanical bowel preparation and oral antibiotics before elective colorectal surgery with surgical site infection: a network meta-analysis. *AMA Netw Open.* 2018;1(6):e183226.

Chapter 11

Right Hemicolectomy: Robotic-Assisted Technique

Michael R. Marco and Alessio Pigazzi

DEFINITION

Robotic Colectomy

- Robotic colectomy is a minimally invasive surgery nearly identical to laparoscopic colectomy. However, the surgeon is using robotic instruments and controlling them from a nearby computer console instead of operating with laparoscopic instruments bedside.

Incidence of Adopting Robotic Surgery Techniques

- Since its approval by the FDA for abdominal and general surgery in 2000 robotic surgery has become a new frontier in minimally invasive surgery. The first robotic right hemicolectomy for cecal diverticulitis was first reported in 2001.[1]
- Initially the rate of adopting robotic surgery was low with only minimal increase in the rate of robotic surgery from 0.5% in 2009 to 2.3% in 2012.[2] This could be partly due to the learning curve, although recently there have been more systematic training programs designed specifically for residents, fellows, and surgeons, which helped in adopting this new technology by many surgeons.[3]

Pros and Cons of Robotic Surgery for Right Hemicolectomy

Pros

- A steady camera, fully controlled by the surgeon with improved 3D visualization, giving depth perception of the operative field.
- It has articulating wrists with 180° articulation, 540° rotation, and eliminates the surgeon's tremor. These characteristics lead to easier manipulation, enhanced dexterity, and precise control of complex movements especially in narrow spaces with up to 40% reduction in the time taken to perform a task.[4,5]
- Robotic platform can help the surgeons in performing more complex tasks during right hemicolectomy such as:
  - Intracorporeal anastomosis: A recent meta-analysis that included 4450 patients who underwent minimally invasive right hemicolectomy (73.1% laparoscopic approach, 26.9% robot-assisted approach) showed improved outcomes with intracorporeal anastomosis. The extracorporeal anastomosis group had significantly higher odds of conversion to open surgery (OR 1.87, 95% CI 1-3.45, P = .046), total complications (OR 1.54, 95% CI 1.05-2.11, P = .007), anastomotic leakage (AL) (OR 1.95, 95% CI 1.4-2.7, P = .003), surgical site infection (SSI) (OR 1.69, 95% CI 1.4-2.6, P = .002), and incisional hernia (OR 3.14, 95% CI 1.85-5.33, P < .001) compared to the intracorporeal group.[6] Although robotic surgery is not associated with better outcomes compared to laparoscopic surgery, recent meta-analysis showed that there might be benefit for robotic surgery when they included the intracorporeal anastomosis in the analysis.[7,8]
  - Complete mesocolic excision: It is another technically challenging task that could be associated with better oncological outcome particularly in stage II and III colon cancer.[9] The robotic group showed a statistically significant reduction in conversion rate (0% vs 6.9%, P = .01) but a longer operative time (279 vs 236 min, P < .001) compared with the laparoscopic group.[10]

Cons

- Higher costs
- Longer operative time.
  - One could argue that the easier tasks done robotically do not justify the increase in cost, especially that there are no prospective trials to prove better outcomes with robotic surgery.[11,12]
  - On the other hand, the longer operative time shortens with surgeon's experience and the easier docking for the newer robotic versions like the Xi.
  - A recent retrospective study showed that the total instrument costs of robotic surgery was higher than those of the laparoscopic instruments ($2565.37 for robotic compared with $1507.50 for laparoscopic surgery). However, the author concluded that the average difference in cost of care was calculated as A$1276.13 and A$464.43 less in the robotic with intracorporeal and extracorporeal anastomosis, respectively. This is because the robotic group had a significantly earlier time for return of bowel function (2 vs 4 days, P < .001) and shorter length of stay (3 vs 5 days, P < .001) and fewer complications.[13] Clearly, more randomized trials are needed because most of the data available are retrospective and the level of evidence is low.

PATIENT HISTORY AND PHYSICAL FINDINGS

Indication of Robotic Surgery for Right Hemicolectomy

- Indications
  - Right colon cancer
  - Appendectomy
  - Benign disease affecting the right colon such as right colon diverticulitis or inflammatory bowel disease. Even though the data to support the safety of robotic surgery in inflammatory bowel disease is scarce, the robot is being used more often in inflammatory bowel disease due to its popularity nowadays among surgeons.[14] However, one must pay extra attention while using robotic surgery with inflamed tissue because of the potential loss of haptic feedback.
- Contraindications
  - Inability to tolerate pneumoperitoneum, positioning either in Trendelenburg or reverse Trendelenburg due to associated patients' comorbidities
  - Extensive intra-abdominal adhesions

SURGICAL MANAGEMENT

Preoperative Planning

- Preoperative planning is a critical step to have a successful outcome regardless of the technique used to perform the surgery.
- First step is to have a thorough history and physical examination with special emphasis on cardiac and pulmonary problems as well as previous surgeries to identify patients that cannot be candidates for robotic surgery.
- Preoperative medical optimization and risk stratification are indicated similar to any other surgeries.
- It is very important to perform a complete workup of the disease with blood work including complete blood count, chemistry panel, routine coagulation profile and type and screen.
- Good preoperative localization of either the tumor, diverticulitis, or IBD (inflammatory bowel disease) by means of computed tomography (CT) scan, and colonoscopy.
- In our practice we do not prefer preoperative India ink marking for right colon lesions because it obscures the planes of tissue and interfere with identifying the proper mesocolic plane. Instead we use intraoperative colonoscopy liberally if needed to identify the lesion.
- Reviewing the vascular anatomy on the CT preoperatively is critical and could potentially avoid inadvertent vascular injury during minimally invasive surgery especially because of the variable anatomy of the right colon vasculature.[15]
- In our practice, we use mechanical and chemical bowel preparation on the day prior to surgery in the form of clear liquid diet, MiraLAX and antibiotics. This uniformly results in a clean colon, which is mandatory for intracorporeal anastomosis and intraoperative colonoscopy.
- Patients usually receive preoperative heparin subcutaneous 5000 units, preoperative prophylactic antibiotics in the holding area, unless contraindicated.

- Having a team experienced and well familiar with the robotic platform is a key for a successful surgery. This team includes an anesthesiologist, surgical assistant, experienced scrub nurse, and circulating staff. The experienced bedside robotic nurse can significantly decrease the operative time by quick troubleshooting of the robotic issues like arms collision and also can effectively assist the surgeon in the operative steps. A standard set of open instrumentation including vascular instruments should be always available in the room.

Positioning

- A large operating room is required to have enough space for the DaVinci robot with its four arms, surgeon console, second console for trainees, a monitor stack, and the colonoscopy tower if needed.
- Patient is placed in a modified lithotomy position to access the anus if needed for intraoperative colonoscopy.
- Patients should be secured to the table so that they may not slip during the procedures. We use a viscoelastic foam pad with a high coefficient of friction specifically made for patient positioning during laparoscopic and robotic cases. All patients will have both arms tucked with enough padding to minimize pressure on the nerve areas and bony prominence. Foley is routinely placed in all patients.
- The DaVinci robot is docked from the patient's right side. The bedside assistant and surgeon's console are usually on the patient's left side. The scrub technician and the table with the sterile instruments are usually at the patient's foot.
- Paying attention to proper positioning is crucial for a successful and efficient robotic assisted procedure because changing the patient position after docking the robot is cumbersome and prolongs the operating time.

OPERATIVE STEPS

Port Placement and Exploratory Laparoscopy

- Pneumoperitoneum is established through the Veress needle in the left upper quadrant with subsequent direct insertion of the 8-mm camera port. The camera port is placed about two fingerbreadths to the left of midline, midway between the xiphoid and the pubis as shown in (**FIGURE 1**). Port#1 is an 8-mm trocar that is placed one handbreadth cephalad and lateral to the camera. Port#2 is an 8-mm trocar that is placed one handbreadth caudal and lateral to the camera. Port#3 is an 8-mm trocar that is placed high in the subxyphoid region or sometimes in the suprapubic region according to the surgeon's preference. A 12-mm assistant port can be placed midway between port #1 and #2 and one handbreadth lateral to both of them. The assistant port can be used for stapling, additional retraction, and passing sutures.
- Once entrance into the abdomen is gained, and a laparoscopic view deems that the patient anatomy is feasible to a minimally invasive approach as well as to lyse adhesions if needed.
- This step might decrease the operative time used for adhesiolysis done robotically.

- Next the table should be rotated to the left and in Trendelenburg position by approximately 15° to 20° just enough to expose the right colon mesentery. The robotic cart is docked at the patient's right flank, and ports placed in the left abdomen as described below (**FIGURE 1**). A monopolar scissors is placed in Arm#3, Camera in Arm#2, and fenestrated bipolar grasper is placed in Arm#1. Needle holder is placed in Arm#4 when needed for the anastomosis part.

Identification and Ligation of the Ileocolic Vessels

- Our preferred approach is medial to lateral approach. First the cecum is held and retracted up to stretch and identify the ileocolic vessels (**FIGURE 2**).
- We enter the retroperitoneum behind the ileocolic vessels and create the space between Toldt fascia and the mesentery of the right side of the colon at the base of the ileocolic vessels. The duodenum is exposed once we get into that plane and pushed down (**FIGURE 3**). The ileocolic vessels are skeletonized close to the junction with the superior mesenteric vessels. The fat and lymphatic tissue over the superior mesenteric vein (SMV) will be removed with the specimen.
- We dissect above the loose areolar tissue plane of the SMV. The ileocolic artery and vein are divided between hemoclips (**FIGURE 4**).

90 SECTION II SURGERY OF THE COLON, APPENDIX, RECTUM, AND ANUS

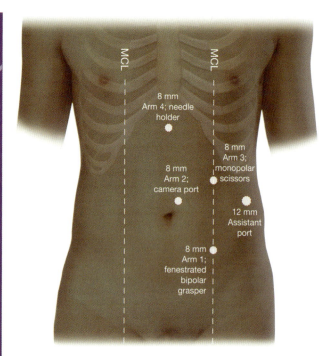

FIGURE 1 • Right colectomy port placement: *Ports # 1,2, 3, and 4* are 8-mm robotic ports. *Assistant port* is a 12-mm laparoscopic assistant port. MCL, Midclavicular.

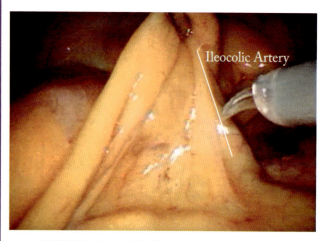

FIGURE 2 • Identification of the ileocolic vessels.

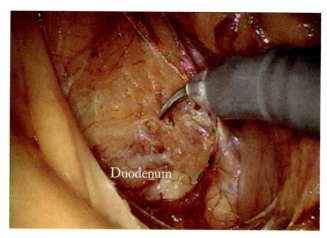

FIGURE 3 • Dissection of the retroperitoneal plane and identification of the duodenum.

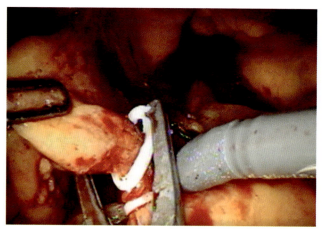

FIGURE 4 • Clipping of the ileocolic vessels.

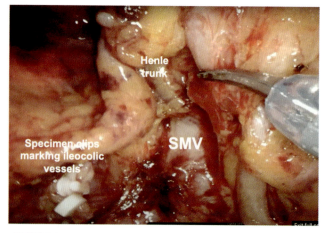

FIGURE 5 • Loose areolar plane of dissection above the SMV.

Dissection of the Retroperitoneal Plane and Identification of the Duodenum

- We then perform a medial to lateral mobilization lifting all the limb for areolar tissue from the SMV medially and superiorly toward the head of the pancreas and the duodenum (FIGURE 5).
- While paying attention to drop the duodenum and head of the pancreas gently from the mesocolic tissue without injuring them. We continue the medial to lateral dissection all the way till we reach the white line of Toldt laterally. Usually, the ureter and gonadal vessels are covered by Toldt fascia if dissection is carried in the correct plane without violating the retroperitoneal Toldt fascia.

Mobilization of the Proximal Transverse Colon and Hepatic Flexure

- Next the omentum is retracted cephalad, and the assistant will pull the colon in a caudal direction to expose the avascular plane between the omentum and the transverse colon in the mid transverse colon area.
- The omentum is separated from the colon using scissors or vessel sealer from medial to lateral in the avascular plane. This maneuver will open the lesser sac and we confirm the proper dissection plane by identifying the back of the stomach. The transverse colon is freed all the way to the hepatic flexure.

Identification of Trunk of Henle and Ligation of the Middle Colic Vessels

- We then resume our dissection above the SMV lifting all areolar tissue from the SMV. We continue dissection in a cephalad direction till we identify the trunk of Henle. Usually, it can be identified by following the anterior superior pancreaticoduodenal vein on top of the head of the pancreas.
- Surgeons must be very cautious while dissecting in this area because injury to any of these veins can lead to substantial bleeding that could be difficult to control. We identify the right gastroepiploic vessels and gastroepiploic nodes that are usually preserved unless lymph nodes look pathologically enlarged or there is a malignant tumor in the hepatic flexure.
- We continue dissecting cephalad till the lesser sac is entered and we connect the plane that we had been dissecting underneath the transverse colon mesentery. The middle colic trunk is usually identified in this area and the right branch of middle colic vessels are divided using vessel sealer or hemoclips.
- For hepatic flexure or proximal transverse colon tumors, we do partial omentectomy by taking down the attachments of the right-sided omentum from the gastroepiploic arcade.

Mobilization of the Right Colon and Terminal Ileum

- We will then take down the attachments of the right side of the colon to the undersurface of the liver, the hepatic flexure, and the right colic gutter. Eventually the terminal ileum will also be lifted from the retroperitoneal attachments.
- The mesentery of the terminal ileum and the mesentery of the mid transverse colon will be divided using vessel sealer. The terminal ileum and the transverse colon were divided with a robotic or laparoscopic stapler with 60-mm load. The specimen will be temporarily placed over the liver.

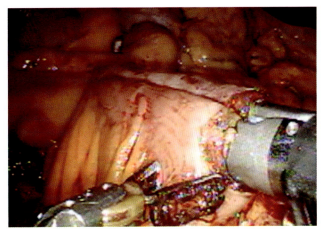

FIGURE 6 • Intracorporeal anastomosis: creating the common channel using a linear stapler.

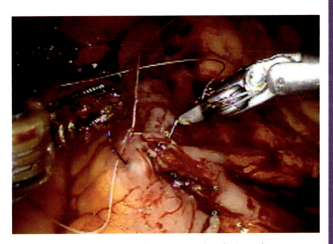

FIGURE 7 • Intracorporeal anastomosis: closing the common enterotomy using 3-0 absorbable stitches.

Intracorporeal Anastomosis, Reinspection, and Closure

- Our preference is to do intracorporeal isoperistaltic side-to-side ileocolic anastomosis. The ileum and transverse colon are aligned for the anastomosis and we confirm that the small bowel mesentery is not twisted.
- After creating the enterotomy and colotomy using monopolar scissors, the common channel is created using a linear stapler with a 60-mm load to minimize bleeding from the staple line (**FIGURE 6**).
- The common enterotomy is then closed using two layers of 3-0 absorbable stitches in a continuous fashion (**FIGURE 7**). Hemostasis is checked then the specimen is then extracted from a Pfannenstiel incision.

PEARLS AND PITFALLS

Overcoming the loss of tactile feedback	■ Paying attention to the visual cues with regard to tension and manipulation of the tissues. And avoiding excess tension as soon as the surgeon has enough exposure. Extra care must be taken to handle tissue gently, especially when the bowel is friable as seen in acute ulcerative colitis and Crohn disease patients. ■ Conceptualizing the spatial relationships of robotic instruments and reposition safely without direct visualization. ■ Minimizing external collision and optimizing range of motion of robotic arms by mentally visualizing the spatial relationships of the robotic arms.
Laparoscopic skills	■ Expert laparoscopic skills prior to the utilization of the robotic technology can facilitate the acquisition of the above tasks.
Robotic methods	■ Hybrid laparoscopic and robotic methods can sometimes save time by performing some tasks laparoscopically and allow one docking.
Vasculature anatomy	■ Critical understanding of the right colon vasculature anatomy and reviewing the vessels anatomy on the preoperative CT scan can minimize vascular injuries.
External clashing	■ Avoiding collision by external clashing can be done by placing ports at least one handbreadth or 10 cm apart.

POSTOPERATIVE CARE

- All patients will be on ERAS protocol unless contraindicated.
- This includes minimizing narcotics by using other multimodal pain regimens and transversus abdominis plane (TAP) block in the preoperative and postoperative settings.
- Patients will have their diet advanced as tolerated on postoperative day 0.
- All cancer and IBD patients will be discharged home on deep venous thrombosis (DVT) prophylaxis for 3 weeks unless contraindicated due to high risk of thromboembolic events.

COMPLICATIONS

- Complication of robotic right hemicolectomy is similar to other techniques of colectomy including bleeding and leakage.
- Because the robotic dissection field is limited, missed duodenal and small bowel injury can occur if the robotic surgeon is not paying attention.
- In order to avoid this complication:
  1. Keep in mind that the principles of laparoscopic surgery such as triangulation and visualization as they continue to apply with robotic surgery
  2. Make sure you maintain adequate visualization of the surgical field. Instruments should always be in the field of view.
- If duodenal or small bowel injury is noted, it can be repaired with intracorporeal suturing primarily.
- A traction injury or a thermal injury can occur and small thermal burns can easily be missed. All diathermy dissection should be performed only under direct vision.

REFERENCES

1. Weber PA, Merola S, Wasielewski A, Ballantyne GH. Telerobotic-assisted laparoscopic right and sigmoid colectomies for benign disease. *Dis Colon Rectum.* 2002;45(12):1689-1694; discussion 1695.
2. Moghadamyeghaneh Z, Hanna MH, Carmichael JC, Pigazzi A, Stamos MJ, Mills S. Comparison of open, laparoscopic, and robotic approaches for total abdominal colectomy. *Surg Endosc.* 2016;30(7):2792-2798.
3. Schreuder HWR, Wolswijk R, Zweemer RP, Schijven MP, Verheijen RHM. Training and learning robotic surgery, time for a more structured approach: a systematic review. *BJOG.* 2012;119(2):137-149.
4. Gómez Ruiz M, Lainez Escribano M, Cagigas Fernández C, Cristobal Poch L, Santarrufina Martínez S. Robotic surgery for colorectal cancer. *Ann Gastroenterol Surg.* 2020;4(6):646-651.
5. Moorthy K, Munz Y, Dosis A, et al. Dexterity enhancement with robotic surgery. *Surg Endosc.* 2004;18(5):790-795.
6. Emile SH, Elfeki H, Shalaby M, et al. Intracorporeal versus extracorporeal anastomosis in minimally invasive right colectomy: an updated systematic review and meta-analysis. *Tech Coloproctol.* 2019;23(11):1023-1035.
7. Genova P, Pantuso G, Cipolla C, et al. Laparoscopic versus robotic right colectomy with extra-corporeal or intra-corporeal anastomosis: a systematic review and meta-analysis. *Langenbeck's Arch Surg.* 2021;406(5):1317-1339.
8. Hannan E, Feeney G, Ullah MF, et al. Robotic versus laparoscopic right hemicolectomy: a case-matched study. *J Robot Surg.* 2022;16(3):641-647.
9. Zurleni T, Cassiano A, Gjoni E, et al. Surgical and oncological outcomes after complete mesocolic excision in right-sided colon cancer compared with conventional surgery: a retrospective, single-institution study. *Int J Colorectal Dis.* 2018;33(1):1-8.
10. Spinoglio G, Bianchi PP, Marano A, et al. Robotic versus laparoscopic right colectomy with complete mesocolic excision for the treatment of colon cancer: perioperative outcomes and 5-year survival in a consecutive series of 202 patients. *Ann Surg Oncol.* 2018;25(12):3580-3586.
11. Solaini L, Bazzocchi F, Cavaliere D, Avanzolini A, Cucchetti A, Ercolani G. Robotic versus laparoscopic right colectomy: an updated systematic review and meta-analysis. *Surg Endosc.* 2018;32(3):1104-1110.
12. Park JS, Choi GS, Park SY, Kim HJ, Ryuk JP. Randomized clinical trial of robot-assisted versus standard laparoscopic right colectomy. *Br J Surg.* 2012;99(9):1219-1226.
13. Ahmadi N, Mor I, Warner R. Comparison of outcome and costs of robotic and laparoscopic right hemicolectomies. *J Robot Surg.* 2022;16(2):429-436.
14. Renshaw S, Silva IL, Hotouras A, Wexner SD, Murphy J, Bhan C. Perioperative outcomes and adverse events of robotic colorectal resections for inflammatory bowel disease: a systematic literature review. *Tech Coloproctol.* 2018;22(3):161-177.
15. Wu C, Ye K, Wu Y, et al. Variations in right colic vascular anatomy observed during laparoscopic right colectomy. *World J Surg Oncol.* 2019;17(1):16.

Chapter 12 Transverse Colectomy: Open Technique

Y. Nancy You

DEFINITION

- The transverse colon is the segment of the abdominal colon between the hepatic and the splenic flexures. The transverse colon is an intraperitoneal organ of variable length, bound by the two flexures, which are secondarily retroperitoneal areas of the colon typically fixed in position.
- The main blood supply to the transverse colon is the middle colic vessels. The transverse colon, with transverse mesocolon and middle colic vessels, lies in intimate proximity to the lesser sac, which is in turn bound by the quadrate lobe of the liver, the stomach, the pancreas, and the omentum. The operative surgeon must be fully familiar with these anatomic relations in order to avoid injury to these nearby structures.
- Transverse colectomy is a relatively uncommon procedure, as pathology in the proximal transverse colon is often addressed by an extended right hemicolectomy, whereas pathology in the distal transverse colon is often addressed by an extended left hemicolectomy.
- Indications for transverse colectomy may be broadly divided into benign and malignant reasons.
- Benign diseases with pathology focally located within the segment of the transverse colon represent the most natural indication for transverse colectomy. Examples may include focal inflammatory processes, localized trauma, or local perforation.
- Transverse colectomy for primary malignancies of the transverse colon has been controversial.[1] Because of the varying contributions to the lymphatic drainage of the transverse colon cancer from the ileocolic, the right colic, and the left colic blood vessels, extended right or extended left hemicolectomy has been preferred over segmental transverse colectomy for primary tumors of the transverse colon.[2]
- Transverse colectomy may be required as a part of a curative en bloc resection of a noncolonic malignancy arising from a nearby organ due to the close proximity of the transverse colon to other structures around the lesser sac. Surgeons must be cognizant of anatomic relations in order to safely carry out the intended operation.

DIFFERENTIAL DIAGNOSIS

- Endoscopic tissue biopsy is a key step in the diagnostic workup of patients with both benign and malignant diseases involving the transverse colon.
- In patients presenting with a locally advanced tumor mass that obliterates the lesser sac and involves adjacent organs such as the stomach, the pancreas, and the transverse colon, care must be undertaken to differentiate malignancies of the colonic origin vs those that arose from adjacent organs but involves the transverse colon secondarily. Tissue diagnosis by biopsy should be secured in order to execute the optimal treatment regimen according to the primary malignancy.

PATIENT HISTORY AND PHYSICAL FINDINGS

- The goals of preoperative assessment should include determining whether urgent vs elective intervention is needed, facilitating intraoperative planning, and assessing the benefits vs risks toward a sound surgical decision.
- The patient should be examined for fitness to undergo an operation through a detailed assessment of patient's medical history, performance status, medication regimens, other medical needs, and psychosocial competency.
- Symptoms such as abdominal cramping, difficulty with passage of stool or flatus, bleeding, or severe pain should be queried. Conditions that would necessitate urgent/emergent rather than elective surgical intervention must be ruled out. Patients with an obstructing transverse colonic lesion and a competent ileocecal valve can rapidly develop a closed loop obstruction with high risks for ischemic colon and perforation and must be attended to emergently (**FIGURE 1**).
- Elements of prior surgical history that may present intraoperative difficulties such as previous stomach, pancreas, or colonic operations, and prior antecolic or retrocolic bowel bypass reconstructions, must be elicited. Prior operative reports should be obtained and reviewed.

IMAGING AND OTHER DIAGNOSTIC STUDIES

- All patients should ideally undergo both abdominal–pelvic cross-sectional imaging as well as endoscopic examination with possible biopsies.
- Endoscopic examination of the colon should be undertaken preoperatively to confirm the location and the focality of the pathology within the transverse colon (**FIGURE 2**).
  - Endoscopically, the transverse colon can be recognized by the triangular shape of the bowel lumen as well as by the anchoring landmarks of the splenic and hepatic flexures.

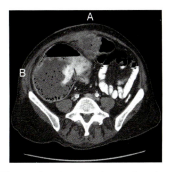

FIGURE 1 • CT scan showing an obstructing transverse colonic lesion (A) in a patient with a competent ileocecal valve. Closed loop obstruction causes massive dilation of the cecum (B). The high risks for ischemia and perforation require emergent surgical intervention.

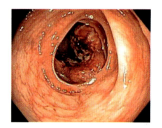

FIGURE 2 • Colonoscopic view of a mass lesion in the transverse colon, which is recognized by the triangular shape of the bowel lumen and the anchoring splenic and hepatic flexures. Histologic diagnosis can be obtained by endoscopic biopsy of the mass.

- If there is any doubt as to whether the lesion will be able to be localized with confidence intraoperatively, then the lesion should be marked with endoscopic tattooing.
- If there is any concern for involvement of adjacent organs, such as the stomach, an esophagogastroscopy should also be performed.[3]
■ Cross-sectional imaging of the abdomen is performed through computed tomography (CT) or magnetic resonance imaging (MRI) scans. Imaging characteristics may supplement histologic data and aid in the differential diagnosis. In addition, percutaneous biopsy may be needed.
- In cases of malignant disease, imaging will help differentiate between colonic and noncolonic origin of the disease.
- Presence of distant metastatic disease and evidence of direct local invasion to adjacent organs should be assessed and appropriate intraoperative management plans should be made.
- Finally, any abnormal-appearing adenopathy along vessels other than the middle colic vascular should be specifically assessed in order to determine whether the particular malignancy would be better managed through an extended right or extended left colectomy rather than a transverse colectomy.

SURGICAL MANAGEMENT

■ Thorough preoperative preparation, confirming that the diagnosis is correct, the indication is appropriate, and that possible intraoperative findings have been anticipated and planned for, is the basis for successful intraoperative management and speedy postoperative recovery.

Preoperative Planning

■ The operative surgeon should thoroughly review the patient's history and diagnostic workup to minimize any unexpected and unplanned for intraoperative finding.
■ Diagnostic biopsy and histologic results should be verified. A malignant diagnosis should be particularly noted in order to help determine the extent of the bowel resection and lymphadenectomy.
■ Documentation from preoperative endoscopy should be reviewed, particularly if the operative surgeon did not perform the procedure. The presence and location of a marking tattoo should be confirmed.
■ Preoperative imaging is used to help anticipate any involvement of the adjacent organs and the possible need for en bloc resection intraoperatively. Any need for additional technical assistance from other surgeons should be planned for.
■ In cases of perforation and anticipated significant intraperitoneal contamination that may render bowel anastomosis unsafe, plans should be made for ostomy marking and education preoperatively.
■ Preoperative bowel preparation, whether antimicrobial and mechanical, mechanical only, or no preparation, is a highly variable practice and is left to the discretion of the practicing surgeon.
■ Prophylactic intravenous antibiotics with coverage against gram-positive, gram-negative, and anaerobic flora of the skin and gut are typically administered prior to incision and continued for the first 24 hours.
■ Prophylaxis against deep venous thrombosis is typically administered prior to incision and during the hospital stay.

Positioning

■ Patients are usually placed in a supine position. If there is any possibility of extending the resection to the left colon or any possible need for intraoperative endoscopy, consideration should be given for placing the patient in lithotomy position.

INCISION AND ABDOMINAL EXPLORATION

- A midline incision extending from the epigastrium to below the umbilicus is made.
- The abdominal cavity is explored for the presence of other pathology not identified by preoperative imaging. In cases of malignant disease, peritoneal lining, omentum, and hepatic and bowel surfaces are inspected and palpated for any evidence of metastatic disease. In women, the pelvic organs, including the ovaries, should be inspected. Any suspicious nodule should be biopsied for pathologic assessment as findings may affect the decision of proceeding to the remaining of the procedure.

OMENTUM DISSECTION AND EXPOSURE OF THE LESSER SAC

- The relationship between the transverse colon pathology and the lesser sac is assessed.
- Exposure to the lesser sac is gained in one of two ways, depending on whether omentectomy is performed or not.
- If disease pathology does not necessitate en bloc omentectomy or if there is desire to preserve as much of the omentum as possible, then greater omentum is retracted cephalad and the transverse colon is retracted caudad. This reveals the avascular plane between the greater omentum and the transverse mesocolon (**FIGURE 3**). The pale yellow omental fat is distinguished from the fat of the appendices epiploicae

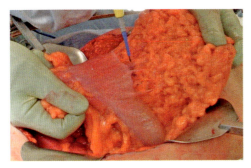

FIGURE 3 • Retracting the greater omentum cephalad and the transverse colon caudad helps reveal the avascular plane between the greater omentum and the transverse mesocolon.

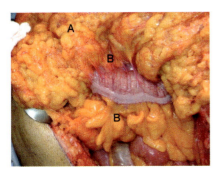

FIGURE 4 • The pale yellow cobblestone fat of the omentum (A) is distinguished from the bright yellow smooth fat of the appendices epiploicae of the transverse colon (B).

of the transverse colon (**FIGURE 4**). As this plane is dissected, the greater omentum is freed from the transverse colon and mesocolon and entrance into the lesser sac is gained. This can be confirmed by visualization of the posterior wall of the stomach dorsally and of the anterior surfaces of the duodenum, pancreas, and transverse mesocolon ventrally.

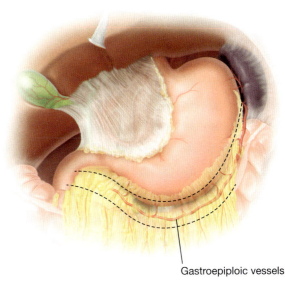

Gastroepiploic vessels

FIGURE 5 • Dissection of the omentum is carried out either proximal (inside of) or distal (outside of) the gastroepiploic artery arcade (*dotted lines*) depending on the extent of the disease, surgeon preferences, and the desire to preserve the gastroepiploic arcade.

- If the disease pathology necessitates en bloc resection of part or all of the omentum, then the gastrocolic ligament should be divided. The gastroepiploic artery arcade is identified along the greater curvature of the stomach. Dissection of the omentum is carried out either proximal (inside of) or distal (outside of) the arcade depending on the extent of the disease, the surgeon preference, and the desire to preserve the gastroepiploic arcade (**FIGURE 5**). The deeper avascular plane of the lesser sac, deep to the omentum but superficial to the transverse mesocolon, is entered. The omentum is thus isolated and divided between clamps.

MOBILIZATION OF THE HEPATIC FLEXURE AND THE SPLENIC FLEXURE

- In order to gain enough mobility of the colon for intraoperative manipulation and to allow for a tension-free anastomosis after resection, it is often necessary to mobilize one or both of the flexures.[4]
- To mobilize the hepatic flexure, attention is turned to the ascending colon. The colon was retracted medially to identify the peritoneal reflection (white line of Toldt). The covering peritoneum of the paracolic gutter is then incised and divided using electrocautery. This avascular tissue plane is followed in a lateral to medial fashion, separating the colonic mesentery from the retroperitoneum. This dissection plane is then carried cephalad toward the hepatic flexure, where division of the lateral peritoneal attachments will free the hepatic flexure. As the dissection is carried medially, care must be taken to avoid injury to the retroperitoneal duodenum (**FIGURE 6**). At this time, this dissection plane should be joined with prior dissection plane of the omentum so that communication to the lesser sac is established.
- To mobilize the splenic flexure, attention is turned to the descending colon. The descending colon is retracted medially to identify the lateral peritoneal attachments in a similar fashion as described in the mobilization of the ascending colon above. The avascular tissue plane is similarly followed and carried cephalad toward the splenic flexure (**FIGURE 7**). The splenocolic ligament is encountered in this process and divided using electrocautery. As the lower pole of the spleen comes into view, care should be taken to divide any adhesion between the omentum and the capsule as to avoid unintended capsular tears with retraction and dissection. Often, numerous adhesions between the omentum and the appendices epiploicae of the colon are encountered, and care must be taken to separate these either by electrocautery or between clamps to avoid bleeding. Finally, additional avascular ligaments to the stomach and/or the pancreas may be encountered and should be divided. After this, entry into the lesser sac is gained. The distal transverse colon and splenic flexure are now completely free of posterior retroperitoneal attachments and are fully mobile.
- After completing the dissections outlined in this step, the lesser sac is exposed completely, and the anterior surfaces of the transverse mesocolon should be in full view (**FIGURE 8**).

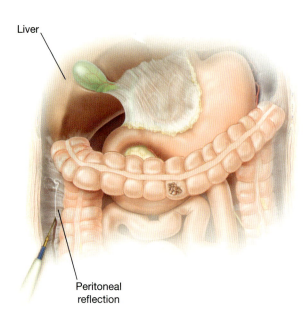

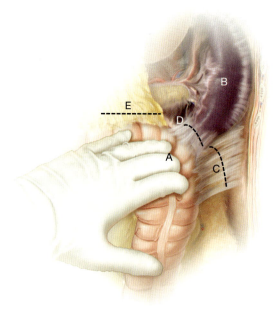

FIGURE 6 • Anatomic relations for mobilization of the hepatic flexure: The ascending colon is retracted medially to identify the lateral peritoneal reflection (white line of Toldt); the covering peritoneum is divided to free the hepatic flexure. The hepatic surface, the gallbladder, the duodenum, and the anterior pancreas' surface are in close proximity, and care must be taken to avoid injury to these organs.

FIGURE 7 • Mobilization of the splenic flexure. The splenic flexure of the colon (*A*) is retracted medially to identify and release the lateral peritoneal attachments. Care is taken to avoid injury to the spleen (*B*). The renocolic ligament (*C*), the splenocolic ligament (*D*), and the gastrocolic ligament (*E*) are identified and subsequently divided. This allows entry into the lesser sac and frees the distal transverse colon and splenic flexure from posterior retroperitoneal attachments.

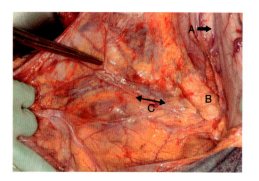

FIGURE 8 • After the lesser sac is exposed completely, posterior wall of the stomach (*A*) and anterior surface of the pancreas (*B*) are visualized. The anterior surfaces of the transverse mesocolon with middle colic vessels (*C*) should be in full view.

ISOLATION AND DIVISION OF THE MIDDLE COLIC VESSELS

- The anatomy of the middle colic artery can be highly variable, and often, it does not present as a single vessel.
- The middle colic vessels can usually be identified by visual inspection or palpation along the transverse mesocolon via the lesser sac (**FIGURE 9**). When proximal ligation is needed, as is in the case for malignant disease, the overlying peritoneum is scored and the vessels should be dissected up to the lower border of the pancreas and ligated at this location (**FIGURE 9**). Care should be taken to avoid avulsion injury to the smaller collateral venous branches from the pancreaticoduodenal arcade and to avoid clamp injury to the pancreatic parenchyma. When the root of the middle colic vessels is identified, the surrounding nodal-bearing mesenteric tissue should be swept toward the specimen side. The vessels can then be isolated and controlled with suture ligature.
- If the middle colic vessels and the lesser sac are involved by the disease pathology and/or obliterated, then the middle colic vessels can be approached from the root of the small bowel mesentery. After the transverse mesocolon is retracted cephalad, the root of the mesentery is exposed. The overlying peritoneum is scored and dissected away to expose the anterior surface of the superior mesenteric artery.[5] The superior mesenteric artery is followed cephalad until the middle colic branches off, and the origin of the middle colic vessels can be isolated at this location (**FIGURE 10**). Extreme care must be undertaken to prevent injury to the underlying superior mesenteric vessels.

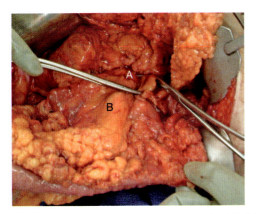

FIGURE 9 • The middle colic vessels (*A*) are identified in the transverse mesocolon (*B*) and then dissected and taken between clamps. When proximal ligation of the middle colic vessel is required, the vessels are transected at the inferior border of the pancreas.

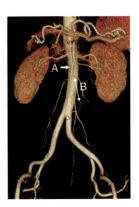

FIGURE 10 • At the root of the small bowel mesentery, superior mesenteric artery (*A*) is followed cephalad until the middle colic branches off (*B*).

BOWEL RESECTION AND ANASTOMOSIS

- After division of the middle colic vessels, the blood supply to the transverse colon is maintained by the marginal artery, which can be found along the entire colon.
- The length of the bowel resection is determined by the extent of disease pathology and by the extent of the vascular supply. In cases of benign inflammatory disease, a margin of normal, healthy colon should be present for reanastomosis. In cases of primary malignancy of the transverse colon, a minimum gross negative margin of 5 cm proximal and distal to the tumor should be present.
- Once the points of proximal and distal bowel resection are identified, the presence of pulsatile blood supply to the cut ends via the marginal artery should be verified. If adequate blood supply cannot be confirmed, the length of the resection must be extended to points where blood supply is present.
- In most cases, bowel continuity is immediately reestablished. However, in cases of gross peritoneal contamination, gross inflammation, grave systemic illness, and others, the safety of a bowel anastomosis may be questioned, and creation of an end colostomy with either a mucous fistula or a long distal blind limb may be wise. A second-stage procedure can be performed for delayed reanastomosis.
- Once the decision for immediate bowel anastomosis is made, the mesenteric orientation is checked to ensure that there is no twisting.
- The bowel anastomosis can be performed in a variety of ways, depending on the surgeon's preference. The most common methods include a hand-sewn end-to-end technique or a stapled side-to-side (functional end-to-end) technique.
- Using the hand-sewn technique, the divided ends of the colon are aligned end to end. The anastomosis is created in two layers, with an outer layer of interrupted sutures placed into the seromuscular layer of the bowel wall and an inner layer of running suture placed full thickness, incorporating the bowel mucosa (**FIGURE 11**).
- In the stapled technique, the ends of the bowel are divided with a linear stapler. These divided ends of the colon are then aligned side to side. Small enterotomies are made typically by excising a corner off each staple line, allowing the jaws of the linear stapler to be inserted and the stapler to be fired (**FIGURE 12**). The area of the enterotomy through which the stapler has been inserted is then closed either by sutures or by a second firing of the stapler. Staple lines are inspected for hemostasis. Areas of crossing staple lines may be imbricated with interrupted suture in a Lambert fashion.
- If there is well-vascularized omentum nearby, it may be patched over the anastomosis to help future contain any anastomotic leakage postoperatively.
- The size of the mesenteric defect between the right and left colon should be assessed. Small- and moderate-sized defects should be closed to prevent internal hernia and any mesenteric twisting. Typically, if the middle colic vessels had been ligated at their origins, the defect is large and closure is not necessary.

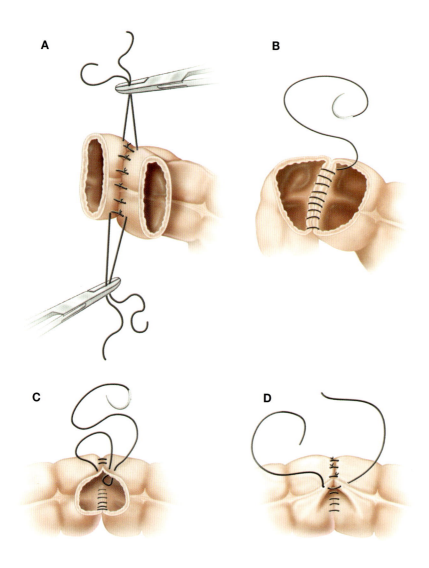

FIGURE 11 • In a hand-sewn end-to-end colocolonic anastomosis, the divided ends of the colon are aligned (A); the anastomosis is typically created in two layers, with an outer layer of interrupted sutures and an inner layer of running suture (B-D).

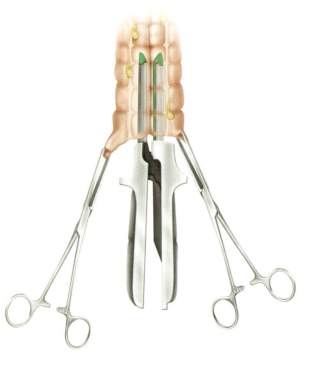

FIGURE 12 • In a stapled side-to-side (functional end-to-end) colocolonic anastomosis, the ends of the bowel are aligned side to side. Small enterotomies are made by excising a corner off each staple line, allowing the jaws of the linear stapler to be inserted into each lumen. The stapler is fired.

ABDOMINAL CLOSURE

- The abdominal fascia is closed after placing any remaining omentum between the bowel loops and the incision if possible. The skin incision is closed using absorbable subcuticular suture or staples. Abdominal drain is not placed.

PEARLS AND PITFALLS

Diagnostic and preoperative assessments	■ Any pathology outside of the transverse colon, transverse mesocolon, and middle colic vessels should be assessed on preoperative imaging, and an extended right or an extended left hemicolectomy should be performed if necessary. ■ In patients presenting with a large tumor mass, anatomic relations to the pancreas, duodenum, stomach, and mesenteric vessels should be carefully accessed. ■ Endoscopic and/or percutaneous tissue biopsy should be obtained to help differentiate malignancies of colonic vs noncolonic origin to allow for optimal treatment planning. ■ Patients presenting with an obstructing transverse colonic lesion and a competent ileocecal valve require emergent surgical attention to avoid perforation secondary to a closed loop large bowel obstruction. ■ The potential need for an ostomy in cases where bowel anastomosis may not be safe should be anticipated to allow for preoperative ostomy marking and education.
Omental dissection and exposure of the lesser sac	■ Exposure to the lesser sac can be gained with or without an omentectomy. ■ The pale granular yellow of the omental fat can be distinguished from the bright, smooth yellow of the fat of the colonic appendices epiploicae to help identify the avascular dissection plane.
Mobilization of the hepatic and/or splenic flexure	■ The surgeon should not hesitate to mobilize either or both of the flexures, as it often greatly facilitates intraoperative manipulation and facilitates a tension-free bowel anastomosis.
Isolation and ligation of the middle colic vessels	■ When the root of the middle colic vessels is approached through the lesser sac, injury to the small veins at the inferior border of the pancreas should be avoided. ■ When the root of the middle colic vessels is approached from the root of the small bowel mesentery, injury to the superior mesenteric vessels should be avoided.
Bowel resection and anastomosis	■ A transverse colectomy can be easily converted to an extended right or an extended left hemicolectomy if needed by intraoperative findings. ■ In some cases, immediate bowel anastomosis may not be safe, and an end colostomy can be made with either a mucous fistula or a long distal blind limb for delayed reanastomosis.

POSTOPERATIVE CARE

- Patients should receive routine postoperative care including adequate analgesia, aggressive pulmonary toilet, and early ambulation.
- Patients are typically kept on no more than a clear liquid diet the night of the operation in case there is a need for any emergency intervention and then advanced to a soft diet by the time of discharge.
- An occasional patient may experience diarrhea, which requires initiation of medicinal fiber and/or Imodium for symptom control.

OUTCOMES

- Patients generally tolerate a transverse colectomy well. The risk of anastomotic complications requiring reoperation is less than 5%, and a colostomy is not routinely required.
- Leakage from the colocolonic anastomosis may manifest as peritonitis, colocutaneous fistula, or localized intraperitoneal abscess.

- Patients with clinical signs of sepsis and peritonitis should be managed by prompt return to the operation for reexploration, washout, resection of the prior anastomosis, and creation of end colostomy and mucous fistula.
- Localized abscesses may collect in the subhepatic, subphrenic, and lesser sac spaces. The diagnosis can be made by CT of the abdomen, and clinically stable patients may be managed by percutaneous drainage.
- Superficial wound infection occurs in 10% to 15% of the cases and should be managed by incision and drainage of any subcutaneous abscess.
- Transverse colectomy is not expected to significantly alter bowel function postoperatively.[6] Although some patients may experience more frequent and looser stools during the immediate postoperative period, most patients reported an average of 1 to 2 stools per day and adapt to a normal bowel regimen over 6 to 12 months.

COMPLICATIONS

- Bleeding
- Wound infection
- Anastomotic leak
- Intra-abdominal abscess
- Poor bowel function

REFERENCES

1. Hopkins JE. Transverse colostomy in the management of cancer of the colon. *Dis Colon Rectum*. 1971;14(3):232-236.
2. Gordon PH. Malignant neoplasm of the colon. In: Gorden PH, Nivatvongs S, eds. *Principles and Practice of Surgery for the Colon, Rectum and Anus*. 33rd ed. Informa; 2007:550-553.
3. Stamatakos M, Karaiskos I, Pateras I, et al. Gastrocolic fistulae; from Haller till nowadays. *Int J Surg*. 2012;10(3):129-133.
4. Araujo SE, Seid VE, Kim NJ, et al. Assessing the extent of colon lengthening due to splenic flexure mobilization techniques: a cadaver study. *Arq Gastroenterol*. 2012;49(3):219-222.
5. Tajima Y, Ishida H, Ohsawa T, et al. Three-dimensional vascular anatomy relevant to oncologic resection of right colon cancer. *Int Surg*. 2011;96(4):300-304.
6. You YN, Chua HK, Nelson H, et al. Segmental vs. extended colectomy: measurable differences in morbidity, function, and quality of life. *Dis Colon Rectum*. 2008;51(7):1036-1043.

Chapter 13

Laparoscopic Transverse Colectomy

Govind Nandakumar and Sang W. Lee

DEFINITION

- Transverse colectomy refers to removal of the portion of the colon between the hepatic flexure and the splenic flexure—the transverse colon. This portion of the colon derives its blood supply from the right and left branches of the middle colic vessels in addition to collateral flow from the ileocolic, right colic, and left colic vessels. Transverse colectomy is commonly performed for tumors and/or polyps of this region. An alternative approach to these tumors is to perform an extended right or extended left colectomy. This chapter focuses on laparoscopic transverse colectomy.

PATIENT HISTORY AND PHYSICAL FINDINGS

- A complete history and physical focusing on the underlying pathology is essential. For patients with colon cancer and/or polyps, a detailed surgical history, personal cancer history, and family history is essential.
- Preoperative genetic counseling and testing may be indicated based on age and family history.
- Presence of an inherited cancer syndrome such as familial adenomatous polyposis or hereditary nonpolyposis colon cancer syndrome may require a total colectomy rather than a transverse colectomy.
- During the history and physical examination, it is important to elicit history of prior abdominal surgery, distension, and obstruction prior to making a decision regarding open vs laparoscopic approach.
- History or physical examination suggestive of focal abdominal pain and tenderness are suggestive of abdominal wall invasion. In this cases, a more extensive or open surgical approach may be needed.
- History and physical examination should also evaluate the cardiovascular and respiratory systems to assess the ability to tolerate pneumoperitoneum.
- Nutritional status and recent history of major weight loss should be considered in performing primary anastomosis.

IMAGING AND OTHER DIAGNOSTIC STUDIES

- All patients with colon cancer and/or a polyp should have a complete extent of disease workup including carcinoembryonic antigen, computed tomography (CT) of the abdomen and pelvic, chest X-ray, colonoscopy, and routine preoperative testing.
- The CT should be reviewed carefully to assess potential adjacent organ involvement, metastatic disease, and/or obstructive disease.
- A laparoscopic approach may not be feasible in the presence of massive bowel distension and obstruction.
- Large bulky tumors with a tethered mesentery or adjacent organ involvement may also preclude laparoscopy.

- Colonoscopy for evaluation of the entire colon is important to ensure there are no synchronous lesions proximal or distal to the area of resection.
- For small nonobstructing lesions, endoscopic tattoo marking should be performed prior to surgery.
- Endoscopic tattooing should be performed just distal to the tumor and in three quadrants to facilitate identification of the target lesion during laparoscopic surgery.
- In general, tumors that are identified on CT scan can be readily identified laparoscopically and do not require a tattoo.

SURGICAL MANAGEMENT

Preoperative Planning

- The patient receives a mechanical bowel preparation to facilitate handling of the colon and to facilitate the performance of an intraoperative colonoscopy if required. The need for bowel preparation is controversial. The consequences of a leak may be more significant without preparation. Laparoscopic handling of the colon is easier after mechanical bowel preparation.
- The patient is seen and evaluated by the surgical and anesthesia teams in the preoperative area on the day of surgery.
- Most patients are offered and elect to have an epidural or intravenous catheter for patient-controlled anesthesia.
- A second- or third-generation cephalosporin or ertapenem is used for antibiotic prophylaxis within 1 hour of skin incision and redosed as needed during the procedure. No antibiotics are administered postoperatively.
- Venodyne boots and 5000 units of subcutaneous heparin are used for deep vein thrombosis prophylaxis.

Positioning

- The patient is positioned in a modified lithotomy position with both arms tucked to the sides. It is essential to ensure that all pressure points, fingers, and calves are padded adequately.
- Use of a beanbag and cloth tape allows extreme positioning with decrease in possibility of patient sliding.
- Alternatively, use of gel pads commonly available in the operating room (OR) makes routine taping of patient not necessary.
- Use of shoulder braces should be avoided as they can cause brachial plexus injury.
- Prior to draping, the patient is placed in steep Trendelenburg position and the table is rotated to ensure that the patient is secured well.
- It is essential to ensure that both knees are in line with the torso in order to avoid collision of instruments to patient's thighs when working in the upper quadrants of the abdomen. The abdomen is prepped from the nipples to the midthigh.
- Access to the anus is always maintained for possible intraoperative colonoscopy.
- **FIGURE 1** (laparoscopic setup) shows the OR setup for this procedure. Monitors are placed over the shoulders of the patient so that the surgeon, pathology, and monitors are situated in line.

101

102 SECTION II SURGERY OF THE COLON, APPENDIX, RECTUM, AND ANUS

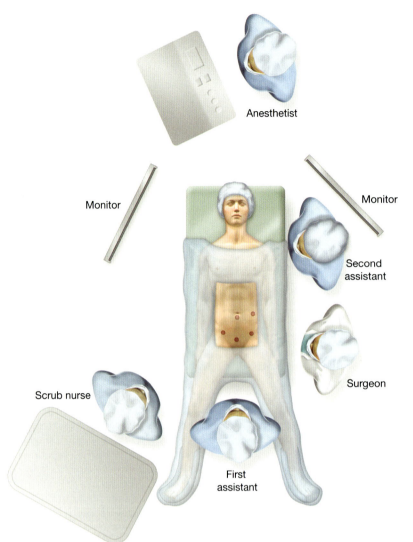

FIGURE 1 • Illustration of the patient, team, and room setup. A modified lithotomy position allows the surgeon or assistant to stand between the legs and to have access to the anus for intraoperative colonoscopy.

SKIN INCISIONS

- A Hasson technique is used to achieve access to the abdomen at the umbilicus.
- Four 5-mm trocars are placed—two on either side of the abdomen lateral to the rectus with one hand breadth between the trocars to avoid instrument conflict. An optional fifth trocar can be placed in the suprapubic area if required for retraction. **FIGURE 2** (trocars) shows the typical trocar placement.

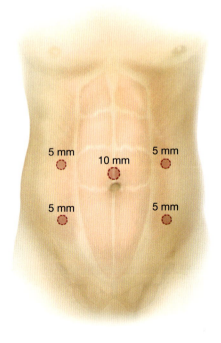

FIGURE 2 • We use this standard configuration of trocar placement for the majority of laparoscopic colon and rectal operations.

LAPAROSCOPIC EXPLORATION

- The abdomen is systematically explored in all four quadrants to look for metastatic disease and/or unexpected pathology.
- Knowledge of the mesenteric anatomy is essential for a successful laparoscopic approach.
- **FIGURE 3** (colon anatomy) shows the colon with its major vascular pedicles. Also depicted is the gastrocolic trunk of Henle that can be a source of bleeding if not recognized during the dissection.
- The right colic vessels commonly originate from the ileocolics (85%).
- The middle colic arteries commonly have more than two branches (55%).

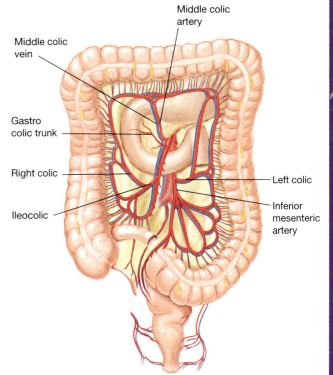

FIGURE 3 • The major vascular pedicles to the colon and the marginal artery that maintains collateral circulation.

PEDICLE LIGATION

- The omentum is retracted upward and placed over the stomach in the upper abdomen to allow for visualization of the transverse colon.
- The ileocolic, middle colic, and left colic vessels are first identified (**FIGURE 4**). Identification of the vascular pedicles is facilitated by traction on the colon to tent the mesentery. Adequate exposure is achieved by grasping each flexure and retracting superiorly and laterally (**FIGURE 5**).
- A window is created in the colon mesentery between the ileocolic and middle colic vessels. With appropriate traction and countertraction, the retromesenteric dissection is continued superiorly, medially, and laterally into the lesser sac (**FIGURE 6**).
- Care is taken to protect the duodenum, head of the pancreas, and the superior mesenteric artery (SMA) and superior mesenteric vein during the dissection.
- The middle colic vessels can be divided at the common trunk or divided individually after bifurcation (**FIGURE 7**). There is significant variation in the anatomy of the middle colic trunk.
- Our practice is to use a bipolar vessel-sealing device to divide the pedicles, but clips and staplers are also options to divide the pedicles. It is important to ensure that the SMA and superior mesenteric vein are protected from injury during

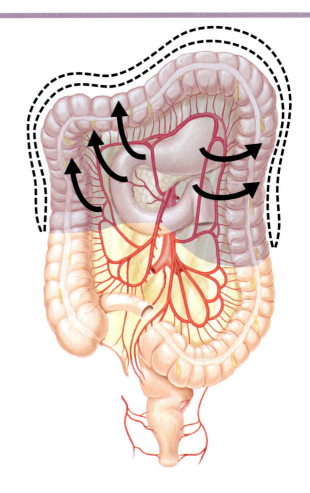

FIGURE 4 • Appropriate traction on the colon in the direction of the *arrows* exposes the mesentery and allows for identification of the major vascular pedicles.

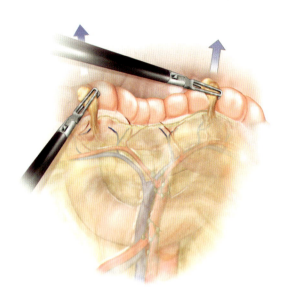

FIGURE 5 • Cephalad and lateral traction is used to visualize the middle colic vessels.

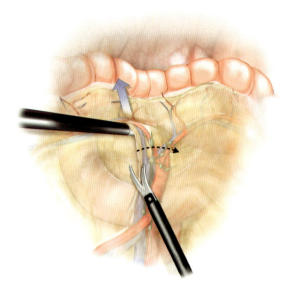

FIGURE 6 • A window is created to the right of the middle colic vessels.

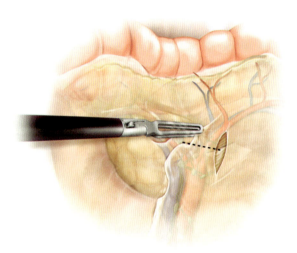

- dissection and transection of the middle colic pedicles, and that sufficient cuff of the vascular pedicle is retained to control bleeding should the vessel sealers fail.
- Strong anterior traction on the transverse colon mesentery optimizes middle colic dissection and decreases the likelihood of inadvertent injury to SMA.

FIGURE 7 • After adequate mobilization and protection of the duodenum and pancreas, the middle colic vessels are divided.

RETROMESENTERIC DISSECTION

- Right retromesenteric dissection
  - Laterally, the dissection is carried to the white line of Toldt and the hepatic flexure (**FIGURE 8**).
  - Medially, the dissection is carried to the root of the middle colic vessels and anterior to the head of the pancreas and the duodenum (**FIGURE 9**). The gastrocolic venous trunk is often encountered during this dissection and can be a source of bleeding if not recognized and controlled (**FIGURE 10**).
  - Superiorly, the dissection is carried cephalad to the transverse colon wall.
  - The remaining attachments to the liver are taken down (**FIGURE 11**).
- Left retromesenteric dissection
  - A similar dissection is carried out on the left side, creating a window between the left colic and middle colic vessels (**FIGURE 7**).
  - Laterally, the dissection is carried to the white line of Toldt and the splenic flexure of the colon (**FIGURE 12**).
  - Medially, the dissection is carried to the root of the middle colic vessels.

Chapter 13 **LAPAROSCOPIC TRANSVERSE COLECTOMY** 105

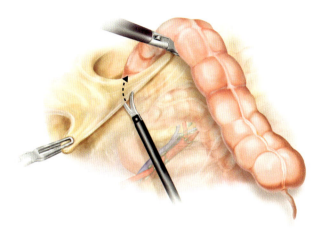

FIGURE 8 • The lateral attachments of the colon are taken down, ensuring there is no thermal injury to the bowel.

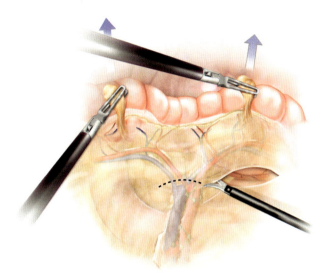

FIGURE 9 • Dissection of the middle colic vessels.

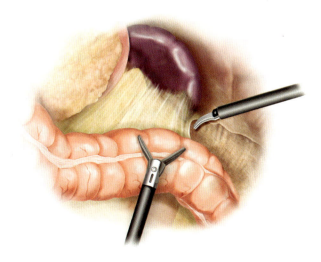

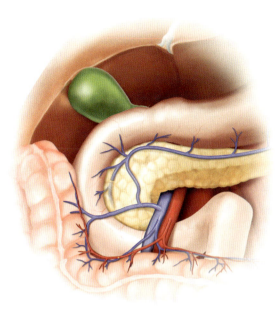

FIGURE 10 • Early identification and control of the gastrocolic trunk prevents bleeding and injury to the superior mesenteric vein.

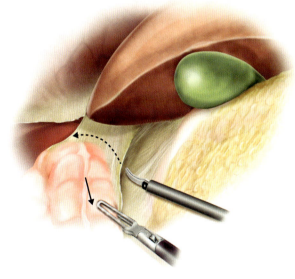

FIGURE 11 • Remaining attachments of the hepatic flexure of the colon to the liver are taken down. The dissection is facilitated by working close to the colon.

FIGURE 12 • Splenic flexure mobilization requires takedown of the splenocolic ligament.

- Superiorly, the dissection is carried to the inferior border of the pancreas and continued along the avascular plane between the left colon mesentery and the tail of the pancreas (**FIGURE 13**).
- At this point, the colon mesentery should be completely mobilized. The transverse colon is only held by the lateral attachments, the omentum, and the pedicles.

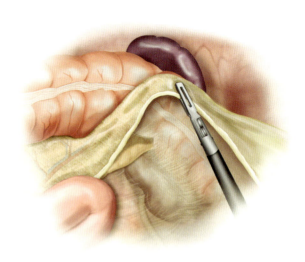

FIGURE 13 • To achieve adequate mobilization, the posterior attachments along the inferior border of the pancreas need to be dissected with entry into the lesser sac.

RELEASE OF LATERAL ATTACHMENTS AND THE OMENTUM

- The omentum is next taken off the transverse colon (**FIGURE 14**). The lateral attachments are taken down on both the sides. The dissection should be started in the midtransverse colon where the two leaves of the greater omentum are fused together. Visualization of the posterior wall of the stomach ensures that the surgical dissection is in the proper plane into the lesser sac. It is important to protect the colon from thermal injury during this portion of the dissection.

- In addition to mobilizing the transverse colon, the right colon, with the hepatic flexure, and the left colon, with the splenic flexure, need to be fully mobilized as well. This will allow for specimen extraction and the creation of a tension-free anastomosis (**FIGURE 15**).

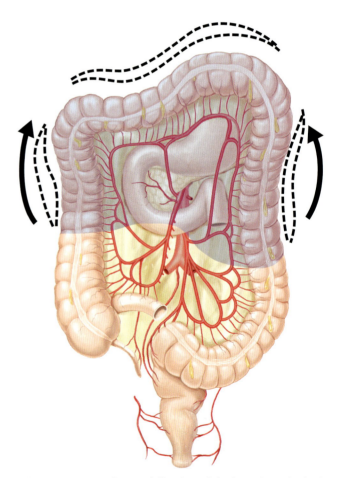

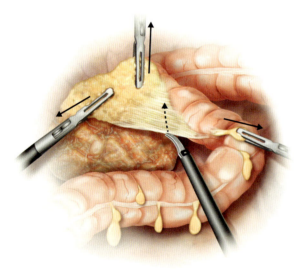

FIGURE 14 • The omentum is dissected off the transverse colon. The omentum is left on the colon around the tumor to ensure an en bloc resection. Early entry into the lesser sac and identification of the posterior wall of the stomach facilitates an efficient dissection.

FIGURE 15 • Complete mobilization of the hepatic and splenic flexures allows for safe specimen extraction and tension-free anastomosis.

SPECIMEN EXTERIORIZATION AND ANASTOMOSIS

- The periumbilical incision is commonly extended as an extraction site and a wound protector is placed (**FIGURE 16**).
- The mobilized transverse colon is exteriorized. Any remaining mesentery is divided.
- A linear stapler is used to divide the colon proximal to the hepatic flexure and distal to the splenic flexure as shown (**FIGURE 16**).
- The specimen is either sent for gross examination or opened in the OR to ensure that adequate margins (5 cm for cancer) were obtained.

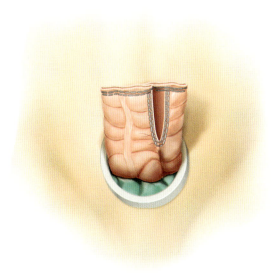

FIGURE 17 • Side-to-side functional end-to-end stapled anastomosis through a wound protector is illustrated.

- If the lesion is located laterally, an extended right or left hemicolectomy with additional pedicles can be taken as needed.
- A side-to-side functional end-to-end stapled anastomosis or a hand-sewn anastomosis can be fashioned based on the preference of the surgeon (**FIGURE 17**).
- The colon is replaced in the peritoneal cavity, and the operative area is examined for hemostasis.
- If there is concern for bleeding, the pneumoperitoneum can be reestablished prior to closure.
- Routine closure of the colonic mesenteric defect is not necessary as complications are minimal.[1]
- The extraction site fascial opening is closed, the trocars are removed under direct visualization, and the skin incision is closed.

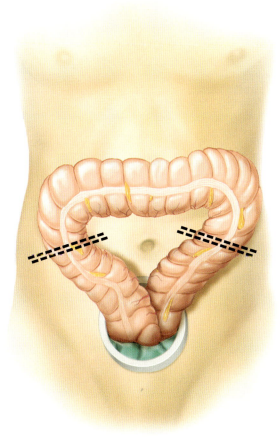

FIGURE 16 • Periumbilical incision with wound protector to extract specimen.

PEARLS AND PITFALLS

Indications	■ Extended right or left hemicolectomies may be more appropriate for tumors located closer to the flexures. ■ Laparoscopy may not be feasible in obstructing tumors with massive bowel distension or tumors with extensive local invasion. History of prior surgeries is not an absolute contraindication to laparoscopy.
Placement of incisions (trocars)	■ Place trocars lateral to the rectus and at least 7-8 cm between each trocar to avoid clashing of instruments. ■ The extraction incision is usually at or superior to the umbilicus.
Positioning	■ Thighs should be parallel to the floor and knees in line with the torso to prevent collision of the instruments with the knees.
Laparoscopic retraction, manipulation, and dissection	■ Care should be taken when dissecting over the head of the pancreas to avoid causing bleeding from the gastrocolic venous trunk of Henle. ■ The SMA and superior mesenteric vein should be protected during middle colic vessels ligation. ■ Bipolar energy devices may not be effective in sealing calcified vessels. Endoloops should be available to control unexpected bleeding. ■ Vessel-sealing devices can lead to lateral spread of thermal energy, and the colon should be protected during dissection. ■ Intraoperative colonoscopy is useful if the exact location of the tumor is unclear. ■ A hand access port can serve as a useful adjunct to complete difficult and challenging dissections (see Chapter 13).
Anastomosis	■ Complete mobilization of both flexures is essential for a tension-free anastomosis. ■ A tension-free anastomosis minimizes postoperative anastomotic leaks. ■ Inadequate mobilization of the splenic flexure can lead to traction injury of the spleen. ■ In cases where there is tension, an extended right colectomy is safer as the small bowel is freely mobile. ■ A wound protector is useful in minimizing contamination and limiting the length of the extraction incision.

POSTOPERATIVE CARE

- The patient is sent to the postsurgical unit and is usually given sips after recovery from anesthesia. Diet is advanced on postoperative day 1 to clear liquids and solids after passing flatus.
- The Foley catheter is removed on day 1 and oral pain medications are started once the patient tolerates solid food.
- The patient is usually discharged on day 3 or 4 when the patient is on oral pain medications, tolerating a diet, and passing flatus.

OUTCOMES

- Large multicenter randomized trials have validated the oncologic safety and potential short-term benefits of laparoscopic surgery for colon cancer.[2,3] Transverse colon cancers were not included in these major trials.
- Smaller retrospective studies have concluded that the oncologic outcomes for laparoscopic treatment of transverse colon cancer are equivalent to the open approach. They also reported some potential short-term benefits.[4,5,6]
- There are limited data on laparoscopic transverse colectomy for benign lesions.
- Laparoscopic transverse colectomy is technically challenging and may carry a higher incidence of conversion to open surgery during the procedure.[7]
- This procedure is best performed by surgeons experienced with open resections of the transverse colon and with significant laparoscopic colorectal experience.

COMPLICATIONS

- Bleeding
  - A medial to lateral dissection approach allows early identification and control of the major vessels and may avoid bleeding.
  - It is important to remain in the avascular plane between the mesentery and retroperitoneum. Significant oozing is a sign that the dissection may be too anterior into the mesentery or too posterior into the retroperitoneum.
  - Clips and endoloops are rarely required with modern energy and vessel-sealing devices but should be easily available to control bleeding, especially in patients with calcified vessels.
  - Postoperative abdominal hemorrhage can be managed with repeat laparoscopic exploration.
  - Postoperative intraluminal hemorrhage is best managed with carbon dioxide colonoscopy and endoluminal control.
- Splenic injury
  - It is safest to dissect toward the spleen rather than to retract the colon away from the spleen and cause a traction injury.
  - Complete mobilization of the splenic flexure will avoid traction injury during the extracorporeal portion of the operation.
  - Splenic injury can usually be managed with pressure and hemostatic agents.
  - Occasionally, with uncontrollable bleeding or with injury to the hilum, splenectomy may be required.

- Anastomotic leak
  - A tension-free anastomosis is facilitated by complete mobilization of both flexures.
  - Pulsatile blood flow is confirmed at the mesenteric transection line to ensure adequate blood supply to the anastomosis.
  - If the proximal margin is devascularized, conversion to an extended right hemicolectomy with an ileocolonic anastomosis may be safer.
  - Small postoperative anastomotic leaks may be managed nonoperatively with intravenous antibiotics and percutaneous drainage as needed.
  - Larger leaks with peritonitis or contamination will likely require proximal diversion.
  - In extreme cases, the anastomosis may need to be taken down and converted to an end stoma.
- Serosal or full-thickness injury to the bowel
  - Careful dissection with attention to the possibility of lateral thermal spread is important.
  - The duodenum should be completely dissected off the mesentery and protected prior to pedicle ligation.
  - The small and large bowels are also at risk for puncture or shear injury during insertion of laparoscopic instruments.
- Deep and superficial surgical site infection
- Early and later incisional hernia formation

REFERENCES

1. Cabot JC, Lee SA, Yoo J, et al. Long-term consequences of not closing the mesenteric defect after laparoscopic right colectomy. *Dis Colon Rectum.* 2010;53(3):289-292.
2. Bonjer HJ, Hop WC, Nelson H, et al. Laparoscopically assisted vs open colectomy for colon cancer: a meta-analysis. *Arch Surg.* 2007;142(3):298-303.
3. Nelson H. Laparoscopic colectomy: lessons learned and future prospects. *Lancet Oncol.* 2009;10(1):7-8.
4. Kim HJ, Lee IK, Lee YS, et al. A comparative study on the short-term clinicopathologic outcomes of laparoscopic surgery versus conventional open surgery for transverse colon cancer. *Surg Endosc.* 2009;23(8):1812-1817.
5. Lee YS, Lee IK, Kang WK, et al. Surgical and pathological outcomes of laparoscopic surgery for transverse colon cancer. *Int J Colorectal Dis.* 2008;23(7):669-673.
6. Schlachta CM, Mamazza J, Poulin EC. Are transverse colon cancers suitable for laparoscopic resection? *Surg Endosc.* 2007;21(3):396-399.
7. Simorov A, Shaligram A, Shostrom V, et al. Laparoscopic colon resection trends in utilization and rate of conversion to open procedure: a national database review of academic medical centers. *Ann Surg.* 2012;256(3):462-468.

Chapter 14 Transverse Colectomy: Hand-Assisted Laparoscopic Surgery Technique

Daniel Albo

DEFINITION

- Transverse colectomy refers to removal of the portion of the colon between the hepatic and the splenic flexures. The transverse colon derives its blood supply primarily from the middle colic vessels. In addition, the transverse colon receives collateral blood flow from the left and right marginal arcades (marginal artery of Drummond and arch of Riolan, respectively).
- Hand-assisted laparoscopic surgery (HALS) is a minimally invasive surgical approach that uses conventional laparoscopic-assisted (LA) surgery techniques but with the addition of a hand-assisted device that allows for the introduction of one of the surgeon's hands into the surgical field. The hand-assisted device is placed at the projected specimen extraction site. HALS in colorectal surgery retains all of the same advantages of conventional LA surgery over open surgery, including less pain, faster recovery, lower incidence of wound complications, and reduction of cardiopulmonary complications, especially in the obese and in the elderly.
- HALS has significant advantages over conventional LA colorectal surgery, including the following:
  - Reintroduces tactile feedback into the field
  - Shorter learning curves; easier to teach
  - Shorter operative times and lower conversion to open rates
  - Allows for the insertion of multiple ports through the hand-assisted device
  - Allows for the introduction of laparotomy pads into the field (helps keeping the small bowel and omentum out of the way, particularly in the obese)
  - Higher usage rates of minimally invasive surgery

DIFFERENTIAL DIAGNOSIS

- Focal inflammatory processes, localized trauma, or local perforation.
- Colon cancer located in the midtransverse colon. Cancers located at the flexures may necessitate extended right or left hemicolectomies in order to ensure adequate lymphadenectomy.
- Other tumors locally extending into the transverse colon (ie, gastric, pancreatic, adrenal tumors, sarcomas) may necessitate en bloc transverse colectomy when resecting the primary tumor to achieve negative margins.

PATIENT HISTORY AND PHYSICAL FINDINGS

- Patients with colon cancer generally present with occult bleeding and anemia. Patients may also present with high-grade obstructing symptoms (crampy abdominal pain and constipation). More advance tumors may present with a complete large bowel obstruction. If these patients have a competent ileocecal valve, they develop a closed loop large bowel obstruction and present with severe right lower quadrant abdominal pain and abdominal distention secondary to a massive colonic dilation proximal to the obstructing lesion. These patients should be taken to the operating room emergently. Unopposed, this will ultimately cause an ischemic perforation of the cecum leading to a catastrophic fecaloid peritonitis and potential oncologic contamination of the abdominal cavity leading to carcinomatosis.
- A detailed personal and family history of colorectal cancer, polyps, and/or other malignancies should be elicited. Physical examination should include a routine abdominal examination, noting any previous incisions.

IMAGING AND OTHER DIAGNOSTIC STUDIES

- A full colonoscopy with documentation of all polyps should be performed. Lesions that are unresectable endoscopically and/or are suspicious for cancer should be tattooed to facilitate localization during surgery. If there is any concern for involvement of adjacent organs, such as the stomach, an esophagogastroscopy should also be performed.
- A computed tomography (CT) scan of the chest, abdomen, and pelvis evaluates for potential metastases. In patients with a large bowel obstruction, the CT scan shows dilation of the right colon and cecum, collapse of the distal colon, and a paucity of fluid and gas in the small bowel (**FIGURE 1**).
- A preoperative carcinoembryonic antigen level is obtained.

SURGICAL MANAGEMENT

Preoperative Preparation

- Clinical trials have shown no need for mechanical bowel preparation.
- Intravenous cefoxitin is administered within 1 hour of skin incision.

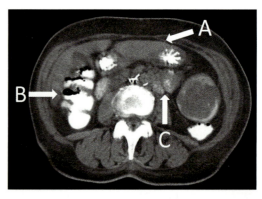

FIGURE 1 • Computed tomography scan shows a large obstructing colon cancer in the transverse colon *(A)* with dilation of the cecum *(B)* and a paucity of fluid and gas in the small bowel *(C)*.

- Use hair clippers if needed and chlorhexidine gluconate skin preparation.
- Preoperative time-out and briefing is performed.

Equipment and Instrumentation
- 5-mm camera with high-resolution monitors.
- 5-mm clear ports with balloon tips. They hold ports in the abdomen and minimize their intra-abdominal profile during surgery.
- Atraumatic graspers and laparoscopic endoscopic scissors.
- A blunt tip, 5-mm energy device.
- 60-mm linear reticulating laparoscopic staplers with vascular and tan loads.
- We use the GelPort hand-assisted device due to its versatility and ease of use. This device allows for the introduction/removal of the hand without losing pneumoperitoneum.

Patient Positioning and Surgical Team Setup
- This is the single most critical determinant of success in laparoscopic colorectal surgery (**FIGURE 2**).
- Place the patient on a supine position, with the arms tucked and padded (to avoid nerve/tendon injuries). The patient is taped over a towel across the chest without compromising chest expansion.
- The surgeon starts at the patient's right lower side with the scrub nurse to the surgeon's right side. The assistant stands at the surgeon's left side.
- Align the surgeon, the ports, the targets, and the monitors in straight line. Place monitors in front of the surgeon and at eye level to prevent lower neck stress injuries.

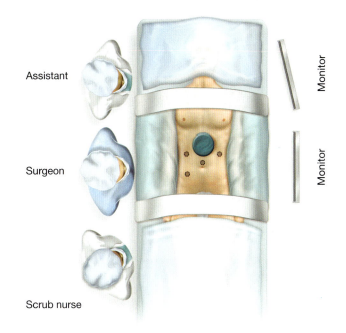

FIGURE 2 • Patient and team setup.

- Avoid unnecessary restrictions to potential team movement around the table. All energy device cables exit by the patient's upper left side. All laparoscopic (gas, light cord, and camera) elements exit by the patient's upper right side.

PORT PLACEMENT AND OPERATIVE FIELD SETUP

- Insert a GelPort through a 5- to 6-cm epigastric incision. This incision will be also used for specimen extraction, transection, and anastomosis. Placement in the epigastric area greatly facilitates dissection of the middle colic vessels through a supramesocolic approach (see step 7).
- Insert three 5-mm working ports in the right upper, right lower, and left upper quadrants. Insert a 5-mm camera port above the umbilicus. Triangulate the ports so the camera port is at the apex of the triangle. This avoids conflict between the instruments and prevents disorientation ("working on a mirror").

OPERATIVE STEPS

- Our HALS transverse colectomy operation is highly standardized and it consists of nine steps:
    - Transection of the inferior mesenteric vein (IMV)
    - Medial to lateral dissection of the descending mesocolon
    - Transection of the left colic artery
    - Mobilization of the sigmoid off the pelvic inlet
    - Mobilization of the descending colon
    - Mobilization of the splenic flexure
    - Mobilization of the right colon
    - Transection of the middle colic vessels (supramesocolic approach)
    - Extracorporeal transection and anastomosis

Step 1: Transection of the Inferior Mesenteric Vein

- This is the critical "point of entry" in this operation. At the level of the ligament of Treitz, the IMV is easy to visualize and is far from critical structures that can be injured during its dissection (no iliac vessels or left ureter nearby). This will be the only time when a true virgin tissue plane is entered. Every step will set up the following ones, opening the tissue planes sequentially.
- The patient is placed on a steep Trendelenburg position with the left side up. Using the right hand, move the small bowel into the right upper quadrant (RUQ) and the transverse colon and omentum into the upper abdomen. If necessary, place a laparotomy pad to hold the bowel out of the field of view

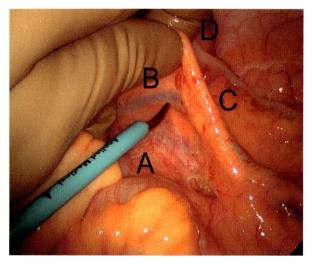

FIGURE 3 • Step 1: Key anatomy. Ligament of Treitz *(A)*. Inferior mesenteric vein (IMV) *(B)*. Left colic artery *(C)* as it separates from the IMV and goes toward the splenic flexure of the colon *(D)*.

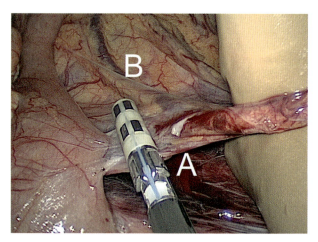

FIGURE 4 • Step 1: Transection of the inferior mesenteric vein *(A)* cephalad of the left colic artery *(B)*.

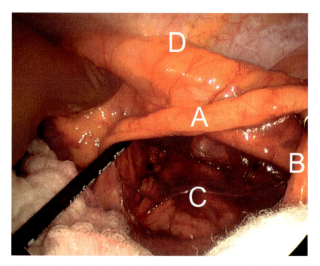

FIGURE 5 • Step 2: Medial to lateral dissection of the descending mesocolon. The surgeon is holding the splenic flexure upward. Notice that there is a laparotomy pad on the field holding the small bowel out of the way and helping provide excellent exposure. The left colic artery is located in the medial edge of the descending mesocolon *(A)*. Inferior mesenteric artery *(B)*. Gerota fascia *(C)*. Descending colon *(D)*.

especially in obese patients. This pad can also be used to dry up the field and to clean the scope tip intracorporeally. Make sure that the circulating nurse notes the laparotomy pad in the abdomen on the white board.

- Identify the critical anatomy: IMV, ligament of Treitz, and left colic artery (**FIGURE 3**).
- If there are attachments between the duodenum/root of mesentery and the mesocolon, transect them with laparoscopic scissors. This will allow for adequate exposure of midline structures.
- Pick up the IMV with the left hand. Dissect under the IMV and in front of Gerota fascia with endoscopic scissors, starting at the level of the ligament of Treitz and proceeding toward the inferior mesenteric artery (IMA). The assistant provides upward traction with a grasper.
- Transect the IMV cephalad of the left colic artery (which moves away from the IMV and toward the splenic flexure of the colon) with the 5-mm energy device (**FIGURE 4**), thus preserving intact the left-sided marginal arterial arcade and maintaining the blood supply to the descending colon segment.

Step 2: Medial to Lateral Dissection of the Descending Mesocolon

- The surgeon's hand and the assistant's grasper retract the IMV/left colic pedicle at the cut edge of the descending mesocolon upward toward the anterior abdominal wall. They then dissect the plane between the mesocolon and Gerota fascia (readily identified by the transition between the two fat planes) with a 5-mm energy device (**FIGURE 5**). We like to dissect this space by gently pushing the retroperitoneum down with the blunt tip of the 5-mm energy device.
- Dissect caudally under the IMV/left colic artery toward the takeoff of the left colic artery off the IMA. Dissect laterally until you reach the lateral abdominal wall. This will greatly facilitate step 5. Dissect superiorly between the splenic flexure and the tail of the pancreas. This will greatly facilitate step 6.

Step 3: Transection of the Left Colic Artery

- Identify the critical anatomy: The "letter T" formed between the IMA and its left colic and superior hemorrhoidal artery (SHA) terminal branches (**FIGURE 6**).
- Holding the SHA up with the left hand, dissect the plane along the palpable groove between the SHA and the left iliac artery using laparoscopic scissors and a 5-mm energy device. Preserve the sympathetic nerve trunk intact in the retroperitoneum. Identify the left ureter in front of the left iliac artery and psoas muscle and medial to the gonadal vessels before transecting anything (**FIGURE 7A**).
- Dissect with your thumb and index finger around and behind the IMA (**FIGURE 7B**).
- Visualize the letter "T" formed between the IMA, the left colic artery, and the SHA (**FIGURE 7A**). Transect the left

colic artery as it takes off the IMA with the energy device (**FIGURE 7C**). The surgeon can now complete the dissection of the mesocolon off the retroperitoneum in a superior to inferior direction down to the level of the pelvic inlet. This will greatly facilitate steps 4 and 5.

Step 4: Mobilization of the Sigmoid off the Pelvic Inlet

- The surgeon pulls the proximal sigmoid colon medially with the left hand and the assistant pulls the distal sigmoid colon medially with a grasper (**FIGURE 8A**). Transect the lateral sigmoid colon attachments to the pelvic inlet with laparoscopic scissors in your right hand. Stay medially, close to the sigmoid and mesosigmoid to avoid injuring the left ureter (**FIGURE 8B**). You should readily enter the retroperitoneal dissection plane dissected during the previous step.
- Dissect caudally until reaching the left side of the Douglas pouch.

Step 5: Mobilization of the Descending Colon

- Retract the descending colon medially with your left hand. Transect the white line of Toldt up to the splenic flexure using endoscopic scissors or energy device with your right hand through the left-sided port. You should readily enter the retroperitoneal dissection plane dissected during step 2.

Step 6: Mobilization of the Splenic Flexure

- Place the patient on reverse Trendelenburg position with the left side up to help displace the splenic flexure down out of the left upper quadrant.
- With the assistant pulling the transverse colon downward with a grasper, the surgeon lifts the stomach up with their left hand and transects the gastrocolic ligament in between the stomach and transverse colon using a 5-mm energy device through the RUQ port site (**FIGURE 9A**). This allows for entrance into the lesser sac and provides for an excellent view of the splenic flexure.
- Transect the gastrocolic ligament (from medial to lateral) with the 5-mm energy device, staying close to the transverse colon and avoiding the spleen. Proceed laterally to the splenic flexure.
- Because the dissection performed in step 2 completely separated the splenic flexure of the colon from the retroperitoneum, the surgeon can now slide their right hand under the splenic flexure, holding the splenic flexure up with the index finger "hooked" under the splenocolic ligament. This allows for an easy transection of the splenocolic ligament with an energy device (**FIGURE 9B** and **C**). The left colon should be now fully mobilized to the midline.

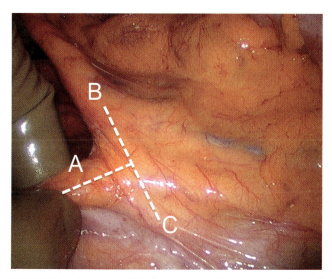

FIGURE 6 • Step 3: Critical anatomy. The letter T formed between the inferior mesenteric artery (A) and its left colic artery (B) and superior hemorrhoidal artery (C) terminal branches.

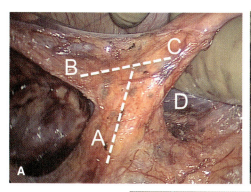
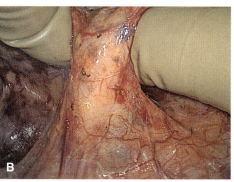
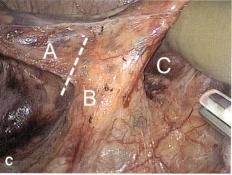

FIGURE 7 • Panel **A**, The "letter T" dissected: inferior mesenteric artery (IMA) (A), left colic artery (B), superior hemorrhoidal artery (C). Notice the left ureter (D) in the retroperitoneum. Panel **B**, The IMA is now completely encircled. Panel **C**, Level of transection of the left colic artery (A) as it branches off the IMA (B). Notice the left ureter (C) in the retroperitoneum. The dotted line shows where the left colic artery will be transected at its origin off the IMA.

114 SECTION II SURGERY OF THE COLON, APPENDIX, RECTUM, AND ANUS

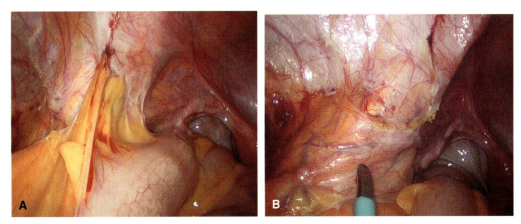

FIGURE 8 • Step 4. Panel **A,** Medial traction on the sigmoid exposes its lateral attachments to the pelvic inlet. Panel **B,** After the sigmoid mobilization is completed, the left ureter is visualized as it crosses over the left iliac artery.

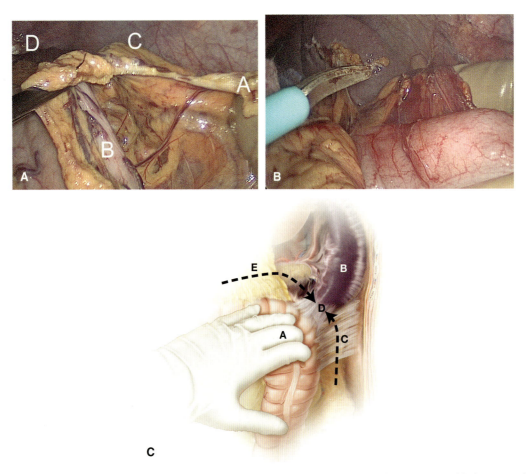

FIGURE 9 • Mobilization of the splenic flexure. Panel **A,** The partially transected gastrocolic ligament is visible between the transverse colon (A) and the stomach (B). Notice the excellent view of the lesser sac laterally toward the splenic flexure of the colon (C) and the spleen (D). Panel **B,** The surgeon is "hugging" the splenic flexure with their hand and "hooking" their index finger under the splenocolic ligament allowing for an excellent exposure and transection of this ligament with an energy device. Panel **C,** Splenic flexure mobilization. The surgeon retracts the splenic flexure of the colon (A) downwards and medially, exposing the attachments of the splenic flexure to the spleen (B). The phrenocolic (C) and splenocolic (D) ligaments are transected in an inferior to superior and lateral to medial direction. The gastrocolic ligament (E) is then transected in a medial to lateral direction, until both planes of dissection meet and the splenic flexure is fully mobilized.

Chapter 14 TRANSVERSE COLECTOMY: HAND-ASSISTED LAPAROSCOPIC SURGERY TECHNIQUE   115

Step 7: Mobilization of the Right Colon

- Standing at the left side of the table, the surgeon completes the transection of the gastrocolic ligament until reaching the hepatic flexure of the colon using a 5-mm energy device.
- At this point, the hepatocolic ligament is readily visible. Slide your right index finger under it, hold it upward, and transect it with a 5-mm energy device.
- Proceeding on a superior to inferior dissection, transect to the right white line of Toldt with laparoscopic scissors. Fully mobilize the ascending colon off the retroperitoneum with the 5-mm energy device. This dissection should proceed from a lateral to medial as well as from a superior to inferior direction. Stay in front of the duodenum, the head of the pancreas, and Gerota fascia.

Step 8: Transection of the Middle Colic Vessels (Supramesocolic Approach)

- Dissection and transection of the middle colic vessels can be one of the most daunting maneuvers in colorectal surgery. Traditionally, these vessels are approached inframesocolically by dissecting the root of the mesotransverse colon at the intersection with the root of the mesentery where the venous anatomy is extremely variable and complex. The superior mesenteric vein (SMV) and its branches, and the gastrocolic venous trunk of Henle and its branches, surround the middle colic vessels. Venous tears tend to travel distally to the next major tributary. In terms of the SMV and the gastrocolic trunk of Henle, this next "tributary" is the portal vein confluence, which lies in a retroperitoneal plane for which you do not have control at this time.
- In order to prevent potentially devastating bleeding complications during the dissection and transection of the middle colic vessels, we have developed a supramesocolic approach to these vessels. The hand-assisted technique greatly facilitates the performance of this technique and makes it very safe.
- The superior aspect of the transverse mesocolon is now readily visible, with the middle colic vessels easily palpable as they cross the third portion of the duodenum in the midtransverse colon (**FIGURE 10**). With the assistant pulling down on the transverse colon downward with a grasper, the surgeon "picks up" the middle colic vessels supramesocolically with their right thumb and index finger. Using their left hand, the surgeon now dissects under the middle colic vessels with the 5-mm energy device, completely encircling the middle colic vessels with the thumb and index finger. With great exposure and control, the surgeon now transects the middle colic vessels with the 5-mm energy device.
- During this approach, the transverse mesocolon separates the SMV and the gastrocolic venous trunk of Henle from the middle colic vessels shielding them and, thus, greatly reducing the potential risk of serious venous injuries. It also allows for a very high transection of the middle colic vessels and, therefore, a great lymphatic nodal capture.
- Prior to the extracorporeal mobilization, we transect the right colic vessels intracorporeally (**FIGURE 11**). Hold the transverse colon up with the right hand; while the assistant retracts the right colon anteriorly and laterally, expose the right-sided vascular arcade that connects the right branches of the middle colic vessels with the right colic vessels (the arch of Riolan). You can now safely transect the right colic vessels at its origin from the ileocolic vessels.

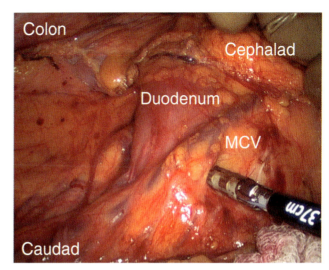

FIGURE 10 • Supramesocolic transection of the middle colic vessels (MCV). The MCV are readily visualized at this point through a supramesocolic approach as they cross over the third portion of the duodenum. This allows for a safe dissection and transection with a 5-mm energy device.

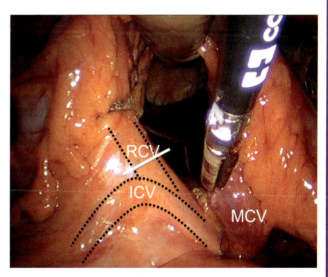

FIGURE 11 • Transection of the right colic vessels. The surgeon is holding the transverse colon (with the right-sided vascular arcade along its mesenteric border) up. The *solid white line* shows where to transect the right colic vessels (RCV) as they branch off the ileocolic vessels (ICV). Transected middle colic vessels (MCV).

Step 9: Extracorporeal Transection and Anastomosis

- Deliver the transverse colon through the epigastric incision with the wound protector in place to minimize the chance of wound infection and oncologic contamination of the wound. Should there be any tension, reintroduce the colon into the abdominal cavity and mobilize the right and/or left colon more laparoscopically. Excessive traction during this step can lead to troublesome vascular injuries on mesenteric structures.
- Transect the colon extracorporeally proximal to the hepatic flexure and distal to the splenic flexure with a linear 60-mm endostapler with tan loads (**FIGURE 12**). The transverse colon specimen contains the middle, right, and left colic pedicles.

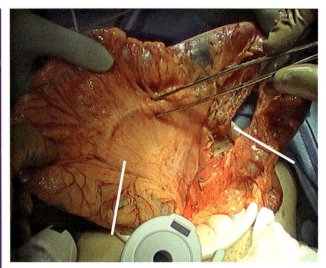

FIGURE 12 • Extracorporeal mobilization and transection. The specimen is exteriorized without any tension. The *white solid lines* show where to transect the colon proximal and distal to the hepatic and splenic flexures, respectively. The tattooed target in the midtransverse colon and the vascular arcade (arch of Riolan) are readily visible.

- At this point, we perform an extracorporeal, anatomic side-to-side, colocolonic anastomosis with a 60-mm linear endostapler using a vascular load (**FIGURE 13**). We avoid using the stapled colonic ends in the anastomosis to prevent potential ischemia at the staple lines intersection. The anastomosis

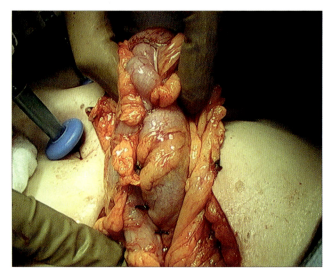

FIGURE 13 • Extracorporeal stapled side-to-side colocolonic anastomosis. The anastomosis is tension-free and has excellent blood supply.

should be tension-free and have an excellent blood supply. We do not close the anastomotic mesenteric gap to prevent potential damage to its blood supply.
- The anastomosis is reintroduced into the abdominal cavity. After changing gloves, all ports are removed. Wounds are closed with absorbable sutures and sealed off with Dermabond. We place a bilateral subcostal nerve block with bupivacaine for postoperative analgesia purposes.

PEARLS AND PITFALLS

Setup	▪ Proper patient, team, port, and instrumentation setup is critical.
Operative technique	▪ Point of entry: IMV at the ligament of Treitz. ▪ Complete every step. Each step sets up the next ones sequentially. ▪ Vascular dissection to visualize the letter T of the IMA and its SHA and left colic branches; identify left ureter prior to left colic transection. ▪ Supramesocolic approach to the middle colic vessels is critical to prevent serious venous injuries.
Pitfall: dissecting anterior to the SHA	▪ Solution: Identify "groove" between left common iliac artery and SHA and dissect in between the two vessels.
Pitfall: tension during extraction of the specimen	▪ Reintroduce the colon into the abdominal cavity and mobilize the right and/or left colon further. Tension during the extraction phase can lead to serious bleeding problems.

POSTOPERATIVE CARE

- Postoperative care is driven by clinical pathways that include the following:
  - Pain control: Intravenous acetaminophen for 24 hours (start in the operating room) followed by intravenous ketorolac for 72 hours (if creatinine is normal). The subcostal nerve block greatly reduces the need for narcotics.
  - Deep vein thrombosis (DVT) prophylaxis with enoxaparin starting within 24 hours of surgery.
  - No additional antibiotics, judicious use of intravenous fluids.
  - No nasogastric tube. Remove Foley catheter on postoperative day 1.
  - Early ambulation, diet ad lib, aggressive pulmonary toilet.
  - Targeted discharge: postoperative day 3.

OUTCOMES

- HALS leads to improvements in short-term outcomes, including less pain, faster recovery, shorter hospital stay, and lower incidence of cardiac/pulmonary complications when compared to open surgery.
- When compared to conventional laparoscopy, HALS results in higher usage rates of minimally invasive surgery, shorter learning curves, lower conversion rates, shorter operative times, and shorter hospital stays.
- For cancer resection, minimally invasive surgery oncologic outcomes are at least comparable to those of open surgery.

COMPLICATIONS

- Wound infections and hernias are markedly reduced vs open surgery.
- Anastomotic leak rates should be below 5%.
- Ureteral injury: critical to identify the left ureter prior to vascular transection.
- DVT: low risk with use of DVT prophylaxis.
- Cardiac and pulmonary complications: significantly reduced compared to the open surgery approach.

SUGGESTED READINGS

1. Orcutt ST, Marshall CL, Balentine CJ, et al. Hand-assisted laparoscopy leads to efficient colorectal cancer surgery. *J Surg Res.* 2012;177(2):e53-e58.
2. Orcutt ST, Marshall CL, Robinson CN, et al. Minimally invasive surgery in colon cancer patients leads to improved short-term outcomes and excellent oncologic results. *Am J Surg.* 2011;202(5):528-531.
3. Wilks JA, Balentine CJ, Berger DH, et al. Establishment of a minimally invasive program at a VAMC leads to improved care in colorectal cancer patients. *Am J Surg.* 2009;198(5):685-692.
4. Marcello PW, Fleshman JW, Milsom JW, et al. Hand-assisted laparoscopic vs. laparoscopic colorectal surgery. A multicenter, prospective, randomized trial. *Dis Colon Rectum.* 2008;51:818-828.
5. Kim HJ, Lee IK, Lee YS, et al. A comparative study on the short-term clinicopathologic outcomes of laparoscopic surgery versus conventional open surgery for transverse colon cancer. *Surg Endosc.* 2009;23(8):1812-1817.
6. Lee YS, Lee IK, Kang WK, et al. Surgical and pathological outcomes of laparoscopic surgery for transverse colon cancer. *Int J Colorectal Dis.* 2008;23(7):669-673.
7. Schlachta CM, Mamazza J, Poulin EC. Are transverse colon cancers suitable for laparoscopic resection?. *Surg Endosc.* 2007;21(3):396-399.

Chapter 15 | Left Hemicolectomy: Open Technique

Saul J. Rugeles and Luis Jorge Lombana

DEFINITION

- Left hemicolectomy is defined as the resection of the left colon in which the extent of resection must correspond to the distribution of the lymphovascular drainage of the inferior mesenteric vein and artery, having as the result negative borders on histopathologic studies, along with in block extirpation of the lymphovascular tissue of the colon with a minimum number of 12 lymph nodes available to be evaluated by a histopathologic study.[1]

DIFFERENTIAL DIAGNOSIS

- Most of the patients with left colon tumors must have a cancer histologic diagnosis before being taken to surgery.
- However, there are cases in which the biopsies of the tumor taken by colonoscopy do not identify the presence of a neoplasia. In these cases, it is recommended to take another biopsy set. If a second set is not diagnostic, it is recommended to proceed with the colectomy and obtain the pathologic study from the surgical specimen.
- Other differential diagnoses for left colon cancer that may necessitate left hemicolectomy include complicated diverticular disease with stenosis/perforation/fistulae, intraluminal foreign bodies with an inflammatory reaction, neoplastic invasion from adjacent organs (especially ovaries), inflammatory bowel disease, and colonic endometriosis.

PATIENT HISTORY AND PHYSICAL FINDINGS

- The patient's medical record must be complete, including a detailed description of signs and symptoms; medical history, with special attention to the evolution of symptoms; food intake and weight changes; and a thorough physical examination, including rectal examination. The abdomen must be carefully examined to search for lumps, carcinomatosis, or ascites. The lymphatic nodal basins must be examined as well.
- Family history of colon, gastrointestinal, breast, endometrial, and prostate cancer is especially important to allow for the identification of possible cases of familiar colon cancer.
- The clinical evaluation must include a subjective global assessment of nutritional status to identify the patients who may benefit from perioperative nutritional therapy.[2]
- The physiologic risk of the patient must be evaluated according to their age, intercurrent diseases, fragility scales and type of surgery, following the institutional preoperative evaluation guidelines.

IMAGING AND OTHER DIAGNOSTIC STUDIES

- Carcinoembryonic antigen (CEA): The baseline preoperative result is an independent variable for survival[1] and postsurgical control must be obtained as an assessment for complete tumor resection. CEA levels will also help with postoperative cancer surveillance.
- Abdominal computed tomography is the most sensitive and specific test for the detection of intra-abdominal metastases.[1]
- Chest computed tomography is the most sensitive and specific test to detect mediastinal and lung metastases.[1]
- Total colonoscopy: Regardless of the primary localization of the tumor, every patient should have a complete colonoscopy study whenever possible, because 2% to 9% of the patients may have synchronous tumors elsewhere in the colon and rectum.[1] The colonic enema with double contrast may be used when colonoscopy is not feasible.

SURGICAL MANAGEMENT

Preoperative Planning

- The type of procedure must be thoroughly discussed with the patient and family. This includes the possibility of a temporary or permanent colostomy.
- Left hemicolectomy is a major surgery that has potential for significant postoperative morbidity and mortality. This needs to be disclosed to the patient while obtaining an informed consent for the procedure.
- There is controversy about the effectiveness and need of mechanical preparation of the bowel before colon resections.[3-5] We prefer to use a "mild" preparation with 2 days of liquid diet and polyethylene laxatives the day before the surgery, achieving the evacuation of large fecal residues.
- In the operating room, before initiating the anesthetic act, it is desirable to follow a checklist in which every professional involved in the surgical act must participate. This checklist should include at least patient identification, type of surgery, type of anesthesia, allergies, expected events during the surgery, the need for blood components, prophylactic antibiotic, surgical devices availability, and potential adverse events and their prevention.

Positioning

- The surgery is performed with the patient in a supine position. The arms should ideally be tucked to the sides, allowing freedom of movement for the surgical team. If one extended arm is required, it should be placed at an angle of 90° and the right arm is preferred.
- If a colorectal anastomosis with a circular stapler is assumed, the patient should be in the lithotomy position. In this case, one must ensure that the patient's thighs maintain a horizontal plane with the patient's abdomen, for them not to interfere with the surgeon's arms (**FIGURE 1**). The lower extremities' position in the brackets must protect them from neuropraxia or vascular injury.
- The surgical team setup is shown in **FIGURE 2**.
- The surgical table must allow inclinations in every way, which will be necessary to expose regions with difficult access, such as the splenic flexure of the colon.

Chapter 15 LEFT HEMICOLECTOMY: OPEN TECHNIQUE 119

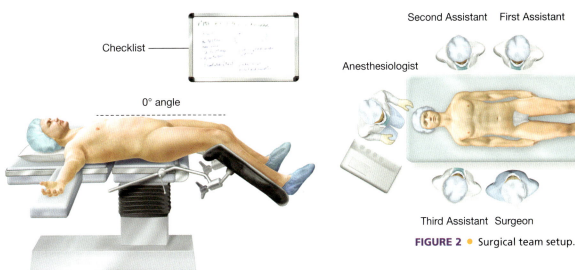

FIGURE 1 • Correct position of the patient in the operating table. Note the horizontal position of the thighs to ensure free movement of surgeon's arms and hands.

FIGURE 2 • Surgical team setup.

- The patient must be secured to the surgical table adequately to prevent body displacements with position changes of the surgical table.

LAPAROTOMY, REVISION OF PERITONEAL CAVITY, AND SURGICAL FIELD PREPARATION

- A midline supra- and infraumbilical laparotomy is performed, carrying the incision down to the pubis, which will improve pelvic exposure. Once the abdominal cavity is opened, it is advisable to protect the wound edges from bacterial and cellular contamination by placing an Alexis wound protector or similar device (**FIGURE 3A** and **B**).
- Following this, one should explore the abdominal cavity, emphasizing the search for liver metastases and synchronous colon tumors, especially in patients in which the total colonoscopy was not possible due to an obstructive tumor.

- Next, the small bowel is displaced toward the right upper quadrant of the abdomen and contained using pads and abdominal rolls. We prefer not to eviscerate the intestines because this increases manipulation of the intestines and therefore increases the possibility of postoperative ileus. In order to achieve good pelvic and distal descending colon exposure, the patient is placed in a Trendelenburg position. A slight inclination of the surgical table toward the right can be helpful. Placement of a Bookwalter retractor facilitates operative exposure.
- The exact location of the left colon tumor is identified and the extent of colonic and lymphovascular pedicle resection is defined (**FIGURE 4**).

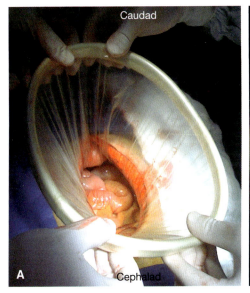
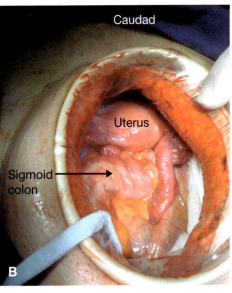

FIGURE 3 • **A** and **B**, The Alexis® retractor has been placed to protect the wound from fecal and tumoral contamination.

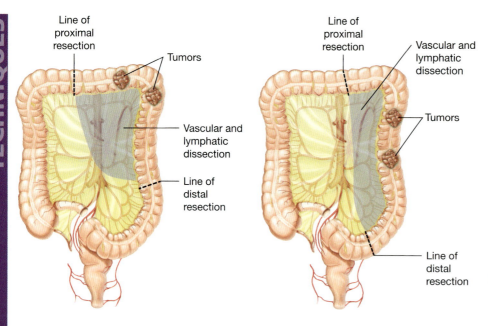

FIGURE 4 • Levels of colon and lymphovascular pedicle resection in accordance to tumor localization.

LATERAL TO MEDIAL MOBILIZATION OF THE LEFT COLON, IDENTIFICATION OF RETROPERITONEAL FASCIA, AND PRESERVATION OF RETROPERITONEAL STRUCTURES

- The sigmoid colon is retracted medially, and the lateral peritoneal fold is exposed down to the pelvic ring (**FIGURE 5**). The identification of the exact site to make peritoneal division is crucial to enter the correct fascial plane.[6]

- Peritoneal sectioning is initiated with the monopolar electrocautery in a cephalocaudal direction. This sectioning must enter in the fusion fascia between the mesocolon and the retroperitoneal fascia. This fusion fascia is identified as a loose avascular tissue with a "foamy" appearance (**FIGURE 6**). If the correct plane is found, the left ureter, left gonadal vessels, and other retroperitoneal structures will lay behind the retroperitoneal fascia protected from surgical injuries (**FIGURE 7**)

- The dissection must proceed now in a cephalad direction, staying in front of Gerota fascia, which should be preserved intact. The descending colon mesentery is elevated. At the end of this maneuver, the descending colon mesentery will be raised, containing the inferior mesenteric artery (IMA) and its branches and the inferior mesenteric vein and its tributaries (**FIGURE 8**).

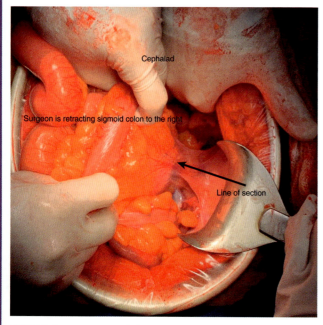

FIGURE 5 • Traction of the sigmoid to the right exposes the exact place to divide the lateral peritoneum.

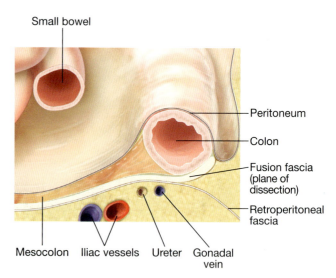

FIGURE 6 • Axial view of the right dissection plane to enter the fusion fascia.

Chapter 15 LEFT HEMICOLECTOMY: OPEN TECHNIQUE 121

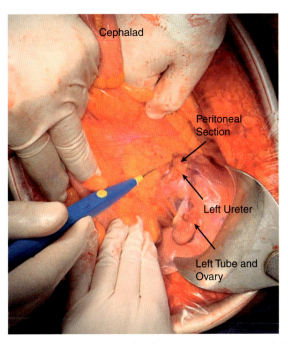

FIGURE 7 • The peritoneum has been sectioned and the fusion fascia is encountered, exposing the left ureter.

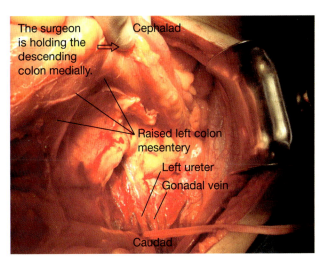

FIGURE 8 • The left colon mesentery has been raised. The retroperitoneal structures are exposed.

MOBILIZATION OF THE SPLENIC FLEXURE: DUAL (MEDIAL AND LATERAL) APPROACH

- At this time, a full mobilization of the splenic flexure is performed. This maneuver can be challenging, because the splenic flexure can have a very deep location in the left upper quadrant of the abdomen.
- To enhance exposure and facilitate dissection, the patient is placed in a reverse Trendelenburg position, with the left side rotated slightly upward.
- The lateral peritoneum sectioning is continued from the initial incision in a cephalic direction as far as possible, avoiding excessive traction of the splenic flexure in order to prevent splenic lacerations. This dissection must be done with electrocautery to see the thin retroperitoneal and fusion fascias. It is very important to maintain dissection in the correct plane between retroperitoneal fascia and the left colon mesentery to avoid injuries to the vasculature of the colon and bleeding in the retroperitoneum. When the splenic flexure is reached, the section of the splenocolic ligament must be done close to the colon to maintain the dissection in the right plane.
- The final approach to the splenic flexure should be complemented with another point of dissection that is initiated in the transverse colon to the left of the middle colic vessels. At this point, the gastrocolic ligament is transected, entering the lesser sac (**FIGURE 9**). The gastrocolic ligament is then transected from medial to lateral with a monopolar scalpel or with a bipolar vessel-sealing device, leaving the greater omentum attached to the surgical specimen.
- With a combined traction of the transverse and descending colon, it is now easier to expose the splenocolic ligament, allowing for its transection with a monopolar scalpel or with a bipolar vessel-sealing device (**FIGURE 10**). The left colon is now fully mobilized all the way to the midline.

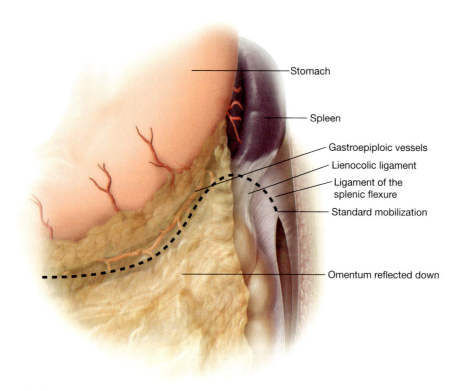

FIGURE 9 • The gastrocolic ligament will be transected, starting to the left side of the middle colic vessels and proceeding from medial to lateral and around the splenic flexure of the colon, under the spleen, and until the previous lateral dissection is reached.

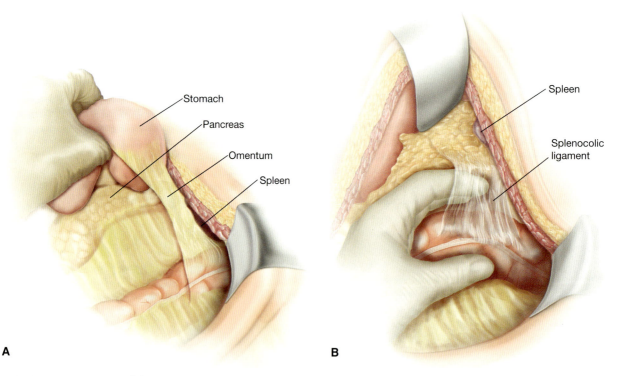

FIGURE 10 • **A-C,** Exposure of the splenocolic ligament. Once the medial and lateral dissection planes are connected, the splenocolic ligament is easily visualized and is now ready to be transected.

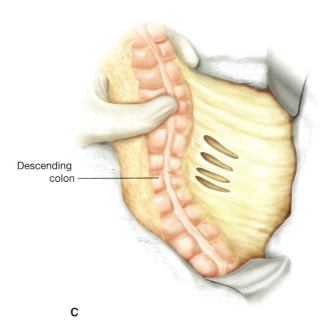

C

FIGURE 10 • *(continued)*

LATERAL TO MEDIAL DISSECTION AND VASCULAR ISOLATION

- The sigmoid and descending colon are retracted laterally, and the peritoneum is sectioned in a vertical direction from the ligament of Treitz to the pelvic inlet, anterior to the aortic artery pulse. At this time, it is possible to see a slight hematoma behind the root of colonic mesentery, product of the previously described lateral dissection. Sectioning the loose tissue in the mesentery root (under the superior hemorrhoidal vessels) communicates the medial and lateral dissection planes (**FIGURE 11**).

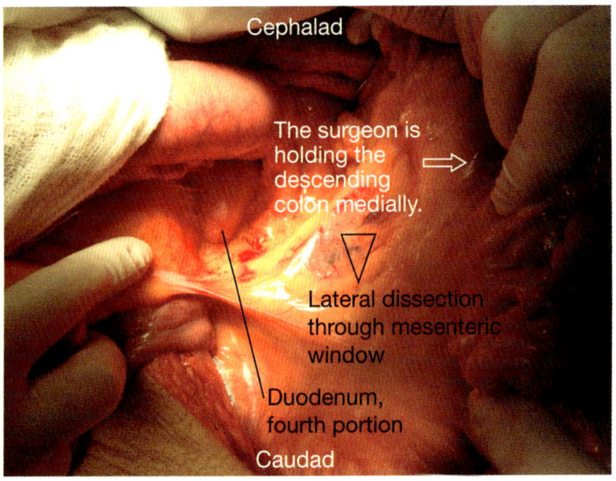

- Lateral to the fourth portion of the duodenum and below the inferior pancreatic border, it is possible to identify the inferior mesenteric vein. The inferior mesenteric vein is then ligated and divided (**FIGURE 12**).

- On this anatomic plane, one should continue sectioning the mesentery in a caudal direction, remaining 1 cm in front of the aorta in order to preserve the abdominal sympathetic plexus (hypogastric trunk). In almost every patient, it is possible to observe the hypogastric trunk as it traverses over the promontory. The hypogastric trunk divides into the right and left hypogastric trunk, which can be identified in the right and left posterolateral pelvis, respectively (**FIGURE 13**). These nerves must be preserved in order to avoid pelvic organs autonomic dysfunction postoperatively.

FIGURE 11 • Medial view of dissection. The fourth portion of duodenum is seen in the surgeon's left and the assistant is retracting the left colon laterally. Notice the slight hematoma behind the root of the colonic mesentery in the right, indicating the zone of previous dissection under the superior hemorrhoidal vessels.

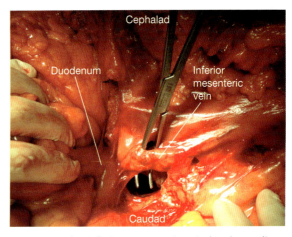

FIGURE 12 • The inferior mesenteric vein has been dissected and is ready to be transected.

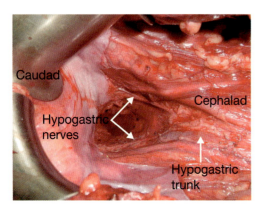

FIGURE 13 • View of sympathetic plexus and origin of the left and right hypogastric nerves.

- The IMA, identified a few centimeters above the aortic bifurcation, is ligated and divided. In proximal tumors, this division can be performed at the origin of left colic artery in order to preserve the IMA, sigmoidal vessels, and superior hemorrhoidal arteries intact. This ensures preservation of a well-vascularized sigmoid colon for the anastomosis, without compromising the oncological extent of the lymphadenectomy (**FIGURE 14**).

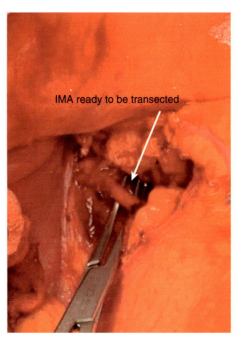

FIGURE 14 • The inferior mesenteric artery (IMA) has been carefully dissected and is ready to be transected.

COLON EXTRACTION AND ANASTOMOSIS

- At this time, a colon segment from the distal transverse colon down to the rectosigmoid junction could be taken to the midline and externalized through the laparotomy incision without tension (**FIGURE 15**). The transection points are chosen based on the oncologic margins needed, ensuring an adequate capture of the appropriate lymphovascular pedicles (**FIGURE 4**). In thin patients, it is possible to feel the pulse of the marginal artery near the points of transection. In more obese patients, or if the pulse is not palpable, the presence of a normal color in the colon is a good indicator of adequate perfusion on the colonic segments to be used for the anastomosis.
- If the extension of the resection allows preserving the sigmoid colon, a side-to-side transverse colon–sigmoid anastomosis with a mechanical stapler is advisable (**FIGURE 16A** and **B**). If the sigmoid colon has to be included in the resection specimen, then an end-to-end colorectal anastomosis with circular stapler via a transanal route must be performed (**FIGURE 16C** and **D**). It is critical that the anastomosis is tension-free; full mobilization of the splenic flexure ensures that this is possible.

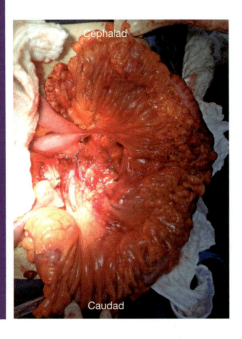

FIGURE 15 • The left colon is now fully mobilized and is exteriorized through the surgical incision. Full mobilization of the splenic flexure will ensure a tension-free anastomosis.

Chapter 15 LEFT HEMICOLECTOMY: OPEN TECHNIQUE   125

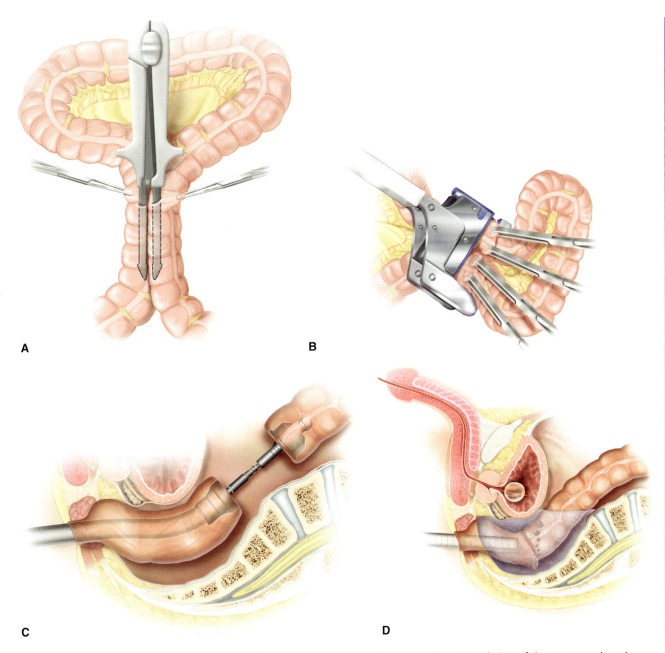

FIGURE 16 • Anastomosis. **A,** Side-to-side stapled transverse colon–sigmoid anastomosis. **B,** Completion of the anastomosis and resection of the left colon specimen with a thoracoabdominal (TA) stapler. **C,** End-to-end stapled colorectal anastomosis. **D,** Completed colorectal anastomosis tested under water. Air bubbles identified during insufflation of the anastomosis would indicate an anastomotic leak.

FINAL REVIEW AND CLOSURE OF THE PERITONEAL CAVITY

- Once the anastomosis is completed, the surgical bed must be reviewed to identify and control small bleeding retroperitoneal points, which are frequent. The anastomosed colon is left in the retroperitoneum. The gap in the posterior peritoneum is closed with a running absorbable suture. The rest of the abdominal cavity is checked, the surgical pads are counted, and the abdominal cavity is closed in the usual way.

SECTION II SURGERY OF THE COLON, APPENDIX, RECTUM, AND ANUS

PEARLS AND PITFALLS

Patient position	An improper position with hip flexion will make it difficult to maneuver during the whole procedure. Make sure the patient's thighs are completely horizontal.
Retroperitoneal fascia misidentification	This is a critical step in this operation. The section of the lateral peritoneum must be located close to the colon to identify the retroperitoneal and fusion fascias.
Identification of the left ureter and other retroperitoneal structures	The left ureter must be kept behind retroperitoneal fascia to avoid injuries. If you have to resect the left ureter (for T4 tumors), the ureter must be identified and repaired.
Splenic flexure mobilization	It is usually the most challenging step of this operation. It must be done with patience, good lighting, and using the dual (medial and lateral) approach previously described.
Tension-free anastomosis	Full mobilization of the splenic flexure is critical for a tension-free anastomosis. Anastomotic tension can lead to anastomotic leaks.

POSTOPERATIVE CARE

- Fluid resuscitation with Ringer lactate to maintain a urinary output of 0.5 to 1 mL/kg/h without overhydration.
- Pain control with patient-controlled analgesia or epidural analgesia. Avoid use of opioids as much as possible.
- Early oral intake and patient mobilization.
- Early removal of bladder catheter (24 hours after surgery).
- Venous thrombosis prophylaxis according to guidelines.
- Routine use of nasogastric tube is not recommended.
- No postoperative antibiotics are needed.

OUTCOMES

- The patient's prognosis depends on the tumor staging, which is determined by the histopathologic study of the specimen (pTNM).[7]
- Some patients will require adjuvant chemotherapy according to the tumor stage.[8]

COMPLICATIONS

- Surgical site infection
- Hematomas
- Anastomotic leak
- Peritonitis
- Prolonged postsurgical ileus
- Incisional hernia

REFERENCES

1. Otchy D, Hyman N, Simmang C, et al. Practice parameters for colon cancer. *Dis Colon Rectum.* 2004;47:1269-1284.
2. Weimann A, Braga M, Harsany L, et al. ESPEN guidelines on enteral nutrition: surgery including organ transplantation. *Clin Nutr.* 2006;25: 224-244.
3. Zhu QD, Zhang QY, Zeng QQ, et al. Efficacy of mechanical bowel preparation with polyethylene glycol in prevention of postoperative complications in elective colorectal surgery: a meta-analysis. *Int J Colorectal Dis.* 2010;25(2):267-275.
4. Fry DE. Colon preparation and surgical site infection. *Am J Surg.* 2011;202(2):225-232.
5. Ramírez JM, Blasco JA, Roig JV, et al. Enhanced recovery in colorectal surgery: a multicentre study. *BMC Surg.* 2011;11:9.
6. Makio M. *Laparoscopic Colorectal Cancer Surgery.* Springer Science+Business Media; 2017.
7. Link KH, Sagban TA, Mörschel M, et al. Colon cancer: survival after curative surgery. *Arch Surg.* 2005;390:83-93.
8. Van Cutsem E, Oliveira J. Colon cancer: ESMO clinical recommendations for diagnosis, adjuvant treatment and follow-up. *Ann Oncol.* 2008;19(suppl 2):ii29-ii30. doi:10.1093/annonc/mdn077

Chapter 16 Left Hemicolectomy: Laparoscopic Technique

Erik Paul Askenasy

DEFINITION

- A "left hemicolectomy" can be a nebulous term because three colonic segments lie in the left abdomen: the splenic flexure, the descending colon, and the sigmoid colon. At times, this can lead to consternation during surgical planning or even intraoperatively. Remembering that the location of the pathology guides the extent of colonic resection as well as the associated vascular and regional lymph nodes can provide much needed clarity. Additionally, understanding the vascular anatomy of the left colon and its common variations is essential for a well-vascularized, oncologically appropriate, and tension-free anastomosis.
- The left colon develops embryologically from the hindgut and contains three segments: the splenic flexure, the descending colon, and the sigmoid colon. The splenic flexure is located in the left upper quadrant and is supplied by antegrade flow from the left branch of the middle colic artery as well as retrograde flow from the left colic artery. Griffith's point is typically found in the splenic flexure and refers to the watershed area between these two arteries and represents a circulatory communication between the superior and inferior mesenteric arteries. The descending colon lies in between the sigmoid colon and the splenic flexure and is supplied by the left colic artery. Finally, the sigmoid colon is located in the left lower quadrant and is supplied by the sigmoidal arteries, branches of the inferior mesenteric artery (IMA) after the takeoff of the left colic artery. In this chapter, we will focus on the splenic flexure and the descending colon.
- A surgeon must be ready for "surprises" when entering the abdomen for a lesion in the descending colon, because there can be wide variation between the location of the target lesion as reported during flexible colonoscopy and the actual location found during surgery. The exact type and extent of resection will be dictated by the lymphovascular pedicles associated with the location of the target lesion (**FIGURE 1**).
- Laparoscopic surgery provides many advantages to the patient, including the following[1-4]:
  - Less pain
  - Faster return to work
  - Quicker return of bowel function
  - Lower risk of incisional hernias
  - Shorter hospital stay

DIFFERENTIAL DIAGNOSIS

- Common indications for laparoscopic left hemicolectomy:
  - Cancer of the splenic flexure or descending colon
  - Adenomatous polyps of the splenic flexure or descending colon not amenable to endoscopic resection
  - Diverticular disease and its sequelae, including colovesicular or colovaginal fistulas
  - Inflammatory bowel disease with stricture, bleeding, or fistula formation

PATIENT HISTORY AND PHYSICAL FINDINGS

- Most patients with early-stage colon cancer are asymptomatic, with lesions found on colonoscopy performed for screening purposes or secondary to a positive fecal occult blood test.

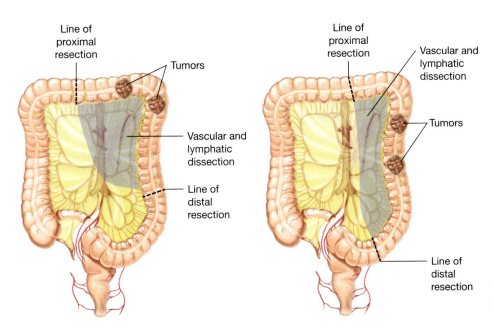

FIGURE 1 • Extent of lymphovascular pedicle resection based on the location of the primary tumor.

128 SECTION II SURGERY OF THE COLON, APPENDIX, RECTUM, AND ANUS

- Late-stage colon cancer can present with abdominal pain, unexplained weight loss, melena, iron deficiency anemia, or a change in bowel habits. Obstructive symptoms are typically secondary to circumferential tumors.
- Patients with uncomplicated diverticulitis report episodic pain in the left lower quadrant of the abdomen associated with fever, changes in bowel habits, and/or bloating.
- The spectrum of symptomatology for complex diverticulitis can be as benign as those for uncomplicated diverticulitis but can progress to localized or even generalized peritonitis.
- Inflammatory bowel disease can cause chronic inflammation leading to structuring of the colon with resultant changes in bowel function such as bloating or obstructive symptoms.
- Patients with neoplastic or inflammatory fistulae into adjacent organs, such as the bladder or vagina, can present with pneumaturia, fecaluria, or fecaloid vaginal discharge.
- A thorough family history of colon or rectal cancer, polyps, and/or other malignancies should be elicited.
- Physical examination should include the following:
  - Abdominal examination, focusing on localized tenderness, masses, and previous scars
  - Digital rectal examination to assess for blood as well as sphincter function

IMAGING AND OTHER DIAGNOSTIC STUDIES

- A full colonoscopy is essential. If a lesion is identified and it is suspicious for malignancy, the area should be tattooed distally to aid with intraoperative localization.
- In malignancy, a triple-phase computed tomography (CT) chest/abdomen/pelvis scan is performed to evaluate for metastases and locoregional extent of disease as well as to delineate the vascular anatomy. A preoperative carcinoembryonic antigen level should also be obtained as a baseline tumor marker for postoperative cancer surveillance purposes.
- In diverticulitis, a routine CT abdomen/pelvis scan with intravenous (IV) contrast is obtained.

SURGICAL MANAGEMENT

Preoperative Preparation

- Although preoperative bowel preparation is controversial, we routinely use a modified Nichol's prep (oral as well as antibiotic bowel prep), as it makes the bowel easier to handle and lowers postoperative infection rates.
- Immune boosting supplements are given.
- Chlorhexidine shower the evening prior to surgery.
- NPO after midnight except sugar-free clear liquids until 2 hours prior to surgery.
- Carbohydrate loading is performed at home as well as in the preoperative area.

- Premedication with acetaminophen.
- Alvimopan is administered in appropriate patients.
- Normothermia maintained with Bair Hugger (36-37 °C) perioperatively.
- Euglycemia maintained perioperatively.
- 2 to 3 g of Cefazolin (based on patient weight) and 500 mg of Flagyl are administered within 1 hour of skin incision.
- Hair clippers are used to clear the field.
- Abdominal blocks are administered (transversus abdominis + posterior rectus sheath, vs quadratus lumborum).
- Chlorhexidine is used for skin preparation; Betadine is used for perineal preparation.
- Narcotic sparing drips are prepared (dexmedetomidine, lidocaine, magnesium sulfate, ketamine, etc) according to institution-specific enhanced recovery protocols.
- Preoperative time-out and briefing.

Equipment and Instrumentation

- One Hasson trochar, one 12-mm port, and two 5-mm ports
- A 10-mm, 30 or 45° camera (may use 5 mm if quality of camera is acceptable)
- Atraumatic bowel gaspers, laparoscopic endoscissors, and a 5-mm energy device

Patient Positioning and Surgical Team Setup

- For pathology proximal to the mid-descending colon, the patient is placed on a supine position. Otherwise, the patient is placed on a lithotomy position.
- Both arms are tucked and padded. Wide silk tape is applied over two towels across the patient's chest in an "X" figure to secure the patient (**FIGURE 2B**).
- The patient is positioned such that the anus is easily accessible.
- The legs are placed in Allen stirrups, making sure the heels are flush against the base. Pressure points are padded posteriorly and laterally.
- The thighs are positioned parallel with the floor to minimize encroachment on the surgeon's right operating arm (**FIGURE 2C**).
- Draping is performed to allow for easy access to the perineum.
- The surgeon starts at the patient's right lower side with the assistant to their left. The assistant drives the camera while the surgeon uses both working ports (**FIGURE 2A**).
- A single monitor is needed and located on the patient's left side, across from the surgeon and at or slightly below eye level.
- All laparoscopic cables should come in from the patient's upper left side. All energy devices, Bovie, and suction should come in from the patient's upper right side. This setup prevents cluttering of the field and facilitates movement of the team around the table.

Chapter 16 **LEFT HEMICOLECTOMY: LAPAROSCOPIC TECHNIQUE** **129**

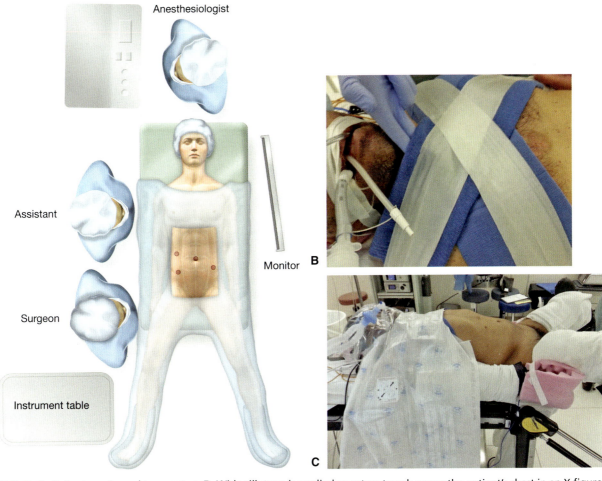

FIGURE 2 • **A,** Patient, ports, and team setup. **B,** Wide silk tape is applied over two towels across the patient's chest in an X figure to secure the patient. **C,** The thighs are positioned parallel with the floor to minimize encroachment on the surgeon's right operating arm.

PORT PLACEMENT AND OPERATIVE FIELD SETUP

- A Hasson trochar is placed at the umbilicus. This serves as the camera port as well as the extraction site. If the pathology is located in the distal descending colon, a 12-mm port is placed in the right lower quadrant and a 5-mm port is placed in the right midquadrant. If the pathology is more proximal, then the two right abdominal ports are shifted cephalad a few centimeters (**FIGURE 2A**).
- A 5-mm port can be placed in the left lower quadrant to aid with takedown of the white line of Toldt and with the splenic flexure mobilization.
- If the vascular pedicle is taken with a 5-mm energy device, then the 12-mm port can be changed to a 5-mm port.

OPERATIVE STEPS

- Although slight adjustments may be necessary based on the exact location of the lesion, laparoscopic surgery for lesions in the splenic flexure or in the descending colon should be standardized to maximize operative efficiency, following these sequential steps:
    - Placement of the omentum above the transverse colon
    - Transection of the inferior mesenteric vein (IMV)
    - Transection of the left colic artery or the IMA (depending on pathology location)
    - Medial to lateral dissection of the descending mesocolon
    - Transection of the gastrocolic ligament and entrance into the lesser sac
    - Transection of the white line of Toldt
    - Mobilization of the splenic flexure
    - Extracorporeal resection and anastomosis vs intracorporeal anastomosis depending on preference
    - Closure of abdominal wounds

Step 1: Placement of Omentum above the Transverse Colon

- The patient is placed in a steep Trendelenburg position and rotated to the right. Omental attachments to the pelvis are taken down with an energy device. The omentum is then placed over the transverse colon and into the left upper quadrant (**FIGURE 3**).

130   SECTION II SURGERY OF THE COLON, APPENDIX, RECTUM, AND ANUS

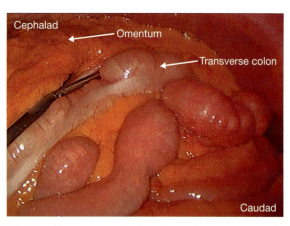

FIGURE 3 • The omentum is placed over the transverse colon.

Step 2: Transection of the Inferior Mesenteric Vein

- The IMV serves as the gateway to the retroperitoneum. Entering this plane in the correct location will facilitate the rest of the operation. The small bowel is swept to the right and the ligament of Treitz is exposed. If necessary, a Ray-Tec sponge can be placed into the abdomen to assist with exposure. It is important to have the circulating nurse mark all Ray-Tec sponges on the operating room (OR) board and account for them in the final count.
- The IMV, located lateral to the ligament of Treitz, and the left colic artery are identified (**FIGURE 4A**).
- Start by picking up the IMV just lateral to the ligament of Treitz and dissect under it with either hot scissors or an energy device.

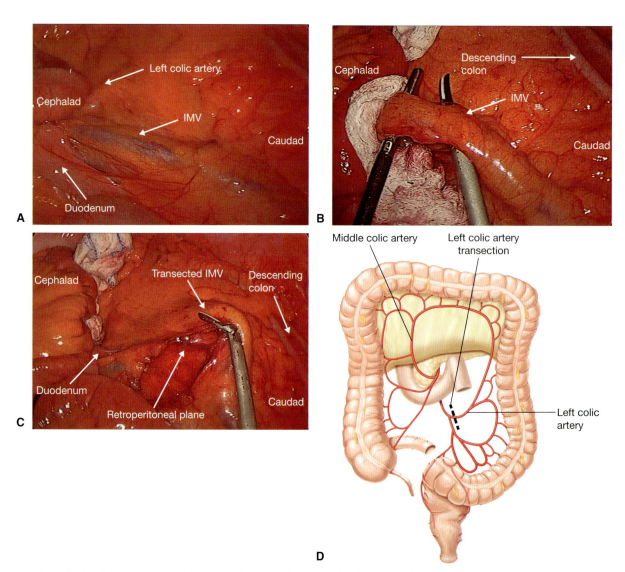

FIGURE 4 • **A,** The inferior mesenteric vein (IMV), located lateral to the ligament of Treitz, and the left colic artery are identified. **B,** The IMV is transected by the ligament of Treitz with an energy device. **C,** The transected IMV is retracted anteriorly and the retroperitoneal plane is created. **D,** The bare area of mesentery between the left colic artery and the middle colic artery distribution. Care must be taken to avoid injuring the marginal artery. In splenic flexure lesion cases, the left colic is transected at its origin from the inferior mesenteric artery (*dotted line*).

- Encircle the IMV and transect it with either a stapler or an energy device at the inferior border of the pancreas (**FIGURE 4B**).
- Lift up on the cut IMV and begin exposure of the retroperitoneal plane (**FIGURE 4C**).
- There is a "bare area" of mesentery between the left colic artery and the middle colic artery. Using an energy device, take this mesentery 1 cm from the lateral edge of the duodenum as far lateral as it is safe. Care must be taken here to avoid angling up toward the colon and risk injuring the marginal artery (**FIGURE 4D**).

Step 3: Transection of the Left Colic Artery or the Inferior Mesenteric Artery

- Proceeding with the dissection caudally, the left colic artery can be readily identified branching off the IMA. For splenic flexure lesions, transection of the left colic artery at its origin of the IMA using an energy device or stapler provides an adequate lymphovascular pedicle (**FIGURES 4D** and **5A**).
- Lesions located in descending colon frequently require inclusion of the sigmoid in the specimen, necessitating a high IMA transection to perform an adequate lymphadenectomy.
- In these patients, the mesodescending colon is dissected caudally until the left colic artery is appreciated and the retroperitoneal plane is created.
- The groove in between the superior hemorrhoidal artery (SHA) and the left iliac artery is identified. The surgeon elevates the SHA and incises the peritoneum under it using hot scissors or an energy device.
- The avascular retroperitoneal plane is swept down bluntly and the left ureter and gonadal vessels are identified and pushed posteriorly into the retroperitoneum. Care is taken to avoid injury to any nerves (hypogastric sympathetic plexus) in this area and they are swept down off the mesocolon. This retroperitoneal dissection plane is carried in a cephalad direction until all that remains between the superior and inferior dissections is the IMA.
- Lifting up on the IMA and its terminal branches, the SHA and the left colic artery will form what appears to be a letter "T" (**FIGURE 5A**). The IMA is then transected at its origin off the aorta with a vascular load stapler or can be taken with an energy device per surgeon preference (**FIGURE 5B**).

Step 4: Medial to Lateral Dissection of the Descending Mesocolon

- The retroperitoneal plane, dissection of which was initiated during the IMV transection step, is now easily accessible. The surgeon completes dissection of this space, avascular plane, located between Gerota fascia posteriorly and the descending mesocolon anteriorly, by holding the mesocolon up with a grasper while pushing the retroperitoneum down bluntly with an energy device (**FIGURE 6**). If needed, an additional 5-mm port is placed in the right upper quadrant for the assistant to help retract the mesocolon anteriorly.
- The retroperitoneal plane is continued until the abdominal wall is reached laterally and until the splenic flexure reached superiorly. The inferior extent of the retroperitoneal dissection depends on the location of the pathology. For lesions at the splenic flexure where the IMA has been left intact, the retroperitoneal dissection continues distally until further dissection is prohibited by the IMA. For lesions at the distal descending colon, where the IMA has been transected, the dissection continues until the pelvic inlet is reached.
- Care much be taken when dissecting cranially in the retroperitoneal plane to avoid dissecting inferior to the pancreas. The pancreas should be left in the retroperitoneal space and the

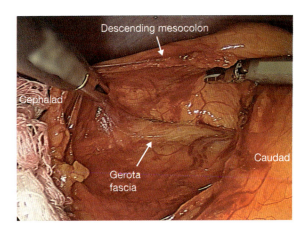

FIGURE 6 • Completion of the medial to lateral dissection. The dissection proceeds in the plane located between the descending mesocolon anteriorly and Gerota fascia posteriorly.

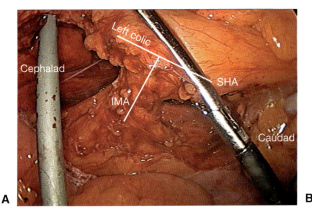
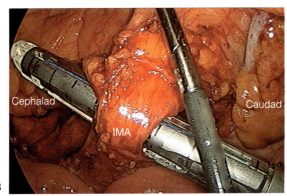

FIGURE 5 • **A,** The "letter T." The inferior mesenteric artery (IMA) and its terminal branches, the superior hemorrhoidal artery (SHA) and the left colic artery, form what looks like a letter T. **B,** High IMA transection with linear vascular load stapler.

mesocolon should be dissected off on the anterior aspect of the pancreatic tail. If done correctly, the lesser sac space is entered and full mobilization of the splenic flexure is facilitated.

Step 5: Transection of the Gastrocolic Ligament and Entrance to the Lesser Sac

- The transverse colon is retracted downward and the stomach is retracted superiorly, exposing the gastrocolic ligament. The gastrocolic ligament is then transected medially with an energy device until the lesser sac is entered.
- Transection of the gastrocolic ligament then proceeds along the distal transverse colon until the splenic flexure is reached (**FIGURE 6**). Care must be taken to avoid inadvertent injury to the colon.

Step 6: Transection of the White Line of Toldt

- The descending colon is now only attached to the lateral abdominal wall by the lateral peritoneal attachments (the white line of Toldt). Medial retraction of the descending colon allows for good exposure of these lateral peritoneal attachments.
- Standing on the right side of the table, the surgeon then takes down the white line of Toldt using hot scissors.
- Alternatively, the surgeon can move in between the patient's legs, place a 5-mm port in the left lower quadrant, and transect the white line of Toldt moving up the left gutter, until reaching the splenic flexure of the colon.

Step 7: Splenic Flexure Mobilization

- The splenic flexure is now encountered. The patient is placed on a reverse Trendelenburg position, helping bring the splenic flexure into view.
- The surgeon and the assistant retract the splenic flexure inferiorly and medially, exposing the splenocolic and phrenocolic ligaments. These ligaments are then transected with a 5-mm energy device (**FIGURE 7**).
- If full mesocolic dissection above the pancreas was performed previously, this can significantly help simplify this occasionally taxing step.
- The splenic flexure and descending colon are now completely free of any attachments and fully mobilized.

Step 8: Extracorporeal Resection and Anastomosis

- The pneumoperitoneum is evacuated and a 4- to 5-cm midline incision is made, centering on the Hasson trochar site at the level of the umbilicus.
- A small Alexis retractor is placed to protect the wound from infection and oncologic contamination. The colon is delivered into the operating field (**FIGURE 8A**). There should be no tension along mesenteric structures during the delivery of the specimen.
- The mesentery of the proximal and distal colon segment is taken in between clamps or with an energy device to the colonic wall. To ensure a well-vascularized anastomosis, the clamp is briefly taken off the marginal artery on the proximal colon side to ensure pulsatile flow or intraoperative fluorescein testing can also be used.
- The proximal and distal margins are circumferentially cleared of excess fat and Kocher clamps are placed on the proximal and distal margins of the resection.

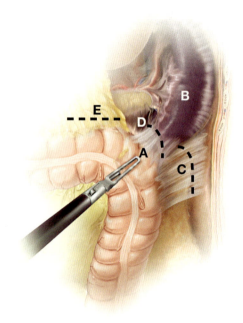

FIGURE 7 • Mobilization of the splenic flexure. The phrenocolic *(C)*, splenocolic *(D)*, and gastrocolic *(E)* ligaments are transected. A, splenic flexure of the colon; B, spleen.

- A no. 10 blade scalpel is used to transect the proximal and distal colon and the specimen is passed off the field. Bleeding mucosal edges should be noted in the proximal and distal colonic segments.
- Two Allis clamps are used to hold the proximal and distal colonic segments up. Using an Asepto and a poole sucker, the open colon ends are irrigated, suctioned, and cleaned of debris as needed.
- The anastomosis is fashioned in a single layer with a running double-armed 4-0 Maxon suture and placed back into the abdomen (**FIGURE 8B**).
- Once the anastomosis is delivered back into the abdominal cavity, the Alexis retractor is twisted and tied with umbilical tape around the Hasson port and the abdomen is re-insufflated to inspect the anastomosis (**FIGURE 8C**).
- The omentum is placed over the anastomosis. Closure of the mesenteric defect is not routinely performed.
- If a 12-mm right lower quadrant port was used, this is closed with an inlet closure device, the 5-mm ports are taken out under direct visualization, and the pneumoperitoneum is evacuated.

Step 9: Closure of Abdominal Wounds

- Gown and gloves are changed in an effort to prevent wound infections.
- Four clean towels are used to square off the surgical field.
- Separate closing instruments, suction, and Bovie tip are used.
- The abdominal fascia is closed with absorbable suture and the skin is closed with staples.

Chapter 16 LEFT HEMICOLECTOMY: LAPAROSCOPIC TECHNIQUE

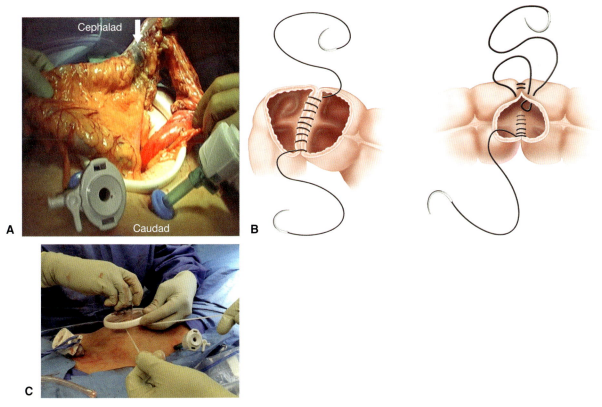

FIGURE 8 • **A,** Extracorporeal mobilization of the colon. Notice the tattooed target area in the splenic flexure of the colon (*arrow*). **B,** Extracorporeal hand-sewn, end-to-end anastomosis. **C,** Once the anastomosis is delivered back into the abdominal cavity, the Alexis retractor is twisted and tied with umbilical tape around the Hasson port and the abdomen is reinsufflated to inspect the anastomosis.

PEARLS AND PITFALLS

Preoperative imaging	■ Carefully review the CT scan as well as the colonoscopy report to determine whether the patient can be in a supine or lithotomy position. ■ Determine if ureteral stent placement will be necessary.
Positioning	■ Lithotomy position: Make sure that the legs are well padded to avoid injury to the lateral peroneal nerves.
Operative technique	■ The IMV at the ligament of Treitz is the "gateway" to the retroperitoneum. ■ Medial to lateral dissection of the retroperitoneal plane. ■ Sweep ureter and gonadal vessels into the retroperitoneum. ■ Identify the letter T before IMA or left colic artery transection. ■ Facilitate splenic flexure takedown by placing a 5-mm left lower quadrant port and by standing in between the legs. ■ Make sure to free splenic flexure from all attachments to ensure full mobilization of the descending colon; this will ensure a tension-free anastomosis.
Pitfall: avoiding injury to the marginal artery	■ Once the IMV has been transected, the mesenteric bare area travels superiorly and medially about 1 cm from the lateral edge of duodenum until the middle colic is appreciated. Resist the temptation to continue toward the colon wall, resulting in injury to the marginal artery.
Pitfall: leaving retroperitoneal structures attached to the colonic mesentery	■ A common pitfall is to perform the retroperitoneal dissection one layer too deep, thereby leaving retroperitoneal structures (tail of the pancreas, left ureter, and gonadal vessels) attached to dorsal surface of the colonic mesentery. This could lead to serious injury of these structures while transecting the mesocolon. Additionally, this will significantly limit the mobility of the colon, which may result in anastomotic tension.

SECTION II SURGERY OF THE COLON, APPENDIX, RECTUM, AND ANUS

Pitfall: floppy descending or sigmoid colon	▪ The lateral and splenic attachments are left for last. This allows the colon to be tethered up to the abdominal wall. If this colon still is not cooperative, place a 5-mm port in the right upper quadrant for the assistant to elevate the colon.
Pitfall: leaving the peritoneum of the lateral abdominal wall on the colon	▪ Another location where it is easy to enter the wrong plane is during the takedown of the lateral colon attachments. ▪ The correct plane is immediately adjacent to the colon wall; stay medially during this phase of the dissection.

POSTOPERATIVE CARE

- An enhanced recovery after surgery pathway is used, which includes the following:
  - Deep vein thrombosis (DVT) prophylaxis with Lovenox starting in the morning of postoperative day (POD) 1
  - No additional antibiotics are required.
  - Pain control:
    - Tylenol scheduled q6h (first dose in the OR); maximum dose: 4 g/d
    - Robaxin scheduled q6h, starting in the post anesthesia care unit (PACU)
    - Although nonsteroidal anti-inflammatory drug use is debatable, Naproxen BID scheduled if creatinine allows
    - Gabapentin TID prn
    - Dilaudid 0.3 mg IV q3 hour prn
  - Alvimopan (Entereg) twice a day until return of bowel function.
  - Only labs needed are hemoglobin/hematocrit (H/H) and basic metabolic panel on POD1 unless clinically indicated.
  - Diet.
    - Patient leaves the OR without a nasogastric tube.
    - Okay for full liquid diet after leaving PACU.
    - Advance diet to soft diet on POD1 unless bloated.
    - Patient does not need to pass gas or have a bowel movement prior to advancing diet.
    - SLIV POD1 if doing well.
  - Encourage early ambulation—POD0 when arrives to floor.
  - Foley: If placed, remove at the end of case or POD1
  - Discharge: For patients that had surgery in the morning with stable vitals, examination, and labs, we have been sending them home that evening regardless of whether bowel function has returned. Otherwise, discharge on POD1 or POD2.

OUTCOMES

- Laparoscopic surgery leads to improvements in short-term outcomes, including a faster recovery, shorter hospital stay, and less pain.
- There is no difference in oncologic outcomes between laparoscopic and open surgery.

COMPLICATIONS

- Ureter injury: prevented by clear visualization of the retroperitoneal plane.
- Sexual dysfunction (retrograde ejaculation): prevented by careful preservation of hypogastric sympathetic plexus located at the sacral promontory.
- Wound infection: decreased incidence by careful attention to surgical technique.
- DVT: prevented by initiating sequential compression device therapy prior to anesthetic induction and timely initiation of pharmacologic prophylaxis.

REFERENCES

1. Juo YY, Hyder O, Haider AH, et al. Is minimally invasive colon resection better than traditional approaches? First comprehensive national examination with propensity score matching. *JAMA Surg.* 2014;149(2):177-184.
2. Kuhry E, Schwenk W, Gaupset R, et al. Long-term outcome of laparoscopic surgery for colorectal cancer: a Cochrane systematic review of randomized controlled trials. *Cancer Treat Rev.* 2008;34(6):498-504.
3. Liang Y, Li G, Chen P, et al. Laparoscopic versus open colorectal resection for cancer: a meta-analysis of results of randomized controlled trials on recurrence. *Eur J Surg Oncol.* 2008;34(11):1217-1224.
4. Bennet CL, Stryker SJ, Ferreira MR, Adams J, Beart RW. The learning curve for laparoscopic colorectal surgery. Preliminary results from a prospective analysis of 1194 laparoscopic-assisted colectomies. *Arch Surg.* 1997;132(1):41-44.

Chapter 17

Left Hemicolectomy: Hand-Assisted Laparoscopic Technique

Kristen D. Donohue, Brendan F. Scully, and Daniel L. Feingold

DEFINITION

- Left hemicolectomy is defined as a segmental resection of the splenic flexure colon with its mesentery including the left colic artery and the left branch of the middle colic artery. This operation, most commonly performed for neoplasia is, in general terms, a mirror image of a right colectomy whereby the colon is mobilized and the mesentery is dissected out and transected, allowing exteriorization of the loop of colon. During left colectomy for cancer, the adjacent greater omentum is usually resected en bloc with the colon.
- The straight laparoscopic approach to splenic flexure lesions can be challenging, especially in cases with a large neoplasm, colonic obstruction, significantly elevated body mass index or difficult splenic flexure ("extreme" flexure). In these circumstances, the hand-assisted laparoscopic surgery (HALS) approach to left hemicolectomy may prove advantageous over a pure laparoscopic approach.
- HALS is a minimally invasive surgical approach that uses conventional laparoscopic-assisted (LA) surgery techniques with the addition of a hand-assist device (placed in the projected specimen extraction site) that allows for the introduction of a hand into the surgical field. HALS in colorectal surgery retains all of the same advantages of conventional LA surgery over open surgery, including less pain, faster recovery, lower incidence of wound complications, and reduction of cardiopulmonary complications, especially in the obese and in the elderly.
- Advantages of HALS over conventional LA colorectal surgery include:
  - Reintroduces tactile feedback into the field
  - Shorter learning curves; easier to teach
  - Shorter operative times and lower conversion to open rates
  - Higher utilization rates of minimally invasive surgery

PATIENT HISTORY AND PHYSICAL FINDINGS

- Prior surgical history can influence the approach to left colectomy
  - Prior colon resection
    - Previous colectomy may affect the remaining colonic blood supply as well as reach for the anastomosis and can influence the operative plan regarding what bowel segment will be used for the anastomosis.
  - Prior endoluminal stenting
    - Decompression of an obstructing tumor of the splenic flexure helps to avoid a two-stage approach to colectomy and facilitates HALS resection, but stenting can be associated with an inflammatory or desmoplastic reaction that can make the subsequent dissection difficult.
  - Extensive intra-abdominal surgery
    - Extensive or dense adhesions may prohibit a minimally invasive approach.
  - Prior gastric or bariatric surgery, in particular, can distort the anatomy and make for challenging dissection for left colectomy.
  - Prior abdominoplasty
    - May limit intra-abdominal domain afforded by the pneumoperitoneum and can jeopardize the ability to complete a laparoscopic left colectomy.
- Morbid obesity or an abundance of intra-abdominal adipose tissue may hinder a minimally invasive approach.

IMAGING AND OTHER DIAGNOSTIC STUDIES

- Contrast-enhanced cross-sectional imaging of the abdomen and pelvis, typically performed for cancer staging purposes, is useful for planning the surgery in terms of accurately localizing the tumor and determining the site of the hand port. Imaging can also alert the surgeon to a potentially difficult splenic flexure takedown (extreme flexure, significant colon looping, bulky colon neoplasia adjacent to the spleen, etc).
- Colonoscopy to evaluate the proximal colon. In addition, endoscopy permits accurate tumor localization with submucosal tattooing.

SURGICAL MANAGEMENT

Preoperative Planning

- Colonoscopy, pathology reports, and relevant cross-sectional imaging should be reviewed.
- Intraoperative carbon dioxide (CO_2) colonoscopy should be available in the operating room for localization purposes (if necessary) as well as for assessing the integrity of the anastomosis.
- Mechanical bowel preparation facilitates intraoperative colonoscopy in cases where preoperative localization fails and the addition of oral antibiotics to the preparation helps reduce postoperative infectious complications.
- In cases of neoplasia, the operative plan should be to perform a cancer operation regardless of whether the colonoscopy biopsies fail to demonstrate malignancy.
- In general, segmental splenic flexure resection does not require left ureteral stenting, but this may be helpful in certain circumstances.
- Enhanced recovery protocols, used routinely for elective colectomy (described elsewhere in this textbook), and a discussion regarding colonic perfusion assessment with fluorescence angiography are beyond the scope of this chapter.

Positioning

- For HALS left hemicolectomy, the authors prefer to use padded split-leg position and rely on elastic wraps to secure the patient's legs to the operating room table (**FIGURE 1**). This allows the surgeon or an assistant to stand between the patient's legs during the procedure and facilitates intraoperative colonoscopy. Split-leg positioning may be preferable to

135

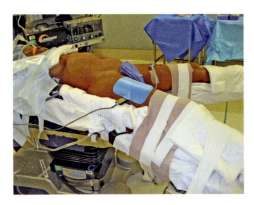

- stirrups as the legs are maintained in a neutral position and pressure-related nerve injuries are minimized.
- The patient should be secured to the operating room table with a chest strap and a nonslip traction pad, as extreme positioning is often necessary.
- The right arm should be padded and tucked in a neutral position to allow access to the patient.
- An orogastric tube helps keep the stomach decompressed during the operation.

FIGURE 1 • Patient positioning. We prefer a split-leg position to allow the surgeon to operate from between the legs and to minimize potential leg injuries.

TECHNIQUES

ENTERING THE ABDOMEN AND INITIAL EXPOSURE

- A Pfannenstiel or lower midline incision is created for hand-port placement (**FIGURE 2A**). A 5-mm camera port is placed in the supraumbilical midline, and 5-mm working ports are placed in the right lower quadrant and left lower quadrant positions.
- In cases where the IMA pedicle is not dissected, placing the hand port in the supraumbilical position facilitates dissection, extraction, and anastomosis (**FIGURE 2B**). The camera port in these cases is positioned caudal and to the left of the umbilicus. When utilizing a supraumbilical hand port, the surgeon typically stands at the patient's right hip and places the left hand through the hand access port and uses the energy device introduced through one of the 5-mm working ports. With this approach, the assistant usually stands between the legs to control the camera and retracts using one of the 5-mm working ports.
- In patients with prior abdominal surgery, laparoscopic access can be created by cut-down or Veress needle technique in a presumed safe location. This allows laparoscopic evaluation of abdominal wall adhesions, which can be lysed prior to creating the hand-port access. Alternatively, adhesions can be lysed in an open fashion through the hand-port incision; the surgeon's ability to perform adhesiolysis in this fashion may be limited. Inability to lyse these adhesions can jeopardize the laparoscopic approach.
- The patient is placed in steep Trendelenburg with the table tilted right side down.
- The greater omentum is draped over the transverse colon and liver. The small bowel is retracted out of the pelvis and toward the right upper quadrant of the abdomen, exposing the sigmoid and left colon mesentery (**FIGURE 3**).

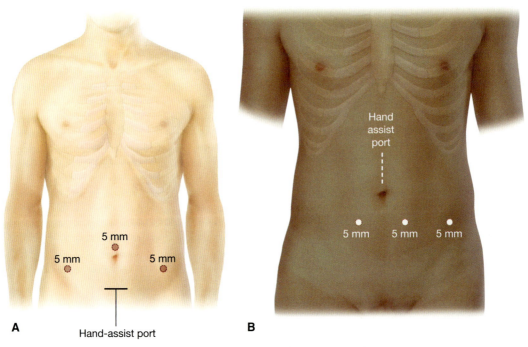

FIGURE 2 • A and B, Port placement options.

Chapter 17 LEFT HEMICOLECTOMY: HAND-ASSISTED LAPAROSCOPIC TECHNIQUE 137

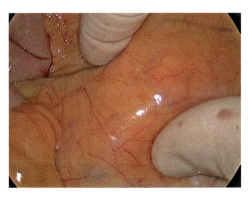

FIGURE 3 • Left colon mesentery.

- A laparotomy pad placed intra-abdominally through the hand port aids in the retraction of the small bowel and in maintaining exposure. This also facilitates cleaning the scope without having to remove the scope from the abdomen. To reduce the chance of a retained pad, a hemostat is placed on the surgeon's gown, signifying that a pad is in the belly. When the pad is removed (typically just prior to specimen extraction), the hemostat is removed from the gown. If the surgeon goes to remove their gown with the hemostat still in place, the team is alerted that there may be a retained foreign body in the patient.
- A 30° angled scope is used at the discretion of the surgeon. Angled scopes enable the surgeon to look over the horizon (particularly useful during splenic flexure takedown) and improves laparoscopic access to the field by allowing the scope to be held away from the dissection.
- While surgeons develop a personalized step-wise approach to performing this operation, the specific order of the steps in any given patient's operation is influenced by the anatomy and the difficulty of the operation.

MESENTERIC DISSECTION, MEDIAL TO LATERAL

- The sigmoid colon and its mesentery are mobilized in order to permit a tension-free extracorporeal extraction and the creation of a tension-free anastomosis. In cases where this degree of mobilization is not required, these steps may be omitted.
- The surgeon stands at the patient's right hip, and the assistant stands at the right shoulder holding the camera inserted through the umbilical port. The inferior mesenteric artery (IMA) pedicle is elevated with the surgeon's right thumb and index finger (**FIGURE 4**) and is retracted toward the patient's left hip. The surgeon uses an energy device through the right lower quadrant port to dissect dorsal to the IMA and its superior hemorrhoidal terminal branch (**FIGURE 5**). The aortic bifurcation, common iliac arteries, and sacral promontory are helpful anatomic landmarks and are appreciated prior to starting the dissection. The peritoneum beneath the pedicle is scored to the level of the sacral promontory.

- Palpating the left common iliac artery located underneath the mesosigmoid and the sacral promontory helps orient the surgeon (**FIGURE 6**).
- Care is taken to preserve the hypogastric nerves, located dorsal to the superior hemorrhoidal vessels, intact.
- The retromesenteric plane is developed by sweeping the retroperitoneum down (dorsally) and elevating the mesentery upward toward the anterior abdominal wall (**FIGURE 6**). The plane is developed laterally toward the side wall, superiorly over Gerota fascia and toward the tail of the pancreas, and

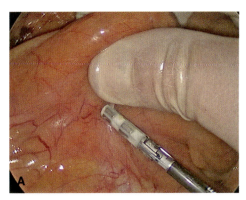

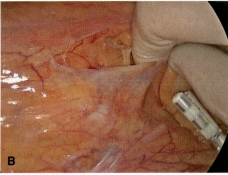

FIGURE 4 • Grasping the IMA pedicle. The IMA and its terminal branch, the superior hemorrhoidal artery, are elevated off the retroperitoneum with the surgeon's right thumb and index finger.

FIGURE 5 • A and B, Scoring the peritoneum to enter the retromesenteric plane. The plane of dissection proceeds along the dorsal aspect of the superior hemorrhoidal vessels.

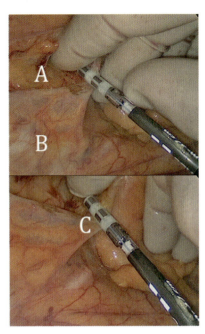

FIGURE 6 • Palpating the right (A) and left (B) common iliac as well as the sacral promontory (C) helps orient the surgeon.

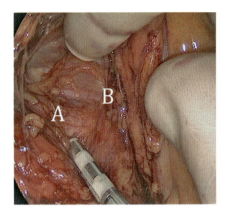

FIGURE 7 • Retromesenteric dissection. The left ureter (A) and the left gonadal vessels (B) are identified and preserved intact in the retroperitoneum.

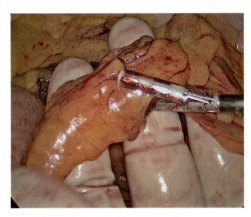

FIGURE 8 • Dividing left colic artery.

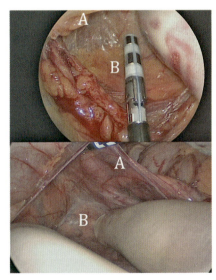

FIGURE 9 • Further retromesenteric dissection. This dissection is carried along the plane located between the mesocolon (A) and Gerota fascia (B).

caudally toward the presacral space. As this is a bloodless embryological tissue plane of dissection, bleeding is usually caused being in the wrong plane of dissection either into the overlaying mesentery (anteriorly) or into the retroperitoneum (posteriorly). Recognizing that you are not in the actual embryonic fusion plane allows you to adjust the dissection and reenter the correct plane. The proper tissue plane is visualized as the transition between the two different fat planes of the mesocolon anteriorly, and the retroperitoneum (Gerota fascia) posteriorly.

- The left ureter and gonadal vessels are identified and preserved by sweeping these structures down into the retroperitoneum (**FIGURE 7**).
- With the hand supinated within the retromesenteric space, a mesenteric window is created between the main sigmoidal artery and the left colic artery. The takeoff of the left colic artery off the IMA is then divided with the energy device (**FIGURE 8**) while ensuring the left ureter is preserved in the retroperitoneum. Tumor localization should be confirmed (by intraoperative colonoscopy, if needed) prior to vessel ligation and committing to the resection.
- Once the left colic artery is transected, the retromesenteric space opens up, allowing further dissection in this plane laterally and cephalad. This dissection is carried along the plane located between the mesocolon and Gerota fascia (**FIGURE 9**).
- The patient is then placed in reverse Trendelenburg position with the table tilted right side down while the surgeon stands between the patient's legs and the assistant stands at the patient's right hip.
- The assistant holds the camera and, using an atraumatic grasper through the right-sided port, retracts the left transverse colon cephalad. The surgeon orients themselves by palpating the aorta and visualizing the ligament of Treitz (**FIGURE 10**). The surgeon, with the left hand in the abdomen and the energy device through the left-sided port, carefully enters the retromesenteric plane medial to the inferior mesenteric vein (IMV) by incising the peritoneum longitudinally along the dorsal aspect of the IMV (**FIGURE 11**).

Chapter 17 LEFT HEMICOLECTOMY: HAND-ASSISTED LAPAROSCOPIC TECHNIQUE   139

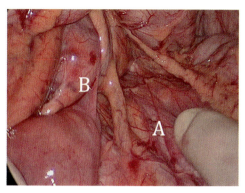

FIGURE 10 • Medial-to-lateral dissection at the IMV. The surgeon orients themselves by palpating the aorta *(A)* and visualizing the ligament of Treitz *(B)*.

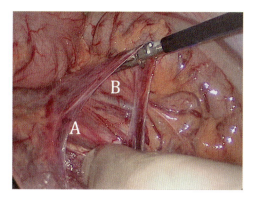

FIGURE 11 • Medial-to-lateral dissection at the IMV. Care is taken to avoid injuring the left ureter *(A)* and gonadal vessels *(B)*.

- Care is taken to avoid injury to the proximal small bowel in this dissection. Taking down the ligament of Treitz and opening up the paraduodenal recess should be done with cold laparoscopic scissors to prevent thermal injury to the proximal small bowel.
- The medial-to-lateral dissection at the IMV level is the cephalad extension of the medial-to-lateral plane that had been already dissected at the level of the IMA. Elevating the colon mesentery off the retroperitoneum allows the two retromesenteric spaces to meet. When mobilizing the plane at the IMV, care should be taken not to enter the plane too deeply as this can injure the ureter, gonadal bundle, or other retroperitoneal structures.
- The IMV is then divided with the energy device at the cephalad extent of the dissection.
- The retromesenteric plane is then further developed cephalad to the inferior edge of the pancreas and laterally over the left kidney toward the splenic flexure, effectively separating already the splenic flexure of the retroperitoneum. This will greatly facilitate the splenic flexure mobilization later during the operation.

SPLENIC FLEXURE MOBILIZATION

- The patient is then placed in an even steeper reverse Trendelenburg position; this delivers the plane of dissection closer to the hand port.
- The assistant retracts the greater omentum, and the surgeon's left hand applies countertraction to expose the bloodless plane between the omentum and the transverse colon (**FIGURE 12**). The omentum is released from the transverse colon and the lesser sac is entered at the midline. The dissection proceeds across the omentum and gastrocolic ligament proceeds laterally, as far as possible, exposing the splenocolic ligament (**FIGURE 13**). The splenocolic ligament is then transected with the energy device.
- In difficult splenic flexure releases, it is helpful to utilize alternating approaches across the lesser sac and up the left paracolic gutter (bidirectional approach). This dissection creates a knuckle in the splenic flexure anatomy that accentuates the remaining tethering attachments that require division.
- In cancer resections, the omentum adherent to the area of the cancer is resected en bloc.
- Care is taken to avoid injury to the short gastric vessels, stomach, pancreas, and spleen.

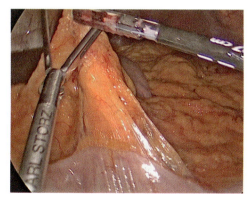

FIGURE 12 • Splenic flexure mobilization. The assistant retracts the greater omentum while the surgeon retracts the transverse colon.

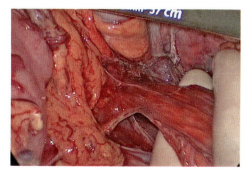

FIGURE 13 • Mobilization of the splenic flexure: exposure of the splenocolic ligament. This ligament will be transected with the energy device.

LATERAL TO MEDIAL DISSECTION

- The descending colon has already been mobilized during the medial-to-lateral dissection of the mesocolon as described previously, and now the colon is only tethered to the left gutter by the lateral peritoneal attachments. While the assistant retracts the colon by grasping an epiploic appendage medially, the surgeon releases the colon from the sidewall using the energy device (**FIGURE 14**). This dissection should immediately enter the retromesenteric dissection plane. Lateral dissection is continued superiorly until the lesser sac dissection is met and the splenic flexure is fully released.

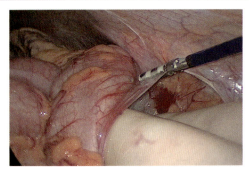

FIGURE 14 • Lateral to medial dissection.

DISSECTION OF THE TRANSVERSE COLON MESENTERY

- The surgeon's supinated left hand underneath the mesentery exposes a clear space in the transverse mesocolon at the inferior border of the pancreas. Opening this mesenteric window facilitates the dissection to release the left transverse mesocolon from its retroperitoneal attachment (**FIGURE 15**).
- The left branch of the middle colic artery is dissected out and divided at the base of the mesentery with the energy device. The anatomy of the middle colic artery is variable, and more than one branch may need to be taken. The left colon is now fully mobilized (**FIGURE 16**).

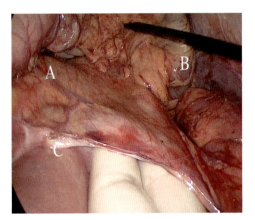

FIGURE 15 • Dissection of the transverse colon mesentery. The transverse colon mesentery along the inferior border of the pancreas (A) between the spleen (B) and the ligament of Treitz (C) is exposed.

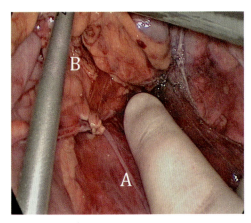

FIGURE 16 • Full mobilization of the left colon is achieved. After complete mobilization of the left colon to the midline, Gerota fascia (A) and the tail of the pancreas (B) can be visualized.

ASSESSMENT OF REACH

- Prior to exteriorization, the left upper quadrant is inspected and hemostasis is ensured. Each site of mesenteric vessel ligation is inspected as well.
- The intra-abdominal laparotomy pad is retrieved.
- The hand port is removed, and the colon is exteriorized through a wound protector.
- Appropriate levels of transection are identified and the colon is divided with a linear stapler in open fashion, per usual. The specimen is oriented by a stitch to aid pathologic evaluation and is delivered off the field.
- Reach is assessed and no tension should be appreciated. If needed, the hand port can be replaced and further mobilization can be performed.

ANASTOMOSIS

- The anastomosis is created in stapled or hand-sewn fashion in iso- or antiperistaltic orientation at the discretion of the surgeon (**FIGURE 17**).
- The authors advocate creating an omental pedicle laparoscopically (when possible) and draping this over the anastomosis.
- The mesenteric defect is broad and is not typically closed.
- Gentle, sequential anal dilation using standard EEA sizers can relax the anal sphincter complex in the setting of a colo-colonic anastomosis.

Chapter 17 LEFT HEMICOLECTOMY: HAND-ASSISTED LAPAROSCOPIC TECHNIQUE

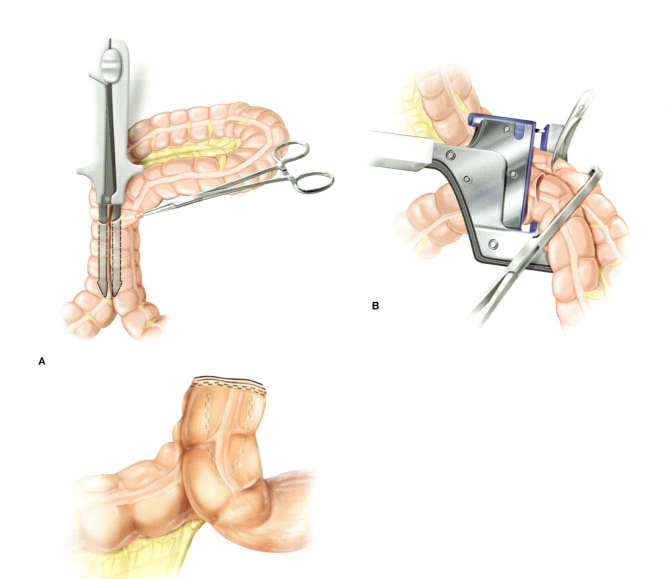

FIGURE 17 • Creating the colocolonic side-to-side anastomosis. **A,** A common channel is created in side-to-side fashion. **B,** The anastomosis is completed and the specimen is delivered. **C,** The completed anastomosis.

PEARLS AND PITFALLS

Inadequate reach	The splenic flexure is not completely released or the transverse mesocolon is not freed from the inferior border of pancreas. Rarely, the hepatic flexure may need to be released as well. If you cannot achieve adequate reach with a segmental resection, consider an extended right colectomy and utilize an ileocolic anastomosis.
Inability to exteriorize the colon	Persistent attachments to the retroperitoneum or omentum need to be taken down.
Inability to identify left ureter	Retromesenteric dissection too deep into the retroperitoneum or the ureter is adherent to the mesenteric side of the dissection. Find the ureter at the level of the left colic artery instead of at the IMA.

Tumor not confidently localized	Evaluate the sigmoid colon and proximal colon and perform on-table CO_2 colonoscopy, if needed.
Proximal colon ischemic after mesenteric division	Inadequate collateral colonic blood supply via the marginal artery requires further resection back to healthy colon.
Dissection not progressing	Place additional 5-mm working port(s) or convert to open procedure.
Poor access to the splenic flexure	Place the patient in even steeper reverse Trendelenburg and tilt the table left side up.
Splenic bleeding	Use the laparotomy pad to control the bleeding while the team prepares an energy device or absorbable hemostatic agents. Convert to open procedure if unable to achieve hemostasis.

POSTOPERATIVE CARE

- Enhanced recovery after surgery pathway recommendations are described elsewhere in this textbook.
- Remove the bladder catheter the morning after the operation to reduce the risk of urinary tract infection. These patients generally recover similarly to patients who have undergone right colectomy.
- Avoid immediate postoperative nasogastric tubes.
- Encourage early and progressive ambulation and pulmonary toilet.
- Utilize deep vein thrombosis prophylaxis.
- Trial regular diet intake as patients tolerate rather than waiting for flatus or the first bowel movement.
- Utilize multimodal analgesia by incorporating nonnarcotic medications (ketorolac, acetaminophen, etc) and regional blocks (transversus abdominis plane, erector spinae, rectus sheath, etc) to help reduce narcotic use and minimize the incidence and duration of postoperative ileus.

OUTCOMES

- Minimally invasive colectomy is associated with shorter in-hospital convalescence and less narcotic use compared with open surgery.[1]
- For cancer resection, laparoscopic colectomy oncologic outcomes are similar to those of open resection.[1-3]
- Hand-assisted colectomy, as compared with straight laparoscopy, shortens operative times without increasing length of hospital stay or narcotic use.[4]

- Oncologically, extended resections beyond a segmental colectomy do not significantly improve outcomes, although there is ongoing debate regarding the preferred approach.[5]

COMPLICATIONS

- Anastomotic dehiscence is a potential complication after any bowel anastomosis is created. This can be minimized by ensuring adequate blood supply and eliminating tension across the anastomosis.
- Extraction site wound infections can be minimized by using National Surgical Quality Improvement Program (NSQIP) approved protocols and wound protectors.

REFERENCES

1. The Clinical Outcomes of Surgical Therapy Study Group. A comparison of laparoscopically assisted and open colectomy for colon cancer. *N Engl J Med.* 2004;350(20):2050-2059.
2. Guillou PJ, Quirke P, Thorpe H, et al. Short-term endpoints of conventional versus laparoscopic-assisted surgery in patients with colorectal cancer (MRC CLASICC trial): multicentre, randomized controlled trial. *Lancet.* 2005;365:1718-1726.
3. Jayne DG, Thorpe HC, Copeland J, et al. Five-year follow-up of the Medical Research Counsel CLASICC trial of laparoscopically assisted versus open surgery for colorectal cancer. *Br J Surg.* 2010;97:1638-1645.
4. Marcello PW, Fleshman JW, Milsom JW, et al. Hand-assisted laparoscopic vs. laparoscopic colorectal surgery. A multicenter, prospective, randomized trial. *Dis Colon Rectum.* 2008;51:818-828.
5. Manceau G, Alves A, Meillat H, Benhaïm L, et al. What is the optimal elective colectomy for splenic flexure cancer: end of the debate? *Dis Colon Rectum.* 2022;65:55-65.

Chapter 18

Left Hemicolectomy: Robotic-Assisted Technique

Navin Rajindra Changoor and Mark Soliman

DEFINITION

- Robotic-assisted left hemicolectomy involves resection of the distal transverse, splenic flexure, and descending and sigmoid colon with the assistance of a robotic surgery platform such as the da Vinci system. Robotic-assisted approaches allow the patient to have reduced pain, faster return of bowel function, reduced length of hospital stay, lower overall cost of care, improved cosmesis, lower hernia rates, and quicker return to work.[1-3]

DIFFERENTIAL DIAGNOSIS

- Patient undergoing a left hemicolectomy may have any one of the following:
  - Colon cancer
  - Diverticulitis
  - Crohn disease
  - Diverticular bleeding

PATIENT HISTORY AND PHYSICAL FINDINGS

- Symptoms of bowel obstruction such as nausea, vomiting, distension, constipation, and obstipation should prompt urgent intervention.
- Patients should be evaluated for any comorbidities that would need optimization prior to surgery.
- In obese patients, a thorough pulmonary evaluation should be performed to anticipate potential underlying medical conditions, such as chronic obstructive pulmonary disease, that could complicate ventilation during Trendelenburg positioning.
- Constitutional symptoms of unexpected weight loss or loss of appetite may be early signs of metastatic disease and may prompt further workup.
- Abdominal examination with a focus on abdominal obesity, abdominal folds, and previous scars is important as this will aid in operative planning.

IMAGING AND OTHER DIAGNOSTIC STUDIES

- Computed tomography of the chest, abdomen, and pelvis should be obtained for tumor staging prior to cancer operations.

- Preoperative complete colonoscopy and possible tattooing can confirm tumor location and exclude secondary pathology.

SURGICAL MANAGEMENT

Key Steps

- Position the patient
- Access the abdomen, establish pneumoperitoneum, and place ports
- Position the small bowel
- Initiate dissection
- Identify, skeletonize, and divide the inferior mesenteric artery (IMA)/inferior mesenteric vein (IMV)
- Splenic flexure
- Lateral mobilization
- Divide the rectosigmoid colon
- Select proximal transection point and divide the mesentery
- Assess perfusion
- Colorectal anastomosis
- Leak test

Preoperative Planning

- Enhanced recovery after surgery (ERAS; described in Chapter 52) protocols/pathways have contributed significantly to preoperative optimization. ERAS includes prehabilitation, nutritional supplements, patient education, and inclusion of a mechanical bowel preparation with oral antibiotics.

Positioning

- The patient is placed in a low lithotomy position with padded stirrups and arms tucked at the sides. The patient's legs are placed in Allen stirrups with the knees at 100° to 120° of flexion to avoid conflict between the thighs and the robotic arms and instruments. All extremities are padded to avoid neurovascular injuries.
- The assistant surgeon should be on the right side of the patient and can help with retraction, suctioning, and irrigation as needed.
- The scrub tech is also on the right side next to the assistant surgeon.

DOCKING

- The Xi robotic cart can move the robotic arms 360° around the center and can be easily docked to either side of the patient but should ideally be docked on the left side. Targeting enables alignment and proper position of the arms.

TROCAR PLACEMENT

- The abdomen is entered via an optical trocar entry technique in the right upper quadrant. The robotic ports are placed in a linear arrangement along a line between the left upper and right lower quadrant (see **FIGURE 1**). Each port is placed equidistant from each other about a hand's breadth from each other to avoid instrument conflict. This line can be adjusted to move more vertically or more horizontally depending on different colon anatomy, which can help facilitate splenic flexure reach.

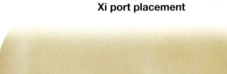
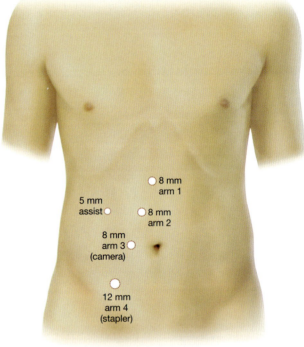

FIGURE 1 • Port placement for the da Vinci Xi robot.

POSITIONING THE SMALL BOWEL

- The patient is positioned in a Trendelenburg position and with the left side up to allow for gravity assist and proper exposure of the left colon and its mesentery. The small bowel is swept out of the pelvis to expose the root of the left colon mesentery. The rectosigmoid colon is retracted anteriorly to tent up the entire mesentery in a straight line (**FIGURE 2**).

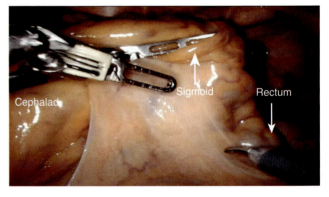

FIGURE 2 • Sigmoid colon mesentery tented upward.

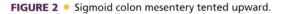

DISSECTION

- Using a monopolar scissors, the peritoneum overlying the base of the mesentery is scored at the peritoneal groove on the right side of the lateral mesorectum at the sacral promontory, along the inferior border of the superior hemorrhoidal vessels and up to the inferior border of the IMA (**FIGURE 3**). If the dissection proceeds in the correct plane, the CO_2 pneumoperitoneum will aid in the dissection (pneumodissection) and will help to identify the avascular embryological tissue planes and separate the colonic mesentery from the retroperitoneum planes.
- Using the monopolar scissors or vessel sealer, the plane between the sigmoid/left colon mesentery and the

Chapter 18 LEFT HEMICOLECTOMY: ROBOTIC-ASSISTED TECHNIQUE   145

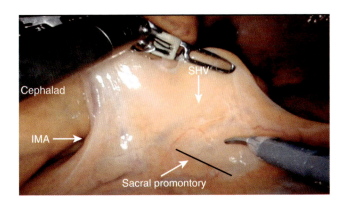

retroperitoneal structures is developed bluntly from medial to lateral. This dissection continues upward until the inferior mesenteric artery and vein are completely mobilized, the left ureter is identified close to the mesenteric root (inferior to the IMA, the left ureter is located in the retroperitoneum medially to the left gonadal vessels), the hypogastric nerves are identified and preserved, and the lateral peritoneal reflection is reached.

FIGURE 3 • Preparing to initiate dissection along the peritoneal groove over the sacral promontory (black line). IMA, inferior mesenteric artery; SHV, superior hemorrhoidal vessel.

IMA/IMV LIGATION

- The entire pedicle is encircled and high ligation of the IMA and IMV is performed with the robotic vessel sealer after being individually dissected and skeletonized (**FIGURES 4** and **5**). The IMV can be ligated near the IMA or higher up near the duodenum (**FIGURE 6**). This is primarily dictated by the reach of the colon to the rectum to perform a tension-free anastomosis.

Splenic Flexure Mobilization and Lateral Attachments

- The dissection is continued from medial to lateral toward the splenic flexure, mobilizing the descending colon mesentery off Gerota fascia (**FIGURE 7**). If the splenic flexure is mobilized for a tension-free anastomosis, the inferior border of the distal pancreas should be recognized to maintain the dissection plane anterior to the pancreas (**FIGURE 8**). The

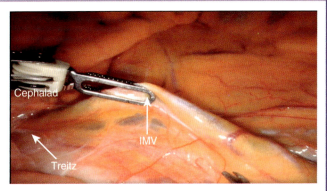

FIGURE 6 • Identification of the IMV next to the ligament of Treitz. After circumferential dissection, the IMV will be divided with a vessel sealer energy device.

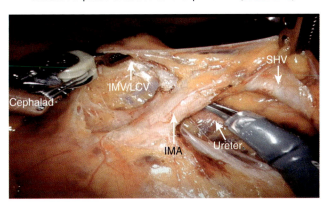

FIGURE 4 • Isolation of the IMA pedicle. IMA, inferior mesenteric artery; IMV, inferior mesenteric vein; LCV, left colic vessels; SHV, superior hemorrhoidal vessels.

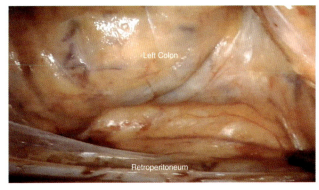

FIGURE 7 • Medial to lateral mobilization after dividing the IMA pedicle.

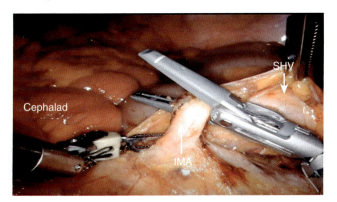

FIGURE 5 • Division of the IMA with the robotic vessel sealer.

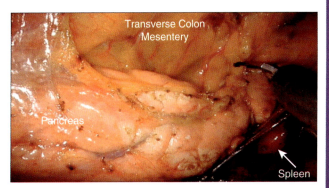

FIGURE 8 • Medial to lateral mobilization of the mesocolon exposing the tail of the pancreas.

sigmoid and descending colon is now retracted medially to divide a thin remaining layer of peritoneum along the line of Toldt. This dissection continues from lateral to medial toward the splenocolic ligament. Alternatively, the lesser sac is entered from medially and the omentum and splenocolic ligament are divided starting from the distal transverse colon.

DIVIDE THE RECTOSIGMOID COLON

- Upon complete mobilization of the descending colon and the splenic flexure, the peritoneum lateral to the rectosigmoid junction is scored and a window created using blunt dissection along the posterior wall of the colon (**FIGURE 9**). This allows transection of the rectosigmoid colon with a robotic stapler through the right lower quadrant port (**FIGURE 10**).

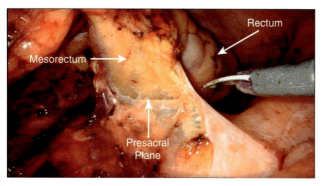

FIGURE 9 • Mobilization of the rectosigmoid junction.

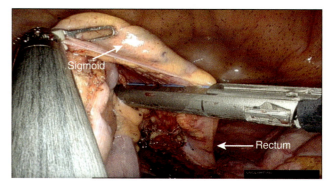

FIGURE 10 • Intracorporeal transection of the rectosigmoid junction.

SELECT PROXIMAL TRANSECTION POINT AND DIVIDE THE MESENTERY

- A proximal transection point is chosen based on the divided IMA pedicle. The remaining mesentery is divided to the planned proximal transection. Bowel perfusion can be optimally visualized with indocyanine green injection and the infrared mode of the robotic camera.

COLORECTAL ANASTOMOSIS

- There are numerous techniques for the colorectal anastomosis. They can be broadly classified into intracorporeal and extracorporeal. The completed anastomosis is checked for perfusion using indocyanine green injection, and a hydropneumatics leak test is performed (**FIGURES 11-13**).
- For an extracorporeal anastomosis, the transected colon is brought out through the proposed extraction site with either periumbilical or Pfannenstiel incision and the colon is divided extracorporeally at the proximal transection point. The specimen is passed off the field and the proximal colon is prepared with the anvil of the circular stapler, placing it into the descending colon and secured with a purse string suture. An end-to-end or end-to-side anastomosis to the rectum is then created with the circular stapler.
- For an intracorporeal anastomosis, the stapler port is enlarged and the is anvil introduced into the abdomen. A colotomy is made on the specimen side just distal to the final proximal

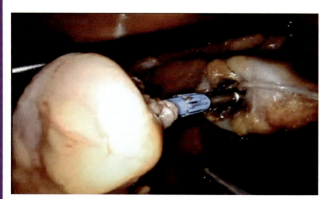

FIGURE 11 • Coupling the anvil and EEA stapler for the colorectal anastomosis.

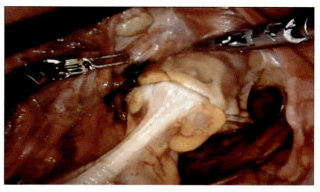

FIGURE 12 • Completed colorectal anastomosis.

Chapter 18 LEFT HEMICOLECTOMY: ROBOTIC-ASSISTED TECHNIQUE 147

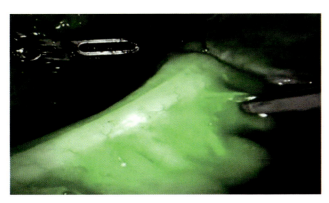

FIGURE 13 • Perfusion assessment using indocyanine green.

transection site and the anvil is advanced to the anterior wall of the descending colon after incising the wall over the tip of the anvil. The anvil spike should be placed approximately 5 cm from the planned proximal transection site. The initial colotomy site is then closed with a running suture and the colon transected with the robotic stapler just proximal to this closure. Alternatively, the anvil is introduced with the anvil spike attached to a looped silk suture. The anvil is then placed through an enterotomy with the tip aiming distally. The enterotomy is closed with a running suture and the robotic stapler is used to transect the colon just proximal to this. It is important that the staple line includes the silk suture attached to the anvil spike. This can be then pulled out of the staple line to position the anvil for an end-to-end anastomosis.

PEARLS AND PITFALLS

Instrument collisions	▪ A common issue when trocars are suboptimally placed too close to each other in relation to the target organ. Adjustment of the robotic arms and elbow joints can improve the instrument movement, but if this fails then repositioning of the trocars may be the best next step.
Morbid obesity	▪ In morbidly obesity patients, the thickened mesentery makes it significantly difficult to safely identify, isolate, and divide the inferior mesenteric artery/vein and left colic vessels. In addition, small bowel loops can be difficult to mobilize out of the pelvis and the needed Trendelenburg positioning may not be tolerated by the patient.
Colon length	▪ Colon length can be obtained by the following maneuvers: ▪ High ligation of the IMA close to the junction to the aorta allows significant length to be obtained after mobilization of the descending colon mesentery off of the retroperitoneum and Gerota fascia. ▪ High ligation of the inferior mesenteric vein is performed close to the duodenum and a medial to lateral splenic flexure mobilization at the inferior border of the pancreas if there is still inadequate. ▪ Omentum can be taken off the transverse colon for additional length. ▪ The middle colic vessels can then be clamped to check for adequate perfusion of the colon with Firefly technology before middle colic vessel division.

POSTOPERATIVE CARE

- Patients are admitted to the hospital, encouraged to ambulate on post operative day 0, encouraged to use incentive spirometry and prophylactic anticoagulation.
- Patients are started on a full liquid diet and then advanced rapidly to low-fiber diet by postoperative day 1 if they continue to do well.
- Multimodal pain management strategies are utilized in order to avoid narcotic pain medications.
- Patients are ready for discharge by postoperative day 1 to 3.

COMPLICATIONS

Ureteric Injury

- This most commonly occurs during ligation of the IMA on failing to recognize the ureter being pulled up onto the left colon mesentery. Identifying the ureter and ensuring it is adequately pushed down onto the retroperitoneum prior to dividing the IMA pedicle is the best technique to avoid such a complication.

Bleeding

- Bleeding can be encountered at the mesenteric root. The third arm can be used to immediately occlude the root proximally to allow time to suction and identify the exact source. Control of the root can be obtained with a vessel loop or in some cases suturing. Early conversion and laparotomy is sometimes necessary.
- Intraluminal anastomotic bleeding is not uncommon and can occur early postoperatively. In most cases this type of bleeding will stop spontaneously but may require flexible sigmoidoscopy for control of bleeding.

Anastomotic Leak

- Intraoperative leaks are due to technical complications in most cases. It is important to ensure a tight proximal purse string, while avoiding asymmetry in the bowel thickness that is drawn into the anvil base. Additional care should be taken to prevent any diverticuli from being included in the staple line. Once a leak is identified intraoperatively then the anastomosis is taken down with further distal transection and reanastomosis.

REFERENCES

1. Lacy AM, García-Valdecasas JC, Delgado S, et al. Laparoscopy-assisted colectomy versus open colectomy for treatment of non-metastatic colon cancer: a randomised trial. Lancet. 2002;359(9325):2224-2229.
2. Casillas MA Jr, Leichtle SW, Wahl WL, et al. Improved perioperative and short-term outcomes of robotic versus conventional laparoscopic colorectal operations. Am J Surg. 2014;208(1):33-40.
3. Lacy AM, Delgado S, Castells A, et al. The long-term results of a randomized clinical trial of laparoscopy-assisted versus open surgery for colon cancer. Ann Surg. 2008;248(1):1-7.

Chapter **19**

Sigmoid Colectomy: Open Technique

Anish Jay Jain, Shiva Seetahal, Tolulope A. Oyetunji, and Wayne A. I. Frederick

DEFINITION

- A sigmoidectomy is the resection of the sigmoid colon to the level of the rectosigmoid junction. The extent of the lymphadenectomy will be determined by the indication (benign vs malignant disease).
  - Focal segmental sigmoid resection for benign disease can be accomplished by dividing the sigmoidal vessels close to the bowel wall, without the need for a high pedicle transection. A complete sigmoidectomy with lymphadenectomy (described in this chapter) includes transection of the inferior mesenteric artery (IMA) at its origin and resection of the proximal superior hemorrhoidal vessels (SHV) and sigmoidal branches.
- Laparoscopic techniques for sigmoid colectomies have grown increasingly popular as surgeons become more comfortable with the technique and data demonstrate multiple benefits (shorter length of stay, less postoperative pain, reduced incisional hernias, etc) compared to the open technique. However, it is still imperative that surgeons are comfortable with the open technique as preoperative contraindications and intraoperative difficulties to/with the laparoscopic approach do occur.

DIFFERENTIAL DIAGNOSIS

- Indications for sigmoidectomy include the following:
  - Polyps
  - Diverticular disease (ie, complicated diverticulitis, perforation, fistulae, etc)
- Other indications include sigmoid volvulus, ischemic or infectious colitis, and trauma.

PATIENT HISTORY AND PHYSICAL FINDINGS

- Most patients with early-stage colon cancer are asymptomatic. Disease is found on colonoscopy performed for screening purposes or for workup of an anemic patient or a patient with a positive fecal occult blood test.
- Late-stage colon cancer can present with abdominal pain, unexplained weight loss, melena, iron deficiency anemia, or changes in bowel habits. Obstructive symptoms are typically secondary to circumferential tumors.
- Patients with uncomplicated sigmoid diverticulitis report episodic pain in the left lower quadrant associated with fever, changes in bowel habits, and/or bloating.
- The spectrum of symptomatology for complex diverticulitis can be as benign as those for uncomplicated diverticulitis but can progress to localized or even generalized peritonitis.
- Patients with neoplastic or inflammatory erosion (fistula) into adjacent organs, such as the bladder or vagina, can present with pneumaturia, fecaluria, or fecaloid vaginal discharge.
- A thorough family history of colon or rectal cancer, polyps, and/or other malignancies should be elicited.

- The physical examination should include the following:
  - Focused abdominal examination, including notation of abdominal scars.
  - Digital rectal examination, focused on assessment of sphincter function.
  - Rigid proctoscopy for all patients with sigmoid polyps or cancer reported by endoscopy to be within 20 cm from the anal verge. This will allow for confirmation of the site of the lesion, which oftentimes may not coincide with the endoscopy report. This information may alter the surgical and oncologic approach. It is not uncommon for patients thought to have sigmoid adenocarcinoma based on colonoscopic findings to actually have rectal adenocarcinoma on rigid proctoscopy examination. The latter patients would need to have a low anterior resection operation and, potentially, could benefit from neoadjuvant therapy.
  - Rigid proctoscopy should NOT be performed in patients presenting with acute diverticulitis or perforation to avoid worsening of a microperforation by air insufflation.

IMAGING AND OTHER DIAGNOSTIC STUDIES

- Carcinoembryonic antigen (CEA): The baseline preoperative result and postsurgical control must be obtained as an assessment for complete tumor resection. Absolute CEA presurgical value is an independent variable for survival.
- Contrast-enhanced abdominal computed axial tomography is the most sensitive and specific test for detection of intraabdominal metastases. It is also helpful in diverticulitis cases to evaluate for the extent of diverticular disease and for the possible presence of peridiverticular abscess, stricture, and/or fistula.
- Chest computed axial tomography is the most sensitive and specific test to detect mediastinal and lung metastases.
- Complete colonoscopy: Regardless of the primary location of the tumor, every patient should have a complete colonoscopy study whenever possible, since 2% to 9% of the patients may have synchronous tumors elsewhere in the colon and rectum. Preoperative colonoscopic tattooing (distal to the target lesion) greatly aids in the localization of the tumor intraoperatively.
- A colonic enema with double contrast may be used in patients in whom colonoscopy is not possible. Virtual colonoscopy (computed tomography colonography) is also an option for those that cannot undergo colonoscopy.

SURGICAL MANAGEMENT

Preoperative Planning

- The patient should be mechanically bowel prepped preoperatively with the GoLYTELY solution in combination with oral antibiotics the day before.

- The nil per os (NPO) status is then effective after midnight.
- The necessary radiologic and laboratory examination should be verified and reviewed accordingly.
- Patient should be consented appropriately for the procedure.
- We typically do not place preoperative stents for patients undergoing sigmoid colectomy for resolved diverticulitis. However, if there is any concern regarding potential difficulty in identification of the ureter, ureteral stenting should be considered.
- Appropriate perioperative intravenous antibiotic prophylaxis is given on induction.
- Consideration should be given to intravenous steroid supplementation if the patient is steroid dependent.
- Subcutaneous low molecular weight heparin is given on induction. Mechanical venous thromboembolism prophylaxis is initiated in all patients.
- A preoperative briefing with the entire surgical team is conducted. Items discussed include patient identification, type of surgery, type of anesthesia, expected events during the surgery, the need for blood components, prophylactic antibiotic, surgical devices availability, and potential adverse events and their prevention.

PATIENT POSITIONING AND OPERATING TEAM SETUP

- The patient should be placed in a standard supine position for induction of anesthesia.
- Following induction and securing of the endotracheal tube, a Foley catheter should be inserted.
- The patient is then placed in a low lithotomy position (**FIGURE 1**). The thighs are placed parallel to the ground to prevent interference with the movement of the arms and the placement of a retractor. Special care should be given to the positioning of the patient's legs in the stirrup devices; adequate padding of all pressure points and symmetrical positioning can minimize sliding of the patient during gravity-assisted maneuvers and prevent neurovascular injury to the lower extremities during the procedure.
- The arms should be tucked at the sides with appropriate padding on all pressure points to afford the surgeons adequate space during the procedure and to prevent neurovascular injuries to the upper extremities during the procedure.
- Once the patient has been positioned and secured to the operating table, the rectum should be irrigated with saline solution using a piston syringe in order to evacuate remnant stool and bowel prep fluid.
- The patient can then be prepped and draped. The drape should have an opening that allows for easy access to the perineum without disrupting the sterile field of the abdomen.
- The surgeon stands to the patient's right side, with their first assistant standing to the patient's left side and with the scrub nurse standing to the surgeon's right side. A second assistant, if available, stands between the patient's legs (**FIGURE 2**).

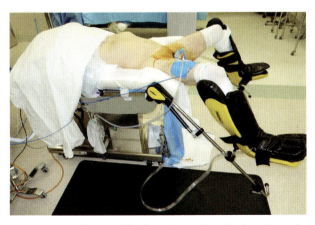

FIGURE 1 • Patient positioning. The patient is placed on a low lithotomy position, with the arms tucked to the side and the legs secured on Yellofin stirrups. Note that the thighs are parallel to the ground to prevent interference with the movement of the arms by the operating team. All pressure points are padded to prevent neurovascular injuries.

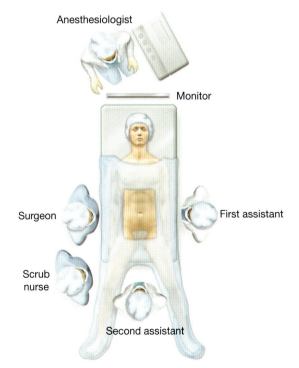

FIGURE 2 • Operating team setup. The surgeon stands to the patient's right side, with their assistant standing to the patient's left side and with the scrub nurse standing to the surgeon's right side. A second assistant, if available, stands between the patient's legs.

LAPAROTOMY, INSPECTION, AND SURGICAL FIELD PREPARATION

- A midline laparotomy incision from the umbilicus to the pubis is usually sufficient to begin the procedure. Additional access can be gained by extending the incision cranially toward the xiphoid process as necessary. Care should be taken to stay within the midline of the rectus sheath (linea alba) on opening.
- In patients with previous abdominal surgery, adherent bowel can complicate entry into the peritoneal cavity and meticulous dissection may be warranted. If possible, it might be easier to gain access into the abdomen by going above the previous midline scar where adhesions may be less tenuous.
- Upon entry into the peritoneal cavity, moistened laparotomy pads are to be placed around the to serve as wound protectors and reduce the likelihood of wound infection.
- A self-retaining retractor (eg, a Balfour or Bookwalter retractor) can then be placed for adequate exposure.
- A careful and thorough examination of the abdominal cavity is critical. Evidence of metastatic disease or carcinomatosis must be appreciated before proceeding with the procedure. If present, these significantly impact both management and prognosis.
- The colon should be palpated in cases involving tumors to verify the position of the disease and assess the extent of resection. In procedures for diverticular disease, the state of the entire colon should be investigated, as this may impact the optimal extent of resection.
- Following inspection, if the decision is made to proceed, the small bowel should be eviscerated and packed to the right upper quadrant using a moist laparotomy pad or a moist towel to better facilitate exposure.

LATERAL TO MEDIAL MOBILIZATION OF THE LEFT COLON AND IDENTIFICATION OF THE LEFT URETER

- Once the decision to proceed has been made, the supplying vessels and lymph basins should then be identified. Sigmoid colectomy usually entails resection of the sigmoid arterial supply originating at the IMA and the SHV with the accompanying lymph nodes that reside within that basin. The IMA should be carefully identified along with the path of planned resection along the mesentery; the extent of the planned resection along the length of the sigmoid dictates the degree to which the left colon must be mobilized.
- The patient is placed in a Trendelenburg position with the left side elevated to facilitate exposure.
- Mobilization of the colon is facilitated by retracting the sigmoid colon toward the midline.
- Using a combination of electrocautery and blunt dissection, release the lateral attachments of the sigmoid and descending colon by transecting the line of Toldt (**FIGURE 3**).
- Dissection along the line of Toldt should be largely bloodless, as this is an avascular plane. The dissection should then be extended both proximally along the descending colon toward the splenic flexure and distally toward the rectosigmoid junction.
- The sigmoid and descending colon mesentery is separated from the retroperitoneum using a sharp lateral to medial dissection approach.
- At this point, care should be taken to identify the left ureter and gonadal vessels and ensure that they are kept intact in the retroperitoneum outside of the field of dissection (**FIGURE 4A** and **B**). In the lower abdomen, the left ureter is located medial to the gonadal vessels, closer to the midline.
- Identification of the left ureter may be complicated in cases of diverticulitis where previous inflammation has created extensive adhesions. In such patients, preoperative placement of ureteric stents may be beneficial. It is still imperative to know different techniques for intraoperatively identifying the ureter at this anatomic location. Retrograde tracing starting at the iliac vessels is one option. Another is the elicitation of peristalsis within the true ureter on gentle palpation.

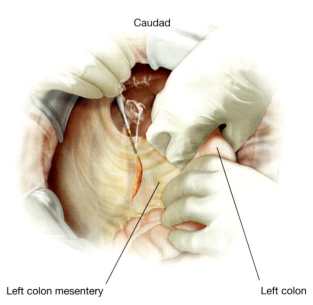

FIGURE 3 • Lateral to medial mobilization of the left colon. With the sigmoid and descending colon retracted medially, the white line of Toldt is transected from the pelvic inlet to the splenic flexure.

Chapter 19 SIGMOID COLECTOMY: OPEN TECHNIQUE   151

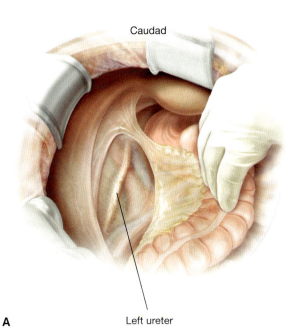
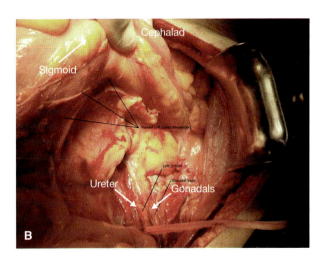

FIGURE 4 • Exposure of the left ureter. The illustration **(A)** shows the view of the operative field from cephalad to caudad direction. The operative picture **(B)** shows a caudad to cephalad view of the field. In the lower abdomen, as the descending and sigmoid mesocolon are separated from the retroperitoneum by the lateral to medial dissection, the left ureter is located medial to the gonadal vessels, close to the midline.

MOBILIZATION OF THE SPLENIC FLEXURE

- Taking down the splenic flexure may be unnecessary on occasions with very redundant sigmoid, but more often, it is required in order to achieve a tension-free anastomosis.
  - A tension-free anastomosis is the most critical element to prevent an anastomotic leak.
- This maneuver can be challenging, because the splenic flexure can have a very deep location in the left upper quadrant of the abdomen. Special attention should be afforded to this part of the operation, as extensive bleeding from splenic capsular injury can be troublesome. Splenic bleeding can usually be addressed using electrocautery, packing, or topical hemostatic agents.
- For this step of the operation, the patient is placed on a reverse Trendelenburg with the left side up position to facilitate operative exposure.
- A bidirectional technique for mobilization of the splenic flexure is used: from the left paracolic gutter upwards, and through the lesser sac from a medial to lateral direction (**FIGURE 5**).
- The lateral peritoneum sectioning is continued from the initial incision in a cephalic direction as far as possible, avoiding excessive traction of the splenic flexure and thus preventing splenic lacerations.
- The splenodiaphragmatic and splenocolic ligaments are transected with a monopolar scalpel or with a bipolar vessel-sealing device (**FIGURE 5**).
- The final approach to the splenic flexure should be complemented with another point of dissection that is initiated in the transverse colon to the left of the middle colic vessels. At this point, the gastrocolic ligament is transected, entering the lesser sac. The gastrocolic ligament is transected from medial to lateral (**FIGURE 5**) with a monopolar scalpel or

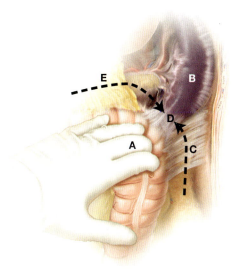

FIGURE 5 • Splenic flexure mobilization. Mobilization of the splenic flexure. The surgeon retracts the splenic flexure of the colon *(A)* downward and medially, exposing the attachments of the splenic flexure to the spleen *(B)*. The phrenocolic *(C)* and splenocolic *(D)* ligaments are transected in an inferior to superior and lateral to medial direction. The gastrocolic ligament *(E)* is then transected in a medial to lateral direction until both planes of dissection meet and the splenic flexure is fully mobilized.

with a bipolar vessel-sealing device, until the lateral plane of dissection is reached.
- Finally, the attachments of the splenic flexure to the tail of the pancreas are divided with electrocautery. The left colon is now fully mobilized all the way to the midline.

INFERIOR MESENTERIC ARTERY TRANSECTION

- With the first assistant's two hands holding the proximal and distal sigmoid colon upward, the root of the mesosigmoid colon is clearly visualized by the primary surgeon from the right side of the table. At the root of the mesentery, the arch of the SHV can be seen and palpated.
- Placing the index finger behind the SHV arch allows the surgeon to incise with electrocautery the right surface of the peritoneum just under the dorsal surface of the SHV.
- This plane of dissection along the dorsal aspect of the SHV is carried distally over the promontory (leading into the presacral space) and proximally up to the origin of the IMA. The IMA is dissected circumferentially at its origin from the aorta.
- The hypogastric nerve is swept down and left intact in the retroperitoneum to avoid autonomic pelvic organ dysfunction postoperatively.
- At this point, the colon mesentery is divided in between the sigmoid and descending colon with a vessel-sealing device, starting from the antimesenteric border and extending toward the origin of the IMA. The marginal arcade is transected along this dissection line close to the colon wall at the proposed anastomosis level.
- The IMA is then ligated between Sarot clamps, incised, and doubly ligated with braided 2-0 suture (**FIGURE 6A** and **B**). High IMA ligation allows for an excellent lymph node harvest.
- It is also paramount to preserve the proximal colonic blood supply intact (the marginal artery of Drummond) in order to have a healthy anastomosis.

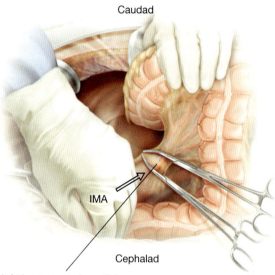
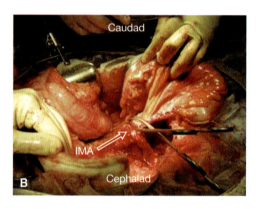

FIGURE 6 • **A** and **B**, Inferior mesenteric artery (IMA) transection. With the assistant holding the sigmoid colon up, the IMA is transected between clamps and will subsequently be ligated with heavy silk sutures.

COLON TRANSECTION

- Following mobilization of the left colon, the sigmoid colon can then be resected.
- We prefer to use the GIA staplers with 60-mm blue cartridges (3.1 mm) for the proximal transection. The proximal transection is performed between the sigmoidal and left colic vessel distribution, between the sigmoid and descending colon segments.
- For the distal transection, we prefer the 90-mm transabdominal (TA) stapler to complete the resection. The distal transection is performed just distal to the rectosigmoid junction (**FIGURE 7**), which can be identified by the splaying of the tinea coli. The remaining specimen mesenteric attachments are transected with a vessel-sealing device.
- For diverticular disease, the extent of the proximal transection is variable, as it depends on the extent of diverticular disease. The distal transection, however, must always be distal to the rectosigmoid junction to ensure that there are no diverticular elements distal to the anastomosis.
- Once this part of the operation has been successfully completed, the specimen can be removed from the operative field and sent to the pathologist for evaluation.

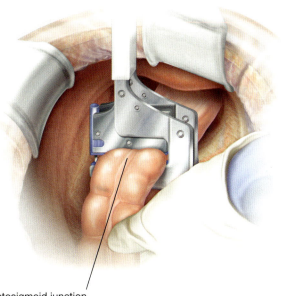
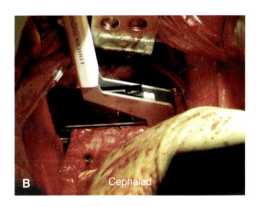

A Rectosigmoid junction

FIGURE 7 • Distal specimen transection. **A** and **B,** The distal transection is performed with a 90-mm TA stapler just distal to the rectosigmoid junction, which can be identified by the splaying of the tinea coli.

ANASTOMOSIS

- There are two options for restoring intestinal continuity—hand-sewn vs stapled anastomosis. We favor a stapled anastomosis whenever possible.
- If a partial (subtotal) sigmoidectomy is all that is needed (as is the case sometimes in diverticulitis cases), then it may be feasible to perform a GIA stapled side-to-side colocolonic anastomosis in contiguity before transecting the specimen (**FIGURE 8A**). The anastomosis is then completed (and the specimen transected) with a TA stapler (**FIGURE 8B**).
- More commonly, however, when the entire sigmoid colon is removed, performing a colorectal anastomosis is best

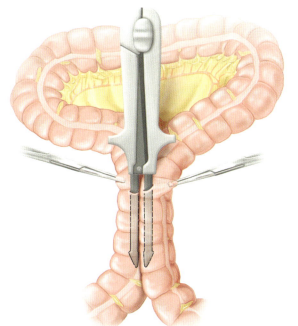
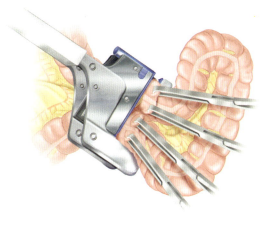

FIGURE 8 • Anastomosis after partial (subtotal) sigmoidectomy. In these cases, it may be feasible to perform a GIA stapled side-to-side colocolonic anastomosis in contiguity before transecting the specimen (**A**). The anastomosis is then completed (and the specimen transected) with a TA stapler (**B**).

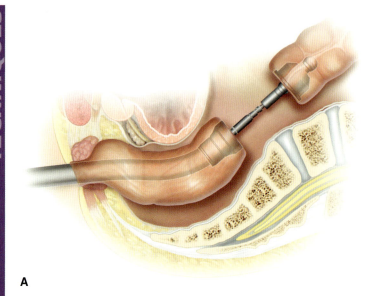

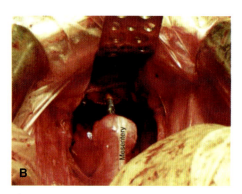

FIGURE 9 • Anastomosis after a full sigmoid resection. **A** and **B,** An end-to-end EEA 29-Fr stapled anastomosis is performed.

achieved by an end-to-end colorectal anastomosis using an end-to-end anastomosis (EEA) stapling device (**FIGURE 9**).
- The size of the stapler selected should be dictated by the caliber of the colon and rectum. If possible, a 28- to 29-Fr size is desirable to reduce the incidence of anastomotic strictures.
- The anvil of the stapler is placed in the descending limb/colon via a colotomy and secured using a purse-string nonabsorbable suture, preferably a 3-0 nylon.
- A well-trained assistant surgeon then moves to the patient's perineum and inserts the stapler into the rectum. The anal canal should be digitally dilated with lubricated fingers before inserting the EEA stapler.
- The anvil is then approximated with stapler under the guidance of the abdominal surgeon and is then fired. Care must be taken to avoid torquing the stapler instrument during the fire maneuver to avoid disrupting the anastomosis.
- The perineal surgeon must then inspect the proximal and distal "donuts" from the stapler. Two intact donuts must be observed; discontinuity in the donuts must raise suspicion for an inadequate anastomosis and should warrant further inspection and possible interrogation of the anastomosis. We do not routinely test the anastomosis, but this may be achieved via transrectal instillation of methylene blue dye and/or air under water (air leak test) (**FIGURE 10**).
- Hand-sewn anastomosis is less common in the modern era, but it is a skill that should reside within the armamentarium of every general surgeon.
- We prefer to perform a double-layered closure starting with full-thickness 3-0 Vicryl sutures through the colon and rectal walls in a running fashion. This is followed by 3-0 Vicryl or 2-0 Silk Lembert sutures through the serosa of the colon and adventitia of the rectum to buttress the anastomosis.
- In patients with a narrow pelvis, maneuvering may be difficult. Interrupted sutures should also be used to reinforce areas of potential leak or inadequate anastomosis following

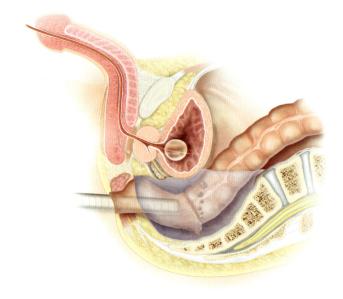

FIGURE 10 • The anastomosis is then tested under water. The presence of air bubbles would indicate an anastomotic disruption, which necessitates a revision of the anastomosis.

stapling. The main danger would be overzealous placement of sutures, leading to ischemia at the anastomotic tissue.
- The role of diverting colostomy or ileostomy has declined in recent years. These are most commonly performed in patients with Hinchey 3 or 4 perforated diverticulitis. Otherwise, they are adjuncts in cases where the integrity of the anastomosis is in question. This may include patients with positive leak tests on table or patients with risk factors for anastomotic breakdown such as steroid use or severe malnutrition. In patients in whom a diverting ostomy is deemed prudent, we prefer a loop ileostomy owing to the relative ease with which these can be reversed later on.

Chapter 19 **SIGMOID COLECTOMY: OPEN TECHNIQUE** **155**

CLOSURE

- Once intestinal continuity has been restored, a final inspection of the abdomen is usually sufficient before closure.
- All packs should be removed and counted, and hemostasis should be complete before fascial closure.
- The fascia is best reapproximated using a running, double-stranded size 0 polydioxanone (PDS) suture.

- The skin can then be closed using skin staples.
- Dry dressings are adequate, although newer vacuum dressings are becoming popular owing to the preponderance for wound infections following colon surgery. We, however, still use the dry dressing and wound infection has not been a problem in our practice.

PEARLS AND PITFALLS

Localizing the target lesion	■ Preoperative colonoscopic tattooing greatly aids in the localization of the tumor intraoperatively. ■ If not available, on-table colonoscopy may be necessary.
Patient position	■ An improper position with hip flexion will make it difficult to maneuver during the whole procedure. Make sure the patient's thighs are parallel to the ground.
Identification of the left ureter	■ Identification of the left ureter is critical prior to vascular transection. ■ In difficult cases, stenting may help identify the ureter. ■ Stents do not decrease ureteral injury but aid in the intraoperative identification of the injury when it happens.
Splenic flexure mobilization	■ May not be necessary in cases with a very redundant sigmoid colon. ■ In most cases, it is required to ensure a tension-free anastomosis.
Anastomosis	■ A tension-free anastomosis is the most critical element to prevent an anastomotic leak. ■ It is also paramount to preserve the proximal colonic blood supply intact (the marginal artery of Drummond) in order to have a healthy anastomosis.

POSTOPERATIVE CARE

- The Foley catheter is left in situ for 24 hours to assess fluid status and because of the increased likelihood of urinary retention following surgery in the pelvis.
- A nasogastric tube is not routinely employed.
- The patient should be monitored closely until fully awake and stable.
- Clear fluids can be started on the evening of surgery.
- Early ambulation is essential.
- Patients should be instructed on the use of incentive spirometry to prevent atelectasis postoperatively.
- Pain control with patient-controlled analgesia or epidural analgesia is required.
- Antibiotics should be discontinued within 24 hours as per protocol.
- Pharmacologic venous thrombosis prophylaxis is instituted according to guidelines.

OUTCOMES

- The patient's prognosis depends on the tumor staging, which is determined by the histopathologic study of the specimen (pTNM).
- Many patients will require adjuvant chemotherapy according to the tumor stage.

COMPLICATIONS

- Wound infections
- Incisional hernias
- Urinary/sexual dysfunction: important to preserve hypogastric nerves and parasympathetic ganglia intact
- Ureteral injury: critical to identify the left ureter prior to IMA transection
- Anastomosis leak: critical to construct a well-vascularized, tension-free anastomosis
- Deep vein thrombosis (DVT): lowers risk with use of adequate DVT prophylaxis
- Cardiac and pulmonary complications
- Pelvic abscess: reduced incidence with placement of an omental pedicle flap in the pelvis
- Perineal wound breakdown is a notorious problem, especially in high-risk patients

DISPARITIES

- As with many other major oncologic operations, there are disparities in outcomes of patients undergoing sigmoidectomy. Major disparities have been noted in terms of race, insurance status, and income.
- Numerous studies have demonstrated racial disparities in postoperative outcomes in Black patients undergoing major

operations, especially oncologic procedures. Disparities are particularly remarkable in Black patients undergoing colectomies and radical prostatectomies. Black patients who undergo colectomies are at increased risk of requiring homologous blood transfusion, in-hospital mortality, prolonged length of stay, and postoperative complications.

- Insurance status also serves as an independent risk factor for postoperative outcomes in patients undergoing any form of colectomies. In fact, Medicaid insurance status can serve as a predictor of increased rates of open colectomies, higher mortality, length of stay, complications, readmission rates, and hospital charges.

- Nationally representative samples of patients undergoing sigmoid colectomies have demonstrated disparities in terms of outcomes and total hospital charges favoring patients within the highest income quartile vs those in the lowest income quartile. When controlling for aforementioned factors (race and insurance status) the disparity in outcomes based on income is insignificant, but the disparity in total hospital charges remains.

SUGGESTED READINGS

1. Bonds AM, Novick TK, Dietert JB, et al. Incisional negative pressure wound therapy significantly reduces surgical site infection in open colorectal surgery. *Dis Colon Rectum*. 2013;56(12):1403-1408.

2. Bothwell WN, Bleicher RJ, Dent TL. Prophylactic ureteral catheterization in colon surgery. A five-year review. *Dis Colon Rectum*. 1994;37(4):330-334.

3. Fang YJ, WU XJ, Zhao Q, et al. Hospital-based colorectal cancer survival trend of different tumor locations from 1960s to 2000s. *PLoS One*. 2013;8(9):e73528.

4. Jafari MD, Halabi WJ, Jafari F, et al. Morbidity of diverting ileostomy for rectal cancer: analysis of the American College of Surgeons National Surgical Quality Improvement Program. *Am Surg*. 2013;79(10):1034-1039.

5. Juo YY, Hyder O, Haider AH, et al. Is minimally invasive colon resection better than traditional approaches?: first comprehensive national examination with propensity score matching. *JAMA Surg*. 2014;149(2):177-184.

6. Neifert S, Ilonzo N, Gribben JL, Leitman IM. Economic disparities in patients undergoing sigmoidectomy. *J Soc Laparoendosc Surg*. 2018;22(4):e2018.00066. doi:10.4293/JSLS.2018.00066

7. Ramos-Valadez DI, Ragupathi M, Nieto J, et al. Single-incision versus conventional laparoscopic sigmoid colectomy: a case-matched series. *Surg Endosc*. 2012;26(1):96-102.

8. Rosato L, Mondini G, Serbelloni M, et al. Stapled versus hand sewn anastomosis in elective and emergency colorectal surgery. *G Chir*. 2006;27(5):199-204.

9. Smith RL, Bohl JK, McElearney ST, et al. Wound infection after elective colorectal resection. *Ann Surg*. 2004;239(5):599-605; discussion 605-607.

10. Sukumar S, Ravi P, Sood A, et al. Racial disparities in operative outcomes after major cancer surgery in the United States. *World J Surg*. 2015;39(3):634-643. doi:10.1007/s00268-014-2863-x

Chapter 20 Sigmoid Colectomy: Laparoscopic Technique

Arden M. Morris

DEFINITION
- Laparoscopic sigmoid colectomy is a laparoscopic procedure that involves complete or partial removal of the sigmoid colon most often with a primary anastomosis, which can be performed intra- or extracorporeally.

DIFFERENTIAL DIAGNOSIS
- Laparoscopic sigmoid colectomy is most often performed to treat colon cancer or diverticulitis but may also be performed to treat a benign neoplasm, which cannot be resected endoscopically, Crohn's or other fistulizing disease, intussusception, sigmoid volvulus, or other obstructive, inflammatory, or infectious conditions.

PATIENT HISTORY AND PHYSICAL FINDINGS
- A complete history should be tailored to the patient's primary diagnosis and should include a description of constitutional symptoms (nausea/vomiting, anorexia, weight loss or gain, fever, diaphoresis, and fatigue), pain (site, quality, timing, and inciting and relieving factors), dietary and bowel habits (constipation, diarrhea, frequency, continence, obstructive symptoms, and bleeding), urinary habits, and sexual function.
- Physical exam includes a description of the presence and quality of distension, tenderness, guarding (voluntary or involuntary), rebound, and organomegaly. It is important to check carefully for evidence of a mass. For the sigmoid colon, this should be specifically checked by using one hand to elevate the left flank and the other hand to palpate the left lower quadrant between the iliac spine and the infraumbilical midline abdomen. The presence of involuntary guarding during this maneuver may indicate inflammation of the sigmoid colon consistent with acute or smoldering diverticulitis.
- A digital rectal exam must be performed preoperatively. The exam should include digital palpation of the coccyx, ischial tuberosities, and levators. The exam should include an assessment of sensation (anal wink), anal sphincter tone, and voluntary contraction (normal vs diminished squeeze and normal relaxation vs paradoxical puborectalis contraction with bearing down).

IMAGING AND OTHER DIAGNOSTIC STUDIES
- There are many options for preoperative diagnostic imaging. For suspected diverticulitis and/or other inflammatory or fistulizing disease, abdominal/pelvis computed tomography (CT) is the most effective means for diagnosis and operative planning. In addition, CT documentation of the presence of diverticulitis is particularly important in the event that the patient's symptoms do not abate postoperatively.
- For neoplastic disease, chest/abdomen/pelvis CT should be performed to identify possible metastases to identify the extent of the tumor if possible.
- Although CT with oral and rectal contrast is useful for both intra- and extraluminal assessment (**FIGURE 1**), a fluoroscopic examination with barium or water-soluble contrast enema is also useful to assess the bowel lumen especially if colonoscopy cannot be performed (**FIGURE 2**).
- In the case of rectal prolapse, defecography exam preoperatively can provide additional information about the extent of sigmoid colon intussusception and the presence of an enterocele or rectocele (**FIGURE 3**).
- Full colonoscopy should be performed preoperatively to assess the proximal colon and to tattoo the colon proximally and distally to neoplastic lesions (**FIGURE 4**).

SURGICAL MANAGEMENT
Preoperative Planning
- Although the use of a full mechanical bowel preparation continues to be debated, at a minimum the sigmoid and rectum should

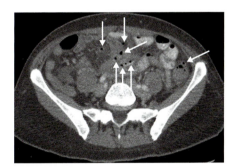

FIGURE 1 • Axial CT scan of the pelvis with diverticulitis and extraluminal gas *(arrows)*.

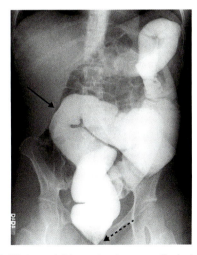

FIGURE 2 • Water-soluble contrast enema displaying a sigmoid volvulus *(block arrow)*. Notice the "omega loop" configuration of the sigmoid volvulus pointing to the right upper quadrant of the abdomen and the "bird's beak" narrowing at the entrance of the pelvis *(dashed arrow)*.

157

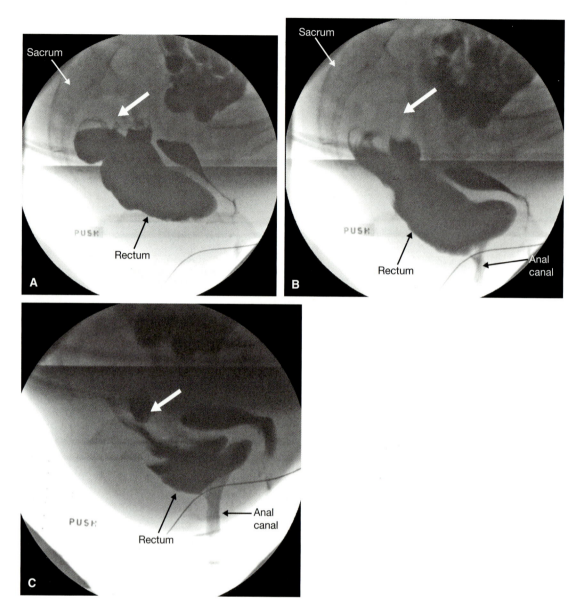

FIGURE 3 • **A-C,** Defecography displaying redundant sigmoid progressively intussuscepting into the rectum *(block arrows)* and thereby causing obstructed defecation.

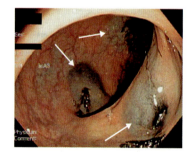

FIGURE 4 • Colonoscopy with submucosal injection of India ink *(arrows)* to mark the area of concern prior to operation. The colon is injected in three separate locations distal to the target lesion in order to maximize intraoperative localization of the target lesion.

be cleansed of stool using enemas the night before and morning of surgery in order to drive an anastomotic stapler through the rectum for reattachment. If a complete mechanical bowel preparation is undertaken, oral antibiotics should be included.

- Although use of laparoscopy has reduced the risk of wound infections among patients undergoing colon surgery, risk of deep-space organ infections remains. Broad-spectrum intravenous antibiotics should be given within 30 minutes prior to the abdominal incision. Intraoperatively, antibiotic redosing should be discussed by the surgeon and anesthesiologist for any operation that lasts 4 hours or longer.
- Risk of deep venous thrombosis is increased among patients with a diagnosis of cancer or inflammatory bowel disease, patients who undergo abdominal or pelvic surgery, and those who have prolonged operations. Patients who undergo

Chapter 20 SIGMOID COLECTOMY: LAPAROSCOPIC TECHNIQUE

laparoscopic sigmoid colectomy fulfill several of these criteria and therefore are at a substantially increased risk of venous thrombosis. To reduce this risk, sequential compression devices should be applied to bilateral lower extremities and initiated *preinduction*, when they are most effective at countering the effects of periinduction venous pooling. After induction, 5000 units of heparin should be delivered subcutaneously.

Patient Positioning

- After endotracheal general anesthesia has been induced, the patient is placed in a split-leg or dorsal lithotomy position and secured in a beanbag, with careful attention to padding the extremities, tucking the right arm at the side, and lowering the thighs to be parallel to the floor if possible. If the hips are flexed, the thighs are higher than the abdomen and can hinder the laparoscopic dissection (**FIGURE 5**).
- Tape the patient across the chest over a towel to secure them to the operating room (OR) table.
- A urinary catheter is placed to decompress the bladder and assist with monitoring urine output during the operation. If the normal anatomic location of the left ureter has been compromised by previous surgery or by an inflammatory condition such as diverticulitis, which can shorten the mesentery and pull the ureter medially, then placement of a ureteral stent or a lighted ureteral stent should be considered.
- An orogastric tube is placed to decompress the stomach.

FIGURE 5 • Patient positioning. The patient is placed on a low lithotomy position with the legs on Yellofin stirrups. The thighs are positioned parallel to the ground to avoid conflict with the surgeon's arms. The patient is placed on a beanbag with both arms tucked and taped to the table over a towel. All pressure points are padded to prevent neurovascular injuries.

- If the mechanical bowel preparation or preoperative enemas are inadequate, the surgeon should perform a rigid sigmoidoscopy to clear the rectum of stool after endotracheal general anesthesia has been induced.
- Most hospitals in the United States now require a robust time-out that includes a verbal statement of the patient's identification, diagnosis, medications and allergies, the planned procedure, and positioning, as well as the names and roles of the operating team and a list of necessary equipment and potential problems.

PORT PLACEMENT AND OPERATING TEAM SETUP

- The surgeon stands to the patient's right side, with the scrub nurse next to them. The assistant stands to the left side of the table (**FIGURE 6**). Two monitors, facing the surgeon and the assistant, are used.
- A 12-mm umbilical incision is created sharply and extended to the level of the fascia. The fascia is elevated with 2-0 Vicryl tacking sutures and then opened sharply. The Hasson port is then placed within the peritoneal cavity and tacking sutures are pulled up and clamped. This will be used as the camera port.
- Insufflation with carbon dioxide (CO_2) at high flow is initiated to an appropriate pressure of approximately 14 mm Hg.
- After inspection of the abdominal cavity with the laparoscope, three additional 5-mm working ports are placed under visualization in the right upper, right lower, and left lower quadrants of the abdomen (**FIGURE 7**).

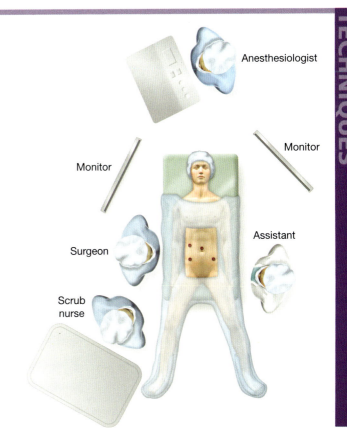

FIGURE 6 • Operating team setup. The surgeon stands to the patient's right side, with the scrub nurse next to them. The assistant stands to the left side of the table. Two monitors, facing the surgeon and the assistant, are used.

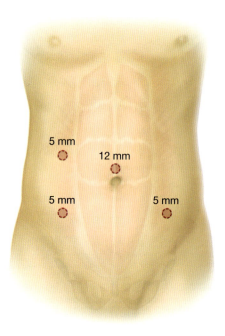

FIGURE 7 • Port placement. A 12-mm camera port is inserted supraumbilically using the Hasson technique. After insufflation of the pneumoperitoneum, three additional 5-mm working ports are placed under visualization in the right upper, right lower, and left lower quadrants of the abdomen.

INFERIOR MESENTERIC ARTERY TRANSECTION

- The sigmoid colon is inspected and, if necessary, adhesions are lysed. The omentum and small intestine are retracted into the right upper quadrant and the operating table is rotated into Trendelenburg and right side down positions as needed for bowel retraction.
- The sigmoid colon is grasped broadly with a bowel grasper and elevated toward the anterior abdominal wall to expose the sacral promontory and the medial peritoneal fold (**FIGURE 8**).
- The peritoneum is incised below (dorsal) the inferior mesenteric artery (IMA) and its terminal branch, the superior hemorrhoidal artery (SHA).
- The dissection is continued from medial to lateral, beginning the separation of the mesocolon and the retroperitoneum, exposing the left ureter and gonadal vessels, which are identified and preserved intact in the retroperitoneum (**FIGURE 9**).
- The IMA is dissected circumferentially. Lifting up on the IMA and its terminal branches, the SHA and the left colic artery, will form what appears to be a letter "T" (**FIGURE 10**).

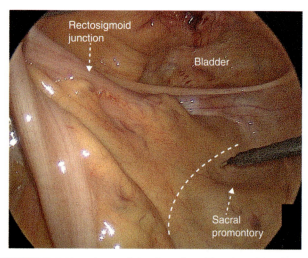

FIGURE 8 • Vascular pedicle dissection. The sigmoid colon is pulled toward the anterior abdominal wall, tenting out the base of its mesentery peritoneum at the sacral promontory. The peritoneum is incised along the root of the mesocolon (dotted line), dorsal to the IMA/SHA arteries, across the promontory, and toward the right posterolateral cul-de-sac.

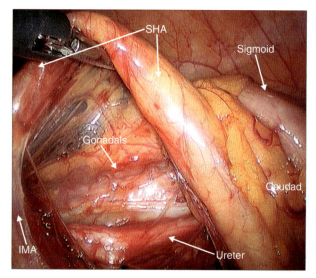

FIGURE 9 • Identification of the ureter. With the SHA, distal to its origin of the IMA, tented up toward the anterior abdominal wall, the mesosigmoid is separated from the retroperitoneum. This exposes the left ureter and gonadal vessels, which are identified and preserved intact in the retroperitoneum.

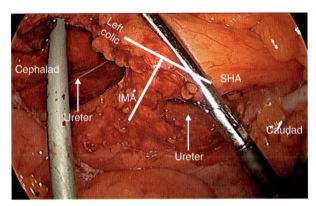

FIGURE 10 • The IMA is dissected circumferentially. Lifting up on the IMA and its terminal branches, the SHA and the left colic artery will form what appears to be a letter "T." The ureter can be seen safely preserved in the retroperitoneum.

- The IMA is then transected at its origin off the aorta with a vascular load stapler (**FIGURE 11**) or an energy device.

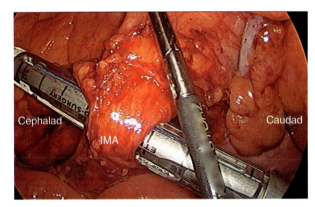

FIGURE 11 • IMA transection. The IMA is then transected at its origin off the aorta with a vascular load stapler.

- The mesentery of the colon is then transected with an energy device, from the IMA stump up to the colon wall, at the level of the planned proximal transection (typically between the sigmoid and descending colon).

MEDIAL TO LATERAL MOBILIZATION

- The sigmoid and descending mesocolon are dissected off the retroperitoneum via a medial to lateral approach (**FIGURE 12**).
- With the assistant helping hold the mesocolon up, the surgeon gently dissects along the transition between the two fat planes (Gerota fascia in the retroperitoneum, dorsally, and the mesocolon, ventrally).

- This dissection is carried laterally to the lateral abdominal wall, inferiorly to the level of the pelvic inlet and superiorly until you separate the tail of the pancreas from the posterior aspect of the splenic flexure. Completion of this step will greatly facilitate all subsequent steps of this operation.
- The left ureter and gonadal vessels should be identified and preserved intact in the retroperitoneum.

FIGURE 12 • Medial to lateral mobilization. The sigmoid and descending mesocolon are dissected off the retroperitoneum via a medial to lateral dissection approach. With the assistant helping hold the mesocolon up, the surgeon gently dissects with an energy device along the transition between the two fat planes (Gerota's fascia in the retroperitoneum, dorsally, and the mesocolon, ventrally). This dissection is carried laterally to the lateral abdominal wall, inferiorly to the level of the pelvic inlet, and superiorly until you separate the tail of the pancreas from the posterior aspect of the splenic flexure. Completion of this step will greatly facilitate all subsequent steps of this operation.

DIVISION OF THE LATERAL PERITONEAL ATTACHMENTS AND MOBILIZATION OF THE SPLENIC FLEXURE

- After completing the medial to lateral portion of the descending colon mobilization from the sacral promontory to the splenic flexure and over Gerota fascia, the lateral sigmoid colon retroperitoneal attachments are divided with scissors (**FIGURE 13**) and/or an energy device.
- The splenic flexure is now encountered. Full mobilization of the splenic flexure (**FIGURE 14**) is often needed in order to ensure a tension-free anastomosis.

- The patient is placed on a reverse Trendelenburg position, helping bring the splenic flexure into view.
- The surgeon and the assistant retract the splenic flexure inferiorly and medially, exposing the splenocolic and phrenocolic ligaments. These ligaments are then transected with a 5-mm energy device (**FIGURE 15**) in an inferior to superior and lateral to medial fashion.
- At this point, it is often easier to start the transection of the gastrocolic ligament medially, entering the lesser sac and proceeding with the transection of the gastrocolic ligament in a medial to lateral dissection (**FIGURE 14**) until the lateral dissection plane around the splenic flexure is encountered.

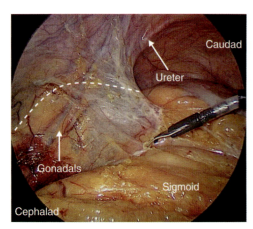

FIGURE 13 • Lateral sigmoid colon mobilization. The lateral retroperitoneal attachments of the sigmoid colon are divided (dotted line), readily entering the previous medial to lateral dissection plane. The left ureter and gonadal vessels are visualized in the retroperitoneum.

- The splenic flexure and descending colon are now completely free of any attachments and fully mobilized toward the midline.
- Mobilization of the splenic flexure is greatly facilitated by having completed the medial to lateral mobilization of the splenic flexure in the previous step.

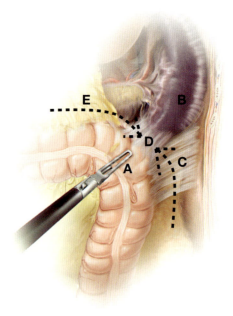

FIGURE 14 • Mobilization of the splenic flexure. The surgeon retracts the splenic flexure of the colon (A) downward and medially, exposing the attachments of the flexure to the spleen (B). The phrenocolic (C) and splenocolic (D) ligaments are transected in an inferior to superior and lateral to medial direction. The gastrocolic ligament (E) is transected in a medial to lateral direction until both planes of dissection meet and the splenic flexure is fully mobilized.

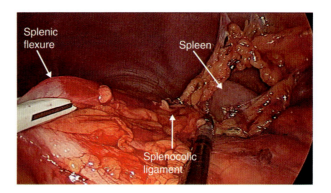

FIGURE 15 • Mobilization of the splenic flexure: transection of the splenocolic ligament.

DIVISION OF THE SIGMOID COLON

- An endostapler is inserted into the 12-mm port and used to divide the sigmoid colon distal to the rectosigmoid junction (FIGURE 16), which can be identified by the splaying of the tinea coli.
- The abdomen is desufflated, the umbilical port is extended to a 4-cm incision, and a wound protector is placed.
- The sigmoid colon is grasped at its transected distal end and pulled through the 4-cm incision to an appropriate location on the descending colon for the proximal side of the anastomosis.
- If an end-to-end colorectal anastomosis will be constructed, a bowel clamp and purse-string device are applied to the descending colon, which is divided to permit removal of the sigmoid colon. The anvil for a size 31-mm end-to-end anastomosis (EEA) stapler is placed in the descending colon and the purse string is drawn up snugly and tied.

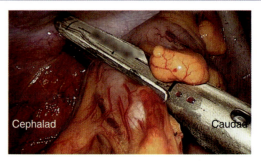

FIGURE 16 • Distal transection. An endostapler is inserted into the 12-mm port and used to divide the sigmoid colon distal to the rectosigmoid junction.

- If a side-to-end anastomosis will be constructed, the descending colon is transected between clamps; the anvil of the EEA stapler device is inserted through the

Chapter 20 SIGMOID COLECTOMY: LAPAROSCOPIC TECHNIQUE

open distal end of the colon and the anvil (with a spear attached to it) is delivered through the antimesenteric aspect of the descending colon approximately 5 cm from the opened distal end. The distal end is closed with a linear stapler.
- The sigmoid colon is removed from the field.

CREATING AND TESTING THE ANASTOMOSIS

- The colon end with the anvil in place is dropped back into the abdomen and the fascial incision is closed. Insufflation with CO_2 is reinitiated.
- With laparoscopic visualization, an EEA stapler is inserted through the anal canal and into the rectum. When the stapler reaches the proximal-most portion of the rectum, the spike is advanced through the rectal wall adjacent to the staple line.
- A grasper is used to remove the spike from the stapler shaft. The spike must be carefully placed in a uniform location in order to avoid losing it within the peritoneal cavity. Using graspers, the spike and anvil are then married (**FIGURE 17A**) and the EEA stapler is closed and deployed (**FIGURE 17B**). The stapler is then removed from the anal canal and the anastomotic donuts are inspected. Two intact donuts should be observed. The spike is removed from the abdomen.
- To test for leakage, the anastomosis is covered with sterile saline and the proximal colon is gently compressed. A rigid or flexible sigmoidoscope is inserted through the anal canal and into the rectum, insufflating the rectum with air until it escapes the anal canal. The staple line is carefully inspected for evidence of air bubbles (**FIGURE 18**). When no air bubbles are seen, the rectum is desufflated and the sigmoidoscope is removed. Air bubbles would indicate an anastomotic leak and would necessitate either revision of the anastomosis and/or performance of a proximal diverting ostomy, depending on the severity of the leak as well as on patient and operative circumstances.

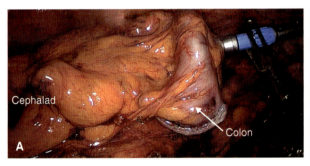 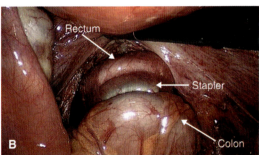

FIGURE 17 • Intracorporeal stapled anastomosis: A side-to-end stapled EEA is constructed. Using graspers, the spike (rectal side) and anvil (colon side) are married (**A**) and the EEA stapler is closed and deployed (**B**), creating the anastomosis.

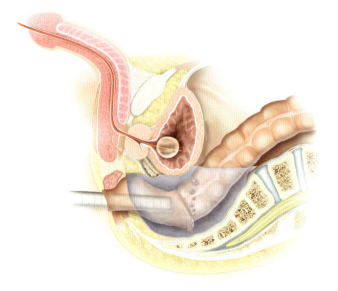

FIGURE 18 • Air leak test. The completed colorectal anastomosis is tested under water. Air bubbles identified during insufflation of the anastomosis indicate an anastomotic leak.

WOUND CLOSURE

- Port sites are closed at the skin in the preferred manner.
- The umbilical fascia closure is inspected and completed if necessary. Subcutaneous tissue is irrigated with sterile saline and skin is closed as desired.

SECTION II SURGERY OF THE COLON, APPENDIX, RECTUM, AND ANUS

PEARLS AND PITFALLS

Preoperative planning	■ For any neoplastic lesion, use of preoperative colonoscopic tattoo can help to avoid resecting the incorrect colon segment. ■ This practice is particularly important for laparoscopic resection as the colon cannot be palpated prior to the first division.
IMA division	■ The nerve plexus adjacent to the IMA takeoff is associated with sexual function in males. Therefore, the dissection should proceed directly beneath the pedicle and extend laterally. ■ Patients should be informed preoperatively that even with great care, it is possible to injure the nerves, which may lead to impaired sexual function.
Anastomosis	■ In some cases, mobilization for a tension-free anastomosis will be facilitated with extra port placement. For example, an additional suprapubic 5-mm port can greatly assist visualization during the mesenteric dissection toward the splenic flexure. ■ If the descending colon is in spasm or if it is difficult to insert a size 31-mm stapler anvil, the bowel can be relaxed with administration of 0.5-1 mg intravenous glucagon in the absence of hypotension. ■ Careful attention to the location of spike placement is of utmost importance. The most common site for placement is the left gutter just distal to dissection. The spike should be removed from the abdomen prior to the air leak test.
Avoiding ureteral injury	■ The ureters must be carefully visualized after the initial mesentery division and again during division of the lateral peritoneal attachments. If there is a concern for ureteral injury, intravenous indigo carmine should be administered, followed by a search for extravasation of blue dye.

POSTOPERATIVE CARE

■ The orogastric tube and any ureteral stents should be removed prior to awakening the patient from anesthesia. Within 24 hours of surgery, the urinary catheter should be removed.

■ Persuasive evidence indicates that an enhanced recovery program of limited intraoperative intravenous fluids, early postoperative ambulation, early feeding, and minimization of narcotic pain medication can lead to a more rapid recovery and earlier discharge. Such early discharge has not been associated with increased risk for readmissions.

OUTCOMES

■ Functional outcomes after laparoscopic sigmoid colectomy may include reduced pain and spasms prior to bowel movements if the patient suffered from an obstructive or inflammatory diagnosis.

■ Although many patients report defecatory urgency and increased frequency in the 30-day postoperative period, in most cases the urgency resolves and frequency declines after 4 to 6 weeks.

COMPLICATIONS

■ Peroneal nerve injury (positioning)
■ Ureteral injury
■ Postoperative bleeding
■ Wound infection
■ Anastomotic leak
■ Anastomotic stenosis
■ Sexual dysfunction
■ Bowel dysfunction (urgency and frequency)

SUGGESTED READINGS

1. Ambrosetti P, Jenny A, Becker C, et al Acute left colonic diverticulitis—compared performance of computed tomography and water-soluble contrast enema: prospective evaluation of 420 patients. *Dis Colon Rectum*. 2000;43(10):1363-1367.
2. Benson AB III, Bekaii-Saab T, Chan E, et al. Localized colon cancer, version 3.2013: featured updates to the NCCN Guidelines. *J Natl Compr Cancer Netw*. 2013;11(5):519-528.
3. Delaney CP, Brady K, Woconish D, et al. Towards optimizing perioperative colorectal care: outcomes for 1,000 consecutive laparoscopic colon procedures using enhanced recovery pathways. *Am J Surg*. 2012;203(3):353-355; discussion 355-356.
4. Hendren S, Morris AM, Zhang W, et al. Early discharge and hospital readmission after colectomy for cancer. *Dis Colon Rectum*. 2011;54(11):1362-1367.
5. Kim EK, Sheetz KH, Bonn J, et al. A statewide colectomy experience: the role of full bowel preparation in preventing surgical site infection. *Ann Surg*. 2014;259(2):310-314.
6. Morris AM, Regenbogen SE, Hardiman KM, et al. Sigmoid diverticulitis: a systematic review. *JAMA*. 2014;311(3):287-297.

Chapter 21

Sigmoid Colectomy: Hand-Assisted Laparoscopic Technique

Daniel A. Anaya and Daniel Albo

DEFINITION

- A sigmoidectomy is the resection of the sigmoid colon to the level of the rectosigmoid junction. The extent of the lymphadenectomy will be determined by the indication (benign vs malignant disease).
- Focal segmental sigmoid resection for benign disease can be accomplished by dividing the vessels close to the bowel wall, without the need for a high pedicle transection. A complete sigmoidectomy (described in this chapter) includes transection of the inferior mesenteric artery (IMA) at its origin and resection of the proximal superior hemorrhoidal artery (SHA) and sigmoidal branches.
- Hand-assisted laparoscopic surgery (HALS) is a minimally invasive surgical approach that uses conventional laparoscopic-assisted (LA) surgery techniques with the addition of a hand-assisted device (placed in the projected specimen extraction site) that allows for the introduction of a hand into the surgical field. HALS in colorectal surgery retains all of the same advantages of conventional LA surgery over open surgery, including less pain, faster recovery, lower incidence of wound complications, and reduction of cardiopulmonary complications, especially in the obese and in the elderly.
- Advantages of HALS over conventional LA colorectal surgery include the following:
  - Reintroducing tactile feedback into the field
  - Shorter learning curves; easier to teach
  - Shorter operative times and lower conversion to open rates
  - Higher utilization rates of minimally invasive surgery

DIFFERENTIAL DIAGNOSIS

- Indications for sigmoidectomy include the following:
  - Polyps
  - Colon cancer
  - Diverticular disease (ie, complicated diverticulitis, perforation, fistulae, etc)
- Other indications include sigmoid volvulus, inflammatory bowel disease, ischemic or infectious colitis, and trauma.

PATIENT HISTORY AND PHYSICAL FINDINGS

- Patients with sigmoid pathology can be asymptomatic, with abnormalities found during screening colonoscopy.
- The most common symptoms are bleeding (occult/anemia or overt), obstruction, and pain.
- The initial history should include the following:
  - Time course of presenting symptoms, including bleeding, constipation, and pain
  - Presence/absence of rectal incontinence
  - History of sexual function (erection and ejaculation for males, dyspareunia for females)
  - Information regarding associated urologic symptoms such as recurrent urinary tract infections, dysuria, pneumaturia, and/or fecaluria, which suggest a possible fistula with the urinary tract
  - Presence of systemic symptoms such as fever and weight loss
  - Previous surgical history, specifically regarding abdominal and/or pelvic surgery
  - Personal and/or family history of prior colon cancer/polyps, inflammatory bowel disease, or diverticular disease
- The *physical examination* should include the following:
  - Focused abdominal examination, including the notation of abdominal scars
  - Digital rectal examination, focused on assessment of sphincter function
  - Rigid proctoscopy for all patients with sigmoid polyps or cancer reported by endoscopy to be within 20 cm from the anal verge. This will allow for confirmation of the site of the lesion, which oftentimes may not coincide with the endoscopy report. This information may alter the surgical and oncologic approach. It is not uncommon for patients thought to have sigmoid adenocarcinoma based on colonoscopic findings to have rectal adenocarcinoma on rigid proctoscopy examination. The latter patients would need to have a low anterior resection operation and, potentially, could benefit from neoadjuvant therapy.
  - Rigid proctoscopy should not be performed in patients presenting with acute diverticulitis or perforation to avoid worsening of a microperforation by air insufflation.

IMAGING AND OTHER DIAGNOSTIC STUDIES

- A complete colonoscopy should be performed to rule out synchronous disease. Regardless of the primary location of the tumor, every patient should have a complete colonoscopy study whenever possible, since 2% to 9% of the patients may have synchronous tumors elsewhere in the colon and rectum.
- For cancer and/or polyps, a tattoo must be placed just distal to the lesion at three different points within the circumference to allow for intraoperative localization of the target.
- A colonic enema with double contrast may be used in patients in whom colonoscopy is not possible. Virtual colonoscopy (computed tomography [CT] colonography) is also an option for those that cannot undergo colonoscopy.
- A contrast-enhanced CT of the abdomen and pelvis is obtained to rule out adjacent organ involvement, to evaluate for extraluminal complications (eg, abscess, fistula), and to

165

rule out metastatic disease in patients with cancer. A CT of the chest completes the metastatic workup.
- A carcinoembryonic antigen (CEA) level is obtained in all cancer cases. The baseline preoperative result and postsurgical control must be obtained as an assessment for complete tumor resection. Absolute CEA presurgical value is an independent variable for survival.

SURGICAL MANAGEMENT

Preoperative Planning

- An informed consent, including discussion of the need for a possible ostomy, is obtained.
- We use an enhanced recovery after surgery clinical pathway (described elsewhere in this textbook) for the perioperative management of all of our colorectal surgery patients.
- A mechanical preoperative bowel preparation may be considered to facilitate the handling of the colon during laparoscopic surgery. Fleet enemas are prescribed to facilitate the performance of the anastomosis.
- All patients should receive preoperative prophylactic antibiotics, following published guidelines. We administer 1 to 2 g of ertapenem based on patient's BMI within 1 hour of surgical incision.
- Pharmacologic deep vein thrombosis (DVT) prophylaxis should be given to patients perioperatively, based on current recommendations and guidelines.

Equipment and Instrumentation

- We use a minimalistic approach to instrumentation, emphasizing a streamlined, efficient, and reproducible approach to our procedures. The entire operation is performed with essentially three instruments (a slotted grasper, am energy device, and a stapler) plus the camera. This approach minimizes clutter, makes the operation more efficient, and maximizes cost-efficiency.
- 5-mm, 30° scope with high-resolution monitors.
- 5- and 12-mm clear ports with balloon tips. They hold ports in the abdomen during instrument exchanges, minimize dripping/condensation on the scope, and minimize intra-abdominal profile/fulcrum effect of the trocars during surgery.
- A blunt tip, 5-mm, 37-cm long energy device.
- A slotted laparoscopic grasper
- 60-mm linear roticulating laparoscopic staplers with vascular and tan cartridges.
- We use the GelPort hand-assisted device due to its versatility and ease of use. This device allows for the introduction/removal of the hand without losing pneumoperitoneum and allows for insertion of multiple ports through the hand-assisted device if necessary. It also allows for the introduction of laparotomy pads into the field, which are very useful to retract bowel/omentum in obese patients and to clean up the field and the scope during the procedure. It is imperative to mark every lap pad introduced into the abdomen on the operating room (OR) board and include them in the final counts to avoid inadvertently leaving a lap pad in the abdominal cavity after the procedure.
- We like to use a disposable three-instrument long pouch to place the energy device and slotted graspers during the procedure. This pouch is placed on the patient's left hip/thigh in between the surgeon and the monitor. This pouch functions like a holster to facilitate an easy and intuitive handling of the two instruments used during the entire operation and allowing the surgeon's eyes to never leave the target in the monitor.

Patient Positioning and Operating Room Setup

- A preoperative briefing with the entire surgical team is conducted. Items discussed include patient identification, type of surgery, type of anesthesia, expected events during the surgery, the need for blood components, prophylactic antibiotic, surgical devices availability, and potential adverse events and their prevention.
- A dedicated, highly trained team in laparoscopic concepts is paramount. Critical members of this team concept are the scrub nurse, the circulating nurses, the assistants, and the anesthesia team members. I cannot emphasize enough the importance of a total team concept in accomplishing the highest level of performance during laparoscopic surgery.
- Proper patient position and OR setup is critical for successful performance of minimally invasive surgery (**FIGURE 1**).
- The patient is placed in a modified lithotomy position using Yellofin stirrups with the heels firmly planted in the stirrups to avoid having the patient slide with gravity assist maneuvers during the procedure.
- Pressure-bearing areas in the calf and lateral legs are padded to prevent DVTs and lateral peroneal nerve injury.
- The patient's toes, knee, and contralateral shoulders are aligned.
- The thighs are placed parallel to the ground to prevent conflict with the surgeon's arms.
- The patient's buttocks are placed at the edge of the table to allow for smoother introduction of the end-to-end anastomosis (EEA) stapler at time of reconstruction. The coccyx should be readily palpable off the edge of the table.
- Both arms are tucked at the sides, with padding added to protect against neurovascular injuries.

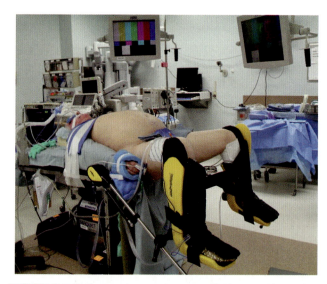

FIGURE 1 • Patient and operating room (OR) setup. The patient is placed in a modified lithotomy position with the thighs parallel to the floor and the arms tucked. The patient is secured to the OR bed using a chest tape-over-towel technique.

Chapter 21 SIGMOID COLECTOMY: HAND-ASSISTED LAPAROSCOPIC TECHNIQUE   167

- The patient is taped to the table across the chest over towels to avoid slipping. The shoulders are padded to avoid neurovascular injuries.
- All laparoscopic elements (CO_2 line, camera, light cord) exit through the right upper side. All energy device cords exit through the upper left side. This allows for a clutter-free working space for the operative team.

Team Positioning and Draping

- The patient is prepped with chlorhexidine and draped to facilitate easy access to the perineum.
- The surgeon stands at the patient's right lower side, with the assistant to their left side and the scrub nurse to their right side (**FIGURE 2**).
- Two monitors are placed in front of the team at eye level and slighted tilted upward (to avoid ergonomic injury to the surgeon's lower neck/brachial plexus) on the patient's left side.
- There are four important principles that we follow for all laparoscopic cases: alignment, triangulation, a flat horizon, and gravity assist.
- Alignment involves the placement of the team, ports, target lesion, and monitors in straight lines of vision.
- Triangulation involves the creation of an imaginary triangle, where the surgeon's hands/instruments/trocars are at the angles in the base of the triangle, and the target lesion is located at the apex of the triangle. The camera bisects this triangle and, in laparoscopic surgery, is always in front of the hands of the surgeon. This is in contrast to open surgery, where the surgeon's hands are in front of the eyes.
- The concept of horizon is a fundamental difference between laparoscopic and open surgery. In open surgery, the surgeon looks down into the field. In laparoscopic surgery, the surgeon looks to their front, introducing the concept of the horizon. It is imperative that the camera operator maintains a flat horizon in front of the operator to avoid disorientation. This is particularly important with the use of angled scopes (ie, a 30° scope).
- Extreme gravity assist maneuvers are critically important in laparoscopic surgery to keep the bowel and omentum away

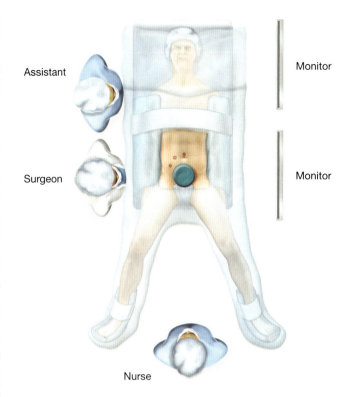

FIGURE 2 • Team and monitor setup. The surgeon stands at the patient's right lower side with the assistant to their left and the scrub nurse to their right. The monitors are placed in front of the team at eye level.

from the operative field and to provide optimal exposure. To accomplish this while avoiding the patient sliding during the procedure, the patient needs to be secured to the table, so the table and the patient move as one. Padding on all pressure points is imperative to avoid neurovascular injuries to the extremities during the procedure.

PORT PLACEMENT

- Insert the GelPort through a 5- to 6-cm Pfannenstiel incision (**FIGURE 3**). One of the main advantages of HALS is that it uses the extraction site incision necessary in colorectal surgery procedures during the entire operation instead of just using it at the end of the procedure. This allows for the introduction of the surgeon's hand without losing pneumoperitoneum insufflation at various portions of the operation, reintroducing tactile feedback for the surgeon, making the operation much more efficient.
- The size of this incision in centimeters is usually 1 to ½ cm less than the surgeon's glove size. Make this incision as long as you need it to be comfortable during the operation; the size of the extraction size has no impact on any meaningful perioperative outcome.
- This incision will be also used for specimen extraction. The Pfannenstiel incision (as opposed as vertical extraction site incisions) results in better cosmesis, lowers the incidence of wound infections and hernias, and allows for more working space between the hand and the instruments.
- Ports: Insert a 5-mm working port in the right upper quadrant (RUQ), a 12-mm working port in the right lower quadrant, and a 5-mm camera port above the umbilicus. These three ports are triangulated, with the camera port at the apex of the triangle. This setup avoids conflict between the working instruments and the camera and prevents disorientation (avoids "working on a mirror") (**FIGURE 3**).

TECHNIQUES

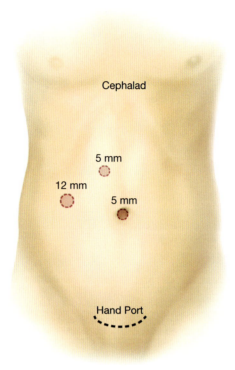

FIGURE 3 • Port placement. The hand port is inserted through a 6-cm Pfannenstiel incision at the projected extraction site. A 5-mm camera port is inserted supraumbilically. A 5-mm and a 12-mm working port are inserted in the right upper and right lower quadrants, respectively.

OPERATIVE STEPS

- All of our operations are process-driven and highly standardized to maximize efficiency, quality, and cost-efficiency. We divide the operations in well-defined, sequential steps. Every step has a single strategic objective (it is the name of the step), a clear beginning and end, and a critical anatomy that is required to be identified.
- We believe that this stepwise approach makes it easier to teach and learn these complex operations. In fact, it is designed to strip down all complexity and to shorten the learning curve of the surgeon.
- Every step opens the planes of dissection that are necessary for the steps that will follow, flowing "downstream" and opening the planes of dissection sequentially always in front of the operator. This way, the only time that the surgeon encounters a virgin tissue plane is at the very beginning of the operation. We call this first step the point of entry.
- The ideal point of entry has three characteristics: it is easy to find, has minimal to no anatomical variations, and minimizes potential injury to other structures around it during its performance. In order to simplify our operations we use only two potential points of entry for all our laparoscopic colorectal surgeries. For all resections to the left side of the middle colic vessels, we use the inferior mesenteric vein (IMV) as the point of entry.
- Our HALS sigmoidectomy operation consists of nine steps:
    1. Transection of the IMV
    2. Transection of the IMA
    3. Medial to lateral dissection of the mesocolon
    4. Sigmoid colon mobilization off the pelvic inlet
    5. Lateral descending colon mobilization
    6. Mobilization of the splenic flexure
    7. Intracorporeal distal transection
    8. Extracorporeal proximal transection
    9. Intracorporeal anastomosis

Step 1: Transection of the Inferior Mesenteric Vein

- This is the critical "point of entry" in this operation. We favor it over starting at the IMA level due to the IMV's constancy in location, the ease of its visualization by the ligament of Treitz, and the absence of structures that can be harmed around it (no iliac vessels, left ureter, or hypogastric nerve nearby). This will be the only time during the operation when a virgin tissue plane is entered. Every step will set up the following ones, opening the tissue planes sequentially.
- The patient is placed on a steep Trendelenburg position with the left side up. Using the right hand, move the small bowel into the RUQ and the transverse colon and omentum into the upper and right abdomen. If necessary, place a laparotomy pad to hold the bowel out of the field of view, especially in obese patients. This pad can also be used to dry up the field and to clean the scope tip intracorporeally. Make sure the circulating nurse notes the laparotomy pad in the abdomen on the white board.
- Identify the critical anatomy: IMV, ligament of Treitz, and left colic artery (**FIGURE 4**).

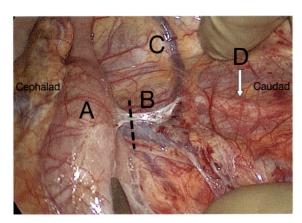

FIGURE 4 • Step 1: Key anatomy. Ligament of Treitz *(A)*. Inferior mesenteric vein (IMV) *(B)*. Left colic artery *(C)* as it separates from the IMV and goes toward the splenic flexure of the colon. The left ureter *(D)* is located far from the IMV transection point *(dotted lines)*.

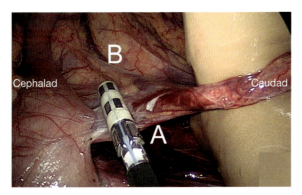

FIGURE 5 • Step 1: The surgeon holds the inferior mesenteric vein *(A)* anteriorly with their right hand and transects it cephalad of the left colic artery *(B)* with a 5-mm energy device.

- If there are attachments between the duodenum/root of mesentery and mesocolon, transect them with laparoscopic scissors or energy device. This will allow for adequate exposure of midline structures.
- Pick up the IMV/left colic artery with the right hand. Incise the peritoneum under the IMV/left colic artery and dissect in front of Gerota fascia with the energy device, starting at the level of the ligament of Treitz. Proceed with the dissection caudally toward the IMA. The assistant provides upward countertraction with a grasper.
- Transect the IMV with the energy device (**FIGURE 5**) cephalad of left colic artery, which moves away from the IMV and toward the splenic flexure of the colon, with the 5-mm energy device, thus preserving intact the left-sided marginal arterial arcade and preserving the blood supply to the anastomosis.

Step 2: Transection of the Inferior Mesenteric Artery

- Identify the critical anatomy: the "letter T" formed between the IMA and its left colic and superior SHA terminal branches (**FIGURE 6**).
- Using the hand, the aorta is identified and tracked down to the level of its bifurcation. The IMA will originate 1 to 2 cm proximal to this level.

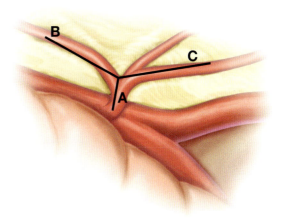

FIGURE 6 • Step 2: Critical anatomy. Identify the letter T formed between the inferior mesenteric artery *(A)* and its left colic artery *(B)* and superior hemorrhoidal artery *(C)* terminal branches.

- Using your thumb, palpate the groove between the left common iliac artery pulse and the SHA. Use your index finger to encircle the SHA and pick it up, turning it into an arch. The SHA fold is thicker than the inexperienced surgeon may think. A common mistake during this portion of the operation is to think that the SHA fold is too thick, wrongly thinking that you are instead under the left common iliac artery and the left ureter. This results in a too shallow dissection plane superficial to the SHA and, therefore, entering the wrong plane into the mesocolon, resulting in troublesome bleeding and disorienting the surgeon.
- Holding the SHA up with the right hand, dissect the plane along the palpable groove between the SHA and the left iliac artery using an energy device. After scoring the peritoneum under the SHA, use a 5-mm energy device to dissect (by gently pushing downward toward the retroperitoneum) along the avascular plane located between the meso-descending colon, anteriorly, and the retroperitoneum, posteriorly. This avascular plane can be identified by the transition between the two distinctive fat planes.
- Preserve the sympathetic nerve trunk intact in the retroperitoneum. Identify the left ureter, located in front of the left iliac artery and psoas muscle and medial to the gonadal vessels, before transecting any structure (**FIGURE 7**). If you are directly on the psoas muscle, chances are that you left the left ureter attached to the dorsal surface of the mesocolon; bring it down into the retroperitoneum gently using blunt dissection with the energy device.
- If you cannot identify the ureter, try dissecting superior to inferior, starting from the IMV plane of dissection and moving caudally behind the IMA. If you still cannot find it, perform a lateral to medial mobilization of the sigmoid colon toward the midline. In this latter scenario, you will encounter the left gonadal vessels first, lateral to the left ureter.
- You can now visualize the dissected letter "T" (**FIGURE 7**). Dissect with your thumb and index finger around and behind the IMA. With the left ureter safely preserved in the retroperitoneum, transect the IMA at its origin with a vascular load stapler (**FIGURE 8**, *dotted line*). This ensures excellent lymph

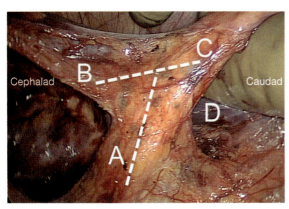

FIGURE 7 • Step 2: The letter T dissected: inferior mesenteric artery (IMA) *(A)*, left colic artery *(B)*, and superior hemorrhoidal artery (SHA) *(C)*. Notice the left ureter *(D)* in the retroperitoneum. The IMA takeoff is just cephalad from the aortic bifurcation *(dotted lines)*. The thumb and index finger are lifting the SHA off the groove located anterior to the right common iliac artery.

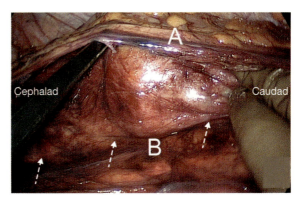

FIGURE 9 • Step 3: Medial to lateral dissection of the descending mesocolon. The surgeon's hand is holding the descending mesocolon and colon anteriorly *(A)*, separating them from Gerota fascia and other retroperitoneal structures *(B)*. The dissection proceeds along the transition between the two distinct fat planes *(arrows)*.

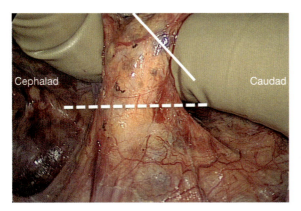

FIGURE 8 • Step 2: The inferior mesenteric artery (IMA) is now completely encircled and will be transected at its origin *(dotted line)* with a stapler or energy device. Alternatively, the vascular transection can be done at the takeoff of the superior hemorrhoidal artery and sigmoidal vessels *(solid line)*, preserving the IMA and left colic vessels intact and ensuring prograde blood flow into the descending colon.

node harvest and great exposure for step 3. The presence of the hand in the abdomen allows for a safe control of what could be serious bleeding from the IMA stump off the aorta should the staple line fail.

- Alternatively, the vascular transection can be done at the takeoff of the SHA and sigmoidal vessels (**FIGURE 8**, *solid line*), preserving the IMA and left colic intact and ensuring prograde blood flow into the descending colon segment that will be eventually used for the anastomosis. The drawback is that this makes the medial to lateral dissection step somewhat more challenging because the IMA will keep the mesocolon tethered to the retroperitoneum.

Step 3: Medial to Lateral Dissection of the Descending Mesocolon

- The surgeon's right hand and the assistant's grasper hold the descending mesocolon up, creating a working space between the mesocolon and the retroperitoneum (**FIGURE 9**). The plane between the mesocolon and Gerota fascia, readily identified by the transition between the two fat planes, is dissected bluntly in a downward direction toward the retroperitoneum with the 5-mm energy device.
- Dissect caudally toward the pelvic inlet; this will greatly facilitate performance of step 4.
- Dissect laterally until you reach the lateral abdominal wall; this will greatly facilitate performance of step 5.
- Dissect cephalad, under the splenic flexure of the colon, until reaching the inferior border of the pancreas. This is critical for an easy mobilization of the splenic flexure during step 6.

Step 4: Sigmoid Colon Mobilization off the Pelvic Inlet

- The surgeon pulls the sigmoid colon medially, exposing the lateral sigmoid colon attachments (**FIGURE 10A**). Transect the attachments between the sigmoid and the pelvic inlet with laparoscopic scissors or energy device in your left hand, staying medially, close to the sigmoid and mesosigmoid, to avoid injuring the ureter/gonadal vessels.
- Dissect caudally until reaching the entrance to the left pelvic inlet.
- The left ureter and gonadal vessels, dissected in step 3, should be visible (**FIGURE 10B**).

Step 5: Lateral Descending Colon Mobilization

- Retract the descending colon medially with your left hand. Transect the white line of Toldt up to the splenic flexure using endoscopic scissors. You should readily enter the retroperitoneal dissection plane dissected during step 3 (**FIGURE 11**).

Step 6: Splenic Flexure Mobilization

- Place the patient on reverse Trendelenburg position with the left side up to help displace the splenic flexure down out of the left upper quadrant.
- The key to an easy splenic flexure mobilization is to have completed the separation of the splenic flexure off the retroperitoneum during the medial to lateral mobilization (step 3).

Chapter 21 SIGMOID COLECTOMY: HAND-ASSISTED LAPAROSCOPIC TECHNIQUE 171

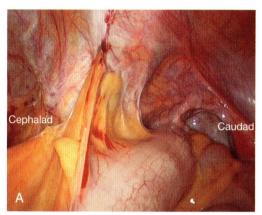

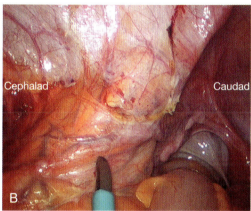

FIGURE 10 • Step 4. **A,** Medial traction on the sigmoid exposes its lateral attachments to the pelvic inlet. **B,** After the sigmoid mobilization is completed, the left ureter is visualized as it crosses over the left iliac artery.

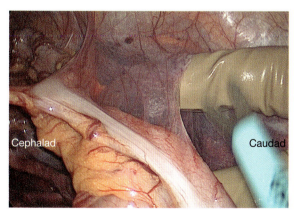

FIGURE 11 • Step 5: Transection of the lateral descending colon attachments. Notice that the hand has entered the retroperitoneal dissection plane previously dissected during step 3.

- We use a bidirectional dissection approach to the splenic flexure mobilization, with an upward lateral dissection along the left gutter and a medial to lateral dissection along the lesser sac meeting around the splenic flexure (**FIGURE 12**).
- The medial to lateral phase of the splenic flexure mobilization is started by entering the lesser sac at the midline. With the assistant pulling the transverse colon downward with a

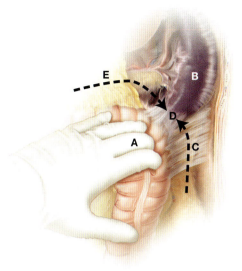

FIGURE 12 • Step 6: Mobilization of the splenic flexure. The surgeon retracts the splenic flexure of the colon (A) downward and medially, exposing the attachments of the flexure to the spleen (B). The phrenocolic (C) and splenocolic (D) ligaments are transected in an inferior to superior and lateral to medial direction. The gastrocolic ligament (E) is transected in a medial to lateral direction, until both planes of dissection meet and the splenic flexure is fully mobilized.

grasper, the surgeon lifts the stomach up with their left hand, exposing the gastrocolic ligament. Transect the omentum and the gastrocolic ligament in between the stomach and transverse colon using a 5-mm energy device through the RUQ port site (**FIGURE 13A**). This allows for easy entrance into the lesser sac and provides for an excellent view of the splenic flexure.

- Transect the gastrocolic ligament (from medial to lateral) with the 5-mm energy device, staying close to the transverse colon and avoiding the spleen. Proceed laterally toward the splenic flexure. Care must be taken to avoid inadvertent injury to the colon.
- At this point, a superior to inferior and lateral to medial dissection around the splenic flexure is performed. Because the medial to lateral dissection performed in step 3 completely separated the splenic flexure of the colon from the retroperitoneum, the surgeon can now slide their right hand under the splenic flexure, connecting the two planes of dissection around the flexure, with the index finger "hooked" under the splenocolic ligament. This allows for an easy transection of the splenocolic ligament with an endoshears or energy device (**FIGURE 13B**).
- Attachments of the splenic flexure to the pancreas are transected and the splenic flexure is now fully mobilized to the midline.

Step 7: Intracorporeal Distal Transection

- Dissect the rectosigmoid junction circumferentially. The rectosigmoid junction can be identified by the splaying of the tenia coli. Transect the upper mesorectum with the 5-mm

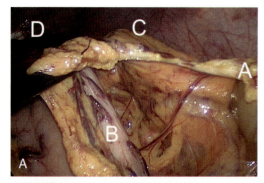

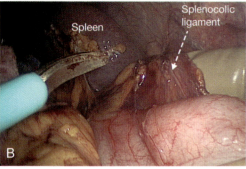

FIGURE 13 • Step 6: Mobilization of the splenic flexure. **A,** The partially transected gastrocolic ligament is visible between the transverse colon *(A)* and the stomach *(B)*. Notice the excellent view of the lesser sac laterally toward the splenic flexure of the colon *(C)* and the spleen *(D)*. **B,** The surgeon is "hugging" the splenic flexure with their right hand and is "hooking" their index finger under the splenocolic ligament, allowing for an excellent exposure and transection of this ligament with an energy device.

- energy device at the level of the projected distal bowel transection.
- While pulling on the sigmoid upward with the left hand, transect the bowel intracorporeally just distal to the rectosigmoid junction with a linear Endo GIA stapler device (**FIGURE 14**).
- At this point, transect the mesocolon between the sigmoid and left colic vessels with the 5-mm energy device. Start at the stapled IMA stump on the specimen side, and move up toward the colon wall, transecting the left colic artery (at its origin, off the IMA stump) and the marginal artery (close to the colon wall).

Step 8: Extracorporeal Proximal Transection

- Deliver the sigmoid and descending colon through the Pfannenstiel incision site with the Alexis wound protector in place to protect the wound from oncologic/infectious contamination.
- There should be absolutely no tension during the extraction of the specimen. Otherwise, mesenteric tears that could lead

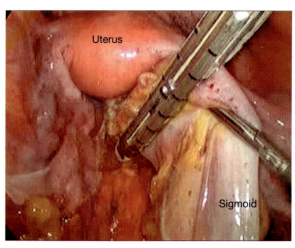

FIGURE 14 • Step 7. The intracorporeal distal transection is performed with a linear stapler just distal to the rectosigmoid junction.

to troublesome bleeding may occur. If there is tension during the extraction phase, completely mobilize the splenic flexure if you have not done so already.
- Transect the colon between Kocher clamps between the sigmoidal and left colic vessel distribution, at the point where the mesocolon was previously transected intracorporeally during the previous step. Send the specimen to the pathologist for evaluation.
- Now place the anvil of a 29-mm EEA stapler device into the descending colon and exteriorize it through the antimesenteric border with the spike approximately 5 cm proximal to the open end of the colon. Close the distal end of the descending colon with a linear stapler cartridge.
- Reintroduce the descending colon with the anvil in place into the abdomen in preparation for the anastomosis. Close the hand access port and re-insufflate the pneumoperitoneum.

Step 9: Intracorporeal Colorectal Anastomosis

- You are now ready to perform the intracorporeal side-to-end colorectal anastomosis (**FIGURE 15**).
- The assistant introduces the 29-mm EEA stapler device into the rectum and opens the spear through the rectal stump, anterior to the staple line, under direct laparoscopic visualization.
- Making sure the mesentery is facing medially and that there are no twists in the bowel, the two ends of the stapler are brought together and the stapler is closed, while avoiding any additional tissue to slip in between the two ends. Once fully closed, the stapler is fired and the EEA carefully pulled back out of the rectum.
- To ensure that the anastomosis is intact, we check for the two donuts to be complete and subsequently test the anastomosis by insufflating it under water, ensuring that it is airtight (**FIGURE 16**).

Chapter 21 SIGMOID COLECTOMY: HAND-ASSISTED LAPAROSCOPIC TECHNIQUE 173

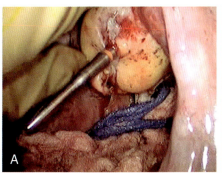
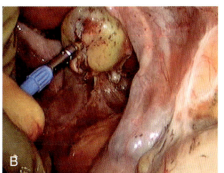
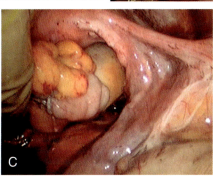

FIGURE 15 • Step 9. An intracorporeal side-to-end colorectal anastomosis is performed with a 29-mm end-to-end anastomosis stapler. The spear is brought out anterior to the rectal stump staple line **(A)** and is connected with the anvil previously placed in the descending colon **(B),** and the anastomosis is completed by firing the stapler **(C)**.

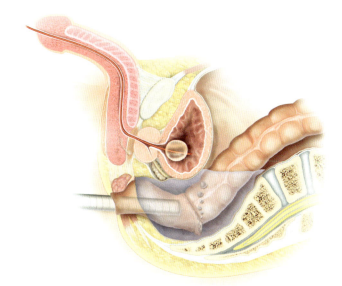

FIGURE 16 • The completed colorectal anastomosis is tested under water. Air bubbles identified during insufflation of the anastomosis indicate an anastomotic leak.

WOUND CLOSURE

- The Pfannenstiel incision is closed using a running 2-0 Vicryl suture from the posterior rectus sheet and a running no. 1 polydioxanone (PDS) suture for the anterior rectus sheet. All skin incisions are closed with 4-0 PDS subcuticular sutures. Dermabond is applied to seal off all wounds.
- We retowel the field with clean towels and change gown and gloves, Bovie electrocautery, suction cannulas prior to wound closure in an effort to minimize wound infections.
- We do not routinely use drains.

174 SECTION II **SURGERY OF THE COLON, APPENDIX, RECTUM, AND ANUS**

PEARLS AND PITFALLS

Indications	■ For benign cases, a segmental sigmoid resection, with vascular transection close to the bowel wall may be enough. ■ For malignant cases, a complete sigmoidectomy with a high vascular pedicle transection is necessary to ensure adequate lymphadenectomy.
Operative approach	■ A HALS approach improves minimally invasive surgery utilization, reduces conversions, and shortens OR times. ■ A standardized, stepwise approach leads to higher efficiency and quality.
Positioning	■ Gravity assist maneuvers allow for good visualization and exposure. ■ Secure the patient to the table, while protecting all pressure-baring areas. ■ Make sure that all anesthesia lines and monitors are working appropriately after positioning the patient; there will be limited access to the arms during the procedure. ■ Avoid unnecessary clutter of cables/lines; open the working space for the operating team.
Port placement	■ Align the surgeon, trocars, target, and monitor in straight lines. ■ Triangulate all ports aiming to the target. ■ Place the hand access port in a Pfannenstiel location.
Vascular transection	■ Transection of the IMV is the SAFEST point of entry for this operation. ■ A high IMA transection facilitates the medial to lateral dissection and ensures an excellent lymphadenectomy. ■ It is essential to identify the left ureter above prior to IMA transection.
Mesenteric dissection	■ A complete medial to lateral dissection of the mesentery is critical to facilitate all subsequent steps of this operation. ■ A medial to lateral dissection technique maximizes the advantages of laparoscopic instruments and is preferred to a lateral to medial approach.
Distal transection	■ The distal transection is easier to perform intracorporeally than extracorporeally. ■ The distal transection is performed just distal to the rectosigmoid junction, identified by the splaying of the taenia coli.
Intracoporeal anastomosis	■ A tension-free anastomosis is critical to avoid anastomotic leaks. ■ Preserve the marginal artery of Drummond to ensure good perfusion of the descending colon segment. ■ Always test the integrity of the anastomosis, and be ready to repair or redo it if a leak is identified.

POSTOPERATIVE CARE

■ Fast-track or enhanced recovery after surgery (ERAS) programs have shown to expedite postoperative recovery and to minimize postoperative complications following colon surgery. No postoperative antibiotics are used. DVT prophylaxis with heparin products is used routinely.
■ We do not use a nasogastric tube.
■ Remove the Foley catheter on the first postoperative day.
■ Encourage early ambulation, minimize postoperative use of narcotics, and promote early feeding as tolerated.
■ Patients usually meet criteria for discharge on postoperative days 3 to 4.

OUTCOMES

■ The outcomes following HAL sigmoidectomy are excellent.
■ HAL colectomy is associated with all the short-term outcome benefits of conventional laparoscopic surgery over open surgery, including less postoperative pain, earlier return of bowel function, and shorter length of stay.
■ HAL colectomy is associated with a higher usage rate and a lower rate of conversion to an open approach (2%-6% vs 20%-25%) when compared to conventional laparoscopic colectomy.
■ Postoperative complications are equivalent for HAL and conventional laparoscopic sigmoid colectomy.
■ HAL sigmoidectomy for cancer yields similar long-term oncologic outcomes compared to open surgery.

COMPLICATIONS

■ Surgical site infection
■ Anastomotic leak
■ Postoperative bleeding
■ Postoperative small bowel obstruction
■ Urinary retention
■ Dehiscence/hernia
■ Medical complications: DVT/pulmonary embolism, urinary tract infection, myocardial infarction, and so forth

SUGGESTED READINGS

1. Cima RR, Pattana-arun J, Larson DW, et al. Experience with 969 minimal access colectomies: the role of hand-assisted laparoscopy in expanding minimally invasive surgery for complex colectomies. *J Am Coll Surg.* 2008;206:946-952.
2. Jayne DG, Thorpe HC, Copeland J, et al. Five-year follow-up of the Medical Research Counsel CLASICC trial of laparoscopically assisted versus open surgery for colorectal cancer. *Br J Surg.* 2010;97: 1638-1645.
3. Marcello PW, Fleshman JW, Milsom JW, et al. Hand-assisted laparoscopic vs. laparoscopic colorectal surgery. A multicenter, prospective, randomized trial. *Dis Colon Rectum.* 2008;51:818-828.
4. Orcutt ST, Balentine CJ, Marshall CL, et al. Use of a Pfannenstiel incision in minimally invasive colorectal cancer surgery is associated with a lower risk of wound complications. *Tech Coloproctol.* 2012;16(2):127-132.
5. Orcutt ST, Marshall CL, Balentine CJ, et al. Hand-assisted laparoscopy leads to efficient colorectal cancer surgery. *J Surg Res.* 2012;177(2):e53-e58.

6. Orcutt ST, Marshall CL, Robinson CN, et al. Minimally invasive surgery in colon cancer patients leads to improved short-term outcomes and excellent oncologic results. *Am J Surg*. 2011;202(5):528-531.

7. Ozturk E, Kiran RP, Geisler DP, et al. Hand-assisted laparoscopic colectomy: benefits of laparoscopic colectomy at no extra cost. *J Am Coll Surg*. 2009;209:242-247.

8. Wilks JA, Balentine CJ, Berger DH, et al. Establishment of a minimally invasive program at a VAMC leads to improved care in colorectal cancer patients. *Am J Surg*. 2009;198(5):685-692.

9. Zhuang CL, Ye XZ, Zhang XD, et al. Enhanced recovery after surgery program versus traditional care for colorectal surgery: a meta-analysis of randomized controlled trials. *Dis Colon Rectum*. 2013;56(5):667-678.

Chapter 22

Sigmoid Colectomy: Single-Incision Laparoscopic Surgery Technique

Rodrigo Pedraza and Eric Mitchell Haas

DEFINITION

- Single-incision laparoscopic sigmoidectomy is a minimally invasive technique in which a sigmoid colectomy is performed laparoscopically through a single-port device. The entirety of the procedure is accomplished using one sole incision through which all the laparoscopic instruments are placed.
- Reduced port single-incision laparoscopic sigmoidectomy is a modified technique in which the single-port device is placed through a Pfannenstiel incision and an additional port is placed through the umbilicus. This technique is also called "single plus one" sigmoidectomy[1] and is used to facilitate operative exposure, avoid instrument conflict, and benefit from the Pfannenstiel incision—diminished infection, dehiscence, and hernia rates.

PATIENT HISTORY AND PHYSICAL FINDINGS

- Single-incision laparoscopic sigmoidectomy is safe and feasible for essentially all benign and malignant sigmoid diseases requiring resection.[2-4] The most common indications include diverticular disease, cancer, and polyps.
- Patients with diverticular disease typically present with recurrent episodes of diverticulitis or complications such as perforation or obstruction. Left lower quadrant pain and tenderness are commonly encountered and may be accompanied with nausea, vomiting, and fever. Lower gastrointestinal (GI) bleeding is rarely present.
- Cancer and polyps of the sigmoid colon are frequently diagnosed incidentally during screening colonoscopy. Those with large polyps or malignancy may present with hematochezia, bowel obstruction, perforation, or lower abdominal or pelvic pain.
- Single-incision laparoscopic sigmoidectomy is contraindicated in patients who cannot tolerate major abdominal surgical procedures, such as those with severe hemodynamic instability, recent myocardial infarction, or severe thromboembolic event.
- History of prior abdominal surgery may lead to a prolonged procedure due to extensive lysis of adhesions; nonetheless, it is not an absolute contraindication to the use of the single-incision approach.
- The procedure may be performed in patients with high body mass index (BMI). However, the high complexity and high conversion rates make this a less ideal scenario for single-incision sigmoidectomy. In patients with high BMI, conventional multiport or hand-assisted laparoscopic technique may be more suitable.
- Large, bulky tumors may require further incision lengthening during the procedure, losing pneumoperitoneum, thus hindering the ability to complete the case with the single-incision technique. Nevertheless, some single-port devices allow incision lengthening without compromising the pneumoperitoneum.
- Surgeons without experience with single-incision colectomy may encounter technical difficulties. Before offering this approach, competency with conventional multiport and/or hand-assisted laparoscopic techniques is recommended. Additionally, it is suggested that the surgeon becomes proficient in single-incision sigmoidectomy in those with benign disease prior to performing oncologic resections.

IMAGING AND OTHER DIAGNOSTIC STUDIES

- Regardless of the procedure indication, all patients necessitate appropriate preoperative evaluation with endoscopic and radiologic studies.
- For patients with diverticular disease, colonoscopy or flexible sigmoidoscopy is warranted to assess the length of the affected bowel, to determine resection levels, and to confirm the diagnosis. Furthermore, a computed tomography (CT) scan of the abdomen and pelvis is mandatory to evaluate the severity of the pericolonic disease. Some patients with severe active disease demonstrated on the CT scan may benefit from a course of antibiotics or even abscess drainage prior to the procedure.
- If the indication for the sigmoidectomy is a colonic polyp or malignancy, endoscopic tattooing of the lesion is required to ensure proper location during the laparoscopic procedure (**FIGURE 1**).
- For malignant cases, a complete oncologic workup is mandatory. A multidisciplinary approach involving surgeon and medical oncologist is preferable. Lymph node and distant

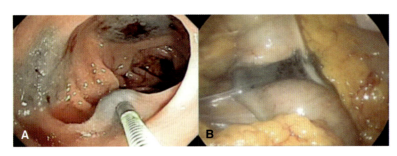

FIGURE 1 • Tattooing the lesion in at least three quadrants of the bowel wall during colonoscopy (**A**) facilitates proper location of the pathology during the laparoscopic approach (**B**).

Chapter 22 SIGMOID COLECTOMY: SINGLE-INCISION LAPAROSCOPIC SURGERY TECHNIQUE   177

organ involvement are evaluated with the CT scan of the abdomen and pelvis and positron emission tomography (PET) scan. Patients with lower tumors in the rectosigmoid junction may need magnetic resonance imaging (MRI) to evaluate tumor local progression into the pelvis and lymph node status.

SURGICAL MANAGEMENT

Preoperative Planning

- Bowel preparation is traditionally achieved through a polyethylene glycol–based laxative solution and oral antibiotics. This practice has recently been called into question. An accepted alternative is the use of a modified bowel preparation with preoperative enema to clear out the distal stool.
- In the operating room and under anesthesia, rigid proctosigmoidoscopy is recommended to ensure the level of the lesion is above the rectum and to ensure that the bowel is clean of fecal matter.
- For noncontaminated cases, prophylactic antibiotics are administered according to the Surgical Care Improvement Project (SCIP) measures.
- If the cases involve active infection such as those with recurrent diverticulitis or perforation, broad-spectrum antimicrobials with gram-negative and anaerobe bacterial coverage are chosen.

Positioning

- The patient is placed in a modified lithotomy position with both arms tucked at the patient's side. The patient is secured with adhesive tape over the chest, without compromising chest expansion (**FIGURE 2**). Antislip rubber pads may be used to further secure the patient to the operating room table. It is imperative to ensure proper and secured positioning, as later in the procedure, Trendelenburg position will be required.
- The optimal modified lithotomy position is achieved with a 25° to 30° thigh flexion and with moderate thigh abduction (**FIGURE 2**). This positioning allows adequate surgeon maneuverability, avoiding conflict with the patient's thighs while affording proper perineal access.
- For abdominal entry, laparoscopic exploration, and lysis of adhesions, the patient is in supine position. In this portion of the procedure, the surgeon and assistant are located on the right and left side, respectively.
- Thereafter, the patient is placed in Trendelenburg position with the left side elevated. The surgeon and assistant are located on the right side of the patient with the laparoscopic monitor on the left (**FIGURE 3**).

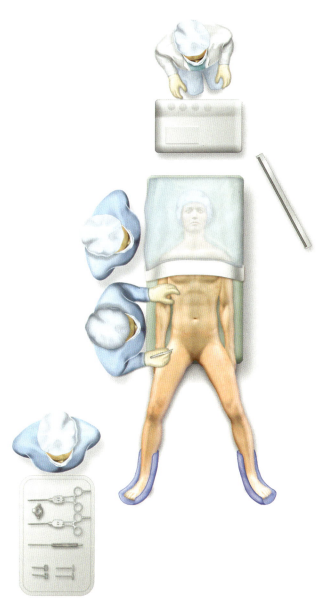

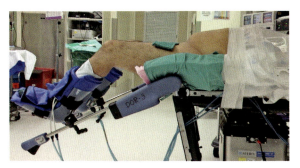

FIGURE 2 • Patient positioning. The patient is placed in a modified lithotomy, 25° to 30° thigh flexion, and with moderate thigh abduction to allow adequate surgeon maneuverability, avoiding conflict with the patient's thighs while affording proper perineal access. It is imperative to further secure the patient to the table—we use adhesive tape over the chest, avoiding compromising chest expansion.

FIGURE 3 • Operative room patient/surgeon configuration for single-incision laparoscopic sigmoid colectomy.

INCISION AND PORT PLACEMENT

- Typically, a 2.5-cm vertical umbilical skin incision is performed (**FIGURE 4**). The umbilical stump is divided, affording fascial lengthening to 4 cm without modifying the skin incision (**FIGURE 4**). Following entry into the abdominal cavity, the single-port device is placed.
- An alternative approach is the abdominal entry using a 4-cm Pfannenstiel incision (**FIGURE 5**). This modification improves cosmetic outcomes while decreasing wound infection and hernia rates. This approach is challenging, as the instruments are in close proximity with the target operative field, limiting maneuverability. Thus, when this approach is used, we favor a single plus one technique using a Pfannenstiel incision with an additional 5-mm incision for the camera in order to avoid instrument conflict (**FIGURE 5**).
- Prior to port placement, a surgical sponge may be introduced into the abdominal cavity to facilitate retraction later in the procedure.
- Port placement varies depending on the single-port device used. Once the port is placed, pneumoperitoneum is created and the laparoscopic camera and instruments are introduced.
- A 30° camera and traditional straight laparoscopic instruments are used. Alternatively, articulated instruments may be employed.
- In order to afford maximal operative reach and to avoid internal and external instrument conflict, bariatric and standard length instruments may be used simultaneously. Moreover, a right-angle light cord adaptor may be used to further decrease conflict.

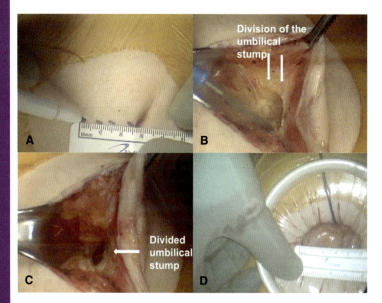

FIGURE 4 • Umbilical incision. **A,** The skin incision is 2.5 cm in length, but after division of the umbilical stump (**B** and **C**), the fascial incision size is lengthened to 4 cm (**D**).

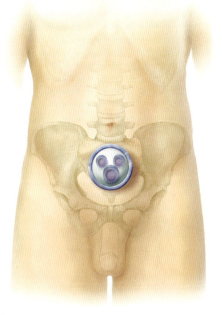
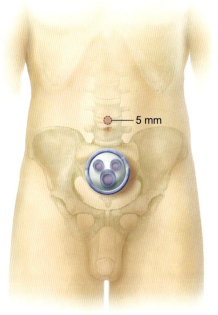

FIGURE 5 • **A,** Pfannenstiel incision port configuration for single-incision laparoscopic sigmoid colectomy. **B,** "Single plus one" technique: The addition of a 5-mm camera port in the umbilicus facilitates steps during the procedure and minimizes instrument and surgeon/assistant conflict.

EXPLORATION AND LYSIS OF ADHESIONS

- The abdominal cavity is thoroughly examined to assess the disease process and, in oncologic cases, to evaluate the presence of metastatic disease.
- If required, lysis of adhesions may be safely performed laparoscopically.

DEVELOPMENT OF THE PRESACRAL PLANE

- With the patient in Trendelenburg position and the left side elevated, the small bowel loops are retracted superiorly and to the right to expose the target operative field. The surgical sponge facilitates small bowel retraction.
- The sigmoid and rectosigmoid junction are identified and retracted anteriorly and laterally (**FIGURE 6**).
- The sacral promontory is identified and the peritoneum is incised medially with either a monopolar or bipolar energy device (**FIGURE 6**). An avascular presacral plane is created and further developed using blunt and sharp dissection

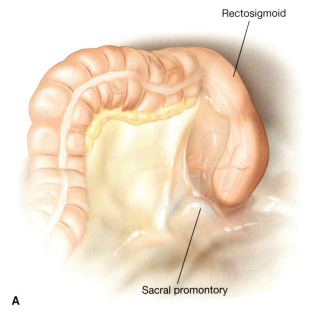
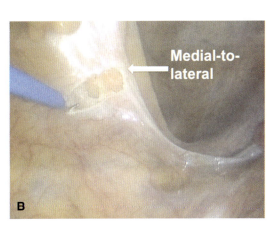
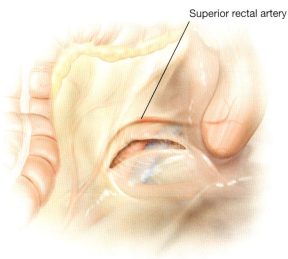
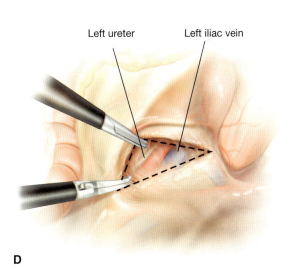

FIGURE 6 • Presacral plane development. **A,** The rectosigmoid is retracted laterally and anteriorly; the sacral promontory is identified as landmark prior to the peritoneal incision. **B,** The peritoneum is incised in a medial to lateral fashion. **C,** The presacral dissection continues and the superior rectal artery is identified. **D,** The plane is further developed using a triangulation technique with one instrument elevating the tissue while the other instruments are carrying out the dissection. Additional critical structures are identified and preserved, including the left ureter and left iliac vein.

with a bipolar tissue-sealing device (**FIGURE 6**). During this dissection, anatomic landmarks include the sacral promontory, superior rectal artery, left ureter, left gonadal vein, and left iliac vein. The concept of single-incision triangulation is used. In this technique, one instrument elevates the tissue anteriorly while the other—from the surgeon's dominant hand—performs dissection in a "hand-over-fist fashion."

- The dissection plane is developed without excessive deep dissection to avoid pelvic plexus injury. Furthermore, it is imperative to identify and to preserve the left ureter.
- Once the presacral plane is fully developed, attention is then drawn to the identification of the left colic artery.

DEVELOPMENT OF THE RETROPERITONEAL PLANE

- Once identified, the left colic artery is grasped and elevated. A peritoneal incision is made medial to the vessel and the retroperitoneal plane is created using either a monopolar or bipolar energy device (**FIGURE 7**).
- The retroperitoneal plane is further developed, making use of the triangulation technique described previously. The dissection is carried out anterior to Gerota fascia, along the inferior border of the pancreas, and moving laterally toward the white line of Toldt. The superior portion of the left ureter is identified and preserved.

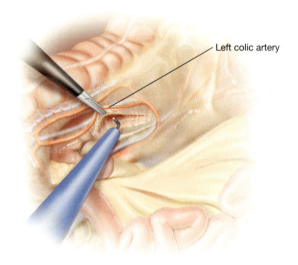

FIGURE 7 • The left colic artery is grasped and elevated. A peritoneal incision is made medial to the vessel and the retroperitoneal plane is created and further developed using a triangulation technique. The dissection is carried out anterior to Gerota's fascia and toward the white line of Toldt.

HIGH VASCULAR DIVISION—THE EAGLE SIGN

- At this point, the left colic and superior rectal arteries are isolated and elevated to readily identify the inferior mesenteric artery (IMA). This maneuver results in the exposure of the "eagle sign." The "body" of the "eagle" is the IMA, the superior "wing" the left colic artery, and the inferior wing the superior rectal artery (**FIGURE 8**). The identification of this sign facilitates appropriate vascular identification and division. The IMA is now safely divided at its origin with a bipolar energy device or linear stapler. The inferior mesenteric vein is then identified and divided. In those with benign disease, a high ligation technique is not required and division takes place at the level of the superior rectal artery.

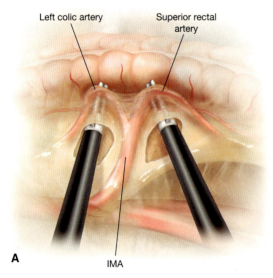
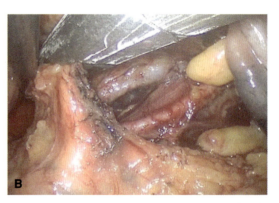

FIGURE 8 • **A,** The eagle sign: The body of the eagle is the inferior mesenteric artery (IMA), the superior wing the left colic artery, and the inferior wing the superior rectal artery. **B,** The IMA is now safely divided at its origin with a bipolar energy device or linear stapler.

LATERAL ATTACHMENTS AND SPLENIC FLEXURE TAKEDOWN

- Some cases may require splenic flexure mobilization to afford a tension-free anastomosis. This is achieved by detaching the gastrocolic ligament at the level of the distal transverse colon, allowing entry to the lesser sac. At this level, the splenocolic ligament is readily taken down, affording a complete splenic flexure mobilization.
- The lateral attachments of the descending colon are taken down from the pelvic brim to the splenic flexure. The descending colon is grasped and retracted medially while the attachments are released with a bipolar tissue-sealing device (**FIGURE 9**).
- In order to fully mobilize the left colon, additional rectosigmoid pelvic attachments are taken down. This also achieves proper upper rectum mobilization, which is beneficial for the specimen division.

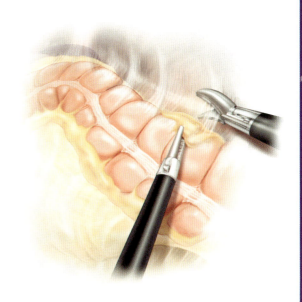

FIGURE 9 • Lateral to medial dissection. The lateral attachments of the sigmoid and descending colon are taken down in an inferior-to-superior direction from the pelvic brim to the splenic flexure, which is readily mobilized if required.

BOWEL DIVISION

- The rectosigmoid is flipped in a medial to lateral direction and its mesentery is divided (**FIGURE 10**). A window is created in the mesentery through which the linear stapler will be placed. The rectosigmoid is then placed in normal anatomic position and it is divided tangentially using a laparoscopic linear stapler.
- The instruments and single-port device are removed and the specimen is exteriorized. The level of the proximal division is chosen and the bowel is divided extracorporeally (**FIGURE 10**).

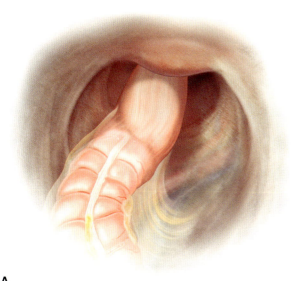

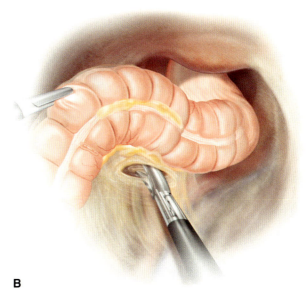

A B

FIGURE 10 • **A,** The rectosigmoid is fully mobilized and ready for division. **B,** A window is created in the mesentery to introduce the stapler in preparation for specimen division. **C,** Rectosigmoid division with a linear stapler. **D,** Extracorporeal mobilization of the bowel for proximal division and preparation for bowel anastomosis.

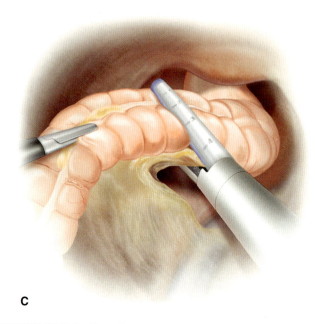
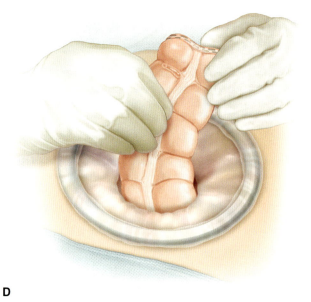

C D

FIGURE 10 • Continued

ESTABLISHMENT OF BOWEL CONTINUITY

- An end-to-end anastomosis is performed with a circular stapler in a traditional fashion.
- We prefer to use a circular stapling device of 29-mm size. Smaller sizes are prone to result in stricture formation and should be avoided, and larger sizes may result in tearing of the bowel wall.
- The anvil of the stapler is introduced into the proximal bowel and is secured with a purse-string suture (**FIGURE 11**). The bowel is introduced back into the peritoneal cavity and the pneumoperitoneum is reestablished.
- The assistant inserts the stapler handle transanally and advances it to the level of the staple line.

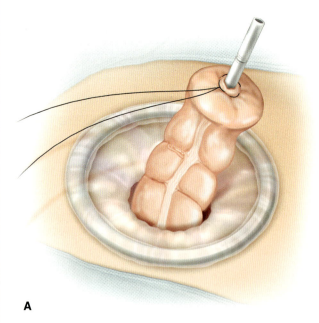
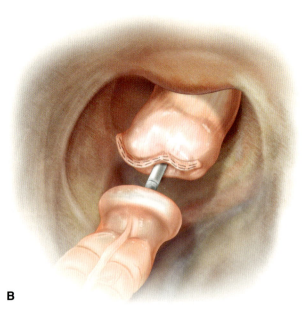

A B

FIGURE 11 • End-to-end colorectal anastomosis. **A,** The anvil of the stapler is introduced and secured into the proximal bowel with a purse-string suture. **B,** After the bowel is reintroduced into the abdomen, the anvil and the handle of the stapler are aligned and the stapler is closed under direct laparoscopic visualization.

Chapter 22 SIGMOID COLECTOMY: SINGLE-INCISION LAPAROSCOPIC SURGERY TECHNIQUE   183

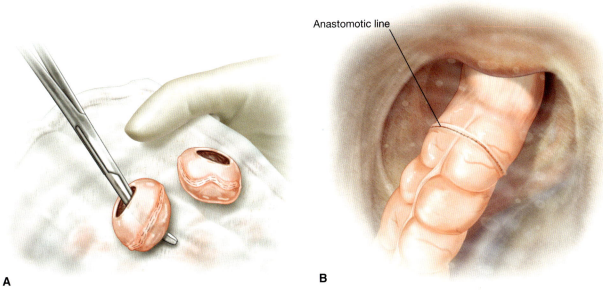

FIGURE 12 • Anastomotic confirmation. **A,** The anastomotic rings are inspected to confirm that they are intact. **B,** An air insufflation test is performed to confirm the absence of anastomotic leak.

- The anvil and the handle of the stapler are aligned and the stapler is closed under direct laparoscopic visualization (**FIGURE 11**). Before performing the anastomosis, it is important to ensure that the bowel is not twisted. Once proper bowel alignment is corroborated, the stapler is fired and then removed transanally.
- Confirmation of a proper anastomosis is performed in three stages. Proctoscopy is performed to visualize the integrity and viability of the anastomosis. The anastomotic rings (donuts) are examined to ensure they are intact circumferentially (**FIGURE 12**). Finally, an air insufflation test is then performed to confirm that the anastomosis is airtight (**FIGURE 12**). If the anastomosis is found to be inadequate, modifications may be required as well as consideration of diversion of the fecal stream, depending on the characteristics of the individual case.

BOWEL DIVERSION

- For cases in which it is unsafe to perform a primary end-to-end colorectal anastomosis, sigmoid resection with end colostomy or, alternatively, anastomosis with a protective loop ileostomy may be performed.

TECHNICAL ALTERNATIVES

- Single-incision laparoscopic sigmoidectomy may be also performed with a lateral to medial dissection approach.
- We favor the medial to lateral approach because it allows identification of critical structures such as the left ureter, facilitating its preservation. Furthermore, we believe that is a more "natural" approach, as the instruments are located in the midline, simplifying the procedure.
- For the lateral to medial approach, the procedure initiates with the release of the lateral attachments of the descending colon, establishment of the retroperitoneal plane, followed by vascular identification and division. Once the sigmoid/left colon is mobilized, the extracorporealization, bowel division, and anastomosis are performed as described previously.

PEARLS AND PITFALLS

Indications	■ Sigmoid diverticulitis, colon cancer, large colon polyps, inflammatory bowel disease.
Preoperative evaluation	■ Colonoscopy with lesion tattooing for polyps and cancer. ■ Abdominopelvic CT scan. ■ PET scan selectively.
Incision	■ 2.5-cm umbilical or 4-cm Pfannenstiel. ■ Single plus one technique: 4-cm Pfannenstiel and 5-mm umbilical port for camera port.
Technique	■ Medial to lateral dissection. Early identification and preservation of the left ureter. ■ Vascular dissection to visualize the eagle sign and high IMA ligation in malignancy. ■ Specimen division with end-to-end anastomosis with 29-mm circular stapler. ■ Proper anastomosis confirmed with proctoscopy, evaluation of anastomotic rings, and air insufflation test.
Postoperative care	■ Patients benefit from the use of a fast-track perioperative protocol.

POSTOPERATIVE CARE

- Postoperative care following minimally invasive colorectal surgery is enhanced with use of a standardized fast-track protocol.[5]
- Orogastric or nasogastric tube is avoided, and diet is resumed with clear liquids 8 to 12 hours after the procedure and advanced with resumption of bowel activity.
- Bladder catheter is removed on postoperative day 1.
- Ambulation is achieved the first night of surgery.
- Postoperative analgesia is accomplished with a combined modality to reduce opioid use. Local infiltration with a long-acting anesthesia can be accomplished with liposomal bupivacaine. Intravenous acetaminophen and nonsteroidal anti-inflammatory drugs can be given in a staggered fashion. Use of opioid can be limited to breakthrough pain, and alvimopan can be used to eliminate the effects of opioids in the GI tract.

OUTCOMES

- Most patients following sigmoid colectomy managed with a fast-track perioperative protocol have an average length of hospital stay of 3 days.[2,4]
- Complications may warrant longer hospital stays and should be managed on an individual basis.
- Hernia rates can be reduced by use of the Pfannenstiel incision vs the umbilical incision.
- Those with malignancies should be placed on oncologic surveillance protocols.

COMPLICATIONS

- Vascular injury with intraperitoneal bleeding
- Ureteral injury
- Sexual and/or urinary dysfunction secondary to autonomic nerve injury
- Prolonged postoperative ileus
- Wound complications (eg, hematoma, seroma, infection, and dehiscence)
- Anastomotic dehiscence
- Intra-abdominal abscess
- Hernia formation

REFERENCES

1. Ragupathi M, Nieto J, Haas EM. Pearls and pitfalls in SILS colectomy. *Surg Laparosc Endosc Percutan Tech*. 2012;22:183-188.
2. Gandhi DP, Ragupathi M, Patel CB, et al. Single-incision versus hand-assisted laparoscopic colectomy: a case-matched series. *J Gastrointest Surg*. 2010;14:1875-1880.
3. Haas EM, Nieto J, Ragupathi M, et al. Single-incision laparoscopic sigmoid resection: a technical video of a standardized approach. *Dis Colon Rectum*. 2012;55:1179-1182.
4. Ramos-Valadez DI, Ragupathi M, Nieto J, et al. Single-incision versus conventional laparoscopic sigmoid colectomy: a case-matched series. *Surg Endosc*. 2012;26:96-102.
5. Vlug MS, Wind J, Hollmann MW, et al. Laparoscopy in combination with fast track multimodal management is the best perioperative strategy in patients undergoing colonic surgery: a randomized clinical trial (LAFA-study). *Ann Surg*. 2011;254:868-875.

Chapter 23

Surgical Management of Complicated Diverticulitis: Perforation and Colovesical Fistula

Scott E. Regenbogen and Lillias Holmes Maguire

DEFINITION

- Diverticulitis is an acute or chronic inflammation and/or infection caused by perforation of a colonic diverticulum. Acute, uncomplicated diverticulitis results from localized inflammation, without perforation, and typically resolves with antibiotics or expectant management.
- Acute complicated diverticulitis includes free perforation with peritonitis or contained perforation with abscess. Chronic manifestations include fistula and stricture. Resection is required for peritonitis or acute inflammation that does not improve with medical therapy, recurrent disease that is life-limiting, fistula, or clinically significant stricture.

DIFFERENTIAL DIAGNOSIS

- The differential diagnosis of left lower quadrant pain, fever, and abdominal tenderness includes diverticulitis, perforated colon cancer, gastroenteritis, stercoral perforation, appendicitis, inflammatory bowel disease, urinary tract infection, aortic dissection or aneurysmal rupture, nephrolithiasis, pelvic inflammatory disease, ovarian torsion, and a variety of other causes of acute abdominal pain.
- Computed tomography (CT) of the abdomen with intravenous and oral contrast is highly sensitive for the diagnosis of inflammation associated with diverticulosis, but cannot exclude other causes of segmental colitis, including perforated neoplasm, ischemia, and Crohn disease. Details of clinical history, family history of colorectal cancer, and previous colon evaluation are helpful in excluding the latter two.
- Except in the emergency setting, malignancy must be excluded, either by endoscopic evaluation or other means, because the principles of oncologic resection, including wide lymphadenectomy and en bloc resection, are typically violated in surgery for benign diverticular disease. Retrospective studies suggest that the likelihood of discovering malignancy on endoscopic examination after diagnosis is significantly higher with complicated disease than with uncomplicated diverticulitis.

PATIENT HISTORY AND PHYSICAL FINDINGS

- Patients with acute diverticulitis typically present with abdominal pain and fever. Because more than 90% of diverticulitis occurs in the sigmoid colon among patients in the Western hemisphere, the symptoms will typically localize to the left lower quadrant.
- Free perforation may present as generalized peritonitis and/or sepsis.
- In the presence of colovesical fistula, the patient may have irritative urinary symptoms or even pneumaturia or fecaluria,

and there may be air or enteral contrast visible in the bladder on a CT scan. Occasionally, patients with colovesical fistula may not report a preceding episode of acute diverticulitis; rather, their initial presentation may be with symptoms of the fistula itself. Passage of urine per rectum is not common with colovesical fistulae from diverticulitis.

- The clinical history should focus on the presence or absence of repeated episodes and symptoms suggesting fistulizing disease—gas or stool in the urine or per vagina.
- In consideration of the differential diagnosis, the examiner should elicit any history consistent with inflammatory bowel disease or ischemic colitis and assess the patient's risk factors for colorectal cancer (age, personal and family history of cancer or polyps, and whether any previous colorectal cancer screening evaluations have been performed).
- Physical examination in the acute setting will reveal localized or generalized abdominal tenderness. Focal guarding in the left lower quadrant is typical. Diffuse rebound tenderness suggests generalized peritonitis from free feculent perforation or purulent peritonitis from abscess rupture. Abdominal wall erythema may suggest incipient colocutaneous fistula. In the chronic setting, patients may have fullness or a palpable mass.

IMAGING AND OTHER DIAGNOSTIC STUDIES

- Typical findings on CT scan of the abdomen include segmental colonic inflammation and pericolonic fat stranding within an area of diverticulosis. There may be extraluminal air or fluid or a contained abscess. Intravenous and oral contrast administration is helpful, although not essential. Rectal contrast is generally unnecessary, except to help with delineating a fistula.
- CT scan is the most sensitive test for diagnosing colovesical fistula (**FIGURE 1**). Other options include contrast enema (**FIGURE 2**), CT or fluoroscopic cystography, cystoscopy, colonoscopy, or oral administration of undigested material (eg, charcoal, poppy seeds) to be observed for in the urine. However, any or all of these diagnostic studies may fail to confirm colovesical fistula, and thus, in some cases, the diagnosis of colovesical fistula may be made based on the presence of pneumaturia and/or fecaluria alone.
- Colonoscopy (**FIGURE 3**) is recommended for evaluation of diverticulitis and colovesical fistula in order to exclude perforated malignancy, which can have similar clinical presentation and radiographic appearance. The presence of malignancy would warrant an oncologic mesenteric lymphadenectomy and en bloc partial cystectomy, whereas the fistula may simply be divided in cases with benign inflammatory etiology. In patient with hematuria and/or a bladder mass on imaging, cystoscopy may be recommended as well.

185

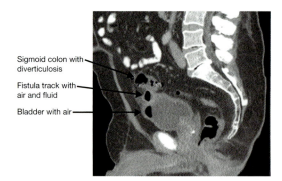

FIGURE 1 • Sagittal computed tomography image demonstrating sigmoid diverticulitis with a fistula track and air in the bladder consistent with colovesical fistula.

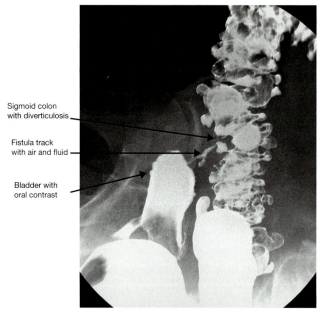

FIGURE 2 • Barium enema demonstrating sigmoid diverticulosis with a fistula track and oral contrast filling the bladder.

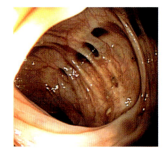

FIGURE 3 • Colonoscopic image of colonic diverticulosis.

SURGICAL MANAGEMENT

- Traditional recommendations for elective colon resection after two episodes of uncomplicated diverticulitis have generally been abandoned. Instead, elective colectomy is recommended on a case-by-case basis, depending on age, comorbidities, severity and frequency of attacks, and the success of medical therapy.
- Elective resection is often advised after recovery from an episode of complicated diverticulitis managed with medical therapy and/or percutaneous drainage.
- Urgent operation may be indicated for free perforation with sepsis.

Preoperative Planning

- When patients present with diffuse peritonitis and sepsis, urgent operation may be required. Broad-spectrum antibiotics should be administered and the patient should be well resuscitated with intravenous crystalloids prior to surgery.
- Every effort should be made before surgery to mark acceptable sites on the abdominal skin for stoma creation bilaterally. Consideration may be given to placement of ureteral stents preoperatively if it can be performed without undue delay.
- Decision-making should be centered on the patient's clinical condition, the severity of pelvic sepsis, the suitability for colorectal anastomosis, and the ability to safely resect the inflammatory segment.
- Options for surgical approach in the emergency setting include the following:
  - Resection with primary anastomosis, with or without diverting loop ileostomy.
  - Resection with end colostomy and rectal stump closure (Hartmann procedure).
  - Proximal diversion without resection.
  - Laparoscopic lavage and drainage has been advocated by some, but recent trials suggesting higher incidence of reintervention, compared with resection, have made lavage a less favored approach.
- Complete colonoscopy in the elective setting should be performed before surgery in order to exclude a perforated malignancy that presented as perforated diverticulitis or synchronous malignancy.
- Cystoscopy and urine cytology may be considered in cases of colovesical fistula if there is suspicion for a primary bladder malignancy.
- Consideration should be given to prophylactic placement of ureteral catheter(s) to assist with identification of the ureter, if it appears to be involved with the inflammatory segment.
- Laparoscopic approaches to complex diverticular disease and colovesical fistula are appropriate in hemodynamically stable patients among surgeons with adequate laparoscopic colorectal surgery skills and training. Hand-assisted and straight laparoscopic techniques have similar short- and long-term reported outcomes.
- If inflammation is severe and there is intention to perform a Hartmann procedure with end colostomy or a colorectal anastomosis with diverting loop ileostomy, the patient should undergo preoperative evaluation and counseling by an enterostomal therapist, including marking suitable locations for a stoma on the abdomen, either unilaterally or bilaterally, if the operative plan will depend on intraoperative findings.
- Mechanical bowel preparation with oral antibiotics is recommended, based on the consensus from a number of retrospective trials, if clinically possible.
- Prophylactic antibiotics to cover skin flora, enteric gram negatives, and anaerobic bacteria should be administered before making the incision.
- Appropriate pharmacologic and/or mechanical prophylaxis for venous thromboembolism is recommended.

Chapter 23 SURGICAL MANAGEMENT OF COMPLICATED DIVERTICULITIS: PERFORATION AND COLOVESICAL FISTULA   187

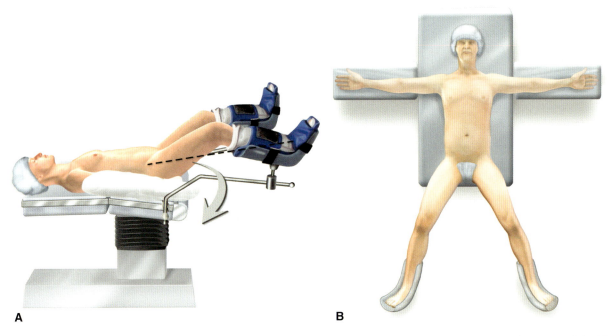

FIGURE 4 • **A,** Modified lithotomy position. Care is taken to ensure that pressure is kept off of the peroneal nerve, and the hips are not excessively extended (*dotted lines* show the appropriate hip angle). **B,** Supine position with legs abducted on a split-leg table.

- For patients with colovesical fistula, a three-way urinary catheter may be used for intraoperative bladder irrigation to evaluate persistent leak after division of the fistula.

Positioning

- The patient is placed in modified lithotomy position (**FIGURE 4A**) or supine with legs abducted on a split-leg table (**FIGURE 4B**) to provide access to the anus.

- If a laparoscopic approach is used, a position-assisting device is recommended to prevent the patient from sliding during positioning changes.
- If stoma markings were performed preoperatively, these should be redrawn with a marker that will remain visible after skin preparation.

TECHNIQUES

LAPAROSCOPIC ELECTIVE SIGMOID COLECTOMY, BLADDER REPAIR

- The video (▶ **Video 1**) depicts the key steps of a laparoscopic sigmoid colectomy for diverticulitis with colovesical fistula.

Abdominal Access and Port Placement

- The abdomen may be accessed via a percutaneous Veress needle or an open Hasson cannula technique.
- Typical port placement is depicted in **FIGURE 5**. A 5- or 12-mm camera port is placed at the umbilicus. Two or three additional working ports are inserted, including a 5-mm port in the right upper quadrant, a 12-mm port in the right lower quadrant (in some cases, may be placed at a potential diverting loop ileostomy site), and a 5-mm port in the left lower quadrant (preferably at a potential colostomy site) or suprapubic position.

Isolation and Division of the Inferior Mesenteric or Superior Hemorrhoidal Artery Pedicle

- In order to gain access to the proximal inferior mesenteric artery (IMA), the greater omentum is elevated over the transverse colon, into the upper abdomen, with the patient in steep Trendelenburg position, with the operating table tilted toward the right. The small bowel is brought to the right upper quadrant and out of the pelvis.
- Elevation of the rectosigmoid mesentery with a grasper through the left lower quadrant port toward the left lower quadrant demonstrates the IMA as a ridge in the sigmoid colon mesentery and exposes a plane between the mesentery and the retroperitoneum on the medial peritoneal fold of the mesentery. With cautery attached to Endo Shears brought through the right lower quadrant port, a long incision is made in the medial peritoneal fold of the mesentery along a clear space seen between the IMA and the retroperitoneum (**FIGURE 6**).
- Through this incision, the left ureter, gonadal vessels, and retroperitoneal tissues are identified and dissected down off of the vessel and the mesentery (**FIGURE 7A**). If the left iliac artery and/or left psoas muscle are exposed, the plane of dissection must be brought more anteriorly. The left ureter is identified definitively by visualizing peristalsis.
- Once the left ureter has been identified and protected in the retroperitoneum, the IMA and its branches, the left colic artery, and the superior hemorrhoidal artery form what appears to be a "letter T," facilitating the identification of these vascular structures (**FIGURE 7B**).

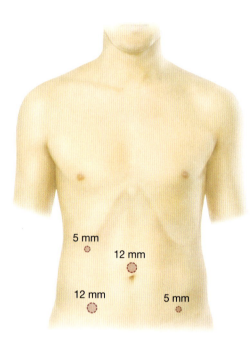

FIGURE 5 • Laparoscopic port placement for sigmoid colectomy. A 5-mm or 12-mm camera port is placed at the umbilicus. Two or three additional working ports are inserted, including a 5-mm port in the right upper quadrant, a 12-mm port in the right lower quadrant, and a 5-mm port in the left lower quadrant or suprapubic position.

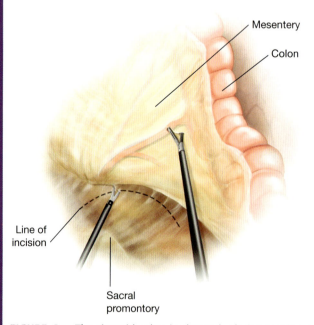

FIGURE 6 • The sigmoid colon is elevated, placing tension on the inferior mesenteric artery (IMA) pedicle, and an incision is made in the medial peritoneal fold dorsal to the IMA (*dotted line*).

- Vascular ligation may take place either at the proximal IMA or at the superior hemorrhoidal artery (SHA). Division of the IMA will allow greater length of mobilization in cases where this is required, but division of the SHA may be adequate in some cases. We use a bipolar vessel-sealing device for vessel ligation (**FIGURE 8A**), but other choices include vascular clips, endoscopic staplers (**FIGURE 8B**), or endoloops. When using an energy device for division, it is advisable to have endoloops available in the room as a backup to control bleeding from the divided pedicle in case of device failure.

Mobilization of the Descending Colon and Splenic Flexure

- The "medial to lateral" dissection of the mesocolon is performed by elevating the divided vascular pedicle, identifying the line of separation between the posterior side of the colon mesentery and Gerota fascia overlying the kidney and retroperitoneum (**FIGURE 9A** and **B**). The retroperitoneal tissues are swept down (dorsally) with a combination of cautery and blunt dissection. This dissection continues laterally to the abdominal side wall and superiorly to the inferior border of the pancreas and the superior edge of the distal transverse colon and splenic flexure. This will greatly facilitate the mobilization of the splenic flexure later during the case.
- The lateral dissection is then performed by retracting the colon medially and dividing the white line of Toldt from the pelvic brim to the splenic flexure. As the dissection continues superiorly, the patient's position is gradually altered, going from steep Trendelenburg toward slight reverse Trendelenburg position. The rightward tilt is maintained. If the medial dissection has been performed completely, there should be only a single tissue layer to divide before meeting the medial plane of dissection.
- At this point, the splenic flexure is mobilized. Full mobilization of the splenic flexure (**FIGURE 10A**) is often needed in order to ensure a tension-free anastomosis.
- The patient is placed on a reverse Trendelenburg position, helping bring the splenic flexure into view. The surgeon and the assistant retract the splenic flexure inferiorly and medially, exposing the splenocolic and phrenocolic ligaments. These ligaments are then transected with a 5-mm energy device (**FIGURE 10B**) in an inferior to superior and lateral to medial fashion.
- At this point, it is often easier to start the transection of the gastrocolic ligament medially, entering the lesser sac and proceeding with the transection of the gastrocolic ligament in a medial to lateral dissection (**FIGURE 10A**) until the lateral dissection plane around the splenic flexure is encountered.
- The splenic flexure and the descending colon are now completely free of any attachments and fully mobilized toward the midline. To check for adequate length, healthy descending colon above the area of inflammation should be able to reach to the pelvis without any tension.
- Mobilization of the splenic flexure is greatly facilitated by having completed the medial to lateral mobilization of the splenic flexure in the previous step.

Chapter 23 SURGICAL MANAGEMENT OF COMPLICATED DIVERTICULITIS: PERFORATION AND COLOVESICAL FISTULA

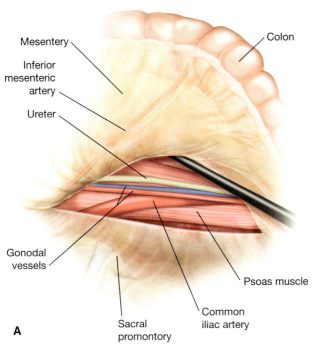
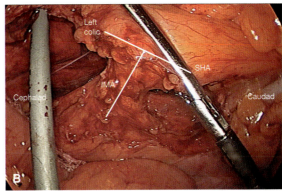

FIGURE 7 • **A,** The mesenteric vessels are isolated by sweeping the retroperitoneal tissues, including the left ureter and gonadal vessels, posteriorly off the mesentery of the sigmoid colon. The left ureter is identified as it crosses under the colon mesentery and is protected in the retroperitoneum. **B,** The inferior mesenteric artery (IMA) and its terminal branches, the left colic artery, and the superior hemorrhoidal artery (SHA) form what appears to be a "letter T," facilitating the identification of these critical vascular structures.

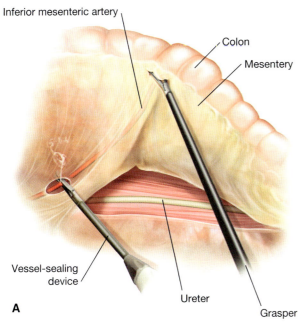
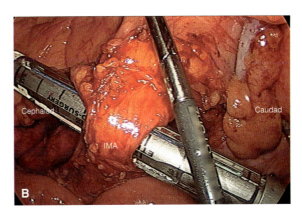

FIGURE 8 • The inferior mesenteric artery (IMA) is encircled at its base and divided with a **(A)** bipolar vessel-sealing device or **(B)** endoscopic stapler, ensuring that the ureter is not ensnared during the division.

SECTION II SURGERY OF THE COLON, APPENDIX, RECTUM, AND ANUS

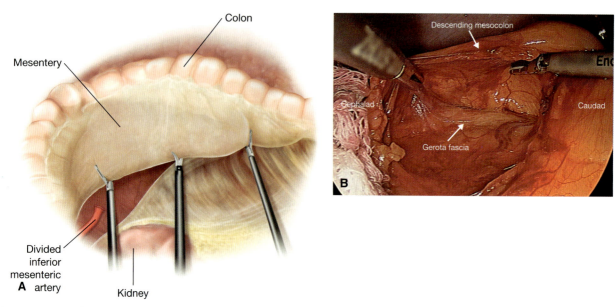

FIGURE 9 • **A** and **B,** A medial to lateral dissection of the mesocolon is performed by elevating the divided vascular pedicle and sweeping the Gerota fascia and retroperitoneal tissues dorsally, laterally to the abdominal wall, and superiorly to the tail of the pancreas and posterior to the splenic flexure of the colon.

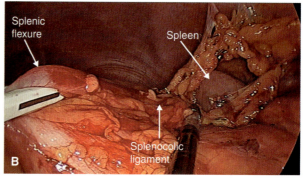

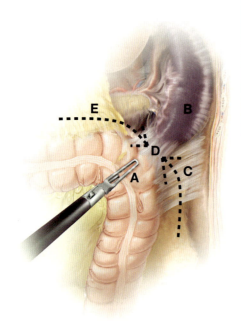

FIGURE 10 • **A,** Mobilization of the splenic flexure. The surgeon retracts the splenic flexure of the colon (*A*) downward and medially, exposing the attachments of the flexure to the spleen (*B*). The phrenocolic (*C*) and splenocolic (*D*) ligaments are transected in an inferior to superior and lateral to medial direction. The gastrocolic ligament (*E*) is transected in a medial to lateral direction until both planes of dissection meet and the splenic flexure is fully mobilized. **B,** Mobilization of the splenic flexure: transection of the splenocolic ligament.

Chapter 23 SURGICAL MANAGEMENT OF COMPLICATED DIVERTICULITIS: PERFORATION AND COLOVESICAL FISTULA

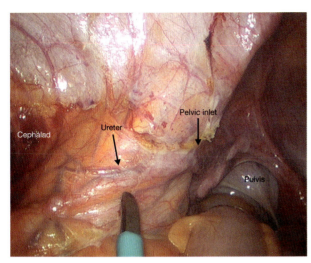

FIGURE 11 • Mobilization of the sigmoid of the pelvic inlet. The left ureter can be seen crossing the left common iliac artery at the level of the left pelvic inlet.

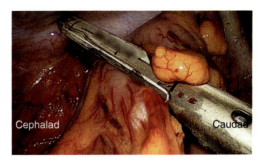

FIGURE 12 • Distal transection. An endostapler is inserted into the 12-mm port and used to divide distal to the rectosigmoid junction.

Mobilization of the Rectosigmoid, Separation, and Repair of the Fistula

- The sigmoid colon typically has attachments to the left side wall at the pelvic inlet. These can be incised with cautery after the ureter has been reidentified, crossing the left common iliac artery at the level of the left pelvic inlet (**FIGURE 11**). Peritoneal incisions down each side of the rectosigmoid to the level of the upper rectum will allow identification of the upper mesorectum.
- The fistula is divided with a combination of sharp dissection and cautery. If it cannot be safely achieved laparoscopically, the extraction incision may be made at this time and separation accomplished by finger fracture using a wound protector or a hand-assisted access port.
- Once the colon and bladder are separated, the bladder may be evaluated by filling the urinary catheter retrograde through the urinary catheter with fluid (we prefer sterile saline with iodine for visualization). Most commonly, there will be no ongoing leak from the bladder, and no repair may be needed. If there is a persistent leak, or if a full-thickness defect is exposed, the bladder may be repaired with one or two layers of absorbable suture material. The closure can also be leak tested by irrigation through the urinary catheter in a similar fashion.
- A closed suction drain may be left in the pelvis if the bladder repair is extensive; but often, the hole in the bladder is quite difficult to identify definitively and drainage is not required for most cases.
- The distal transection is now performed at the level of the upper rectum. The upper rectum is divided distal to the coalescence of the teniae coli by bluntly creating a window between the rectum and mesorectum. The mesorectum is divided at this level using a tissue-sealing device. The upper rectum is then transected either with an endoscopic stapler (**FIGURE 12**) via the right lower quadrant port site or through the extraction incision.

Extraction Incision, Colon Division, and Anastomosis

- The specimen may be extracted through a lower abdominal incision of choice. We prefer a small Pfannenstiel incision with a transverse curvilinear fascial incision.
- An occlusive wound protector may be used, and the specimen is exteriorized through the extraction incision.
- Before division of the bowel, we prefer to clamp the marginal artery distally, then divide it sharply within the mesentery, at a point on the descending colon proximal to the area of inflammation, just beyond the intended point of division. The presence of arterial bleeding from the proximal end indicates adequate blood supply for the future anastomosis.
- The colon is then divided, either with a linear stapler or a purse-string application device.
- A 28 or 31 mm anvil of an end-to-end anastomosis (EEA) device is sewn into the divided end of the colon, and care should be taken to be sure that the mesentery is not twisted as the anvil is brought to the pelvis.
- The handle of the stapler is advanced transanally, up to the rectal staple line, and an end-to-end stapled EEA colorectal anastomosis is performed (**FIGURE 13A**). The resected "donuts" should be examined. The integrity of the anastomosis is tested by insufflating it under water. The presence of an air leak would indicate an anastomotic disruption and would require repair or revision of the anastomosis, with or without proximal diversion (**FIGURE 13B**).

Closure

- If the omentum can be mobilized to the pelvis, it is placed between the anastomosis and the bladder repair as a vascularized soft tissue flap. Alternatively, a peritoneal flap may be raised from the bladder or lower abdomen and secured between the anastomosis and bladder repair.
- The extraction incision is closed in layers. The large laparoscopic ports may be closed from the outside or with the use of a laparoscopic suture passer. The small ports are closed at skin level only.

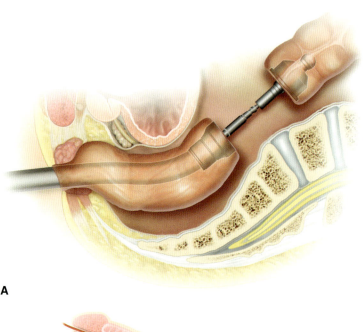

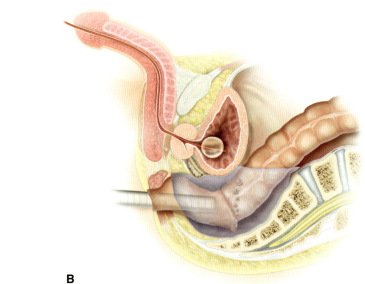

FIGURE 13 • The colorectal anastomosis. **A,** A stapled end-to-end colorectal anastomosis is performed. **B,** The integrity of the anastomosis is tested by insufflating it under water. The presence of an air leak would indicate an anastomotic disruption and would require a revision of the anastomosis.

HARTMANN PROCEDURE AND EMERGENCY SIGMOID COLECTOMY WITH DIVERTING ILEOSTOMY

Abdominal Entry, Containing Contamination

- In an emergency setting, a lower midline laparotomy, occasionally with extension above the umbilicus, facilitates rapid and ample exposure.
- In case of purulent or feculent peritonitis, contamination should first be evacuated and irrigated clear. Often, there will be a contained collection or phlegmon overlying a necrotic perforation. Blunt finger fracture will provide exposure of the perforation, and then contamination should again be contained rapidly. Finger fracture should be performed staying on the colon side to avoid potential iatrogenic injury to organs, such as the bladder or ureter, or blood vessels, such as the iliacs.

Colon Mobilization and Resection

- In hemodynamically unstable patients and others for whom colorectal anastomosis is considered unacceptably high risk, a Hartmann procedure (segmental resection with end colostomy and distal stump closure) is required.
- In hemodynamically stable patients, a primary anastomosis after resection of the diverticulitis segment, with or without diverting ileostomy, may be considered, even in patients who undergo emergency surgery for acute complicated diverticulitis with purulent or feculent peritonitis. The likelihood of long-term stoma-free survival is significantly higher after primary anastomosis than after Hartmann procedure, without significant differences in perioperative morbidity or mortality.

Chapter 23 **SURGICAL MANAGEMENT OF COMPLICATED DIVERTICULITIS: PERFORATION AND COLOVESICAL FISTULA**

- Mobilization for Hartmann procedure should be kept to the minimum necessary. Unlike in elective sigmoidectomy for diverticulitis, it is not essential to resect the rectosigmoid junction or to mobilize the splenic flexure. Rather, the goal should be to resect the grossly perforated colon segment, divide the colon proximal and distal to the acutely inflamed segment, and maintain as much vascular supply as possible for the future colostomy takedown. If primary anastomosis is planned, resection margins should be the same as those for elective resection, and the distal margin should be at or beyond the rectosigmoid junction, so that a colorectal, rather than colocolonic, anastomosis may be constructed.
- For a Hartmann procedure, the descending colon should be mobilized only as much as is required for the divided colon to reach the abdominal wall without tension at the intended colostomy aperture. Excessive mobilization only exposes additional tissue planes into which contamination may extend and establish a future abscess. Mobilization for primary anastomosis may require additional dissection as described for elective resection.
- In a Hartmann procedure, the divided colon/rectal stump can be marked with a permanent suture. The status of the superior hemorrhoidal artery should be documented in the operative report and dissection in the pelvis should be minimized in order to preserve tissue planes for the potential future colostomy closure.
- When an anastomosis and proximal diversion are performed in the emergency setting without mechanical bowel preparation, on-table lavage of the diverted colon may be considered to avoid a long, retained stool-filled segment distal to the ileostomy.
- If malignancy was not excluded with preoperative endoscopic examination, back table examination of the specimen may be performed, and the mucosa examined to evaluate the possibility of a perforated neoplasm.

Abdominal Closure and Stoma Creation

- The colostomy aperture is typically created in the left abdomen, ideally at a site marked preoperatively. Even in the emergency setting, effort should be made to identify and mark potentially problematic skin folds and the contour of the rectus muscles, so that a stoma may be made in an adequate location and brought through the rectus sheath.
- The abdomen is closed in layers. Depending on the extent of contamination, the skin incision may be closed primarily, closed in a delayed primary fashion, closed over gauze wicks, or left open to heal by secondary intention.
- The colostomy is matured in a standard fashion.

PEARLS AND PITFALLS

Indications	- Traditional recommendations for elective resection after two uncomplicated episodes of diverticulitis have generally been abandoned. - Resection is indicated after nonoperative management of complicated diverticulitis, including free perforation, abscess, and fistula. - Free perforation with clinical sepsis is an indication for urgent operation.
Preoperative planning	- Stoma sites should be marked preoperatively, if there is a possibility of colostomy or ileostomy. - Ureteral stent(s) should be considered in cases in which severe retroperitoneal inflammation is suspected based on preoperative imaging. - In elective cases, colonoscopy should be performed preoperatively to exclude a perforated neoplasm. - Mechanical bowel preparation with preoperative oral antibiotics is typically recommended for elective resections. - Appropriate antibiotics and venous thromboembolism prophylaxis should be administered perioperatively.
Choice of operation	- Resection with primary anastomosis, with or without diverting loop ileostomy: for stable patients, with good quality tissues available for anastomosis, without severe soilage in the abdomen/pelvis - Resection with end colostomy and rectal stump closure (Hartmann procedure): for unstable patients, and/or with poor quality tissues available for anastomosis, and/or with severe soilage in the abdomen/pelvis - Proximal diversion without resection: an alternative to a Hartmann procedure in unstable patients and/or difficult to resect disease due to severity of inflammation
Postoperative management	- Postoperative antibiotics are not required in elective cases and are left to surgeon discretion in emergency cases with purulent or feculent peritonitis. - Cystogram may be used to verify repair of bladder fistula prior to removal of urinary catheter.

POSTOPERATIVE CARE

- Postoperative care should include combined analgesia with acetaminophen, nonsteroidal anti-inflammatory medications, narcotics, and/or regional or epidural anesthesia. Mechanical and pharmacologic prophylaxis to prevent venous thromboembolism should be provided. Early mobilization and early enteral feeding are both associated with shorter duration of postoperative ileus and should be encouraged. Routine postoperative nasogastric suction is not recommended.
- Duration of urinary catheterization should be minimized to reduce the risk of urinary tract infection. After repair of colovesical fistula, however, an indwelling urinary catheter

is typically left in place for 5 to 10 days, depending on the complexity of the bladder repair. A cystogram may be performed to confirm an intact repair before Foley catheter removal.

■ Antibiotics are not given postoperatively after elective resection for colovesical fistula but may be continued for a varying duration after urgent operations for frank perforation with purulent or feculent peritonitis.

OUTCOMES

■ The likelihood of recurrent diverticulitis after elective resection is determined largely by the level of anastomosis—less than 5% with a colorectal anastomosis but more than 12% with a colosigmoid anastomosis.

■ Complication rates after a Hartmann procedure are high. The most common complications are wound infection, sepsis, stoma necrosis, and intra-abdominal abscess.

■ Less than half of patients who undergo emergency Hartmann procedure have their colostomy reversed.

COMPLICATIONS

■ Anastomotic leak
■ Abscess
■ Ureteral injury
■ Bowel obstruction
■ Hemorrhage
■ Stoma complications (necrosis, dehiscence, obstruction)
■ Bladder leak

SUGGESTED READINGS

1. Ceresoli M, Coccolini F, Montori G, et al. Laparoscopic lavage versus resection in perforated diverticulitis with purulent peritonitis: a meta-analysis of randomized controlled trials. *World J Emerg Surg.* 2016;11:42.

2. De Moya MA, Zacharias N, Osbourne A, et al. Colovesical fistula repair: is early Foley catheter removal safe? *J Surg Res.* 2009;156(2):274-277.

3. Feingold D, Steele SR, Lee S, et al. Practice parameters for the treatment of sigmoid diverticulitis. *Dis Colon Rectum.* 2014;57(3):284-294.

4. Gustafsson UO, Scott MJ, Schwenk W, et al. Guidelines for perioperative care in elective colonic surgery: Enhanced Recovery After Surgery (ERAS) Society recommendations. *World J Surg.* 2012;37(2):259-284. doi:10.1007/s00268-012-1772-0.

5. Lambrichts DPV, Vennix S, Musters GD, et al. Hartmann's procedure versus sigmoidectomy with primary anastomosis for perforated diverticulitis with purulent or faecal peritonitis (LADIES): a multicentre, parallel-group, randomised, open-label, superiority trial. *Lancet Gastroenterol Hepatol.* 2019;4:599-610.

6. Lee SW, Yoo J, Dujovny N, et al. Laparoscopic vs. hand-assisted laparoscopic sigmoidectomy for diverticulitis. *Dis Colon Rectum.* 2006;49(4):464-469.

7. Liang S, Russek K, Franklin ME. Damage control strategy for the management of perforated diverticulitis with generalized peritonitis: laparoscopic lavage and drainage vs. laparoscopic Hartmann's procedure. *Surg Endosc.* 2012;26:2835-2842.

8. Regenbogen SE, Hardiman KM, Hendren S, et al. Surgery for diverticulitis in the 21st century: a systematic review. *JAMA Surg.* 2014;149(3):292-303.

9. Thaler K, Baig MK, Berho M, et al. Determinants of recurrence after sigmoid resection for uncomplicated diverticulitis. *Dis Colon Rectum.* 2003;46(3):385-388.

Chapter 24

Total Abdominal Colectomy: Open Technique

Tarik Sammour and Andrew G. Hill

DEFINITION

Total abdominal colectomy is defined as the removal of the entire colon, following which the distal ileum is either anastomosed to the rectum or an end ileostomy is created.

DIFFERENTIAL DIAGNOSIS

- Inflammatory bowel disease (IBD), including ulcerative colitis and Crohn disease
- Severe acute colitis (various etiologies)
- Polyposis syndromes, including familial adenomatous polyposis and lynch syndrome
- Slow transit constipation
- Malignancy

PATIENT HISTORY AND PHYSICAL FINDINGS

- Specific history and examination findings will depend on the indication for total abdominal colectomy.
- History of previous abdominal surgery is important, particularly in the setting of IBD. If the patient has had multiple small bowel resections and is at risk of short gut syndrome, then total abdominal colectomy is contraindicated.
- History of baseline continence and pelvic floor function is important.

IMAGING AND OTHER DIAGNOSTIC STUDIES

- Endoscopy: Colonoscopy will have been required to diagnose the disease for which total colectomy is required, and an up-to-date flexible sigmoidoscopy is needed to assess the state of the rectum and ensure it is disease/polyp-free.
- Patients with IBD will, in addition, require small bowel imaging (preferably CT [computed tomography] or MRI enterography) to ensure that the small bowel is free of diseased segments.
- Patients with severe constipation will require a colonic transit study to confirm functional colonic disease.
- Patients with malignancy will require an appropriate staging CT scan and baseline serum carcinoembryonic antigen level.

SURGICAL MANAGEMENT

Preoperative Planning

- The surgeon should obtain informed consent from patient, explaining the procedure, expected recovery, risks, and benefits. Consent should also be obtained for a stoma should this be required.
- The patient's nutritional status should be optimized prior to surgery.
- Preoperative stoma marking should be carried out by a suitably qualified nurse.
- A preoperative sodium phosphate enema is administered.
- Enhanced recovery after surgery (ERAS) perioperative care protocols are applied.[1]
- A midthoracic epidural should be inserted preoperatively, or other forms of regional anesthesia, such as TAPP catheters, should be considered.[2]
- An indwelling catheter should be inserted preoperatively.
- Intravenous antibiotic prophylaxis should be given on induction.[3]
- Consideration should be given to intravenous steroid supplementation if the patient is steroid-dependent.
- Subcutaneous low molecular weight heparin should be given on induction.
- Calf compression stockings should be applied.
- NOTE: Oral mechanical bowel preparation is not routinely recommended.[4]

Positioning

- The patient should be placed supine with their arms out. Ensure the arms are not hyperabducted to avoid brachial plexopathy.
- The patient should be as far down the bed as possible (to provide access to the anus). Ensure the buttocks remain well supported on the bed.
- The legs should be placed in lithotomy braces with adequate padding to avoid neurovascular injuries. Ensure there is no pressure on the common peroneal nerves bilaterally.
- Once the patient is positioned, a digital rectal examination and proctoscopy should be performed to ensure no rectal abnormality.
- The patient skin is prepped and draped from the xiphisternum to the pubis, ensuring access to the anus.
- The surgeon stands on the patient's left side and the first assistant on the opposite side.

INCISION AND ACCESS

- A midline laparotomy is performed.
- A suitable fixed metal laparotomy retractor is inserted.
- After general inspection of the small bowel, this is packed with moist large swab packs into the upper abdominal cavity to enhance operative exposure.

ASCENDING COLON MOBILIZATION

- The ascending colon is mobilized using a lateral to medial approach by medial traction and dissection along the right paracolic gutter using diathermy (**FIGURE 1**).
- Care is taken to identify, and avoid damage to, the right gonadal vessels, right ureter, the duodenum, and head of the pancreas.

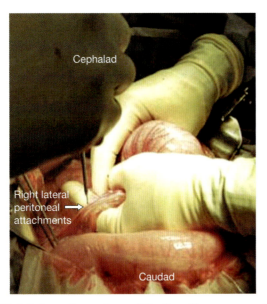
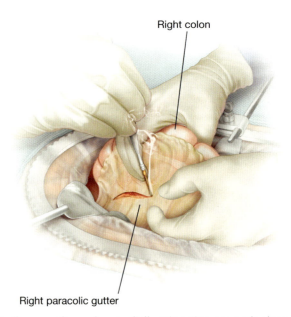

FIGURE 1 • Ascending colon mobilization. The surgeon retracts the ascending colon medially. Dissection proceeds along the right paracolic gutter.

TRANSVERSE COLON MOBILIZATION

- The hepatic flexure is mobilized by dividing the hepatocolic ligament with electrocautery (**FIGURE 2**).
- The greater omentum is retracted superiorly by the assistant, and the transverse colon anteroinferiorly by the surgeon.
- Diathermy is used to separate the greater omentum from the anterior leaf of the transverse mesocolon.
- The mobilization of the splenic flexure is best accomplished by a combination of medial to lateral and lateral to medial dissection approaches.
- The medial to lateral phase of the splenic flexure mobilization is started by entering the lesser sac at the midline (**FIGURE 3A**). The transverse colon is retracted downward and the stomach is retracted superiorly, exposing the gastrocolic ligament. The gastrocolic ligament is then transected medially with an energy device until the lesser sac is entered.
- Transection of the gastrocolic ligament then proceeds along the transverse colon in a medial to lateral direction until the splenic flexure is reached (**FIGURE 3A**). Care must be taken to avoid inadvertent injury to the colon.
- At this point, a superior to inferior and lateral to medial dissection around the splenic flexure is performed (**FIGURE 3B**). The surgeon inserts their right hand behind the splenic flexure (possible due to the previous medial to lateral mobilization step) and hooks their index finger under the splenocolic ligament, gently pulling the splenic flexure down and exposing the splenocolic ligament fully, which is then transected with an energy device (**FIGURE 3B**). The splenocolic ligament is divided as close to the colon as feasible, avoiding undue traction on the spleen.

Chapter 24 TOTAL ABDOMINAL COLECTOMY: OPEN TECHNIQUE 197

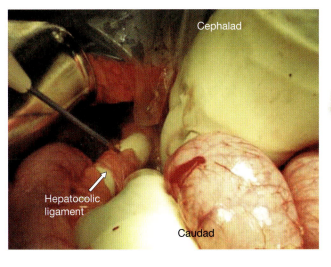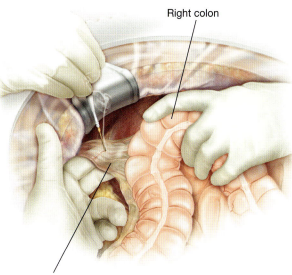

FIGURE 2 • Hepatic flexure mobilization. Gentle traction on the hepatic flexure of the colon exposes the hepatocolic ligament, which is then transected with electrocautery.

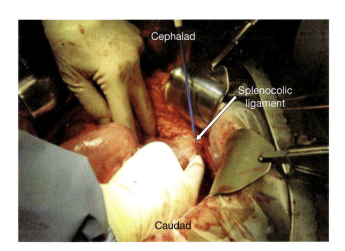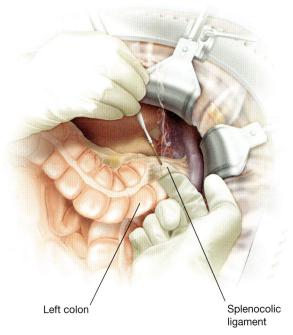

FIGURE 3 • Splenic flexure mobilization. After medial and lateral mobilization of the splenic flexure attachments, the surgeon hooks their right index finger under the splenocolic ligament, providing good exposure and allowing for a safe transection of this ligament.

PROXIMAL DIVISION

- The terminal ileum is mobilized by division of surrounding adhesions.
- The ileocolic pedicle (and right colic if present) is identified and clamped with heavy artery forceps by creating windows on either side with diathermy (**FIGURE 4**).
- The pedicle is divided between the artery forceps and ligated proximally and distally with absorbable braided size 0 ties.
- Alternatively, if the surgeon is certain of the absence of malignancy, then the mesenteric blood supply to the proximal segment can be taken close to the bowel wall.

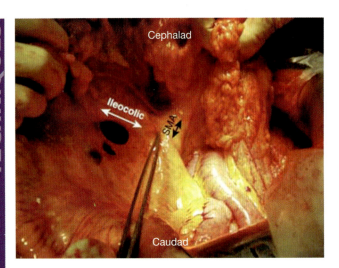 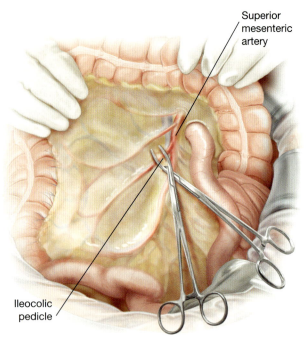

FIGURE 4 • Ileocolic pedicle division. The ileocolic vessels are transected between clamps and will be subsequently ligated with heavy silk sutures. SMA, superior mesenteric artery.

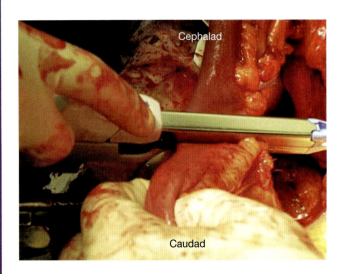 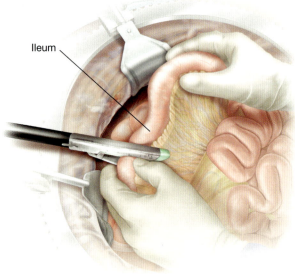

FIGURE 5 • Proximal division. The terminal ileum is transected with a linear stapler.

- The terminal ileum is transected with a single firing of a linear stapler (such as GIA 60-3.5 stapler, or GIA 60-4.8 if the ileum is thickened or inflamed, **FIGURE 5**).
- The ascending colon mesentery is divided from the proximal to distal until the middle colic pedicle is encountered.
- The middle colic pedicle is clamped with heavy artery forceps by creating windows on either side with diathermy.
- The pedicle is divided between the artery forceps and ligated proximally and distally with absorbable braided size 0 ties. Care is taken to avoid injuries to the superior mesenteric artery and vein.

DESCENDING COLON MOBILIZATION

- The descending colon is mobilized using a lateral to medial approach by medial traction of the descending colon and dissection along the left paracolic gutter using diathermy (**FIGURE 6**).
- Care is taken to identify, and avoid damage to, the left gonadal vessels and left ureter (**FIGURE 7**).
- Dissection is stopped at the rectosigmoid junction.

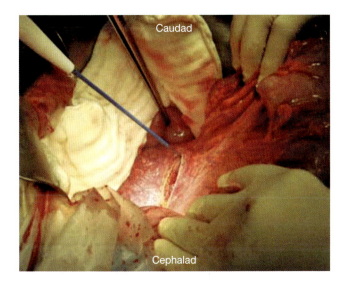
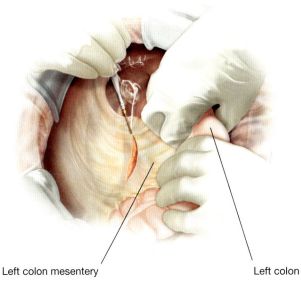

FIGURE 6 • Descending colon mobilization. With the descending colon retracted medially, the lateral peritoneal attachments are transected with electrocautery along the left paracolic gutter.

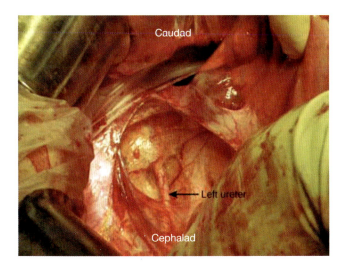
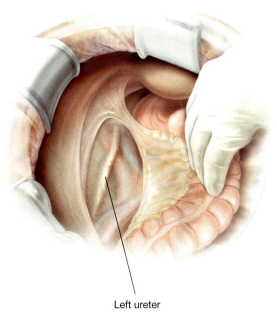

FIGURE 7 • Identification of left ureter. After full mobilization of the descending colon, the left ureter is exposed in the retroperitoneum. The surgeon is retracting the descending colon medially.

DISTAL DIVISION

- The inferior mesenteric pedicle is identified and clamped with heavy artery forceps by creating windows on either side with diathermy.
- The pedicle is divided between the artery forceps and ligated proximally and distally with absorbable braided size 0 ties (**FIGURE 8**).
- Alternatively, if the surgeon is certain of the absence of malignancy, then the mesenteric blood supply to the distal segment can be taken close to the bowel wall.
- The rectosigmoid junction is then divided with a transverse linear stapler (such as a Contour-35 or a TA 60-4.8 stapler, **FIGURE 9**).
- The specimen is removed and sent to the laboratory in formalin.

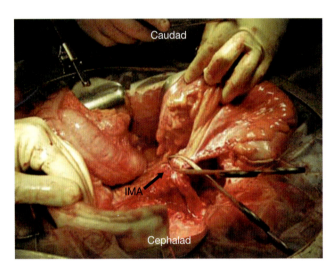
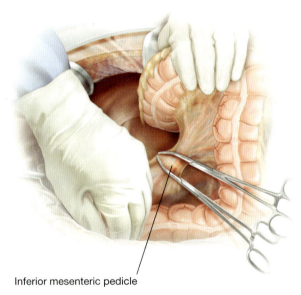

FIGURE 8 • Inferior mesenteric artery (IMA) division. The IMA is transected between clamps and will subsequently be ligated with heavy silk sutures.

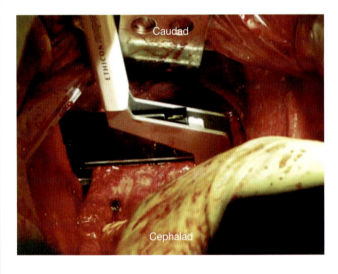
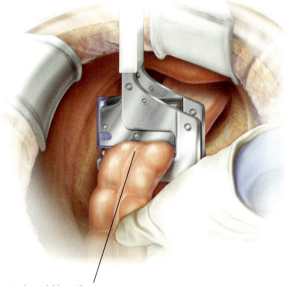

FIGURE 9 • Distal division. Distal transection, at the level of the rectosigmoid junction, is performed with a linear TA stapler device.

Chapter 24 **TOTAL ABDOMINAL COLECTOMY: OPEN TECHNIQUE** 201

ILEORECTAL ANASTOMOSIS

- The distal ileum is inspected to ensure adequate blood supply and length for a tension free ileorectal anastomosis.
- There are several configurations that can be used to join the ileum to the rectum, all of which have various advantages and disadvantages.[5] For the sake of simplicity, a common method is outlined in the section that follows.
- An enterotomy is made with diathermy on the antimesenteric border of the distal ileum, 2 cm proximal to the division staple line.
- The anvil of a circular stapler, the size of which can be established with anal sizers, is inserted into the enterotomy and secured with a purse-string suture (nonabsorbable, monofilament size 0).
- The circular stapler is inserted through the anus and the trocar pushed out through the rectum anterior to the staple line.
- The trocar and the anvil joined, ensuring that the small bowel mesentery is not twisted and the anastomosis is tension-free (**FIGURE 10A**). The stapler is then fired creating a side-to-end ileorectal anastomosis.
- An underwater air leak test is performed by pouring warm water into the pelvis and insufflating air from the below with a proctoscope (**FIGURE 10B**).
- Consideration is given to a covering loop ileostomy if the air leak test is positive, if the patient is malnourished or acutely unwell, or if there are any technical issues with the anastomosis. In more extreme cases, where an anastomosis is undesirable or not possible, an end ileostomy can be fashioned, leaving a closed rectal stump.

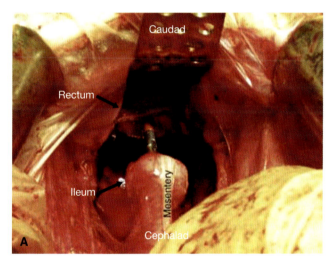
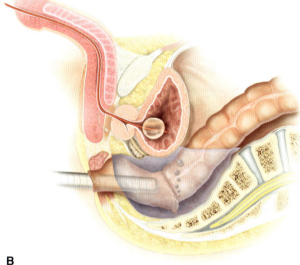

FIGURE 10 • **A,** Ileorectal anastomosis. **B,** The completed ileorectal anastomosis is tested under water. Air bubbles identified during insufflation of the anastomosis indicate an anastomotic leak.

CLOSURE

- Mass fascial closure is performed with size 1 absorbable, monofilament suture.
- Skin is closed with absorbable monofilament subcuticular sutures or staples.
- No intra-abdominal or rectal drains are used.

PEARLS AND PITFALLS

Bleeding from the spleen	Minimizing traction on the splenic flexure is critical to reduce the incidence of splenic tears. If the spleen is torn, hemostatic agents (such as cellulose sheets or fibrin powders) can be used with a swab applying pressure for 5 min to attempt to achieve hemostasis. Ultimately however, if bleeding cannot be stopped, then a splenectomy may be required.
Difficult splenic flexure mobilization	It may be easier to mobilize the splenic flexure by standing between the patient's legs rather than on the patient's right side. The dissection is further helped by repeatedly approaching the splenic flexure bidirectionally proximally and distally until it is freed.

Identification of the ureters	On both sides, the ureters are identified by direct visualization to avoid injury. In their normal anatomical position, they are located on the psoas muscle just lateral to the transverse spinous processes and then pass over the bifurcation of the common iliac arteries to lie on the sacroiliac joints, turning underneath the vas deferens (uterine arteries in females) to enter the bladder. The right ureter is crossed by the right colic artery, ileocolic artery, and gonadal vessels. The left ureter is crossed by the left colic, gonadal vessels, and sigmoid arterial branches. With local invasion or severe inflammation, the ureters can be in a nonanatomical location and more difficult to identify, in which case preemptive ureteric stents (with or without lighting) can help avoid injury.
Management of the rectal stump	In the event that an anastomosis cannot be performed, and an end ileostomy and closed rectal stump are fashioned, it may be desirable to suture the rectal stump to the inferior aspect of the midline wound fascia.[6] This is because, if the rectal stump leaks, a mucous fistula (rather than frank intraperitoneal contamination) will be the result.

POSTOPERATIVE CARE

- ERAS perioperative care protocols are applied.[1]

COMPLICATIONS

- Anastomotic leak (4.4%)[7]
- Pelvic abscess
- Intra-abdominal bleeding
- Adhesive small bowel obstruction (30%)[8]
- Postoperative ileus
- Wound infection
- Cardiopulmonary complications
- Urinary tract infection
- Failure of treatment in IBD (17%-26%)[7]
- Incontinence/diarrhea.
- Overall reduced quality of life compared to general population.[9]

REFERENCES

1. Gustafsson UO, Scott MJ, Hubner M, et al. Guidelines for perioperative care in elective colorectal surgery: Enhanced Recovery After Surgery (ERAS®) Society Recommendations—2018. *World J Surg.* 2019;43(3):659-695.
2. Freise H, Van Aken HK. Risks and benefits of thoracic epidural anaesthesia. *Br J Anaesth.* 2011;107(6):859-868.
3. Rovera F, Dionigi G, Boni L, et al. Antibiotic prophylaxis and preoperative colorectal cleansing: are they useful? *Surg Oncol.* 2007;16(suppl 1):S109-S111.
4. Guenaga KF, Matos D, Wille-Jorgensen P. Mechanical bowel preparation for elective colorectal surgery. *Cochrane Database Syst Rev.* 2011;(9):CD001544.
5. Jolly S, Dudi-Venkata NN, Hanna-Rivero N, et al. Four different ileorectal anastomotic configurations following total colectomy. *ANZ J Surg.* 2020;90(9):1588-1591.
6. Bedrikovetski S, Dudi-Venkata N, Kroon HM, et al. Systematic review of rectal stump management during and after emergency total colectomy for acute severe ulcerative colitis. *ANZ J Surg.* 2019;89(12):1556-1560.
7. Pastore RL, Wolff BG, Hodge D. Total abdominal colectomy and ileorectal anastomosis for inflammatory bowel disease. *Dis Colon Rectum.* 1997;40(12):1455-1464.
8. Nieuwenhuijzen M, Reijnen MM, Kuijpers JH, et al. Small bowel obstruction after total or subtotal colectomy: a 10-year retrospective review. *Br J Surg.* 1998;85(9):1242-1245.
9. Van Duijvendijk P, Slors JF, Taat CW, et al. Quality of life after total colectomy with ileorectal anastomosis or proctocolectomy and ileal pouch-anal anastomosis for familial adenomatous polyposis. *Br J Surg.* 2000;87(5):590-596.

Chapter 25

Total Abdominal Colectomy: Laparoscopic Technique

William C. Chapman Jr. and Matthew G. Mutch

DEFINITION

- Total abdominal colectomy (TAC) is the removal of the abdominal colon, which extends from the cecum to the top of the rectum. The rectosigmoid junction is an intraperitoneal structure identified by the splaying of the teniae coli.
- The procedure is accompanied by either creation of an end ileostomy or an ileorectal anastomosis, often determined by the indication for surgery.
- Minimally invasive techniques for total colectomy, laparoscopic, hand-assisted laparoscopic, or robot-assisted, have been shown to be safe while achieving improved short-term outcomes in comparison to open TAC.

PATIENT HISTORY AND PHYSICAL FINDINGS

- There are several potential indications for a laparoscopic TAC:
  - Colitis
    - Inflammatory bowel disease (IBD): Ulcerative colitis and Crohn disease
      - Refractory to medical management
      - Complications
        - Fulminant colitis
        - Toxic megacolon
        - Stricture
        - Perforation
        - Dysplasia
        - Neoplasm
    - Infectious
  - Colon cancer
    - Synchronous cancers
    - Colon cancer in a patient younger than age 40 years
  - Familial adenomatous polyposis (FAP) with rectal sparing
  - Functional disorders
    - Colonic inertia
    - Neurogenic bowel
- A thorough history and a physical examination are necessary prior to surgery. Prior abdominal surgery is not an absolute contraindication for a laparoscopic approach.
- In IBD patients with colitis, the requirement for surgical intervention is dependent on response to medical management. Assessing the type and duration of previous treatment with immunomodulators and intravenous steroids is therefore critical. Typically, patients that do not achieve significant symptom improvement after 7 days of intravenous steroids are considered refractory to medical management.
- Acute colitis, regardless of etiology, can be safely approached laparoscopically. However, if colitic patients have peritonitis or hemodynamic instability, an open approach may be necessary.

- Normal bowel function ranges from three bowel movements a day to one bowel movement every 3 days. Colonic inertia patients give a long history of constipation that is no longer responsive to laxatives. When the patient gets to the point where their abdominal complaints and bowel function are not responsive to laxatives and their symptoms become intolerable, surgery management should be considered.

IMAGING AND OTHER DIAGNOSTIC STUDIES

- Each indication for surgery has specific evaluations that are necessary to determine optimal treatment and operative approach.
  - Acute colitis
    - Endoscopic examination of the colon is necessary to confirm the diagnosis and extent of disease within the distal gastrointestinal tract.
    - In hospitalized patients, stool culture and toxin analysis to rule out *Clostridium difficile* and cytomegalovirus infections should be performed.
    - Computed tomography (CT) scan or magnetic resonance imaging (MRI) enterography may help evaluate potential significant small bowel involvement in IBD.
  - Colon cancer
    - Pathologic confirmation of adenocarcinoma through tissue biopsy is necessary.
    - Endoluminal evaluation to confirm the number and location of the lesions is necessary. Ideally, the lesion(s) are tattooed with a vital dye to mark the location. It is best to inject the ink distal to the most distal lesion and in at least three different locations around the circumference of the lumen to ensure intraoperative visualization of the tattooed area during laparoscopic surgery.
    - Preoperative staging is completed with a CT scan of the chest, abdomen, and pelvis and a serum carcinoembryonic antigen (CEA) level.
    - Patients younger than age 50 years and/or with a strong family history of colorectal cancer should be considered for genetic counseling.
  - FAP
    - Endoscopy with biopsy and pathologic evaluation confirming the presence of more than 100 adenomatous polyps prompts surgical evaluation.
    - Genetic testing confirming the diagnosis of FAP is desirable, but not all patients with endoscopic findings consistent with FAP will have an identifiable mutation.
    - If the patient is going to be considered for a rectal sparing procedure, the rectum needs to be examined and cleared of all polyps. Only patients with 10 or fewer polyps in the rectum that can be removed or destroyed are eligible for rectal sparing procedures.

203

- Colonic inertia and neurogenic bowel
  - Endoscopic examination of the entire colon is necessary to rule out a mechanical etiology of the patient's constipation.
  - Next, a colonic transit study is necessary to confirm the diagnosis of colonic inertia. During this test, the patient ingests a capsule with 25 radiopaque markers and then undergoes serial plain abdominal x-rays at 3 and 5 days from the time of ingestion. All laxatives and promotility agents must be held. An abnormal examination is when five or more markers are retained in the colon after 5 days. The distribution of the markers is the diagnostic key: Markers scattered throughout the colon are consistent with colonic inertia, whereas accumulation of the markers in the rectum or distal sigmoid colon is suggestive of obstructed defecation or pelvic floor abnormality.
  - Patients should also be evaluated with either a video defecography or dynamic MRI to evaluate for obstructive defecation. If a patient demonstrates evidence of obstructive defecation, they should undergo biofeedback prior to discussing surgery as a definitive treatment option.

SURGICAL MANAGEMENT

Preoperative Planning

- Depending on the operative plan, patients should be marked for optimal siting of a diverting or end ileostomy. Stoma site selection should follow criteria as outlined elsewhere in this text.
- The placement of ureteral stents at the time of surgery is left to the discretion of the surgeon but typically reserved for cases of significant inflammation within the pelvis.

Positioning

- A mechanical bed that is able to place the patient in the extreme gravity-assisted positions is necessary.
- The patient is secured to the bed with a beanbag, a nonslip pad, shoulder braces, or foam pads.

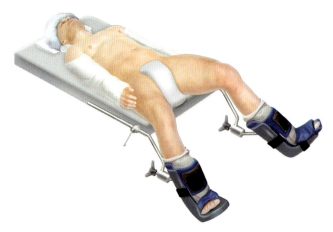

FIGURE 1 • Patient positioning. The patient is placed in lithotomy position with the hips slightly flexed and the legs in Yellofin stirrups. The thighs are placed parallel to the ground to avoid interference with the surgeon's arms and instruments.

- The patient should be placed in the modified lithotomy position with Allen or Yellofin stirrups (**FIGURE 1**). This allows access between the legs to assist with mobilization of the left colon and to the perineum for anastomosis creation.
- The heels are firmly planted on the stirrups to ensure that the patient does not slip and that there are no pressure points along the lateral peroneal nerves or the popliteal vessels during the procedure.
- The thighs are placed parallel to the ground to avoid interference with the surgeon's arms and instruments.
- Both arms are tucked to the patient's side with the thumbs facing up. This allows the surgeon, assistant, and camera driver plenty of room to maneuver during the case.
- A monitor should be placed off the patient's right shoulder during the mobilization of the right and transverse colon.
- A monitor should be placed off the patient's left shoulder for the mobilization of the left colon and splenic flexure.

PORT PLACEMENT AND TEAM SETUP

- There are several options for port placement depending on whether a total laparoscopic surgery or hand-assisted laparoscopic surgery (HALS) is going to be used.
  - Straight laparoscopic approach
    - Camera port—The port is placed in the periumbilical area in equal distance between the xiphoid process and the pubic symphysis (**FIGURE 2A**). The camera should be placed at the apex of the pneumoperitoneum so the widest field of view can be obtained.
    - Working ports—There are two working ports on the right side and two ports on the left side. They should be centered on the camera port, lateral to the rectus muscles, and greater than a hand's width (7 cm) apart.
  - HALS approach
    - Hand port—The hand port is placed in the suprapubic position via either a midline or Pfannenstiel incision (**FIGURE 2B**).
    - Camera port—The camera is placed in the supraumbilical position so that the port does not interfere with the skirt of the hand port.
    - Working ports—A 5-mm working port is placed in both the right and left mid-abdomen. They are placed in equal distance between the hand port and the camera and lateral to the rectus muscle.
  - Team setup
    - For the HALS approach to the right and transverse colon, the surgeon stands on the patient's left side with their left hand through the hand port and right hand manipulating a laparoscopic energy device (such as LigaSure or ultrasonic dissector) through a working port.
    - To mobilize the left colon, the surgeon stands on the patient's right side with right hand inside the

Chapter 25 TOTAL ABDOMINAL COLECTOMY: LAPAROSCOPIC TECHNIQUE 205

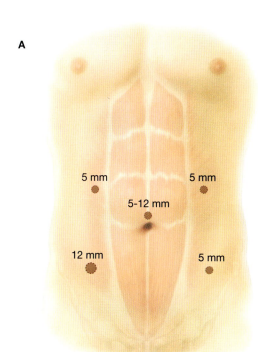
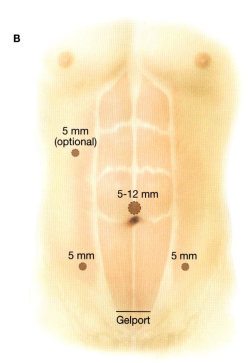

FIGURE 2 • Port placement. **A,** Port placement for a conventional laparoscopic total colectomy. **B,** Port placement for a hand-assisted laparoscopic total colectomy. Note the requirement for a 12-mm port if utilizing a 10-mm camera of endoscopic stapler.

abdomen and left hand manipulating the energy source (**FIGURE 3**). The camera operator stands to the head side of the surgeon.
- The following operative steps are the same whether the procedure is being performed straight laparoscopically or via HALS. For the purpose of this chapter, the HALS approach to the total colectomy operation will be described.
- Equipment
  - Reusable laparoscopic instrumentation—Various reusable laparoscopic instruments are suitable for manipulating the large and small bowel. We prefer nonlocking, atraumatic grasping instruments for the majority of the dissection.
  - Laparoscopic energy devices—TAC requires multiple forms of tissue dissection. While much of the work can be done bluntly in avascular planes, the surgeon will also require vessel-ligating and coagulating capability. Many disposable products exist along these lines and are suitable; in our experience, we prefer to use a scissor connected to monopolar energy and a laparoscopic bipolar device for vessel coagulation.
  - Endoscopic stapler—Depending on vessel and bowel transection preference, surgeons may utilize endoscopic staplers for various portions of laparoscopic TAC. However, many endoscopic bipolar energy devices are now available that are capable of safely sealing the ileocolic, middle colic, and inferior mesenteric artery (IMA) pedicles. When combined with externalization strategies for bowel transection, the need for an endoscopic stapler can often be avoided. Additionally, endoscopic staplers require 10- to 12-mm ports.

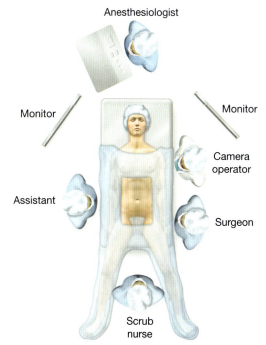

FIGURE 3 • Operating team setup. For the hand-assisted laparoscopic surgery approach to the right and transverse colon, the surgeon stands on the patient's left side with left hand through the hand port while the right hand manipulates the dissection tool or energy device of choice through the left lower quadrant port. During the mobilization of the left colon, the surgeon will stand on the patient's right side, right hand in the abdomen and left hand on the energy source. The camera operator stands to the head side of the surgeon.

TECHNIQUES

MOBILIZATION OF THE RIGHT COLON

- Once the abdomen has been accessed and inspected, the patient is placed in steep Trendelenburg position to pack the small bowel in the right upper quadrant (RUQ). The posterior approach will be described for the mobilization of the right colon. The specific steps of operation are the same for medial to lateral, lateral to medial, and superior to inferior, but the order of the steps is different depending on the approach.
- The goals of this portion of the operation are to access the retroperitoneal plane, identify and sweep the duodenum out of the way, mobilize the right colon mesentery, divide the lateral attachments and omentum, and ligate the vasculature.
- For the posterior approach, the small bowel is placed in the RUQ and the base of the ascending colon mesentery is exposed from the third portion of the duodenum to the cecum (**FIGURE 4**). The ileocolic vessels (ICV) are seen as they cross over the third portion of the duodenum. The patient is not tilted so that the small bowel will stay in the RUQ.
- The middle finger and the thumb grasp the ICV, lifting them off the retroperitoneum. The index finger then sweeps under the mesentery to expose the third portion of the duodenum (**FIGURE 5**). The peritoneum is then scored dorsal to the ICV from the duodenum all the way down to the cecum.
- Once the retroperitoneum is accessed, the duodenum is identified and swept posteriorly. The hand is then placed under the mesentery, palm down, and the ascending colon mesentery is elevated off the retroperitoneum (**FIGURE 6**) through a medial to lateral sweeping dissection approach. The retroperitoneum is bluntly swept down with an energy device.
- This medial to lateral dissection is carried out beyond the colon from the mid-transverse colon, out to the hepatic flexure, and down the ascending colon to the cecum. The more extensively the dissection can be carried laterally, the easier the lateral dissection will be.
- Tension is the key; this is an avascular plane that can be effortlessly dissected with adequate tension. The motion should almost be a swimming-type motion in which tension

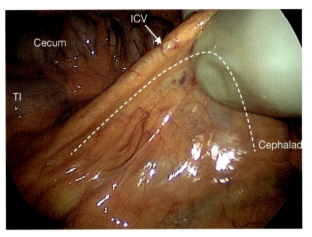

FIGURE 5 • Initiation of the medial to lateral mobilization. With the surgeon holding the ileocolic vessels (ICV) anteriorly, the peritoneum is scored dorsal to the ICV from the duodenum all the way down to the cecum (*dotted line*). TI, terminal ileum.

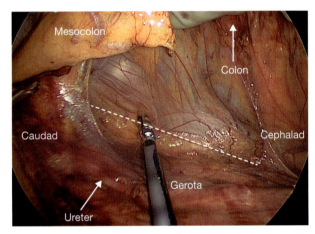

FIGURE 6 • Medial to lateral mobilization of the ascending colon. With the surgeon's hand retracting the colon anteriorly, the ascending mesocolon is separated from the retroperitoneum (Gerota fascia) by sweeping the retroperitoneal tissues dorsally with a 5-mm energy device. This dissection is carried along the transition between the two distinctive fat planes of the mesocolon and Gerota fascia (*dotted line*).

is created, the tissue is swept down, tension is recreated, and the tissue is swept down, over and over.
- Now all that remains are the lateral attachments, which are transected with the laparoscopic energy device up the right gutter (**FIGURE 7**). At this point, the patient is tilted laterally with the right side up so the small bowel will fall to the left upper quadrant (LUQ), further exposing the lateral attachments of the right colon and hepatic flexure.
- Once the cecum is adequately mobilized, the hand is placed back into the abdomen. The left hand is placed under the right colon mesentery and lateral to the colon to expose the lateral attachments, which are divided under tension by the first assistant.
- The right colon and its mesentery are elevated to expose the retroperitoneum and to dissect any remaining retroperitoneal

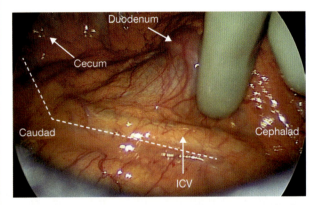

FIGURE 4 • Root of the ascending colon mesentery. The base of the ascending colon mesentery is exposed from the third portion of the duodenum to the cecum. The ileocolic vessels (ICV) are seen as they cross over the third portion of the duodenum. The dissection plane will be initiated along the dorsal aspect of the ICV (*dotted line*).

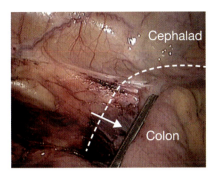

FIGURE 7 • Lateral mobilization of the ascending colon. The white line of Toldt is transected along the right paracolic gutter (*dotted line*). The medial to lateral dissection plane previously dissected is readily entered, facilitating this step of the operation.

attachments. This dissection is carried all the way up to the hepatic flexure.
- At this point, the hand often obstructs visualization. Remove the hand and instead place a 5-mm port through the hand port. With a grasper in the right hand, the cecum is retracted medially, and the energy source in the left hand (passed through the 5-mm port located in the hand port cover) takes down the hepatic flexure.

MOBILIZATION OF THE TRANSVERSE COLON

- The key to mobilizing the transverse colon is accessing the lesser sac. This is accomplished by either dividing the lesser omentum and taking the omentum with the specimen or preserving the omentum by separating it from the transverse colon and its mesentery.
- To resect the omentum, the lateral dissection of the right colon is continued up to the hepatic flexure. The colon is rolled medially and the lateral cut edge of the lesser omentum or hepatocolic attachments are elevated with a laparoscopic instrument. The hepatocolic ligament is then transected with an energy device (**FIGURE 8**). This plane between the omentum, mesentery, and duodenum/stomach is developed, ensuring the duodenum and stomach are swept free; this step is greatly facilitated by the previous medial to lateral dissection step, which already separated the hepatic flexure from the duodenum and the head of the pancreas.

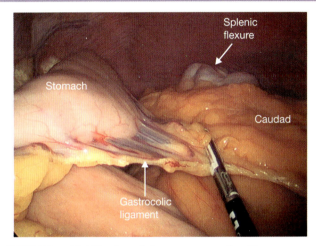

FIGURE 9 • Mobilization of the transverse colon. The gastrocolic ligament is transected from right to left, toward the splenic flexure of the colon, with a bipolar energy device.

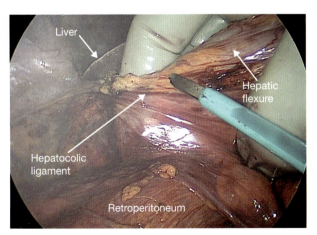

FIGURE 8 • Mobilization of the hepatic flexure. The hepatocolic ligament is transected with a monopolar energy device.

- The gastrocolic ligament is then divided from right to left with an energy device (**FIGURE 9**). This can be a very tedious dissection, as the entire plane tends to be fused, but with good exposure, tension, and patience, the lesser sac is entered. The lesser sac opens up toward the middle of the stomach. Care must be taken to not dissect into the transverse colon mesentery. Once in the lesser sac, the dissection should be carried as far toward the splenic flexure as possible.
- There may be residual attachments of the mesentery to the antrum of the stomach that are taken down by elevating the stomach and pushing the mesentery down.
- With the lesser omentum divided and the lesser sac completely open, the ICV and right colic and middle colic vessels will be easily isolated when it time comes for them to be transected.

TRANSECTION OF THE RIGHT AND MIDDLE MESENTERIC VASCULATURE

- The ICV pedicle is first isolated. The ileocolic pedicle, easily identified because it has been dissected off the retroperitoneum already, is lifted anteriorly. With the ICV pedicle adequately isolated, it can be transected with an energy device (**FIGURE 10**). Transection of the ICV as they cross the third portion of the duodenum ensures that the ICV are transected at their origin without compromising the superior mesenteric vessels, which are located medially in the root of the mesentery.

- Next, the transverse colon is elevated to expose the medial or inferior aspect of the mesentery (**FIGURE 11A**). The surgeon elevates the proximal transverse colon and passes their left hand through the mesenteric defect of the ileocolic pedicle, into the lesser sac, anterior to the pancreas, and encircles the middle colic vessels. The first assistant stands between the legs and via the left lower quadrant (LLQ) port elevates the distal transverse colon and its mesentery. With the middle colic vessels elevated, the base of the mesentery and a bare area should be seen near the ligament of Treitz (**FIGURE 11B**).

- With the transverse colon mesentery elevated, the peritoneum is incised from the bare area on the left (by the ligament of Treitz) to the previously cut edge of the mesentery on the right (**FIGURE 11B**). This allows the individual middle colic vessels to be safely isolated and transected with an energy device. Because of the mobilization and separation of the omentum from the transverse colon mesentery, the vessels can be safely transected without fear of injury to the omentum or stomach.

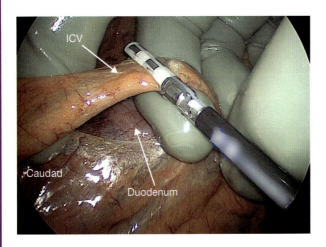

FIGURE 10 • Transection of the ileocolic vessels (ICV). The ICV are transected with the bipolar energy device at their origin as they cross over the third portion of the duodenum.

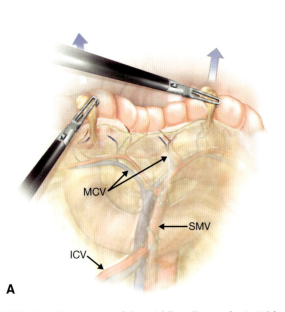
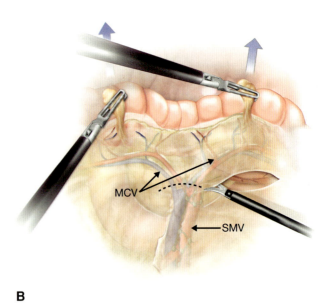

FIGURE 11 • Transection of the middle colic vessels. **A,** With the transverse colon tented upward, the vascular anatomy at the root of the mesentery is identified. The middle colic vessels (MCV) are seen as they originate from the superior mesenteric vessels (SMV). **B,** The root of the mesentery is incised from the bare area on the left (by the ligament of Treitz) to the previously cut edge of the mesentery on the right. This allows the individual MCV to be safely isolated and transected with a bipolar energy device. The *dash line* represents the line for incising the peritoneum over the MCV. ICV, ileocolic vessels.

MOBILIZATION OF THE LEFT COLON

- The patient is placed in a steep Trendelenburg position and tilted left side up, allowing the small bowel and omentum to fall into the RUQ. This exposes the transverse colon and splenic flexure as well as the IMA at its aortic origin and the inferior mesenteric vein (IMV) at the ligament of Treitz.
- The surgeon now moves to the patient's right side and places their right hand in the hand port. The left hand introduces the bipolar energy device through the right lower quadrant (RLQ) 5-mm port and dissection begins.

TRANSECTION OF THE INFERIOR MESENTERIC ARTERY

- The retroperitoneum is accessed at the level of the sacral promontory. The superior hemorrhoidal artery (SHA) is grasped and elevated (**FIGURE 12A**), exposing the IMA and its terminal branches, the SHA, and left colic artery. A wide incision is made in the peritoneum dorsal to this artery (**FIGURE 12B**); the wider the incision, the more the artery can be elevated to obtain better exposure. Because of the curve of the pelvis at this point, the sigmoid mesentery curves up and away from the visual field. Therefore, the retroperitoneal plane is higher than expected, so the more mobile the arterial pedicle is, the easier it is to visualize the correct plane.
- Identification of the left ureter is necessary before the IMA can be ligated (**FIGURE 13**). There are several options for locating the ureter, as detailed below.
    - After mobilization of the SHA as describe earlier, the left ureter can often be found as it drops over the pelvic brim lateral to the IMA-SHA junction.
    - If unable to locate in proximity to the SHA, move into the mid-abdomen. Grasp the IMV and elevate it. Incise the peritoneum dorsal to the IMV, accessing the retroperitoneum. The retroperitoneum is flat in this area, allowing the plane behind the IMV to be carried in a caudad fashion to meet up with the initial plane under the superior rectal artery. The ureter can often be found in the retroperitoneum just dorsal to this plane.
    - If the ureter is still not identified, mobilize the sigmoid and left colon in a lateral to medial fashion. Then investigate the retroperitoneum with the colon medialized.
    - Finally, the top of the hand port can be removed and the left ureter can be located via an open fashion if necessary.
- After the left ureter is identified and swept into the retroperitoneum, the IMA can be isolated at its origin. The index finger elevates the superior rectal artery and the middle finger is used to sweep down the retroperitoneum along the course of the IMA. This motion continues until the bare area is exposed cephalad to the IMA and medial to the IMV.
- It is important to sweep down the retroperitoneal tissue in this area to help preserve the sympathetic plexus around the IMA. Once the IMA is safely isolated and the left ureter is clearly out of harm's way, the IMA can be transected at its origin from the aorta with a bipolar energy device (**FIGURE 14A**) or linear vascular stapler (**FIGURE 14B**).

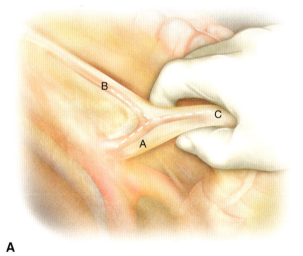
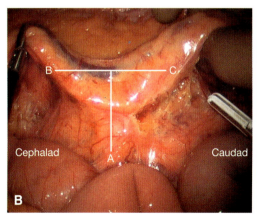

FIGURE 12 • Identification of inferior mesenteric artery (IMA) and its branches. **A,** Grasping the superior hemorrhoidal artery (SHA) anteriorly helps identify the "letter T" formed between the IMA (A) and its left colic artery (B) and SHA (C) terminal branches. The IMA takeoff is just cephalad from the aortic bifurcation. The thumb and the index finger are lifting the SHA off the groove located anterior to the left common iliac artery. **B,** Incision along the dorsal aspect of both the left colic vessels (B) and the SHA (C) allows for safe entry into the retroperitoneal space, helping isolate the IMA (A) at its origin.

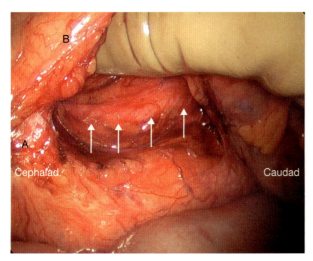

FIGURE 13 • Identification of the left ureter. After the inferior mesenteric artery (IMA) *(A)* and superior hemorrhoidal artery (SHA) *(B)* have been lifted off the retroperitoneum, the left ureter *(arrows)* can be identified and preserved intact. Identification of the left ureter at this stage is critical in order to avoid injuring it during IMA transection.

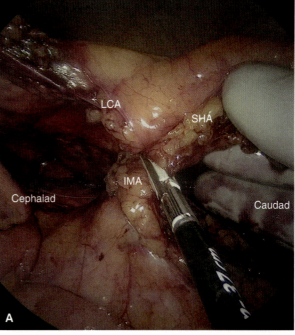

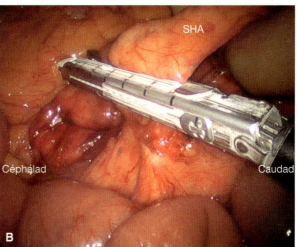

FIGURE 14 • **A** and **B,** Transection of the inferior mesenteric artery (IMA). With the left ureter safely excluded in the retroperitoneum, the IMA is transected with an advanced energy device **(A)** or a linear vascular stapler **(B)** at its origin arising from the aorta prior to branching into the superior hemorrhoidal artery (SHA) and LCA (left colic artery). The surgeon's hand is holding the SHA anteriorly.

TRANSECTION OF THE INFERIOR MESENTERIC VEIN

- The IMV courses parallel to the left colic artery. The previous IMA dissection plane is carried cephalad with a scissor or monopolar energy device (sweeping the retroperitoneal tissues dorsally) until the left colic artery separates from the IMV as it courses toward the splenic flexure at the level of the ligament of Treitz.
- Now that the IMV is elevated off the retroperitoneum, it is isolated at the inferior border of the pancreas and near the ligament of Treitz (**FIGURE 15**). It can be isolated with the same technique used for the IMA: The index finger and the thumb elevate and create tension on the IMV, and the middle finger and/or the dissecting instrument sweeps the retroperitoneum dorsally along the course of the vein.
- A bare area is then created near the inferior border of the pancreas that allows the IMV to be safely isolated.
- Once isolated, it can be safely transected with an energy device (**FIGURE 16**).

Mobilization of the Left Colon

- The left colon mesentery is now dissected off the retroperitoneum using a medial to lateral dissection approach (**FIGURE 17**) all the way out to the lateral abdominal wall.
- The hand is placed palm down under the mesentery to elevate it as a fan-type retractor. The plane is dissected bluntly with an energy device from the sigmoid colon up to the splenic flexure. The further laterally and superiorly the dissection is carried, the easier the lateral dissection and splenic flexure mobilization will be later during the case. Care must be taken during mobilization near the inferior border of the

Chapter 25 **TOTAL ABDOMINAL COLECTOMY: LAPAROSCOPIC TECHNIQUE** 211

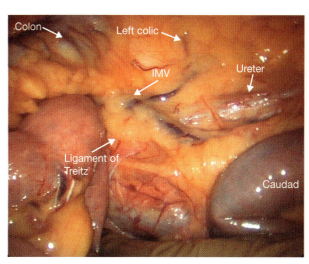

FIGURE 15 • Identification of the inferior mesenteric vein (IMV). The IMV can be identified at the root of the transverse mesocolon at the level of the ligament of Treitz. At this level, the IMV has separated from the left colic artery (which courses away from the IMV and toward the splenic flexure of the colon) and from the left ureter.

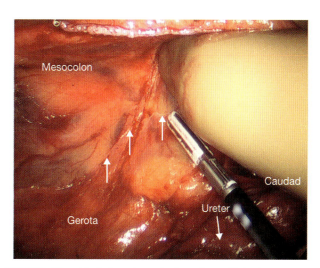

FIGURE 17 • Medial to lateral dissection. With the surgeon holding the mesocolon anteriorly (notice the stapled inferior mesenteric artery stump in between the surgeon's fingers), the retroperitoneal tissues are swept downward (dorsally) with the energy device. The dissection progresses along the potential space between the two fat planes: mesocolon and Gerota (arrows).

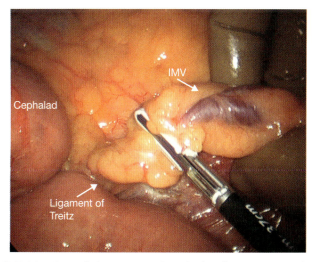

FIGURE 16 • Inferior mesenteric vein (IMV) transection. The IMV is transected at the level of the ligament of Treitz with a bipolar energy device.

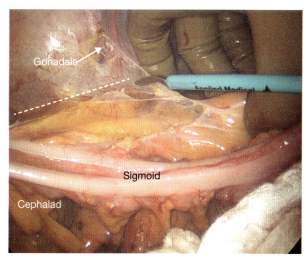

FIGURE 18 • Lateral mobilization of the sigmoid and descending colon. The white line of Toldt (dotted line) is transected with a monopolar scissor. The medial to lateral dissection plane is readily entered, greatly facilitating the lateral mobilization of the descending colon.

pancreas, as it is very easy to carry the dissection deep to the pancreas.
- All that remains at this point are the lateral attachments. First, the hand is used to depress the sigmoid colon to incise the lateral peritoneum (**FIGURE 18**). At this point, it is not uncommon for the hand to obstruct visualization, making it necessary to pass the energy source through the surgeon's fingers or remove the hand altogether from the hand port. The lateral attachments are lysed from the pelvis toward the splenic flexure.
- As the dissection is carried cranially, the surgeon uses a grasper for exposure and the first assistant uses the energy source through the LLQ port to transect the rest of the lateral colon attachments.

MOBILIZATION OF THE SPLENIC FLEXURE

- The mobilization of the splenic flexure is greatly facilitated by the previous transection of the gastrocolic ligament and the previous medial to lateral mobilization of the descending colon.
- The splenic flexure is grasped laterally with the hand and medially with a grasper. Caudal retraction is applied to the colon to identify any remaining attachments between the colon and the diaphragm or spleen. The splenodiaphragmatic and splenocolic ligaments are then transected with an energy device (**FIGURE 19**).
- All that remains are the posterior attachments to the inferior border of the pancreas. Division of these attachments to the midline allows for a full mobilization of the splenic flexure.

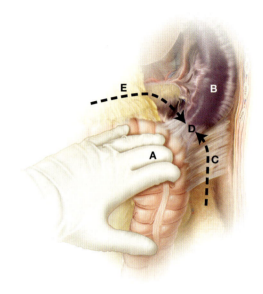

FIGURE 19 • Mobilization of the splenic flexure. The surgeon retracts the splenic flexure of the colon (A) downward and medially, exposing the attachments of the splenic flexure to the spleen (B). The phrenocolic (C) and splenocolic (D) ligaments are transected in an inferior to superior and lateral to medial direction, meeting the previously transected gastrocolic ligament (E) dissection plane around the splenic flexure.

RECTAL TRANSECTION

- Depending on the approach, the rectum can now be prepared for division.
  - HALS
    - Once the colon is completely mobilized and free, it can be extracted through the hand port and the upper rectum can be divided in an open fashion.
    - The colon is extracted by passing the small bowel underneath the colon and its mesentery. The surgeon stays on the patient's right side and the left colon is elevated while the proximal small bowel is fed under the colon and its mesentery. The patient is then tilted left side down to facilitate migration of the small bowel into the LUQ. Once the entire small bowel is passed under the colon, the cecum is grasped and brought out through the hand port. This allows the small bowel to be positioned in the left side of the abdomen, with the cut edge of the small bowel straight and facing to the patient's right side. It is in the correct orientation for an ileostomy or ileorectal anastomosis.
  - Straight laparoscopic approach
    - The top of the rectum is identified by the splaying out of the teniae coli.

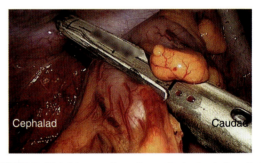

FIGURE 20 • Distal transection. An endostapler is inserted into the right lower quadrant 12-mm port and used to divide the sigmoid colon distal to the rectosigmoid junction.

- The mesorectum is scored at a right angle at the point of distal transection. A window is created between the posterior wall of the rectum and the mesorectum. The rectum is divided with an articulating endoscopic stapler (**FIGURE 20**).
- The mesorectum is then transected at this level with the energy source of choice.
- The colon is then extracted via an LLQ or a suprapubic extraction port.

ILEORECTAL ANASTOMOSIS/END ILEOSTOMY

- The site of the specimen extraction will depend on whether an anastomosis or an end ileostomy is going to be created.
- Ileorectal anastomosis
  - HALS
    - The colon can be extracted via the hand port and the rectum and terminal ileum can be divided in an open fashion.

Chapter 25 TOTAL ABDOMINAL COLECTOMY: LAPAROSCOPIC TECHNIQUE 213

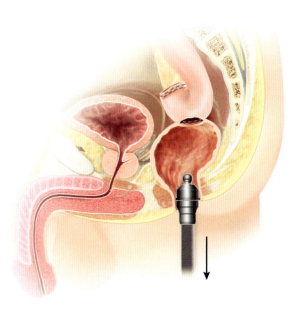

FIGURE 21 • Stapled ileorectal anastomosis. A side-to-end EEA stapled ileorectal anastomosis is constructed using a circular stapler.

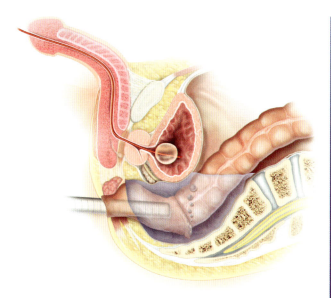

FIGURE 22 • Air leak test. The completed colorectal anastomosis is tested under water. Air bubbles identified during insufflation of the anastomosis indicate an anastomotic leak.

- Once the anvil has been placed in the terminal ileum, a side-to-end, or an end-to-end (EEA) ileorectal anastomosis is created by direct visualization through the hand port or laparoscopically (**FIGURE 21**).
- The entire cut edge of the small bowel mesentery must be visualized to face the patient's right side to ensure there is no twisting.
- The anastomosis is tested under water (air leak test) in standard fashion via the open hand port site (**FIGURE 22**).
- Straight laparoscopic approach
    - A Pfannenstiel or an LLQ incision can be used as the extraction site. If the rectum has been divided, the extraction incision is made and the colon is extracted, starting with the distal transected end.
    - The terminal ileal mesentery is divided.
    - The terminal ileum is divided and a purse string is placed around the anvil of the circular stapler.
    - The ileum is dropped back into the abdomen and the extraction site is closed.
    - Laparoscopically, the stapling cartridge is passed transanally up to the top of the rectal stump.
    - The anvil is reassembled ensuring the small bowel mesentery is not twisted.
    - The anastomosis can be tested with either an air leak test or endoscopic visualization.
- End ileostomy
    - HALS approach
        - The colon is resected and the stoma is created via the open incision of the hand port as described elsewhere in this textbook.
    - Straight laparoscopic approach
        - The colon can be extracted through the ileostomy site, but care must be taken when this approach is used.
            - If the colon is dilated, full of stool, or significantly inflamed, avoid using the stoma site as an extraction site.
            - If the stoma is going to be permanent, realize that in order to get the specimen out, the stoma site may need to be made bigger than usual. This may increase the risk of the patient developing a parastomal hernia.
        - The colon can be extracted via an LLQ or a periumbilical position. Once the colon is extracted and the terminal ileum is divided, it can be dropped back into the abdomen and brought out of the stoma site.
- The ileostomy is then matured in a Brooke ileostomy fashion with absorbable sutures as described elsewhere in this textbook.
- Closure of the abdomen
    - The fascia at all 10-mm port sites or larger should be closed with absorbable suture. The 5-mm port sites are only closed at the skin level.
    - The fascia at the hand port or extraction site can be closed with either interrupted or running stitch of no. 1 slowly absorbable monofilament suture.
    - Prior to skin closure with either staplers or absorbable suture, the subcutaneous tissue is irrigated with antibiotic-containing saline.

PEARLS AND PITFALLS

Options for right colon/mesocolon mobilization	■ Posterior approach: under the small bowel mesentery ■ Medial to lateral: through the right colon mesentery, caudad to the ileocolic pedicle ■ Lateral to medial: incise laterally at the cecum and roll it medially ■ Superior to inferior: enter the retroperitoneum by first dividing the lesser omentum along the hepatocolic ligament
Right colon mobilization: posterior approach	■ If it is difficult to elevate the right colon mesentery and expose the fourth portion of the duodenum, start the dissection at the level of the cecum and work in an inferior to superior direction to mobilize the right colon mesentery.
Right colon mobilization: medial to lateral approach	■ The further the mobilization of the right colon can be carried out laterally, the easier the lateral and hepatic flexure mobilization will be.
Right colon mobilization: superior to inferior approach	■ When trying to enter the lesser sac, roll the right colon medially and elevate the lateral cut edge of the lesser omentum with the grasper. This will allow for direct visualization of this avascular plane, which can be easily dissected in a blunt fashion.
Transection of the middle colic vessels	■ With the lesser sac completely opened and the stomach free of the transverse colon mesentery, the middle colic vessels are free to be safely ligated. ■ When encircling the middle colic vessels, confirm that your hand is on top of the pancreas and ensure that the line of division of the middle colic vessels starts above the ileocolic pedicle, as this ensures that the superior mesenteric artery will not be injured.
Options for mobilization of the left colon/mesocolon	■ Medial approach: This can be started at the level of the sacral promontory or at the level of the IMV. ■ Lateral approach
Four ways of identifying the left ureter	■ A four-step technique was described earlier. Do not spend a lot of time with one approach if you are having difficulty, as the other steps described are necessary to complete the case. Therefore, alternating your approach to identifying the ureter also helps to complete the other steps of the procedure.
Mobilization of the splenic flexure	■ Completing the medial to lateral dissection makes it easier to mobilize the splenic flexure. ■ Be patient when entering the lesser sac. Incise the peritoneum fusing the omentum to the transverse colon and dissect the omentum off the backside of the mesentery one layer at a time.

POSTOPERATIVE CARE

- The patient can begin a liquid diet on the day of surgery. The diet can be advanced as tolerated. Solid food can be safely provided before the resumption of bowel function.
- A urinary catheter should be removed within 24 hours of surgery unless it is needed to assess patient volume status.
- Multimodal pain control combining regional anesthesia (epidural catheters or transversus abdominal plane blocks), IV narcotics, and scheduled oral medications including acetaminophen, NSAIDs such as ketorolac or ibuprofen, and gabapentin has been shown to decrease lengths of stay and postsurgical narcotic use.
- Patients can begin ambulation as early as the day of surgery and by postoperative day 1; they should spend more time out of bed than in it.
- Venous thromboembolism (VTE) prophylaxis is important because of the magnitude of the operation. Low molecular weight heparin (LMWH), subcutaneous heparin, or pneumatic compression boots are all acceptable methods. There are data supporting the use of LMWH for 21 days postoperatively to decrease the risk of VTE.
- For patients with ileostomies, it is important to provide extensive stoma teaching. Points that need to be covered are diet, expected output, measuring of output, and pouching issues.

OUTCOMES

- Laparoscopic TAC for acute colitis is safe, with improved short-term outcomes, decreased hospitalization costs, and no increase in morbidity when compared to open surgery.
- For patients with hereditary nonpolyposis colorectal cancer syndrome (HNPCC) diagnosed with an incident cancer, the risk of developing a metachronous colon cancer is 25%. This high risk is also found in patients younger than age 40 years without a documented mutation in a mismatch repair gene. Therefore, treatment options for resectable colorectal cancer in patients with underlying nonpolyposis colorectal cancer syndrome or those under 40 years should include both segmental resection with annual colonoscopy and TAC with annual proctoscopy.
- Patients with a strong family history of colorectal cancer or documented HNPCC have a significantly lower risk of developing a metachronous colorectal cancer after TAC compared to those patients who underwent a segmental resection.
- HALS and straight laparoscopy have equivalent short-term outcomes for patients undergoing TAC. There was no difference in pain scores, length of stay, return of bowel function, and narcotic usage, but the operative time for the HALS approach was 57 minutes shorter in one study.
- Likewise, additional options in the form of robotic-assisted minimally invasive approach have recently been described.

Chapter 25 **TOTAL ABDOMINAL COLECTOMY: LAPAROSCOPIC TECHNIQUE** **215**

With the latest version of the surgical robot no longer requiring repeated docking and undocking to access multiple areas of the abdomen, more surgeons are utilizing the surgical robot for TAC. While experience remains largely limited, early studies have shown robotic surgery associated with shorter operative times and lengths of stay compared to laparoscopic TACs. Complication profiles were comparable between groups, while costs were significantly higher among the robotic cohort. Overall, current data on robotic outcomes are scant but will likely grow in coming years.

- TAC with ileorectal anastomosis provides an excellent functional outcome and improved quality of life for patients with medically refractory constipation due to colonic inertia.

COMPLICATIONS

- Bleeding
- Anastomotic leak
- Rectal stump leak
- Parastomal hernia
- Pelvic abscess
- Wound infection
- Postoperative ileus
- VTE

SUGGESTED READINGS

1. Chung TP, Fleshman JW, Birnbaum EH, et al. Laparoscopic vs. open total abdominal colectomy for severe colitis: impact on recovery and subsequent completion restorative proctectomy. *Dis Colon Rectum.* 2009;52(1):4-10.
2. Jimenez-Rodriguez R, Quezada-Diaz F, Tchack M, et al. Use of the Xi robotic platform for total abdominal colectomy: a step forward in minimally invasive colorectal surgery. *Surg Endosc.* 2019;33(3):966-971.
3. Lubowski D, Chen FC, Kennedy ML, et al. Results of colectomy for severe slow transit constipation. *Dis Colon Rectum.* 1996;39(1):23-29.
4. Marcello PW, Fleshman JW, Milsom JW, et al. Hand-assisted laparoscopic vs. laparoscopic colorectal surgery: a multicenter, prospective, randomized trial. *Dis Colon Rectum.* 2008;51(6):818-826.
5. Moghadamyeghaneh Z, Hanna M, Carmichael J, et al. Comparison of open, laparoscopic, and robotic approaches for total abdominal colectomy. *Surg Endosc.* 2016;30(7):2792-2798.
6. Ozben V, de Muijnck C, Karabork M, et al. The da Vinci Xi system for robotic total/subtotal colectomy vs. conventional laparoscopy: short term outcomes. *Tech Coloproctol.* 2019;23:861-868.
7. Patton V, Balakrishnan V, Pieri C, et al. Subtotal colectomy and ileorectal anastomosis for slow transit constipation: clinical follow-up at median of 15 years. *Tech Coloproctol.* 2020;24(2):173-179.
8. Sample C, Gupta R, Bamehriz F, et al. Laparoscopic subtotal colectomy for colonic inertia. *J Gastrointest Surg.* 2005;9(6):803-808.

Chapter **26**

Total Abdominal Colectomy: Hand-Assisted Technique

Daniel Albo

DEFINITION

- Total abdominal colectomy is the removal of the abdominal colon, which extends from the cecum to the top of the rectum, following which the distal ileum is anastomosed to the rectum, or an end ileostomy is created.
- Hand-assisted laparoscopic surgery (HALS) is a minimally invasive surgical approach that uses conventional laparoscopic-assisted (LA) surgery techniques with the addition of a hand-assisted device (placed in the projected specimen extraction site) that allows for the introduction of a hand into the surgical field. HALS in colorectal surgery retains all of the same advantages of conventional LA surgery over open surgery, including: less pain, faster recovery, lower incidence of wound complications, and reduction of cardiopulmonary complications, especially in the obese and the elderly.
- Advantages of HALS over conventional LA colorectal surgery include the following:
  - Re-introduces tactile feedback into the field
  - Shorter learning curves; easier to teach
  - Shorter operative times and lower conversion to open rates
  - Higher utilization rates of minimally invasive surgery

DIFFERENTIAL DIAGNOSIS

Indications for HALS total abdominal colectomy:

- Inflammatory bowel disease (IBD)
- Severe acute colitis (various etiologies)
- Polyposis syndromes, including familial adenomatous polyposis and hereditary nonpolyposis colorectal cancer
- Slow transit constipation
- Malignancy

PATIENT HISTORY AND PHYSICAL FINDINGS

- Most patients with colon tumors generally present after an incidental finding during screening colonoscopy, or with occult bleeding and iron deficiency anemia.
- A thorough history and physical examination should include:
  - Previous surgeries (does not preclude a laparoscopic approach)
  - Presence of obstructive symptoms
  - A detailed personal and family history of colorectal cancer, polyps, and/or other malignancies
  - In IBD, the extent of previous medical management, including use of immunomodulators and steroids and response to therapy, is important.
  - Routine abdominal examination, noting any scars.

IMAGING AND OTHER DIAGNOSTIC STUDIES

- A complete colonoscopy should be performed to rule out synchronous disease. Regardless of the primary location of the tumor, every patient should have a complete colonoscopy study whenever possible, since 2% to 9% of the patients may have synchronous tumors elsewhere in the colon and rectum.
- For cancer and/or polyps, a tattoo must be placed just distal to the lesion at three different points within the circumference to allow for intraoperative localization of the target.
- A colonic enema with double contrast may be used in patients in whom colonoscopy is not possible. Virtual colonoscopy (computed tomography [CT] colonography) is also an option for those that cannot undergo colonoscopy.
- A contrast-enhanced CT of the abdomen and pelvis is obtained to rule out adjacent organ involvement, to evaluate for extraluminal complications (eg, abscess, fistula), and to rule out metastatic disease in patients with cancer. A CT of the chest completes the metastatic workup.
- A carcinoembryonic antigen (CEA) level is obtained in all cancer cases. The baseline preoperative result and postsurgical control must be obtained as an assessment for complete tumor resection. Absolute CEA presurgical value is an independent variable for survival.

SURGICAL MANAGEMENT

Preoperative Preparation

- Patients in whom an ileostomy is possible undergo stoma marking by an enterostomal therapist.
- An informed consent, including discussion of the need for a possible ostomy, is obtained.
- We use an enhanced recovery after surgery clinical pathway (described elsewhere in this textbook) for the perioperative management of all of our colorectal surgery patients.
- A mechanical preoperative bowel preparation may be considered to facilitate the handling of the colon during laparoscopic surgery. Fleet enemas are prescribed to facilitate the performance of the anastomosis.
- All patients should receive preoperative prophylactic antibiotics, following published guidelines. We administer 1 to 2 g of ertapenem based on patient's BMI within 1 hour of surgical incision.
- Pharmacologic deep vein thrombosis (DVT) prophylaxis should be given to patients perioperatively, based on current recommendations and guidelines.
- Ultrasound-guided bilateral transversus abdominis plane (TAP) block reduces the need for postoperative narcotics.

Equipment and Instrumentation

- We use a minimalistic approach to instrumentation, emphasizing a streamlined, efficient, and reproducible approach to our procedures. The entire operation is performed with essentially three instruments (a slotted grasper, am energy device, and a stapler) plus the camera. This approach minimizes clutter, makes the operation more efficient, and maximizes cost-efficiency.

216

Chapter 26 **TOTAL ABDOMINAL COLECTOMY: HAND-ASSISTED TECHNIQUE** 217

- A 5-mm, 30° scope with high-resolution monitors.
- 5- and 12-mm clear ports with balloon tips. They hold ports in the abdomen during instrument exchanges, minimize dripping/condensation on the scope, and minimize intra-abdominal profile/fulcrum effect of the trocars during surgery.
- A blunt tip, 5-mm, 37-cm long energy device.
- A slotted laparoscopic grasper.
- 60-mm linear reticulating laparoscopic staplers with vascular and tan cartridges.
- We use the GelPort hand-assisted device due to its versatility and ease of use. This device allows for the introduction/removal of the hand without losing pneumoperitoneum and allows for insertion of multiple ports through the hand-assisted device if necessary. It also allows for the introduction of laparotomy pads into the field, which are very useful to retract bowel/omentum in obese patients and to clean up the field and the scope during the procedure. It is imperative to mark every lap pad introduced into the abdomen on the operating room (OR) board and include them in the final counts to avoid inadvertently leaving a lap pad in the abdominal cavity after the procedure.
- We like to use a disposable three instrument long pouch the place the energy device and slotted graspers during the procedure. This pouch is placed on the patient's left hip/thigh, in between the surgeon and the monitor. This pouch functions like a holster to facilitate an easy and intuitive handling of the two instruments used during the entire operation and allowing the surgeon's eyes to never leave the target in the monitor.

Patient Positioning and Surgical Team Setup

- A preoperative briefing with the entire surgical team is conducted. Items discussed include patient identification, type of surgery, type of anesthesia, expected events during the surgery, the need for blood components, prophylactic antibiotic, surgical devices availability, and potential adverse events and their prevention.
- A dedicated, highly trained team in laparoscopic concepts is paramount. Critical members of this team concept are the scrub nurse, the circulating nurses, the assistants, and the anesthesia team members. I cannot emphasize enough the importance of a total team concept in accomplishing the highest level of performance during laparoscopic surgery.
- Proper patient position and OR setup is critical for successful performance of minimally invasive surgery (**FIGURES 1** and **2**).
- The patient is placed in a modified lithotomy position using Yellofin stirrups with the heels firmly planted in the stirrups to avoid having the patient slide with gravity assist maneuvers during the procedure.
- Pressure-bearing areas in the calf and lateral legs are padded to prevent DVTs and lateral peroneal nerve injury.
- The patient's toes, knee, and contralateral shoulders are aligned.
- The thighs are placed parallel to the ground to prevent conflict with the surgeon's arms.
- The patient's buttocks are placed at the edge of the table to allow for smoother introduction of the end-to-end anastomosis (EEA) stapler at the time of reconstruction. The coccyx should be readily palpable off the edge of the table.

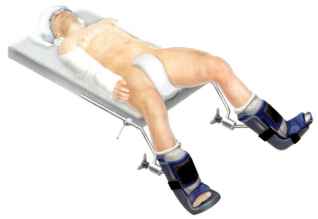

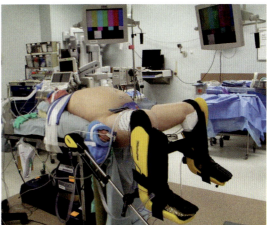

FIGURE 1 • Patient positioning. The patient is on a modified lithotomy position, with the thighs parallel to the ground to avoid conflict with the surgeon's elbows/instruments. The arms are tucked. The patient is secured to the table by taping across the chest over a towel. All pressure points are padded to avoid neurovascular injuries.

- Both arms are tucked at the sides, with padding added to protect against neurovascular injuries.
- The patient is taped to the table across the chest over towels to avoid slipping. The shoulders are padded to avoid neurovascular injuries.
- All laparoscopic elements (CO_2 line, camera, light cord) exit through the right upper side. All energy device cords exit through the upper left side. This allows for a clutter-free working space for the operative team.

Team Positioning and Draping

- The patient is prepped with chlorhexidine and draped to facilitate easy access to the perineum.
- The surgeon starts at the patient's right lower side, with the assistant to their left side and the scrub nurse to their right side or in between the patient's legs (**FIGURE 2**).
- Two monitors are placed in front of the team at eye level and slighted tilted upward (to avoid ergonomic injury to the surgeon's lower neck/brachial plexus) on the patient's left side.
- There are four important principles that we follow for all laparoscopic cases: alignment, triangulation, a flat horizon, and gravity assist.

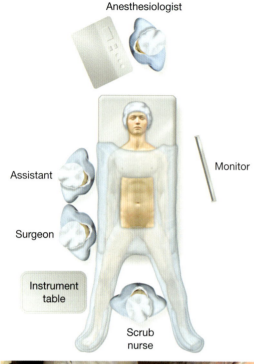

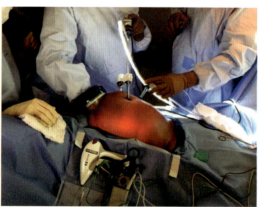

- Alignment involves the placement of the team, ports, target lesion, and monitors in straight lines of vision.
- Triangulation involves the creation of an imaginary triangle, where the surgeon's hands/instruments/trocars are at the angles in the base of the triangle, and the target lesion is located at the apex of the triangle. The camera bisects this triangle and, in laparoscopic surgery, is always in front of the hands of the surgeon. This is in contrast to open surgery, where the surgeon's hands are in front of the eyes.
- The concept of horizon is a fundamental difference between laparoscopic and open surgery. In open surgery, the surgeon looks down into the field. In laparoscopic surgery, the surgeon looks to their front, introducing the concept of the horizon. It is imperative that the camera operator maintains a flat horizon in front of the operator to avoid disorientation. This is particularly important with the use of angled scopes (ie, a 30° scope).
- Extreme gravity assist maneuvers are critically important in laparoscopic surgery to keep the bowel and omentum away from the operative field and to provide optimal exposure. To accomplish this while avoiding the patient sliding during the procedure, the patient needs to be secured to the table, so the table and the patient move as one. Padding on all pressure points is imperative to avoid neurovascular injuries to the extremities during the procedure.
- The energy instruments are placed in a plastic pouch in front of the surgeon to avoid unnecessary instrument transfer during the operation (**FIGURE 2**).

FIGURE 2 • Port placement. The GelPort is placed through a 5 to 6 cm Pfannenstiel incision. Alternatively, the GelPort can be placed on an epigastric location. A 5-mm periumbilical camera port site is inserted. Working ports are inserted in the right upper quadrant, right lower quadrant, and left anterior flank of the abdomen. All ports are triangulated.

PORT PLACEMENT AND OPERATIVE FIELD SETUP

- Insert the GelPort through a 5- to 6-cm Pfannenstiel incision (**FIGURE 3**). One of the main advantages of HALS is that it uses the extraction site incision necessary in colorectal surgery procedures during the entire operation instead of just using it at the end of the procedure. This allows for the introduction of the surgeon's hand without losing pneumoperitoneum insufflation at various portions of the operation, reintroducing tactile feedback for the surgeon, making the operation much more efficient.
- The size of this incision in centimeters is usually 1 to ½ cm less than the surgeon's glove size. Make this incision as long as you need it to be comfortable during the operation; the size of the extraction size has no impact on any meaningful perioperative outcome.

- This incision will be also used for specimen extraction. The Pfannenstiel incision (as opposed as vertical extraction site incisions) results in better cosmesis, lowers the incidence of wound infections and hernias, and allows for more working space between the hand and the instruments.
- Alternatively, the GelPort can also be inserted in the epigastrium, if access to the middle colic vessels is of concern.
- Ports: insert a 5-mm working port in the right upper quadrant, a 12-mm working port in the right lower quadrant, and a 5-mm camera port above the umbilicus. These three ports are triangulated, with the camera port at the apex of the triangle. This setup avoids conflict between the instruments and the camera and prevents disorientation (avoids "working on a mirror"). A third 5-mm working port is inserted in the left anterior flank of the abdomen for the mobilization of the right colon; it can also be valuable for the mobilization of the splenic flexure in patients with deep left upper quadrants.

Chapter 26 TOTAL ABDOMINAL COLECTOMY: HAND-ASSISTED TECHNIQUE 219

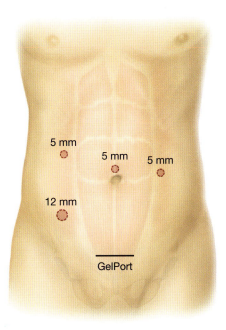

FIGURE 3 • Team setup. The surgeon stands to the patient's right side, with the assistant to their left, and the scrub nurse to their right or in between the patient's legs. The team, ports, targets, and monitors are aligned. Notice the energy devices placed in a pouch in front of the surgeon to minimize instrument transfer.

OPERATIVE STEPS

- All of our operations are process-driven and highly standardized to maximize efficiency, quality, and cost-efficiency. We divide the operations in well-defined, sequential steps. Every step has a single strategic objective (it is the name of the step), a clear beginning and end, and a critical anatomy that is required to be identified.
- We believe that this stepwise approach makes it easier to teach and learn these complex operations. In fact, it is designed to strip down all complexity and to shorten the learning curve of the surgeon.
- Every step opens the planes of dissection that are necessary for the steps that will follow, flowing "downstream" and opening the planes of dissection sequentially always in front of the operator. This way, the only time that the surgeon encounters a virgin tissue plane is at the very beginning of the operation. We call this first step the point of entry.
- The ideal point of entry has three characteristics: it is easy to find, has minimal to no anatomical variations, and minimizes potential injury to other structures around it during its performance. In order to simplify our operations, we use only two potential points of entry for all our laparoscopic colorectal surgeries.
- Our HALS total abdominal colectomy operation consists of 13 steps:
    1. Transection of the inferior mesenteric vein (IMV)
    2. Transection of the inferior mesenteric artery (IMA)
    3. Medial to lateral dissection of the descending mesocolon
    4. Lateral mobilization of the sigmoid and descending colon
    5. Mobilization of the splenic flexure and transverse colon
    6. Mobilization of the hepatic flexure
    7. Supramesocolic transection of the middle colic vessels
    8. Transection of the ileocolic pedicle
    9. Medial to lateral mobilization of the ascending colon
    10. Lateral mobilization of the ascending colon
    11. Intracorporeal distal transection
    12. Extracorporeal mobilization and proximal transection
    13. Intracorporeal ileorectal anastomosis

Step 1: Transection of the IMV

- This is the critical "point of entry" in this operation. We favor it over starting dissection at the IMA level due to the IMV's constancy in location, the ease of its visualization by the ligament of Treitz, and the absence of structures that can be injured around it (no iliac vessels, left ureter, or hypogastric nerve nearby). This will be the only time during the operation when a virgin tissue plane is entered. Every step will setup the following ones, opening the tissue planes sequentially.
- The patient is placed on a steep Trendelenburg position with the left side up. Using the right hand, move the small bowel into the right upper quadrant and the transverse colon and omentum into the upper abdomen. If necessary, place a laparotomy pad to hold the bowel out of the field of view, especially in obese patients. This pad can also be used to dry up the field and to clean the scope tip intracorporeally. Make sure that the circulating nurse notes the laparotomy pad in the abdomen on the white board.
- Identify the critical anatomy: IMV, the ligament of Treitz, and left colic artery (FIGURE 4).
- If there are attachments between the duodenum/root of mesentery and mesocolon, transect them with laparoscopic scissors or energy device. This will allow for adequate exposure of midline structures.
- Pick up the IMV/left colic artery with the right hand. Dissect under (dorsal) the IMV/left colic artery and in front of Gerota fascia with endoscopic scissors or energy device, starting at the level of the ligament of Treitz and proceeding with the

dissection caudally toward the IMA. The assistant provides upward countertraction with a grasper.
- Transect the IMV with the energy device (**FIGURE 5**) cephalad of left colic artery, which moves away from the IMV and toward the splenic flexure of the colon, with the 5-mm energy device.

Step 2: Transection of the IMA

- Identify the critical anatomy: The "letter T" formed between the IMA and its left colic and superior hemorrhoidal artery (SHA) terminal branches (**FIGURE 6**).
- Using the right hand, the aorta is identified and tracked down to the level of its bifurcation. The IMA will originate 1 to 2 cm proximal to this level.
- Holding the SHA up with the right hand, dissect the plane along the palpable groove between the SHA and the left iliac artery using laparoscopic scissors. A wide incision is made in the peritoneum dorsal to the SHA; the wider the incision, the easier the SHA can be elevated to obtain better exposure. After scoring the peritoneum under the SHA, use a 5-mm energy device to dissect by gently pushing the retroperitoneal tissues downward (dorsally) along the avascular plane located between the meso descending colon, anteriorly, and the retroperitoneum, posteriorly. This avascular plane can be identified by the transition between the two distinctive fat planes of the mesocolon and Gerota fascia.
- The SHA fold is thicker than the inexperienced surgeon may think. A common mistake during this portion of the operation is to think that the SHA fold is too thick, wrongly thinking that you are instead under the left common iliac artery and the left ureter. This results in a too shallow dissection plane superficial to the SHA and, therefore, entering the wrong plane into the mesocolon, resulting in troublesome bleeding and disorienting the surgeon.

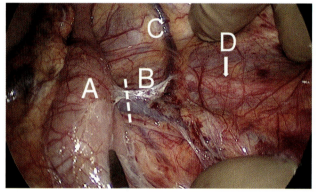

FIGURE 4 • Step 1: Transection of the inferior mesenteric vein (IMV). Key anatomy. A: Ligament of Treitz. B: IMV. C: Left colic artery as it separates from the IMV and goes toward the splenic flexure of the colon. The left ureter *(D)* is located far from the IMV projected transection (dotted lines).

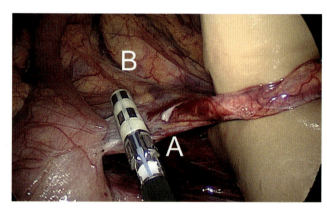

FIGURE 5 • Step 1: Transection of the inferior mesenteric vein (IMV). The surgeon holds the IMV *(A)* anteriorly with their right hand and transects it cephalad of the left colic artery *(B)* with a 5-mm energy device.

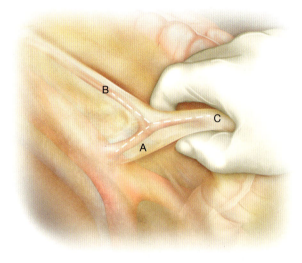

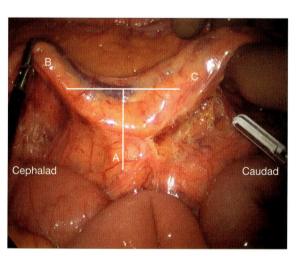

FIGURE 6 • Step 2: Critical anatomy. Identify the "letter T" formed between the inferior mesenteric artery (IMA) *(A)* and its left colic artery *(B)* and SHA *(C)* terminal branches. The IMA takeoff is just cephalad from the aortic bifurcation. The thumb and index finger are lifting the SHA off the groove located anterior to the right common iliac artery.

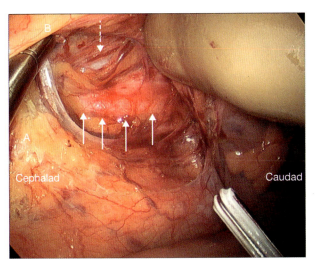

FIGURE 7 • Step 2: Identification of the left ureter and gonadal vessels. After the inferior mesenteric artery (IMA) *(A)* and SHA *(B)* have been lifted off the retroperitoneum, the left ureter (solid arrows) can be identified and preserved intact. Identification of the left ureter at this stage is critical in order to avoid injuring it during the IMA transection. Distal to the takeoff of the IMA, the left gonadal vessels can be identified lateral to the left ureter (dotted arrow).

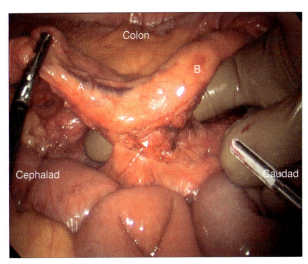

FIGURE 8 • Step 2: Circumferential dissection of the inferior mesenteric artery (IMA). After the left ureter has been identified, the IMA (arrow) is circumferentially dissected at its origin of the aorta. Again, the "letter T" formed between the IMA and it's terminal branches, the left colic artery *(A)* and the SHA *(B)* can be clearly identified.

- Preserve the sympathetic nerve trunk intact in the retroperitoneum. This avoids autonomic dysfunction of the pelvic organs postoperatively.
- Identify the left ureter (**FIGURE 7**), located in front of the left iliac artery and psoas muscle and medial to the gonadal vessels, before transecting anything. If you are directly on the psoas muscle, chances are that you left the left ureter attached to the dorsal surface of the mesocolon; bring it down into the retroperitoneum gently using blunt dissection with the energy device.
- If you cannot identify the ureter, try dissecting superior to inferior, starting from the IMV plane of dissection and moving caudally behind the IMA. If you still cannot find it, perform a lateral to medial mobilization of the sigmoid colon toward the midline. In this latter scenario, you will encounter the left gonadal vessels first, lateral to the left ureter.
- Dissect with your thumb and index finger around and behind the IMA and again visualize the letter "T" formed between the IMA, the left colic artery, and the SHA (**FIGURE 8**).
- With the left ureter safely preserved in the retroperitoneum, transect the IMA at its origin with a vascular load stapler (**FIGURE 9**) or energy device. This ensures excellent lymph node harvest and allows great exposure for the following step. The presence of the hand in the abdomen allows for a safe control of what could be serious bleeding from the IMA stump off the aorta should the staple line fail.

Step 3: Medial to Lateral Dissection of the Descending Mesocolon

- The surgeon's right hand and the assistant's grasper hold the descending mesocolon up, creating a working space between the mesocolon and the retroperitoneum (**FIGURE 10**). The plane between the mesocolon and Gerota fascia, readily identified by the transition between the two fat planes, is dissected bluntly in a downward direction toward the retroperitoneum with the 5-mm energy device.

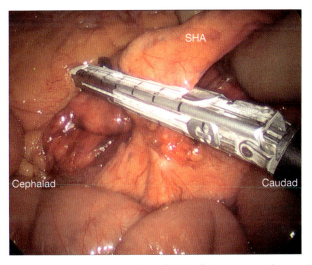

FIGURE 9 • Step 2: Transection of the inferior mesenteric artery (IMA). With the left ureter safely dissected away into the retroperitoneum, the IMA is transected with a linear vascular stapler at its origin of the aorta. The surgeon's hand is holding the SHA anteriorly.

- Dissect laterally until you reach the lateral abdominal wall, caudally toward the pelvic inlet, and cephalad until you separate the splenic flexure from the tail of the pancreas. Completing this step will greatly facilitate performance of Steps 4 and 5.

Step 4: Lateral Mobilization of the Sigmoid and Descending Colon

- The surgeon pulls the sigmoid colon medially, exposing the lateral sigmoid colon attachments (**FIGURE 11A**). Transect the attachments between the sigmoid and the pelvic inlet with laparoscopic scissors in your left hand, staying medially, close to the sigmoid and mesosigmoid, to avoid injuring the ureter/gonadal vessels.

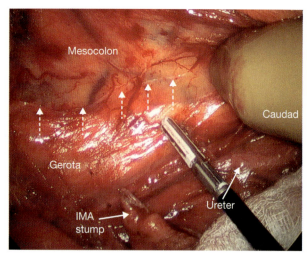

FIGURE 10 • Step 3: Medial to lateral mobilization of the mesocolon. With the surgeon holding the mesocolon anteriorly, the retroperitoneal tissues are swept downward (dorsally) with an energy device. The dissection progresses along the transition of the two fat planes (dotted arrows): mesocolon (anteriorly) and Gerota posteriorly. Notice the stapled inferior mesenteric artery (IMA) stump and left ureter in the retroperitoneum.

- Dissect caudally until reaching the entrance to the left pelvic inlet.
- Retract the descending colon medially with your hand to expose the white line of Toldt. The assistant holds the omentum/bowel out of way.
- Transect the white line of Toldt up to the splenic flexure using endoscopic scissors or energy device (**FIGURE 11B**). You should readily enter the medial to lateral dissection plane dissected during Step 2, greatly facilitating this lateral mobilization of the descending colon.
- Dissect in a cephalad direction until reaching the splenic flexure of the colon.
- The left ureter and gonadal vessels, dissected in Step 3, should be readily visible in the retroperitoneum.

Step 5: Mobilization of the Splenic Flexure

- The patient is now placed on a reverse Trendelenburg position with the left side up to allow the splenic flexure of the colon to come down into the surgical field.
- The mobilization of the splenic flexure is best accomplished by a combination medial to lateral and lateral to medial dissection approaches (**FIGURE 12**). The key to an easy splenic flexure mobilization is to have completed the separation of the splenic flexure off the retroperitoneum during the medial to lateral mobilization (Step 3).
- The medial to lateral phase of the splenic flexure mobilization is started by entering the lesser sac at the midline. The transverse colon is retracted downward and the stomach is retracted superiorly, exposing the gastrocolic ligament. The gastrocolic ligament is then transected medially with an energy device until the lesser sac is entered.
- Transection of the gastrocolic ligament then proceeds along the transverse colon in a medial to lateral direction until the splenic flexure is reached (**FIGURE 12A**). Care must be taken to avoid inadvertent injury to the colon.
- At this point, an inferior to superior (along the left gutter) and lateral to medial (along the lesser sac) dissection around the splenic flexure is performed (**FIGURE 12B**). The surgeon inserts their right hand behind the splenic flexure (possible due to the previous medial to lateral mobilization step) and hooks their index finger under the splenocolic ligament, gently pulling the splenic flexure down and exposing the splenocolic ligament fully, which is then transected with an energy device (**FIGURE 12C**).
- Attachments of the splenic flexure to the pancreas are transected and the splenic flexure is now fully mobilized to the midline.

Step 6: Mobilization of the Hepatic Flexure

- The patient is kept in a reverse Trendelenburg position but with the table now rotated with the right side up to allow the hepatic flexure to come down into the field.
- Standing at the left side of the table, the surgeon retracts the transverse colon downward with their left hand and completes the transection of the gastrocolic ligament until reaching the hepatic flexure of the colon using a 5-mm energy device.
- At this point, the hepatocolic ligament is readily visible. Slide your left index finger under it, hold if upward, and transect it with endoshears or a 5-mm energy device (**FIGURE 13**).

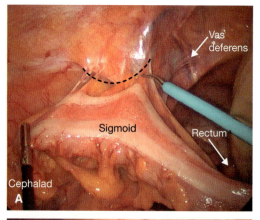

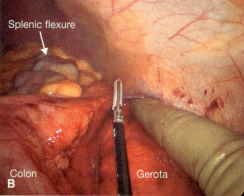

FIGURE 11 • Step 4: Lateral mobilization of the sigmoid and descending colon. **Panel A,** The white line of Toldt (dotted line) is transected with an energy device. **Panel B,** The medial to lateral dissection plane is readily entered, greatly facilitating the lateral mobilization of the descending colon.

Chapter 26 TOTAL ABDOMINAL COLECTOMY: HAND-ASSISTED TECHNIQUE   223

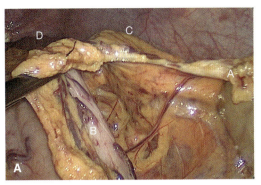

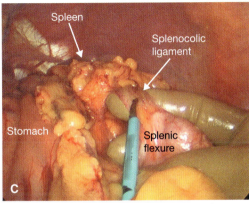

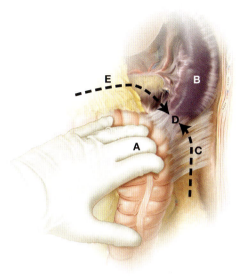

FIGURE 12 • Step 5: Mobilization of the splenic flexure. **Panel A,** The lesser sac, between the transverse colon *(A)* and the stomach *(B)*, is entered. The gastrocolic ligament is transected with an energy device from right to left, toward the splenic flexure of the colon *(C)* until the spleen *(D)* is reached. **Panel B,** The surgeon retracts the splenic flexure of the colon *(A)* downward and medially, exposing the attachments to the spleen *(B)*. The phrenocolic *(C)* and splenocolic *(D)* ligaments are transected in an inferior to superior and lateral to medial direction, meeting the previously transected gastrocolic ligament *(E)* dissection plane around the splenic flexure. **Panel C,** With the surgeon "hugging" the splenic flexure with their right hand, the index finger is hooked under the splenocolic ligament, which is then transected with an energy device

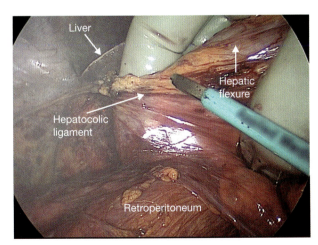

FIGURE 13 • Step 6: Mobilization of the hepatic flexure. Slide your left index finger under the hepatocolic ligament, hold if upward, and transect it with an energy device.

- Proceeding on a superior to inferior dissection and retracting the hepatic flexure downward with your hand separate the hepatic flexure form the second portion of the duodenum and the head of the pancreas with the 5-mm energy device by gently teasing the retroperitoneal tissues down. Take care to avoid avulsing the gastrocolic venous trunk of Henle and its tributaries, which can lead to severe bleeding that is difficult to control.

Step 7: Transection of the Middle Colic Vessels (Supramesocolic Approach)

- Dissection and transection of the middle colic vessels can be one of the most daunting maneuvers in laparoscopic colorectal surgery. Traditionally, these vessels are approached inframesocolically, by dissecting the root of the meso transverse colon at the intersection with the root of the mesentery, where the venous anatomy is extremely variable and complex. The superior mesenteric vein and its branches, and the gastrocolic venous trunk of Henle and its branches, surround the middle colic vessels. Venous tears tend to travel distally to the next major tributary. In terms of the SMV and the gastrocolic trunk of Henle, this next "tributary" is the portal vein confluence, which lies in a retroperitoneal plane for which you do not have control at this time.

- In order to prevent potentially devastating bleeding complications during the dissection and transection of the middle colic vessels, we have developed a supramesocolic approach to the middle colic vessels. The hand-assisted technique greatly facilitates the performance of this technique and makes it very safe.

- The superior aspect of the transverse mesocolon is now readily visible, with the middle colic vessels easily palpable as they cross the third portion of the duodenum in the mid-transverse colon (**FIGURE 14**). With the assistant pulling down on the transverse colon downward with a grasper, the

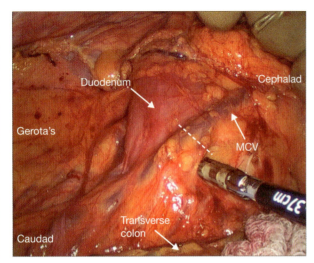

FIGURE 14 • Step 7: Supramesocolic transection of the middle colic vessels (MCV). With the transverse colon retracted caudally, the MCV are readily visualized at this point through a supramesocolic approach as they cross over the third portion of the duodenum. This allows for a safe dissection and high transection (dotted line) with a 5-mm energy device without risking injury to the SMV and gastrocolic venous trunk of Henle.

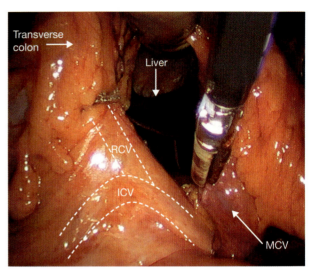

FIGURE 15 • Vascular anatomy after transection of the middle colic vessels (MCV). While pulling upward on the transverse colon, the transected stump of the MCV is observed. The ileocolic vessels (ICV), with its right colic vessels branch (RCV) can be readily identified as they cross over the third portion of the duodenum.

surgeon "picks up" the middle colic vessels supramesocolically with their left thumb and index finger. Using their right hand through the right upper quadrant (RUQ) port side, the surgeon now dissects under the middle colic vessels with the 5-mm energy device, completely encircling the middle colic vessels with the thumb and index finger. With great exposure and control, now the surgeon transects the middle colic vessels with the 5-mm energy device (**FIGURE 14**).

- During this approach, the transverse mesocolon separates the middle colic vessels from the SMV and the gastrocolic venous trunk of Henle from shielding them and, thus, greatly reducing the potential risk of serious venous injuries. It also allows for a very high transection of the middle colic vessels and, therefore, a great lymphatic nodal capture.
- After transection of the middle colic vessels, the ileocolic vessels (ICV) can now be readily identified as they cross over the third portion of the duodenum (**FIGURE 15**).

Step 8: Transection of the Ileocolic Pedicle

- Place the patient on a Trendelenburg position with the right side up to facilitate exposure to the ICV. Place the hepatic flexure back in the RUQ. Move the transverse colon and the omentum into the upper abdomen. Move the small bowel into the left lower quadrant to expose the duodenum and the root of the meso ascending colon. In obese patients, a laparotomy pad may greatly assist in retracting the bowel.
- Grab the ICV as they cross over the third portion of the duodenum with your thumb and index finger and pull them up anteriorly (**FIGURE 16A**).
- With the ICV on stretch, a parallel incision is made with endoshears or energy device underneath (dorsal) to the pedicle (**FIGURE 16B**) extending to the root of the mesentery and the superior mesenteric vein.
- A window is created under the ileocolic pedicle in the avascular plane that separates the pedicle from the retroperitoneum.

- The ileocolic pedicle is isolated and divided close to its origin off the superior mesenteric vessels using an energy device (**FIGURE 16C**).

Step 9: Medial to Lateral Mobilization of the Ascending Colon

- The retroperitoneum is now exposed by the surgeon pulling upward (anteriorly) on the distal transected ICV stump with their left hand while the assistant retracts the meso ascending colon upward (anteriorly) with a grasper.
- Using blunt dissection with a 5-mm energy device, the ascending mesocolon is mobilized off the retroperitoneum by gently sweeping the duodenum and Gerota fascia down (dorsally), utilizing a medial to lateral dissection approach.
- As the dissection proceeds from medial to lateral, and to facilitate exposure, the surgeon's left hand should be pronated and placed underneath the mesocolon, giving upward traction for the retroperitoneal dissection (**FIGURE 17**).
- Mobilization of the right mesocolon is carried out laterally to the abdominal wall, superiorly to the hepatorenal recess and medially exposing the third portion of the duodenum and the head of the pancreas.
- At this point critical structures including the right ureter, the right gonadal vein, and the duodenum are identified and preserved intact in the retroperitoneum.

Step 10: Lateral Mobilization of the Ascending Colon

- The base of cecum is grasped and retracted anteriorly toward the abdominal wall.
- With the ileum on stretch by the assistant, a peritoneal incision is created from the cecum medially along the root of the terminal ileum mesentery (**FIGURE 18A**). You should readily enter the retrocolic space previously created by the medial to lateral mobilization of the ascending mesocolon.

Chapter 26 TOTAL ABDOMINAL COLECTOMY: HAND-ASSISTED TECHNIQUE   225

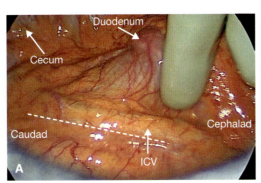
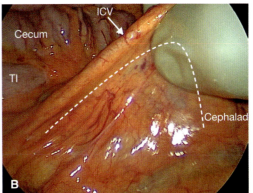
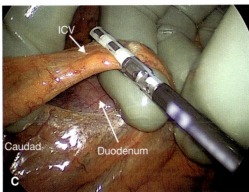

FIGURE 16 • Step 8: Transection of the ileocolic vessels (ICV). **Panel A,** Key Anatomy. The base of the ascending colon mesentery is exposed from the third portion of the duodenum to the cecum. The ICV are seen as they cross over the third portion of the duodenum. The dissection plane will be initiated along the dorsal aspect of the ICV (dotted line). **Panel B,** Initiation of the medial to lateral mobilization. With the surgeon holding the ICV anteriorly, the peritoneum is scored dorsal to the ICV from the duodenum all the way down to the cecum and the terminal ileum (TI) (dotted line). **Panel C,** The ICV are transected at their origin with an energy device.

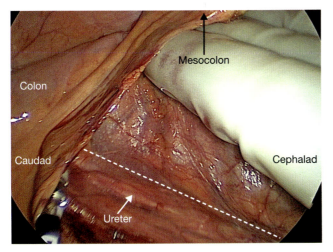

FIGURE 17 • Step 9: Medial to lateral mobilization of the ascending mesocolon. The surgeon, while retracting the ascending mesocolon upward (anterior) with the hand fully pronated and facing upward, separates the ascending mesocolon from the retroperitoneum by dissecting along the transition of the two distinct fat planes (dotted line). The right ureter can be readily identified in the retroperitoneum and is preserved intact.

- The right ureter and the right gonadal vein are most easily identified at this phase of the operation coursing over the right iliac vessels and into the pelvis (**FIGURE 18B**). Lateral and anterior to the psoas muscle, the lateral femoral cutaneous nerve is also frequently identified.

- The white line of Toldt is incised, dividing the only remaining attachments of the ascending colon if the medial to lateral dissection was carried out adequately during the previous step.
- The entire colon is now fully mobilized and ready for transection.

Step 11: Intracorporeal Distal Transection

- Dissect the rectosigmoid junction circumferentially. The rectosigmoid junction can be identified by the splaying of the tinea coli. Transect the upper mesorectum with the 5-mm energy device at the level of the projected distal bowel transection.
- While pulling on the sigmoid upward with the left hand, transect the bowel intracorporeally just distal to the rectosigmoid junction with a linear EndoGia stapler device (**FIGURE 19**).

Step 12: Extracorporeal Mobilization and Proximal Transection

- The entire colon and the terminal ileum are delivered extracorporeally through the Pfannenstiel incision site with the Alexis wound protector in place to prevent infectious and/or oncological soilage of the wound (**FIGURE 20**). There should be absolutely no tension during the extraction of the specimen.
- The terminal ileum is transected at a suitable site between Kocher clamps. The specimen is sent to the pathologist.
- At this point, the anvil of a 28F EEA stapler device is placed through the open end of the terminal ileum and

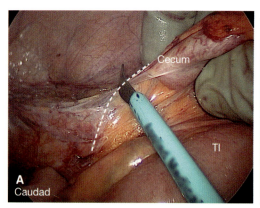
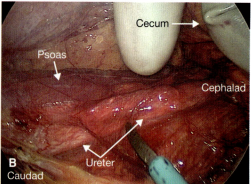

FIGURE 18 • Step 10: Lateral mobilization of the ascending colon. **Panel A,** With the surgeon pulling on the cecum medially and superiorly, a peritoneal incision is created from the cecum medially along the root of the terminal ileal mesentery. **Panel B,** After mobilization of the cecum, the right ureter is readily identified in the retroperitoneum.

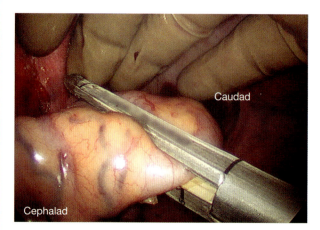

FIGURE 19 • Step 11: Intracorporeal distal transection. The specimen is transected with a linear stapler just distal to rectosigmoid junction, which can be identified by the splaying of the tinea coli.

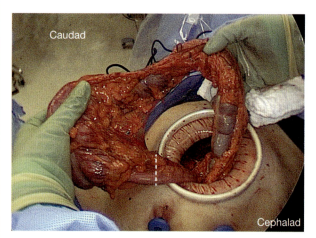

FIGURE 20 • Step 12: Extracorporeal mobilization and transection. The entire colon is extracted without any tension. The distal ileum will be transected along the dotted line between Kocher clamps.

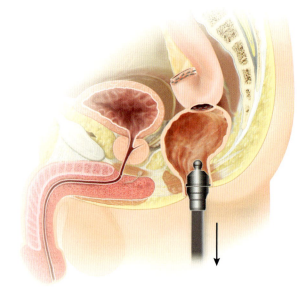

FIGURE 21 • Step 13: Intracorporeal anastomosis. A side-to-end ileorectal anastomosis is constructed with a 28F end-to-end anastomosis stapler device.

Step 13: Intracorporeal Ileorectal Anastomosis

- The terminal ileum, with the anvil in place is re-introduced into the abdominal cavity, the Gelcap is reapplied, and the pneumoperitoneum is re-insufflated.
- The surgeon stands to the patient's right side, with the left hand through the GelPort and with the camera in their right hand through one the right lateral port sites. The patient is placed on a slight Trendelenburg position.
- An experienced assistant introduces the 28F EEA stapler into the rectum and delivers the spear anterior to the rectal stump staple line. The EEA stapler and the anvil are mated (by the surgeon's left hand); the EEA stapler is closed and then fired, creating a side-to-end ileorectal anastomosis (**FIGURE 21**).
- Two intact donuts should be obtained. The distal donut is sent for evaluation as the distal margin. The anastomosis is

is exteriorized with a spear through the antimesenteric border approximately 5 cm from the open end of the ileum. The open end of the terminal ileum is then closed with an endoscopic linear stapler with a 60 mm vascular stapler.

Chapter 26 **TOTAL ABDOMINAL COLECTOMY: HAND-ASSISTED TECHNIQUE** **227**

- inspected to ensure that is tension-free and that it has excellent blood supply.
- Finally, the anastomosis is insufflated under water to ensure that it is airtight. The presence of air bubbles would indicate an anastomotic disruption and should prompt a revision of the anastomosis.

- Alternatively, the distal transection and ileorectal anastomosis can be constructed extracorporeally through the open Pfannenstiel incision site. We find it easier to perform the anastomosis intracorporeally, due to the superior visualization and exposure that laparoscopy provides.

WOUND CLOSURE

- The Pfannenstiel incision is closed using a running 2-0 Vicryl suture from the posterior rectus sheet and a running no. 1 polydioxanone (PDS) suture for the anterior rectus sheet. All skin incisions are closed with 4-0 PDS subcuticular sutures. Dermabond is applied to seal off all wounds.

- We retowel the field with clean towels and change gown and gloves, Bovie electrocautery, and suction cannulas prior to wound closure in an effort to minimize wound infections.
- We do not routinely use drains.

PEARLS AND PITFALLS

Operative approach	<ul><li>A HALS approach improves minimally invasive surgery utilization, reduces conversions, and shortens OR times.</li><li>A standardized, stepwise approach leads to higher efficiency and quality.</li></ul>
Positioning	<ul><li>Gravity-assisted maneuvers allow for good visualization and exposure.</li><li>Secure the patient to the table, while protecting all pressure-baring areas.</li><li>Make sure that all anesthesia lines and monitors are working appropriately after positioning the patient; there will be limited access to the arms during the procedure.</li><li>Avoid unnecessary clutter of cables/lines; open the working space for the operating team.</li></ul>
Port placement	<ul><li>Align the surgeon, trocars, target, and monitor in straight lines.</li><li>Triangulate all ports aiming to the target.</li><li>Place the hand access port in a Pfannenstiel location.</li></ul>
Operative technique	<ul><li>Point of entry: IMV at the ligament of Treitz. Ideal due to its ease of localization and the absence of critical nearby structures that can be injured.</li><li>The medial to lateral dissection steps set up all other steps.</li><li>Visualize the "letter T" and high IMA ligation in malignancy; identify the left ureter prior to IMA transection.</li><li>The supramesocolic approach allows for a much easier and safer transection of the middle colic vessels.</li><li>The ileocolic vessels can be readily identified by the third portion of the duodenum.</li><li>Distal transection and anastomosis: although possible to perform extracorporeally, it is easier to do it intracorporeally (better visualization).</li></ul>
Pitfall: Dissecting anterior to the SHA	<ul><li>Solution: Identify "groove" between left common iliac artery and SHA and dissect in between the two vessels.</li></ul>
Pitfall: Floppy sigmoid difficult to handle	<ul><li>Use the back of the hand as a "shelf" to hold the sigmoid up while picking up the SHA with thumb and index finger.</li></ul>
Pitfall: Cannot identify the left ureter during SHA/IMA dissection	<ul><li>Extend the IMV dissection plane on a superior to inferior direction behind the IMA. If you still cannot find it:</li><li>Mobilize the sigmoid lateral to medial. Distally, the left ureter is located medial to the gonadal vessels.</li></ul>

POSTOPERATIVE CARE

Postoperative care is driven by a clinical pathways that includes the following:

- Pain control: Intravenous acetaminophen for 24 hours (start in the operating room) followed by intravenous ketorolac

for 72 hours (if creatinine is normal). The TAP nerve block greatly reduces the need for narcotics.
- DVT prophylaxis with enoxaparin, starting within 24 hours of surgery.
- No additional antibiotics. Judicious use of intravenous fluids.

- No nasogastric tube. Remove Foley catheter on postoperative day 1.
- Early ambulation. Diet ad lib. Aggressive pulmonary toilette.
- Targeted discharge: postoperative days 3 to 4.

OUTCOMES

- HALS leads to improvements in short-term outcomes, including less pain, faster recovery, shorter hospital stay, and lower incidence of cardiac/pulmonary complications when compared to open surgery.
- When compared to conventional laparoscopy, HALS results in higher utilization rates of minimally invasive surgery, shorter learning curves, lower conversion rates, shorter operative times, and shorter hospital stays.
- For cancer resection, minimally invasive surgery oncologic outcomes are at least comparable to those of open surgery.

COMPLICATIONS

- Wound infections and hernias are markedly reduced with the use of a Pfannenstiel extraction site.
- Urinary/sexual dysfunction: important to preserve hypogastric nerves intact.
- Ureteral injury: critical to identify the ureters prior to vascular transection.
- DVT: low risk with use of DVT prophylaxis.
- Cardiac and pulmonary complications: significantly reduced compared to the open surgery approach.

SUGGESTED READING

1. Cima RR, Pattana-arun J, Larson DW, Dozois EJ, Wolff BG, Pemberton JH. Experience with 969 minimal access colectomies: the role of hand-assisted laparoscopy in expanding minimally invasive surgery for complex colectomies. *J Am Coll Surg*. 2008;206:946-952.
2. Jayne DG, Thorpe HC, Copeland J, Quirke P, Brown JM, Guillou PJ. Five-year follow-up of the Medical Research Counsel CLASICC trial of laparoscopically assisted versus open surgery for colorectal cancer. *Br J Surg*. 2010;97:1638-1645.
3. Marcello PW, Fleshman JW, Milsom JW, et al. Hand-assisted laparoscopic vs. laparoscopic colorectal surgery. A multicenter, prospective, randomized trial. *Dis Colon Rectum*. 2008;51:818-828.
4. Orcutt ST, Balentine CJ, Marshall CL, et al. Use of a Pfannenstiel incision in minimally invasive colorectal cancer surgery is associated with a lower risk of wound complications. *Tech Coloproctol*. 2012;16(2):127-132.
5. Orcutt ST, Marshall CL, Balentine CJ, et al. Hand-assisted laparoscopy leads to efficient colorectal cancer surgery. *J Surg Res*. 2012;177(2):e53-8.
6. Orcutt ST, Marshall CL, Robinson CN, et al. Minimally invasive surgery in colon cancer patients leads to improved short-term outcomes and excellent oncologic results. *Am J Surg*. 2011;202(5):528-531.
7. Ozturk E, Kiran RP, Geisler DP, Hull TL, Vogel JD. Hand-assisted laparoscopic colectomy: benefits of laparoscopic colectomy at no extra cost. *J Am Coll Surg*. 2009;209:242-247.
8. Wilks JA, Balentine CJ, Berger DH, et al. Establishment of a minimally invasive program at a VAMC leads to improved care in colorectal cancer patients. *Am J Surg*. 2009;198(5):685-692.

Chapter 27: Robotic Total Abdominal Colectomy

Dana M. Omer, Jonathan Benjamin Yuval, and Julio Garcia-Aguilar

DEFINITION
- Robotic total abdominal colectomy involves minimally invasive resection of the appendix; cecum; ascending, transverse, descending, and sigmoid colon; along with the associated mesentery and draining lymphatics.
- The operation can be completed with either an end ileostomy or an ileocolic anastomosis.

DIFFERENTIAL DIAGNOSIS
- Although some surgeons use minimally invasive approaches for both emergent and elective total abdominal colectomy, we prefer to limit robotic resections to elective cases.
- The following pathologies are common indications for a nonemergent total abdominal colectomy:
  - Synchronous colon tumors
  - Lynch syndrome with colon cancer
  - Familial adenomatous polyposis with few to no rectal polyps (in select patients)
  - Ulcerative colitis and Crohn's colitis refractory to medical treatment in patients who are not candidates for proctectomy
  - Colonic inertia

PATIENT HISTORY AND PHYSICAL EXAMINATION
- Colonic malignancy is associated with occult or overt alimentary tract bleeding, changes in bowel habits, and unintentional weight loss. Malignancies may be discovered incidentally during a screening colonoscopy without preceding symptoms. The physical exam ranges from normal to palpable abdominal masses. Stage IV peritoneal carcinomatosis can be diagnosed by presence of a Sister Mary Joseph node in the umbilicus or a Blumer's shelf (**FIGURE 1**) in digital rectal examination.
- Ulcerative colitis and Crohn's colitis may be associated with extraintestinal manifestations, such as aphthous oral ulcers, arthritis, and skin manifestations. They may present as colicky abdominal pain, nausea, and extraintestinal manifestations. Rectal inflammation is associated with tenesmus, urgency, incontinence, and frequent passage of blood and mucus.[1]
- Colonic inertia is defined as an inability of the colon to modify stool consistency and inability to move enteric contents from the cecum to the sigmoid at least once every 3 days. Colonic inertia is associated with constipation and bloating. Surgical referral is most common in women around 40 years of age.[2]

IMAGING AND OTHER DIAGNOSTIC STUDIES
- Patients with Lynch syndrome, familial adenomatous polyposis, and other polyposis syndromes should undergo genetic testing and counseling along with their family members.
- Colonoscopy including a tissue biopsy is key in the diagnosis of colon cancer and inflammatory bowel disease and is part of the workup for colonic inertia.
- Colon cancer patients should also undergo a CT scan of the chest, abdomen, and pelvis to rule out distant metastases.
- Additional investigations in the workup for colonic inertia include a transit study (sitz marker study) to confirm slow colonic transit time and a balloon expulsion test to confirm proper anorectal function and rule out obstructed defecation.

SURGICAL MANAGEMENT

Preoperative Planning
- Implementation of Enhanced Recovery after Surgery (ERAS) programs starting in the preoperative period is crucial to preventing infections and other complications, reducing hospital stay and costs, and preserving the quality of life.[3] ERAS protocols are discussed in detail elsewhere in this textbook.
- In elective cases, patients should ideally have bowel preparation with a combination of mechanical preparation and oral antibiotics.[4]
- Patients may require assessment of frailty, medical clearance, and nutritional optimization.[5]
- Ileostomy markings should be made by a wound-ostomy nurse with ostomy care education.
- A complete blood count, basic metabolic panel, and blood typing and screening should be completed. IV access should be prepared in case of need for resuscitation and intraoperative transfusions.
- Alvimopan, an opioid antagonist that does not cross the blood-brain barrier, has been shown to reduce the risk of postoperative ileus if given in the preoperative phase.[6]
- Prophylactic antibiotics should be given prior to incision and should cover enteric organisms.

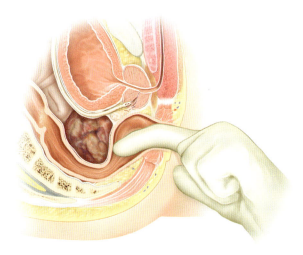

FIGURE 1 • Blumer's Shelf is a physical exam finding on digital rectal exam indicating metastasis into the rectovesical or rectouterine pouch of Douglas.

Positioning and Trocar Placement

- The patient is placed in a modified lithotomy position using stirrups, with the arms tucked and padded along pressure points to avoid neurovascular injury and with a foam belt securing them to the table to avoid sliding during table motion (**FIGURE 2A**).
- The robot boom should be placed between the patient's legs, and the robot arms should be rotated 90° to the right, as it

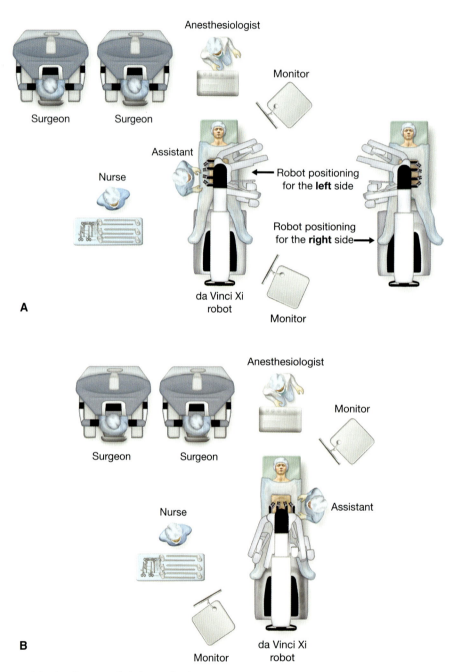

FIGURE 2 • **A,** Patient positioning for a total abdominal colectomy. The patient cart remains between the patient's legs and the boom is rotated based on the steps of the operative field. **B,** Patient positioning for the pelvic dissection. Of note, the boom can be repositioned to work cranially during the isolation and dissection of the middle colic vessels and transverse colon.

is the preferred practice to begin the operation on the vessels of the right colon.
- Efficient trocar placement is crucial in mobilizing the entire colon and minimizing operative time taken up by docking and redocking the robot.
  - As illustrated in **FIGURE 3**, three 8-mm robotic trocars are placed in the left and right upper quadrants and in the left lower quadrant, with an additional 8-mm midline trocar placed 2 to 3 cm superior to the umbilicus for the camera.
  - In the right lower quadrant, a 12-mm trocar is placed to allow passage of a robotic or laparoscopic stapler.
  - Two 5-mm trocars are also placed in each flank for use by the bedside assistant.

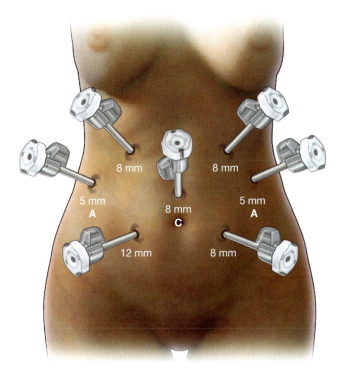

FIGURE 3 • Appropriate port placement is important to maximize efficiency and minimize operative time.

ABDOMINAL ACCESS

- We achieve pneumoperitoneum using a Veress needle through Palmer's point in the left midclavicular line approximately 3 to 5 cm below the costal border, and the abdomen is typically insufflated to 15 mm Hg.
- An 8-mm camera port is inserted through the supraumbilical incision, and the abdominal cavity is explored to assess for adhesions and resectability.
- The remaining trocars are placed under direct vision, and the patient is tilted 12° to 15° to the left and placed in a 12° to 15° Trendelenburg position, depending on the BMI of the patient and displacement of the intra-abdominal organs.
- If present, adhesions are lysed, and the greater omentum is retracted cephalad to expose the transverse colon. The mesocolon is exposed by moving loops of small bowel away from the operative field, typically into the left upper quadrant.
- The robot is then docked (**FIGURE 2A**), and we begin with mobilization of the right colon.

MOBILIZATION OF THE ILEOCOLIC MESENTERY AND RIGHT COLON AND TRANSECTION OF ILEOCOLIC VESSELS (ICVs)

- To expose the ileocolic pedicle, the cecum is retracted anterolaterally, stretching the right mesocolon. The peritoneum is then scored, and an incision is made below the ileocolic vessels.
- Next, the avascular plane between the right mesocolon and the retroperitoneum is identified, and we begin dissection along this plane in a cephalad and lateral direction. The ICVs are dissected and transected at their origin off the superior mesenteric vessels (**FIGURE 4A** and **B**).
- Once the ileocolic pedicle is released, the dissection will continue cephalad along the superior mesenteric vessels, identifying the second and third portions of the duodenum, the pancreatic head, and the middle colic vessels (**FIGURE 5**). It is important to note the anatomical variations in blood supply to the right colon.[7]
- Dissection will continue laterally and cephalad between the mesocolon and the retroperitoneum all the way to the right

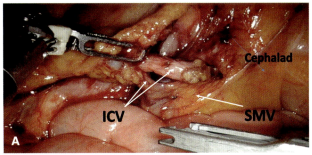
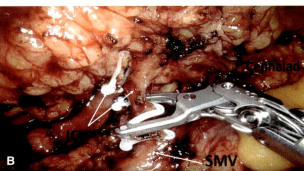

FIGURE 4 • **A** and **B,** Completed vascular dissection of the ileocolic pedicle.

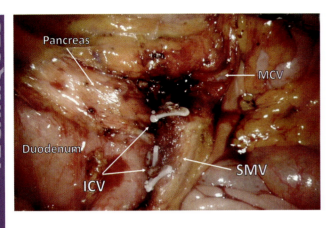

- gutter (laterally), the hepatic flexure (cephalad), and the right side of the transverse colon.
- Next, the right side of the omentum is detached from the transverse colon, and the lateral attachments of the right colon are removed in a cranial-caudal fashion toward the cecum.
- The attachments of the terminal ileum are divided, mobilizing completely the ileocecal region. Finally, the distal ileum is sectioned using the vessel sealer, completing the dissection of the right colon.

FIGURE 5 • Completed vascular pedicle dissection of the right colon with identification of the duodenum and pancreas.

APPROACH TO THE MIDDLE COLIC VASCULATURE

- Isolating the middle colic vessels is key to resecting the transverse colon without injuring the retroperitoneal structures, pancreas, or stomach. The middle colic vessels are best identified following cephalad from the origin the ileocolic pedicle.
- Passing the mesentery of the midtransverse colon over the stomach places the branches of the middle colic vessels under some tension facilitating the identification and dissection.
- Except for tumors located in the midtransverse colon that may require a central ligation of the middle colic vessels, it is easier to dissect and divide right and left branches separately.

- Dividing the areolar tissue around the vessels provides access to the lesser sac over the pancreas completing the mobilization of the right and middle portion of the transverse colon mesentery from the retroperitoneum.
  - This portion of the procedure can often be accomplished with the robot docked toward the right.
  - Occasionally, the boom may need to be redocked and turned 90° to face directly cranially, using the umbilical trocar for the camera and the right and left lower quadrant trocars for the working instruments. The bedside assistant can continue helping with the cephalad traction of the transverse mesocolon from the left side of the patient.

TRANSECTION OF THE INFERIOR MESENTERIC VEIN AND MOBILIZING THE DISTAL TRANSVERSE COLON

- At this point, the robot is redocked, and the arms are now rotated 180° to orient toward the left abdomen and pelvis (**FIGURE 2A** and **B**). The patient is tilted 12° to 15° to the right while remaining in a 12° to 15° Trendelenburg position.
- To mobilize the left colon, we prefer a medial-to-lateral approach, starting with dissection of the inferior mesenteric vein (IMV), which is identified by its proximity to the ligament of Treitz. Lifting the IMV will allow visualization of the plane between Gerota fascia and the mesocolon (**FIGURE 6**). The vessel can be sectioned using a bipolar device.
- The dissection will continue along this plane, resulting in a separation of the lateral retroperitoneum from the mesocolon. Cephalad and medial to the operative field will be the inferior border of the pancreas, where the dissection is continued until the lesser sac is entered (**FIGURE 7**) and followed along the anterior surface of the pancreas toward the hilum of the spleen until the left side of the transverse colon is completely released.
- The left branches of the middle colic vessels are divided next, detaching the transverse colon mesentery from the inferior border of the pancreas.
- Next, the colon is mobilized from the splenic flexure.
  - If the operation entails concurrent resection of the omentum, the lesser sac can be entered by division of the greater omentum outside the gastroepiploic arcade.

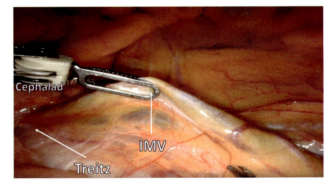

FIGURE 6 • Identification of the IMV lateral to the ligament of Treitz.

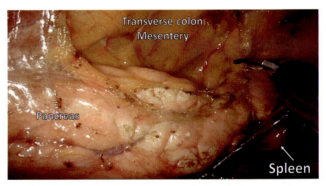

FIGURE 7 • Entering the lesser sac above the inferior border of the pancreas.

- The remainder of the omentum can be divided in the direction of the splenic hilum.
- If the operation does not require omental resection, the greater omentum may be simply detached from the transverse colon in the direction of the splenic flexure.
- The splenocolic ligament is transected with an energy device.

MOBILIZATION OF THE LEFT COLON AND TRANSECTION OF THE INFERIOR MESENTERIC ARTERY

- Once the splenic flexure is released, the inferior mesenteric artery (IMA) is identified by entering the avascular space between the superior rectal vessels and the aortoiliac bifurcation. It is important to preserve the sympathetic nerves as they course close to the aorta and in front of the common iliac arteries.
- The dissection will progress along this plane underneath the mesentery of the sigmoid colon, exposing the left ureter and left gonadal vessels that are left undisturbed in the retroperitoneum (**FIGURE 8**).
- The IMA can be divided between clips using either a vessel sealer or a vascular stapler. The sectioning of the artery is performed approximately 2 cm from its origin to avoid disturbing the autonomic plexuses that run close to the origin of the IMA (**FIGURE 9A** and **B**).
- Once the IMA is sectioned, the mesentery of the sigmoid colon can be bluntly dissected from the retroperitoneum, and the remaining attachments of the descending and sigmoid colon can be removed using sharp dissection moving in a cranial fashion toward the splenic flexure.

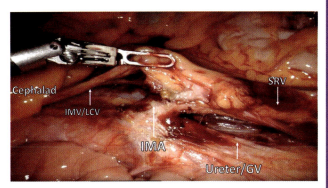

FIGURE 8 • Identification of the left ureter and gonadal vessels during dissection of the IMA.

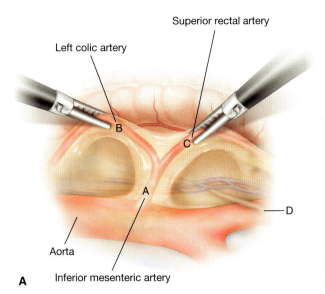

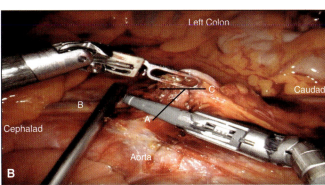

FIGURE 9 • **A,** The T-configuration formed between the IMA (A) and its terminal branches, the left colic (B), and the superior rectal artery (C) is visualized. Notice the left ureter (D) dissected posteriorly in the retroperitoneum. **B,** The IMA is divided at its origin from the aorta with a vessel sealer device.

BOWEL RESECTION AND ANASTOMOSIS

- The final major step of a total abdominal colectomy entails dissection of the upper rectum and mesorectum. We continue the dissection along the IMA and superior rectal pedicle until the mesorectal plane is entered at the level of the sacral promontory (**FIGURE 10**). The mesorectal plane is an avascular tissue plane located between the presacral fascia, posteriorly, and the mesorectal fascia, anteriorly.
- The dissection continues until the superior rectum is mobilized from the mesorectum using the vessel sealer device and subsequently transected using an endoscopic stapler (**FIGURE 11**).
- The robot is undocked, and the proximal rectum is grasped using laparoscopic forceps. A 4- to 6-cm Pfannenstiel incision is created with placement of a wound protector for extraction of the specimen, starting with the divided rectum. The bowel is clamped, divided at the distal ileum, and assessed for twisting.

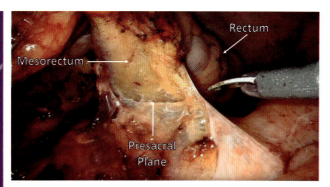

FIGURE 10 • Entering the TME plane in the posterior midline.

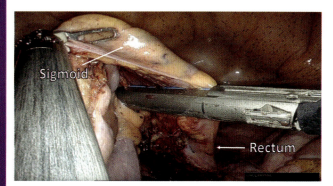

FIGURE 11 • Transection of the rectum.

- The final steps of the procedure involve placement of an anvil from a circular stapler to create an ileorectal anastomosis. The anastomosis is typically created in either a side-to-side isoperistaltic, end-to-side, or end-to-end fashion.
- The distal ileum is replaced into the abdomen along with the anvil, and the Pfannenstiel incision is temporarily closed using either a capped wound protector or a twisting motion to seal the abdomen.

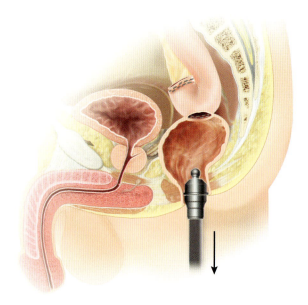

FIGURE 12 • Depiction of a side-to-end ileorectal anastamosis constructed using a circular stapler.

- The pneumoperitoneum is then reinitiated, the robot is docked to complete a tension-free, stapled ileorectal anastomosis (**FIGURE 12**), and the bowel is again checked for twisting. The integrity of the anastomosis is checked using an air leak test. The operative field is assessed for hemostasis, and a pelvic drain is placed posterior to the anastomosis, with extraction in the left lower quadrant trocar site. The robot is undocked, and the pneumoperitoneum is relieved. The fascia and skin incisions are closed.

PEARLS AND PITFALLS

Identification of duodenum and right ureter	Duodenum can be easily identified posterior to the bare area of the mesentery
Identification of the inferior border of the pancreas	Most easily identified at midline where the pancreas is anteriorly raised by the vertebrae
IMA dissection	Avoid traction on the sympathetic nerve plexus, which may lead to sexual dysfunction
Identification of the left ureter and left gonadal vessels	Both medial-to-lateral and lateral-to-medial dissection can be used to identify these structures
Entering the total mesorectal excision plane	It is easiest to identify the correct plane at the posterior midline

Chapter 27 **ROBOTIC TOTAL ABDOMINAL COLECTOMY** **235**

POSTOPERATIVE CARE

- The postoperative course follows the ERAS protocol[3] with the goals of reducing surgical stress, optimizing physiological function, and facilitating recovery. ERAS protocol is described in detail elsewhere in this textbook.
- In the immediate postoperative phase, IV hydration is provided at a maintenance rate using an isotonic solution with the goal of maintaining a euvolemic state. The patient should have fluids discontinued when enteral feeds are tolerated, to avoid salt and volume overload.
- Postoperative nausea and vomiting are managed with a multimodal regimen of antiemetics.
- Nasogastric tube placement is not routine and should be avoided in the absence of ileus or obstruction. Instead, patients should be encouraged to start enteric feeding with clear liquids and advancement as tolerated.
- Reducing the postoperative fasting period allows patients to maintain an anabolic state, avoid postoperative ileus and restore bowel function sooner, and it promotes healing. A sufficient nutritional status facilitates appropriate wound healing and provides support to the immune system in response to infection. A staff nutritionist or dietician can help individualize postoperative management and ensure that the patient receives sufficient caloric intake.
- Postoperative pain is managed in a multimodal approach with a transversus abdominis plane block and nonopioid analgesics such as acetaminophen, ibuprofen, and gabapentin. This may avoid the undesired effects of opiate-based medications, such as sedation, respiratory depression, nausea, vomiting, urinary retention, and ileus.
- Urinary catheters should be removed within 24 hours of surgery.
- Patients should ambulate within 24 hours and may require additional reconditioning with a physical therapist.
- Maintaining normoglycemia may help reduce the morbidity of a colectomy. Insulin can be administered until the patient can tolerate their home medications.
- Follow-up is typically 7 to 10 days after discharge from the hospital.
- Patients treated for cancer should resume oncological surveillance.

OUTCOMES

- The use of robot-assisted surgery has increased rapidly in the United States: over the past 10 years, its use in general surgery increased 24-fold.[8] Compared with laparoscopic surgery, robot-assisted surgery is associated with similar blood loss, similar operative time, better lymph node harvest, and shorter hospital stay.[9,10]
- The benefits of robot-assisted surgery include three-dimensional visualization, stability, and dexterity, allowing surgeons to operate in challenging anatomical spaces.
- Robot-assisted colectomies can facilitate intracorporeal anastomoses.[9]
- Laparoscopic total abdominal colectomy and robotic total abdominal colectomy have similar morbidity and mortality rates; however, the robotic approach is associated with a lower rate of conversion to open colectomy.[9]

COMPLICATIONS

- Surgical site infections are the most common perioperative complication. Management starts in the preoperative phase, with bowel preparation and prophylactic antibiotics targeting colonic bacteria. Superficial site infections may require opening the trocar incision. Deep and organ-space infections can be managed with supplemental percutaneous drainage or surgical drainage.
- Venous thromboembolic disease may be prevented by antithrombotic prophylaxis during hospitalization. Postoperative thromboembolic disease is generally considered provoked and is treated with either a vitamin K antagonist or low-molecular-weight heparin for 3 months. In case of an absolute contraindication to anticoagulation, an inferior vena cava filter can be placed and subsequently removed; there is no benefit to prophylactic filter placement.
- Postoperative ileus is characterized by nausea, vomiting, and abdominal distension in the absence of obstruction. A prolonged ileus (persisting after 5 days) may occur in up to 15% of patients undergoing abdominal surgery. Ileus is typically self-limiting and is managed with supportive care and treatment of the underlying cause.
- The risk of urinary tract infection increases if catheters are kept in place for prolonged periods. Treatment involves removal of the catheter and administration of antibiotics.
- Anastomotic leaks are potentially devastating complications; they tend to present approximately 5 to 7 days after surgery. Risks are associated with the emergent nature of the surgery, patient age, chronic obstructive pulmonary disease, diabetes, steroid use, surgical technique, tension on the suture line, infection or sepsis, ischemia from poor blood supply, and malnutrition. An anastomotic leak may present with low-grade fever; tachycardia; ileus; drainage; abdominal, pelvic, or rectal pain; and peritonitis. Imaging may identify a collection of gas or fluid (or both); in such cases, patients should get volume resuscitation and IV broad-spectrum antibiotics. Management ranges from observation with bowel rest to percutaneous drainage, operative drainage, revision, or diversion.
- Missed injuries most often occur during port placement. Patients present with bleeding or infection, similarly to anastomotic leaks, but these conditions may manifest earlier depending on the size and location of the injury.

REFERENCES

1. Silverberg MS, Satsangi J, Ahmad T, et al. Toward an integrated clinical, molecular and serological classification of inflammatory bowel disease: report of a Working Party of the 2005 Montreal World Congress of Gastroenterology. *Can J Gastroenterol.* 2005;19(suppl A): 5A-36A.
2. McCoy JA, Beck DE. Surgical management of colonic inertia. *Clin Colon Rectal Surg.* 2012;25(1):20-23.
3. Wei IH, Pappou EP, Smith JJ, et al. Monitoring an ongoing enhanced recovery after surgery (ERAS) program: adherence improves clinical outcomes in a comparison of three thousand colorectal cases. *Clin Surg.* 2020;5:2909.
4. Kiran RP, Murray AC, Chiuzan C, Estrada D, Forde K. Combined preoperative mechanical bowel preparation with oral antibiotics significantly reduces surgical site infection, anastomotic leak, and ileus after colorectal surgery. *Ann Surg.* 2015;262(3):416-425; discussion 23-5.

5. Daniele A, Divella R, Abbate I, et al. Assessment of nutritional and inflammatory status to determine the prevalence of malnutrition in patients undergoing surgery for colorectal carcinoma. *Anticancer Res.* 2017;37(3):1281-1287.

6. Winegar B, Cox M, Truelove D, Brock G, Scherrer N, Pass LA. Efficacy of alvimopan following bowel resection: a comparison of two dosing strategies. *Ann Pharmacother.* 2013;47(11):1406-1413.

7. Kuzu MA, Ismail E, Celik S, et al. Variations in the vascular anatomy of the right colon and implications for right-sided colon surgery. *Dis Colon Rectum.* 2017;60(3):290-298.

8. Childers CP, Maggard-Gibbons M. Estimation of the acquisition and operating costs for robotic surgery. *JAMA.* 2018;320(8):835-836.

9. Mlambo B, Shih IF, Li Y, Wren SM. The impact of operative approach on postoperative outcomes and healthcare utilization after colectomy. *Surgery.* 2022;171(2):320-327.

10. Liu H, Xu M, Liu R, Jia B, Zhao Z. The art of robotic colonic resection: a review of progress in the past 5 years. *Updates Surg.* 2021;73(3):1037-1048.

Chapter 28

Colon and Rectal Injury: Primary Repair, Resection and Anastomosis, Colostomy

Louis Jude Magnotti, Devanshi D. Patel, and Martin A. Croce

DEFINITION

- Colon and rectal injuries can follow either penetrating or blunt trauma. The former results from direct penetration of the bowel. The latter is secondary to high-pressure force/compression to the bowel and/or supporting mesenteric blood supply. Both types of injuries can result in partial tears limited to the serosa, full-thickness injuries, or devascularizing injuries leading to bowel ischemia and eventual necrosis.

DIFFERENTIAL DIAGNOSIS

- High suspicion must be maintained when evaluating patients following either penetrating or blunt trauma for associated injuries. Depending on the mechanism, location and trajectory of the inciting injury, solid organs such as the liver, kidney, pancreas, spleen, aorta, or spine may also be affected. Injuries localized to the pelvic region should raise suspicion for concomitant genitourinary injuries.

PATIENT HISTORY AND PHYSICAL FINDINGS

- Any number of signs and symptoms can be present during the initial evaluation of the trauma patient. Complaints of abdominal pain coupled with physical examination findings suggestive of colon or rectal injury can include abdominal tenderness or distention, ecchymosis, rectal wall defect, or blood on digital rectal examination. Hemodynamic instability, peritonitis, or positive adjunct procedures such as focused assessment with sonography for trauma (FAST) or diagnostic peritoneal lavage are indications for exploratory laparotomy.

IMAGING AND OTHER DIAGNOSTIC STUDIES

- Ultrasound or, more specifically, the FAST examination can be utilized for patients with both penetrating and blunt trauma. However, for practical purposes, FAST should be reserved for the evaluation of blunt-injured patients. The perihepatic, perisplenic, and pelvic views are identified and evaluated for free fluid in the evaluation of patients with potential colorectal injuries. A positive finding can aid in decision for operative intervention; however, it is nonspecific for source of injury and should only prompt immediate exploration in the hemodynamically unstable patient.

- Computed tomography (CT) is indicated in the hemodynamically stable patient with signs and symptoms of abdominal injury. The clinician should be looking for findings such as pneumoperitoneum, intramural air, bowel wall thickening, bowel wall enhancement, mesenteric infiltration or stranding, arterial extravasation, fat pad injury, and free fluid in the intra- or retroperitoneal spaces. CT findings of blunt bowel and/or mesenteric injuries can be subtle so all studies must be reviewed with a high degree of suspicion in order to avoid missed injuries and delay intervention.

- CT with administration of rectal contrast (in addition to intravenous) can increase specificity of detecting rectal wall injuries. This technique can be performed quickly and does not significantly distract from further evaluation and treatment.

- Both rigid and flexible proctosigmoidoscopy can aid in identification of both intra- and extraperitoneal rectal injuries. Areas of bleeding, mucosal contusion, or mucosal defect should raise concern for injury and prompt additional intervention.

SURGICAL MANAGEMENT

Preoperative Planning

- Patients with hemodynamic instability, peritonitis, or evisceration require little preoperative planning and should proceed directly to laparotomy.

Positioning

- Patients should be placed in the supine position and with both arms out and prepped from nipples to knees. For suspected rectal injuries, patients may be placed in the lithotomy position to allow for examination under anesthesia and rigid or flexible proctosigmoidoscopy prior to laparotomy as long as the patient remains hemodynamically normal.

- Remove patient from lithotomy and place patient in the supine position prior to laparotomy.

237

OPERATIVE EXPOSURE AND ASSESSMENT FOR INJURY

- Begin with "running the bowel."
- Identify the terminal ileum.
- Inspect the colon and rectum for injury, from the ileocecal valve to the distal intraperitoneal rectum.
- Simultaneously evaluate the mesentery for injury.
- Maintain a high suspicion for missed injury in patients with an odd number of full-thickness penetrating injuries (particularly gunshot wounds).
- Injuries may be subtle, particularly at the mesenteric border.
- Closely inspect even the smallest hematomas for underlying injury.

REPAIR OF COLORECTAL INJURIES

Mesenteric Injuries

- Avoid mass ligation of the mesentery, which may result in bowel ischemia.
- Identify, isolate, and individually ligate bleeding vessels.
- For smaller vessels 4-0 silk ties or suture ligatures are the best.
- For larger vessels 2-0 or 3-0 silk may be used.
- Closely assess bowel surrounding areas of mesenteric injury for vascular compromise.
- In most cases, bowel viability can be determined by visual inspection.
- If bowel viability is in doubt, adjunctive measures may be used.
- Handheld Doppler is preferred because of its ease of use and ready availability in most operating rooms.
- Bowel viability is reliably confirmed by the presence of an audible Doppler signal from the antimesenteric surface of the bowel in question.
- After bleeding is controlled, close the mesenteric defect to prevent internal herniation.
- For devitalizing injuries, perform bowel resection with anastomosis.
- Anastomoses may be stapled or hand-sewn.

Serosal (Partial-Thickness) Injuries

- Repair with interrupted 3-0 silk sutures.
- Orient repairs transversely to minimize luminal narrowing.

Full-Thickness Injuries

- Babcock or other intestinal clamps should be applied to minimize spillage.
- Sharply debride wound margins to remove devitalized tissue if necessary.
- Primary closure is appropriate provided the bowel lumen is not significantly narrowed and the injury encompasses <50% of the bowel circumference.
- If the above is not possible, segmental resection and anastomosis should be performed.
- Orient repairs transversely to minimize luminal narrowing.

TYPES OF REPAIR

Primary Repair

- Closure is performed with either a two-layered repair with an inner layer of 3-0 absorbable suture and outer layer of interrupted 3-0 nonabsorbable suture (silk preferred) or a single layer of full-thickness 3-0 silk interrupted sutures (**FIGURE 1**). (Some surgeons choose a two-layer closure with Vicryl and silk or absorbable and nonabsorbable.)
- Each bite should include a generous portion of serosa with a small portion of mucosa to result in an inverted suture line—an easy way to remember this is to say to oneself—"a good bite of serosa and an Angstrom of mucosa."
- Primary repair of multiple low-grade small bowel injuries is usually preferred because it preserves intestinal length.
- If multiple injuries are contained within a short segment of bowel, resection and anastomosis should be performed instead.

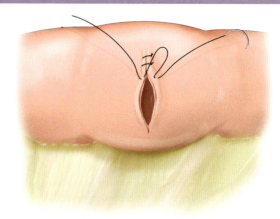

FIGURE 1 • Primary repair of full-thickness colon injury. (Redrawn from Dr. Devanshi D. Patel.)

Chapter 28 **COLON AND RECTAL INJURY: PRIMARY REPAIR, RESECTION AND ANASTOMOSIS, COLOSTOMY**   **239**

COLORECTAL RESECTION WITH ANASTOMOSIS

Dividing the Bowel

- Determine the segment to be resected.
- Identify avascular windows in the mesentery at the proximal and distal margins of the segment to be resected.

- Pinch the mesentery bordering the bowel between the surgeon's thumb and index finger.
- Using a small hemostat, create a window in the mesentery by spreading parallel to the mesenteric vessels so as not to create iatrogenic vascular injury.
- Divide the bowel with a linear cutting stapler.
- Make sure the stapler is oriented parallel to mesentery and angled toward the antimesenteric surface of the bowel that is to remain in situ.

CREATING THE ANASTOMOSIS

Side-to-Side Isoperistaltic (Bayonet) Colocolonic or Colorectal Anastomosis

- Orient the two ends of bowel in an isoperistaltic fashion—antiperistaltic orientation should be avoided as it is nonanatomic and can lead to unintended kinking of the bowel in the postoperative period.
- Near the mesenteric border of the bowel, 3-0 silk stay sutures are placed at the proximal and distal margins of the planned anastomosis.
- Continue with interrupted 3-0 silk suture placement to complete the "back wall" (**FIGURE 2A**).
- Create colotomies parallel to the back row of seromuscular sutures (**FIGURE 2B**).
- The anastomosis should be patulous, but one to two seromuscular stitches should remain distal to each end of the enterotomies to alleviate tension.
- A 3-0 absorbable suture on a tapered needle is used to create the inner layer of the anastomosis.
- Posteriorly, this is done with a running, full-thickness stitch, typically begun at the midpoint of the posterior wall (**FIGURE 2C**).
- The transition from the posterior to the anterior wall of the anastomosis is completed by continuing alternating "inside out" to "outside in" (**FIGURE 2D**).
- After this transition is completed, the above process is completed for the other half of the anastomosis with a second 3-0 absorbable suture until the entire posterior wall of the anastomosis is completed and both stitches are "around the corners."
- The anterior wall is completed with either a simple continuous stitch, a baseball stitch, or a Connell stitch according to the surgeon's preference.
- The key is to ensure mucosal apposition and suture line inversion.
- After this is completed, the two ends of absorbable suture are tied together.
- Complete the anterior second layer by placing interrupted 3-0 silk seromuscular sutures.
- The stay sutures are then tied down.

- Palpate the anastomosis to ensure adequate size.
- Close the mesenteric defect with braided 3-0 absorbable or permanent suture to prevent internal herniation.
- Be careful not to injure the mesenteric vasculature during the mesenteric closure.
- Antiperistaltic colocolonic anastomoses should be avoided as they can be bulky, leading to unwanted kinking of the bowel postoperatively.

End-to-End Colocolonic or Colorectal Anastomosis

- After resection of the injured segment, align the proximal end of the distal bowel with the distal end of the proximal bowel.
- While it is the authors' preference to perform a hand-sewn anastomosis, a side-to-side stapled colonic anastomosis may be performed.
- Regardless of the repair method, enough mobilization of the colonic segments must be performed to ensure a tension-free anastomosis.
- Ensure that the serosa near the mesenteric border on both ends of the bowel has been adequately cleaned to allow for ease of suture placement without compromising anastomotic blood supply.
- Seromuscular 3-0 silk stay sutures are placed at the lateral and medial margins of the planned anastomosis.
- Continue with interrupted 3-0 silk suture placement to complete the "back wall" oriented between both stapled resection lines.
- Create colotomies by removing the stapled resection lines, either sharply or with electrocautery, parallel to the back row of seromuscular sutures.
- As above, ensure that the anastomosis is patulous to prevent stricture.
- A 3-0 absorbable suture on a tapered needle is used to create the inner layer of the anastomosis.
- This is done with a running, full-thickness stitch, typically begun at the midpoint of the posterior wall.
- The transition from the posterior to the anterior wall of the anastomosis is completed by continuing alternating inside out to outside in as one approaches the stay sutures.

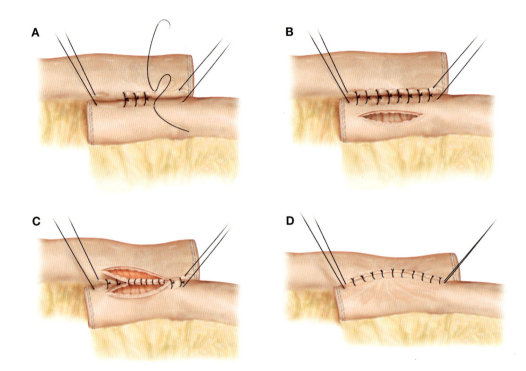

FIGURE 2 • **A,** Securing the posterior wall. **B,** Creating colotomies. **C,** Inner layer secured with running full thickness stitch. **D,** Conversion to outside-in stitch ("baseball" stitch). (Redrawn from Dr. Devanshi D. Patel.)

- After this transition is made, the above process is completed for the other half of the anastomosis with a second 3-0 absorbable suture until the entire posterior wall of the anastomosis is completed and both stitches are around the corners.
- The anterior wall is completed with a simple continuous stitch, a baseball stitch, or a Connell stitch according to the surgeon's preference.
- The key is to ensure mucosal apposition and suture line inversion.
- After this is completed, the two ends of the absorbable suture are tied together.
- Complete the anterior second layer by placing interrupted 3-0 silk seromuscular sutures.
- The stay sutures are then tied down.
- Palpate the anastomosis to ensure adequate size.
- Close the mesenteric defect with braided 3-0 absorbable or permanent suture to prevent internal herniation.
- Be careful not to injure the mesenteric vasculature during the mesenteric closure.

End-to-Side Colorectal (Baker) Anastomosis

- After resection of the injured segment, mobilize sufficient proximal colon along the white line of Toldt such that the colon easily reaches into the pelvis to the rectal stump.
- Clear any additional fatty tissue from the side of the proximal colon.
- The side of the proximal colon should lay tension free against the rectal stump.
- A layer of seromuscular interrupted silk sutures (3-0) should be placed as the back row, below the rectal staple line and below the tinea of the proximal colon.
- The rectal staple line is removed and a colotomy is created on the proximal colon through the tinea (**FIGURE 3A**).
- A running absorbable 3-0 suture is used for the inner layer—full thickness bites, typically performed with two sutures run in opposite directions, with a running Connell for the top layer (**FIGURE 3B** and **C**).
- The anastomosis is then oversewn with 3-0 seromuscular interrupted silks (**FIGURE 3D**).

Chapter 28 COLON AND RECTAL INJURY: PRIMARY REPAIR, RESECTION AND ANASTOMOSIS, COLOSTOMY 241

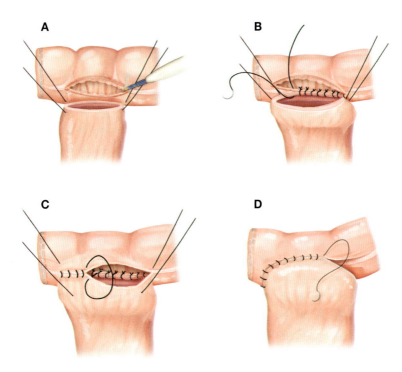

FIGURE 3 • **A,** Removal of rectal staple line and colotomy creation. **B,** Inner layer secured with running full thickness stitch. **C,** Outer layer running Connell stitch. **D,** Seromuscular 3-0 silk interrupted sutures. (Redrawn from Dr. Devanshi D. Patel.)

COLOSTOMY CREATION

- After resection of the distal colon, mobilize sufficient proximal colon along the white line of Toldt such that the colon easily reaches above the skin level without tension.
- Identify target ostomy location on the abdominal wall, typically either above or below the umbilicus at the level of the rectus.
- Create a circular incision at the chosen ostomy site on the abdominal wall down to the level of the anterior rectus sheath (**FIGURE 4A**).
- Incise the anterior rectus sheath in a cruciate fashion.
- Bluntly separate the rectus muscle using a Kelly clamp and handheld retractors.
- Similar to the anterior rectus sheath, incise the posterior rectus sheath in a cruciate fashion.
- Three fingers should easily pass through the intended ostomy site.
- Grasp the resected end of the colon with a Babcock clamp and pull through the abdominal wall in a retrograde fashion (**FIGURE 4B**).
- Care must be taken to maintain proper orientation of the colon so there are no twists in the colon and mesocolon.
- Close the midline fascia in standard fashion.
- If there was any fecal contamination from the injury, the skin should be left open.
- Be sure to protect the skin incision prior to ostomy maturation.
- Remove the staple line from the resected end of the colon with electrocautery (**FIGURE 4C**).
- Mature the colostomy with interrupted full-thickness bites of colon at the edge of the colotomy (small amount of mucosa relative to large seromuscular bite), securing it to the dermis with an absorbable suture (**FIGURE 4D** and **E**).

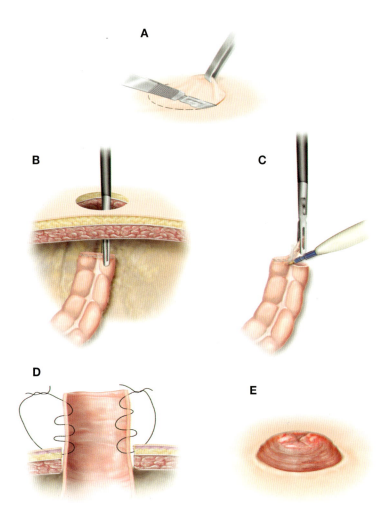

FIGURE 4 • **A,** Circular incision at ostomy site. **B,** Introduction of colon through ostomy site. **C,** Removal of staple line. **D,** Interrupted full thickness sutures through dermis, colon, and colonic end. **E,** Matured colostomy. (Redrawn from Dr. Devanshi D. Patel.)

PEARLS AND PITFALLS

Indications for exploratory laparotomy	■ Hemodynamic instability, evisceration, and peritonitis are clear indications for urgent operative intervention.
Incision	■ Midline laparotomy provides maximum exposure and provides ease of access to evaluate for other sources of solid organ and/or associated injuries.
Damage control	■ Consideration for diversion or second look laparotomy should be based on the patient's hemodynamic status, temperature, pH, blood transfusion requirements, comorbidities, and associated injuries.
Resuscitation	■ Ongoing resuscitation is critical prior to, during, and after the operative period, especially when considering new anastomosis creation.
Definitive procedures	■ Definitive procedures can be performed in the hemodynamically stable patient without significant comorbidities or concern for bowel compromise. Strong consideration for end ostomy vs anastomosis plus proximal diversion (loop ostomy) should be given to those patients with significant pre- and intra-operative transfusion requirements and/or significant medical comorbidities. Ostomy reversal should be delayed until at least 3 months after creation for proximal diversion and up to 6 months for an end ostomy.

Chapter 28 COLON AND RECTAL INJURY: PRIMARY REPAIR, RESECTION AND ANASTOMOSIS, COLOSTOMY

POSTOPERATIVE CARE

- Resuscitation should be continued in the postoperative setting until the patient stabilizes—from a hemodynamic, temperature, and pH standpoint. Nasogastric suction can be utilized until return of bowel function. Early mobilization and enteral feeding should be advanced as appropriate.

OUTCOMES

- Patients who present with hemodynamic instability or with significant comorbidities are at higher risk for increased mortality or morbidity. Overall, most patients can return to normal function preinjury functional status, similar to routine abdominal surgery.

COMPLICATIONS

Anastomotic Leak or Suture Line Failure

- Trauma patients are at increased risk of anastomotic leak or suture line failure. Continued resuscitation plays a vital role in the maintenance of the anastomosis as poor blood flow can severely compromise this portion of the bowel. Careful consideration should be placed on patient selection for definitive repair during the index case.

Intra-Abdominal Abscess

- Multiple factors—mechanism of injury, hemodynamic status, medical comorbidities, age, and sex—contribute to an increased risk of infection in the trauma patient. Contamination of the peritoneal or retroperitoneal space can lead to abscess formation. This should be appropriately and promptly managed with antibiotics and either interventional or operative drainage. A single dose of appropriate prophylactic antibiotic administered prior to operative intervention has been shown to decrease development of intra-abdominal infections.

Fistula

- A fistula is defined as an abnormal passage between two epithelial surfaces and can be a difficult problem to manage postoperatively for both the clinician as well as the patient.

Factors that contribute to formation include large bowel resection, large volume resuscitation, and requirement of multiple operations. Management includes treatment of sepsis if present, maximizing nutrition, correcting fluid and electrolyte abnormalities, and prevention of further wound breakdown. Fistulas can spontaneously close; however, they may require further operative intervention.

Bowel Necrosis

- Unidentified or iatrogenic devitalization of colon or rectal blood supply can result in bowel ischemia and ultimately lead to full-thickness necrosis. Periods of postoperative hypotension increases the risk of bowel compromise. Patients may present with septic shock, and repeat laparotomy is required with likely diversion.

SUGGESTED READINGS

1. Baker JW. Low end to side rectosigmoidal anastomosis; description of technic. *Arch Surg*. 1950;61(1):143-157.
2. Bradley MJ, DuBose JJ, Scalea TM, et al. Independent predictors of enteric fistula and abdominal sepsis after damage control laparotomy: results from the prospective AAST open abdomen registry. *JAMA Surg*. 2013;148(10):947-955. doi:10.1001/jamasurg.2013.2514
3. Burch JM, Brock JC, Gevirtzman L, et al. The injured colon. *Ann Surg*. 1986;203(6):701-711.
4. George SM, Jr., Fabian TC, Voeller GR, Kudsk KA, Mangiante EC, Britt LG. Primary repair of colon wounds. A prospective trial in non-selected patients. *Ann Surg*. 1989;209(6):728-733; 33-4.
5. Gonzalez RP, Turk B. Surgical options in colorectal injuries. *Scand J Surg*. 2002;91(1):87-91.
6. Nakada I, Kawasaki S, Sonoda Y, Watanabe Y, Tabuchi T. Abdominal stapled side-to-end anastomosis (Baker type) in low and high anterior resection: experiences and results in 69 consecutive patients at a regional general hospital in Japan. *Colorectal Dis*. 2004;6(3):165-170.
7. Sharpe JP, Magnotti LJ, Fabian TC, Croce MA. Evolution of the operative management of colon trauma. *Trauma Surg Acute Care Open*. 2017;2(1):e000092.
8. Trust M, Veith J, Brown C, et al. Traumatic rectal injuries: is the combination of computed tomography and rigid proctoscopy sufficient? *J Trauma Acute Care Surg*. 2018;85(6):1033-1037.
9. Weinberg JA, Fabian TC, Magnotti LJ, et al. Penetrating rectal trauma: management by anatomic distinction improves outcome. *J Trauma*. 2006;60(3):508-513; discussion 13-14.

SECTION III: Rectal Resections

Chapter 29

Low Anterior Resection and Total Mesorectal Excision/Coloanal Anastomosis: Open Technique

Konstantinos I. Votanopoulos and Jaime L. Bohl

DEFINITION

- Low anterior rectal resection (LAR) with total mesorectal excision (TME) is defined as the removal of the rectum en bloc with an intact perirectal fascial envelope distal to the cancer-bearing rectal wall. The visceral endopelvic fascia, also known as fascia propria or investing fascia of the mesorectum, is identified by a thin, loose areolar tissue that circumferentially separates the rectum and mesorectum from surrounding pelvic structures. Removal of the rectum with an intact mesorectum ensures complete removal of all lymph nodes and lymphatics that drain the diseased rectum without oncologic contamination of the pelvis at the time of surgery.
- Coloanal anastomosis is the attachment of a mobilized proximal colon segment to the anal canal while preserving the anal sphincter musculature while maintaining a negative distal margin of resection.

DIFFERENTIAL DIAGNOSIS

- This operation is performed primarily for distal rectal cancer when tumor location mandates rectal transection at the level of the pelvic floor (levator ani and puborectalis).

PATIENT HISTORY AND PHYSICAL FINDINGS

- A detailed history should identify locally advanced rectal lesions that are causing bowel obstruction, bleeding, pseudodiarrhea, fecal incontinence, or excessive pelvic or anal pain. Nearly obstructed patients may require a temporary laparoscopic loop sigmoid colostomy prior to neoadjuvant chemoradiation.
- Patients with pain due to fixed tumors in the anal canal and sphincter are not candidates for coloanal anastomosis and require an abdominoperineal resection (APR).
- Prior colon and anorectal surgery, vascular surgery, or sphincter trauma during childbirth may have compromised the vascular supply to the planned colonic conduit or reduce the anal sphincter function.
- Patients with poor functional status or poor fecal control prior to surgery are likely to have reduced quality of life and fecal soiling after surgery. These patients may be best served

with a permanent colostomy rather than a sphincter-sparing coloanal anastomosis.
- Digital rectal examination and rigid proctoscopy should be performed by the lead surgeon prior to the administration of neoadjuvant therapy. Anal sphincter, pelvic floor function, topography of rectal wall involvement, and distance of the distal aspect of the tumor from the dentate line determine the likelihood of sphincter salvage and method of reanastomosis. Submucosal tattooing distal to the rectal tumor identifies the location of clinically regressed tumors after neoadjuvant chemoradiation and is helpful for determining tumor clearance during pelvic dissection.
- A detailed family history is necessary to identify risk of an inherited colon and rectal cancer syndrome as well as risk for metachronous colorectal cancer. We currently screen all young patients (<60 years of age) for Lynch syndrome and refer patients to genetic counseling when they have a positive screen or if they have multiple affected relatives.
- Past medical history should identify patients with cardiopulmonary, liver, or kidney disease not medically suitable for a physiologically demanding operation.

IMAGING AND OTHER DIAGNOSTIC STUDIES

- A complete colonoscopy is obtained to evaluate for potential synchronous lesions that may have to be addressed at the time of surgery.
- Preoperative staging with endorectal ultrasound (ERUS) or rectal protocol magnetic resonance imaging (MRI) determines the need for neoadjuvant chemoradiation. ERUS has a higher sensitivity and specificity for tumor depth rather than lymph node involvement as compared to MRI. MRI allows for assessment of the circumferential margin at the mesorectal envelope.[1]
- As per NCCN guidelines, rectal cancers located at the distal two-thirds of the rectum with T3/T4 wall invasion and/or N+ nodal status will be referred for neoadjuvant treatment to decrease the risk of locoregional recurrence.[2] Additionally, neoadjuvant therapy may lead to tumor shrinkage, increasing the likelihood of sphincter preservation while avoiding exposure of the small bowel, colonic conduit, and

244

Chapter 29 LOW ANTERIOR RESECTION AND TOTAL MESORECTAL EXCISION/COLOANAL ANASTOMOSIS 245

anastomosis to postoperative radiation. Postoperative radiation is associated with increased risk of anastomotic stricture and radiation enteritis.[3]
- We routinely order a contrast-enhanced computed tomography scan of the chest, abdomen, and pelvis to evaluate for distant metastatic disease. Selected patients with liver metastases will be treated with a combination of staged resections and chemotherapy, whereas patients with synchronous peritoneal carcinomatosis will be evaluated for cytoreductive surgery with hyperthermic intraperitoneal chemotherapy.
- Positron emission tomography for the initial staging of rectal cancer rarely alters disease management.[4]
- Carcinoembryonic antigen levels are checked prior to the initiation of neoadjuvant chemoradiation, prior to resection and prior to initiation of adjuvant chemotherapy.

SURGICAL MANAGEMENT

Preoperative Planning

- Patients undergo preoperative counseling and stoma marking by an enterostomal therapist. Counseling allows the patient to understand ostomy care, optimizes stoma placement, and reduces stoma-related complications.[5]
- Placement of ureteral stents can facilitate ureteral identification in the setting of large rectal tumors, inflammation, previous surgery, and pelvic radiation and also increases intraoperative identification of ureteral injuries if they do occur.
- Bowel preparation or enema removes the mechanical obstacle of bowel contents in a narrow pelvis and reduces the tension on an infraperitoneal anastomosis.
- Parenteral antibiotic prophylaxis covering bowel flora is given prior to surgical incision.
- Deep venous thrombosis prophylaxis via sequential compression devices and subcutaneous heparin or low molecular weight heparin (LMWH) prior to surgical incision is administered.
- The surgical tray should include a lighted St. Mark retractor with the longest available blades, a big bite surgical energy device, and laparoscopic cautery and suction.

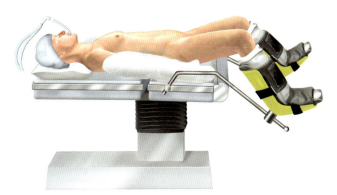

FIGURE 1 • The patient is on a lithotomy position with the patient's hips slightly flexed and the legs completely flexed in Yellofin stirrups.

Positioning

- LAR with coloanal anastomosis requires access to both the pelvis and the perineum. Therefore, patients are placed in a lithotomy position with the hips slightly flexed and the knees completely flexed in Yellofin stirrups. Extra padding is applied on the fibular head and heels to prevent peroneal nerve injury and pressure ulcers. The buttocks are at the edge of the table with the tip of the coccyx accessible. The legs remain adducted during the pelvic dissection but will need to be abducted to allow perineal access during creation of the coloanal anastomosis (**FIGURE 1**).

TECHNIQUES

LOW ANTERIOR RECTAL RESECTION WITH TOTAL MESORECTAL EXCISION

Incision, Abdominal Exploration, and Retraction of the Small Bowel

- A midline laparotomy incision is made from the supraumbilical midline to the pubic bone. The fascia is opened between the rectus muscles. As the incision is opened to the level of the pubic bone, the bladder is mobilized to the left of the incision.
- A careful exploration of the abdominal and pelvic cavity is undertaken to assess for distant metastatic disease and/or unresectable local disease. Attention should be given to the liver, retroperitoneum, aortic and external iliac lymph nodes, as well as peritoneal surfaces. Locally advanced disease may require a diverting colostomy followed by chemotherapy and radiation prior to resection.
- A fixed abdominal retractor, such as a Bookwalter or Thompson retractor, is used for exposure. A laparotomy pad wrapped around the small intestine from the ligament of Treitz to the terminal ileum will prevent loops of small intestine from migrating into the operative field. A midline incision that barely extends above the umbilicus allows for tucking the small bowel under the right abdominal wall.

Mobilization of the Left and Sigmoid Colon, Colonic Mesentery, and Splenic Flexure

- The left colon lateral attachments are incised in a cephalad direction. The areolar plane between the left colonic mesentery and the retroperitoneum is identified and opened. This plane is a few millimeters medial from the peritoneal reflection or white line of Toldt. Developing a plane at the exact edge of the white line of Toldt has the potential of lifting the retroperitoneal structures with subsequent potential ureteral, gonadal vessels, and hypogastric nerve injury.
- The splenocolic, phrenocolic, and renocolic attachments are divided at the splenic flexure. In patients with difficult visualization, the transverse colon is retracted downward and the lesser sac is entered over the midtransverse colon by incising the gastrocolic ligament. Development of this plane in a medial to left lateral direction detaches the omentum from the distal transverse colon so that the medial and lateral planes of dissection can be joined to complete the splenic flexure mobilization (**FIGURE 2**).

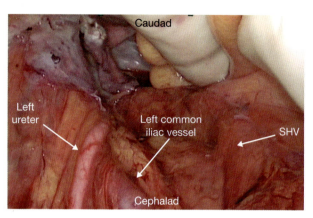

FIGURE 3 • The sigmoid colon and its mesentery have been separated from the retroperitoneum to reveal the left ureter as it crosses the left common iliac vessels. The peritoneal reflection over the left side of the rectum and mesorectum has been incised dorsal to the superior hemorrhoidal vessels (SHV) to allow encircling these vessels prior to ligation.

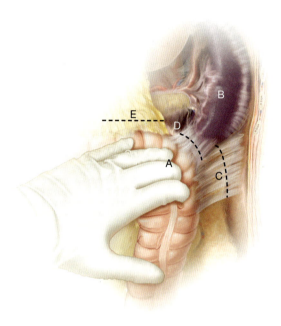

FIGURE 2 • Mobilization of the splenic flexure. The splenic flexure of the colon (A) is retracted medially to identify and release the lateral peritoneal attachments. Care is taken to avoid injury to the spleen (B). The phrenocolic ligament (C), the splenocolic ligament (D), and the gastrocolic ligament (E) are identified and subsequently divided. This dissection can be carried from medial to lateral as well as lateral to medial, until both planes of dissection meet around the spleen.

- The splenic flexure and proximal left colon mesentery are separated from the Gerota fascia. Incomplete mobilization of the splenic flexure results in a short colonic conduit and tension on the colorectal anastomosis, which could then lead to a postoperative anastomotic leak.

Vessel Ligation and Left Ureter Identification

- The separation of the left and sigmoid colon from the retroperitoneum is continued by reversing direction toward the pelvis. The left ureter is identified as it crosses over the left iliac artery and into the pelvis in a way that preserves the retroperitoneal location of the ureter but also identifies the areolar plane that medially extends to the superior hemorrhoidal vessels (SHV) arch (**FIGURE 3**). Lifting the mesosigmoid and placing the index finger behind the SHV arch allows the surgeon to incise with electrocautery the right surface of the peritoneum just under the dorsal surface of the SHV. This plane of dissection along the dorsal aspect of the SHV, as it is carried over the promontory, leads into the presacral tissue plane that will be later developed during the TME. At this point, the mesentery is divided in between the sigmoid and descending colon, starting from the antimesenteric border. The SHV are ligated at the level of their origin from the inferior mesenteric artery (IMA) in order to preserve the left colic pedicle intact. The colon itself is not divided. This prevents

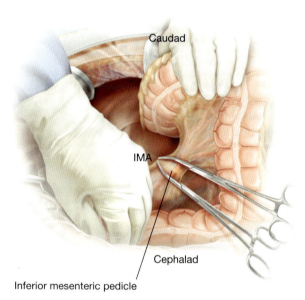

FIGURE 4 • High inferior mesenteric artery (IMA) transection. In coloanal anastomosis cases, the IMA is transected at its origin between clamps in order to obtain maximal mobilization of the colonic conduit.

the colon from dropping into the dissection field during the operation and also allowing for any blood supply deficiencies in the proximal colon to manifest by the end of the dissection and prior to the anastomosis.

- In cases of coloanal anastomosis, a high IMA transection at its takeoff from the aorta is usually performed, to prevent anastomotic tension (**FIGURE 4**). The collateral marginal artery that connects the middle colic artery and the IMA and runs close to the colon provides blood supply to the distal descending colon in these cases.
- Reidentification of the ureter prior to IMA or SHV pedicle ligation ensures the left ureter is safe from injury.
- Additional length of the colonic conduit can be achieved by ligating the inferior mesenteric vein just lateral to the ligament of Treitz.

Chapter 29 LOW ANTERIOR RESECTION AND TOTAL MESORECTAL EXCISION/COLOANAL ANASTOMOSIS   247

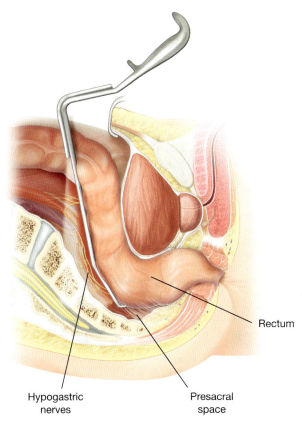

FIGURE 5 • Using a lighted St. Mark retractor, the rectum is retracted anteriorly, exposing the presacral space posteriorly. The hypogastric nerves are exposed and should be swept posteriorly and away from the mesorectum. This begins the superior and posterior portion of the total mesorectal excision.

Posterior Mobilization of the Rectum and Hypogastric Nerve Identification

- A lighted St. Mark retractor is placed posteriorly to the ligated SHV. By retracting the rectum anteriorly, the presacral areolar space is exposed and divided with electrocautery. The hypogastric nerves are identifiable at this location prior to dissecting the presacral space (**FIGURE 5**). These nerves should be swept posteriorly and preserved as they course in a medial to lateral direction along the presacral fascia.
- The presacral dissection plane is bloodless. Proper retraction with the St. Mark retractor assists the surgeon in following the areolar plane between the fascia propria anteriorly and the presacral fascia posteriorly, down to the levator muscles and pelvic floor (**FIGURE 6**).
- Failure to properly expose the presacral space with the lighted St. Mark retractor risks dissecting to far posteriorly and into the presacral venous plexus. Staying on the anterior surface of the areolar plane close to the mesorectal boundary will allow the surgeon to stay in the presacral space, thus avoiding catastrophic bleeding from injured presacral veins.
- Blunt dissection should be avoided at all cause, because it can lead to violation of the mesorectum with the attendant increased risk of locoregional tumor recurrence. It is imperative to adhere to a sharp dissection technique when dissecting around the mesorectum.

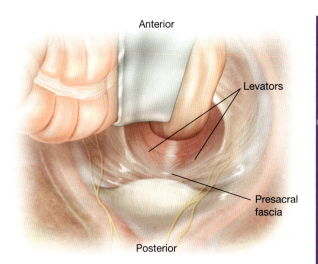

FIGURE 6 • Exposed with the aid of a lighted St. Mark retractor, the presacral plane of dissection should be followed down to the levator muscles and the pelvic floor.

- As the posterior dissection continues laterally, the surgeon must proceed on an anterolateral direction, or in a semicircular fashion, to open the lateral planes. This helps avoiding penetrating through the endopelvic fascia, which holds the hypogastric vein and its branches as well as the parasympathetic plexus attached to the lateral pelvic walls. In this fashion, potentially catastrophic bleeding and severe autonomic dysfunction can be averted.

Division of Lateral Rectal Ligaments

- The lateral rectal ligaments can be taken with cautery or with an energy device. It is not usually necessary to ligate vessels within the lateral stalks except for the middle rectal vessel variants. Identification of the lateral rectal ligaments is achieved by placing the rectum on posterolateral traction between the index and middle fingers in the direction opposite of the lateral rectal ligament to be transected (**FIGURE 7**).

Anterior Mobilization of the Rectum and Proximal Colonic Transection

- Following the areolar tissue circumferentially around the rectum and incising the anterior peritoneal reflection connect the right and left lateral dissections. Once the peritoneal reflection is incised, the dissection continues behind Denonvilliers fascia, which covers the seminal vesicles and prostate (**FIGURE 7**). Dissection anterior to Denonvilliers fascia is associated with annoying bleeding and with an increased risk of parasympathetic nerve damage. This plane is intentionally violated only in anterior tumors that invade into the seminal vesicles or prostate. In these cases, the seminal vesicles and/or part of the prostate have to be resected en bloc with the rectum in order to achieve a clear radial margin.
- In women, the rectovaginal septum is more easily separated from the rectum anteriorly.
- At this point, the colon is transected proximally between the sigmoid and descending colon lymphovascular

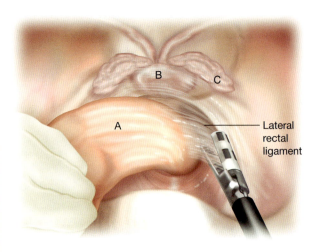

distribution in between Kocher clamps. The transected end of the colon should reach the pubis with ease, ensuring adequate mobilization of the colon conduit for a tension-free anastomosis.

FIGURE 7 • Transection of the lateral rectal ligaments and anterior pelvic dissection. Posterolateral retraction of the rectum (*A*) allows for good exposure of the lateral rectal ligament (the right one is shown here), which can then be transected with cautery or with an energy device. The anterior dissection will then proceed behind Denonvilliers fascia, in the space between the rectum, posteriorly, and the prostate and seminal vesicles (*B* and *C*, respectively), anteriorly.

COLOANAL ANASTOMOSIS: STAPLED TECHNIQUE

- This method is feasible when there is at least 2 cm of rectal stump above the dentate line.
- The rectum is divided above the levators with a contoured stapler. The specimen, including the entire rectum and mesorectum as well as the sigmoid colon, is now fully disconnected and is sent to the pathologist. The pelvis is now empty with good visualization of the pelvic floor (**FIGURE 8**).
- The anvil of a 29 mm end-to-end anastomosis (EEA) is placed in the open end of the descending colon and a purse string is placed around its shaft.
- A 29-mm EEA stapling device is introduced gently into the rectal stump.
- The trocar is brought out through the rectal stump. The elected site of the rectal drum penetration depends solely on creating an exit angle suitable to accept the anvil without the need for further maneuvering of the stapling device itself. Any repositioning of the stapler post exodus of the trocar runs the risk of lateral tear and incomplete rectal stump donut. A long packing forceps is used to push the rectal stump around the trocar penetration point to avoid lateral tearing of the rectal stump (**FIGURE 9**), which could lead to an anastomotic leak.
- The anvil and the EEA stapler are then mated and fired, creating a tension-free coloanal anastomosis (**FIGURE 10A**). Two complete donuts should be obtained; the distal donut should be sent to the pathologist for a frozen section evaluation to ensure the distal margin is negative for cancer. A positive margin may necessitate conversion to an APR. The integrity of the anastomosis is tested by insufflation under water (**FIGURE 10B**). Air bubbles would indicate an anastomotic leak, necessitating a revision of the anastomosis, in addition to a proximal diverting loop ileostomy (depending on the magnitude of the leak).
- The patient is always diverted with a loop ileostomy to protect the anastomosis, and a 19-Fr round drain is placed in the pelvis for no more than 2 to 3 days.

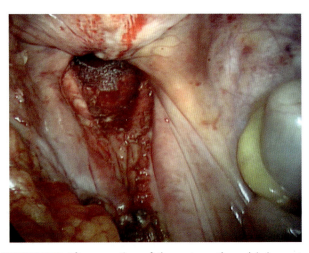

FIGURE 8 • After resection of the rectum, the pelvis is empty, with good visualization of the pelvic floor.

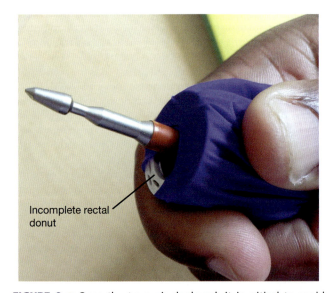

FIGURE 9 • Once the trocar is deployed, it is critical to avoid any movement on the end-to-end anastomosis stapling device to avoid lateral tearing of the rectal stump, which could lead to an anastomotic leak.

Chapter 29 LOW ANTERIOR RESECTION AND TOTAL MESORECTAL EXCISION/COLOANAL ANASTOMOSIS 249

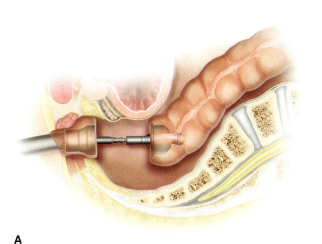
A

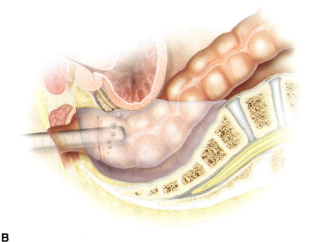
B

FIGURE 10 • Stapled coloanal anastomosis. **A,** An end-to-end anastomosis (EEA) is created with a 29-mm EEA stapler. **B,** The completed colorectal anastomosis is tested under water. Air bubbles identified during insufflation of the anastomosis indicate an anastomotic leak.

COLOANAL ANASTOMOSIS: HANDSEWN TECHNIQUE

Placement of Self-Retaining Anal Retractor

- Eversion of the anal canal with a self-retaining Lone Star anal retractor (**FIGURE 11**), or with two Gelpis, can facilitate surgeon visualization.

Injection of Local Anesthetic With Epinephrine

- The dentate line is identified and the submucosal plane is injected circumferentially with a local anesthetic containing epinephrine. This decreases bleeding and loss of visualization. The distal rectum is divided full thickness sharply transanally above the dentate line (**FIGURE 11**). The distal margin should be sent to the pathologist for a frozen section evaluation to ensure that it is negative for cancer. A positive margin may necessitate conversion to an APR.

Anal Verge Sutures Placed in Four Quadrants

- The 3-0 Vicryl sutures are placed in all four quadrants through the anal mucosa and a small portion of the internal sphincter (outside-in placement). The needles are kept in place and the sutures are tacked down to the Lone Star retractor to keep them secured. These sutures will eventually be placed through the distal colon segment to complete the coloanal anastomosis.

Colonic Conduit Delivery

- A purse-string suture is placed in the open end of the descending colon around an insufflated Foley catheter. The descending colon stump is lubricated and is then delivered to the perineum by slowly pulling the Foley catheter through the open distal rectal stump (**FIGURE 12**). The assistant guides the colonic conduit through the pelvis ensuring adequate colon length, lack of tension on the colonic conduit's blood supply, and orientation without twisting.
- The colonic conduit should easily emerge from the anal canal so the surgeon can see the purse string. This ensures there will be a tension-free anastomosis at the level of the dentate line and allows the surgeon to assess the blood supply of the colonic conduit as it passes through the anal canal. Occasionally, it is necessary to clean a portion of mesenteric fat and appendix epiploicae to prevent its inclusion in the coloanal anastomosis and to debulk a large conduit as it passes through the anal canal.

Colon Anchored With Anal Canal Sutures

- The purse string in the distal colon is amputated, the Foley catheter is removed, and the previously placed four-quadrant distal sutures are now placed full thickness through the open distal colon wall (outside-in placement). The colonic conduit is pushed back up into the anal canal when surgical knots

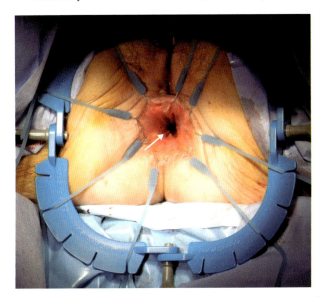

FIGURE 11 • A Lone Star retractor is used to evert the anal canal and to expose the dentate line (*arrow*). The rectum will be transected transanally above the dentate line.

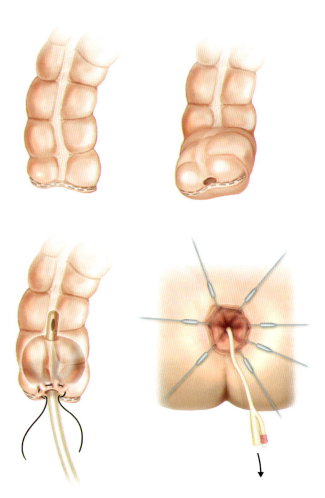

FIGURE 12 • A purse-string suture is placed in the open end of the descending colon around an insufflated Foley catheter. The descending colon stump is lubricated and is then delivered to the perineum by slowly pulling the Foley catheter through the open distal rectal stump.

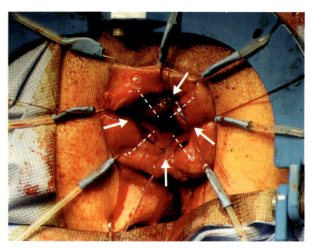

FIGURE 13 • The proximal colon is opened and anchored to the anal canal. The previously placed four-quadrant distal sutures have now been placed full thickness through the open distal colon wall (*arrows*). Placing full-thickness sutures in between these four-quadrant sutures (along the *dotted lines*) will complete the anastomosis.

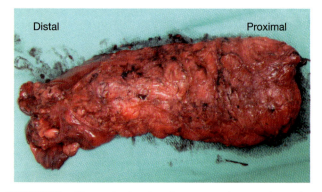

FIGURE 14 • The excised rectum has a smooth posterior surface when the mesorectum is excised intact, with no distal tapering of the mesorectum observed.

are placed to secure the anchoring sutures (**FIGURE 13**). The anchored sutures are kept long and secured with a hemostat outside the anal canal to maintain orientation of the colonic conduit and to guide completion of the coloanal anastomosis.

Completion of Circumferential Anastomosis

- An anal retractor such as a Hill Ferguson or standard Fansler retractor can then be placed through the anal canal and distal colon. Placing interrupted 3-0 Vicryl full-thickness sutures through the colon and anus (inside-out placement) completes the anastomosis (**FIGURE 13**).

En Bloc Removal of the Rectal Specimen

- If a more distal resection is required or if the surgeon prefers to perform a perineal anorectal resection en bloc with the rectal dissection, the surgeon can begin the perineal dissection in the intersphincteric plane, located between the internal and external anal sphincters. This dissection can begin at the dentate line or within the intersphincteric groove at the anal verge. The intersphincteric dissection proceeds proximally to the level of the puborectalis sling of the levators. An abdominal assistant can guide the perineal surgeon to then dissect into the pelvis and connect the two dissection planes. The en bloc rectal and internal anal sphincter dissection can then be passed off the field. The coloanal anastomosis is fashioned as previously described at the level where the intersphincteric dissection began. In cases where the internal anal sphincter is excised, the distal anastomosis should include anal mucosa and parts of the external anal sphincter.[6] The resected specimen should show an intact mesorectum with no tapering on the distal end (**FIGURE 14**).

Loop Ileostomy Creation and Pelvic Drain Placement

- Creation of a loop ileostomy through a previously marked right lower quadrant location diverts stool from the coloanal anastomosis and protects the anastomosis. A 19-Fr round drain is placed behind the anastomosis.

Chapter 29 LOW ANTERIOR RESECTION AND TOTAL MESORECTAL EXCISION/COLOANAL ANASTOMOSIS

PEARLS AND PITFALLS

Mobilizing the left colon	▪ Dissect the plane a few millimeters medial to the white line of Toldt.
Left ureter identification	▪ Complete mobilization of the sigmoid colon mesentery from the retroperitoneum allows identification of the left ureter during proximal IMA ligation.
Mobilization of colonic conduit	▪ High transection of the IMA and transection of the inferior mesenteric vein lateral to the ligament of Treitz elongate the colonic conduit for a tension-free anastomosis.
Posterior mesorectal dissection	▪ Dissecting the areolar plane behind the mesorectum requires the surgeon to lift the rectum anteriorly with a lighted St. Mark retractor. Dissection posterior to this plane risks entry into the presacral venous plexus, which can lead to exsanguinating hemorrhage.
Anterior rectal dissection	▪ Keep dissection behind Denonvilliers fascia unless an anteriorly located tumor necessitates excision to obtain a negative radial margin.
Colonic conduit delivery for anastomosis	▪ Properly orient the colonic conduit so there is no mesenteric twisting or undue tension as it is delivered though the anal canal. Mesenteric fat can be removed from the distal colon to facilitate placement through the canal, but too much dissection can compromise the blood supply of colon and the proximal portion of the anastomosis.
Stapled anastomosis	▪ Avoid maneuvering of the circular stapler after deployment of the trocar. A lateral rectal drum tear extending to the stapler rim will result in an incomplete distal donut and an anastomotic leak.

POSTOPERATIVE CARE

- Prophylactic LMWH is initiated the day of the operation.
- Physical therapy for ambulation is involved on postoperative day (POD) 1.
- Early feeding with clear liquids can increase patient comfort and stimulate return of gastrointestinal motility.
- Bladder dysfunction following deep pelvic dissection is common. We routinely keep a Foley catheter in place for 5 days.
- Although patients wait for return of intestinal function, they can be taught the basics of ileostomy care.
- Patients should be advised that drainage from the rectum could occur despite fecal diversion. A single episode of bloody rectal discharge while the patient is ambulating between PODs 5 and 7 is often an indicator of evacuation of a pelvic fluid collection through the stapler line and does not require further imaging unless the patient shows signs of infection. Persistent rectal drainage that is purulent or bloody should prompt workup for a postoperative complication.

OUTCOMES

- Survival from rectal cancer after multimodality treatment is dependent on disease stage. Overall, 5-year survival is approximately 90% for stage I, 74% to 65% for stage II, and 81% to 33% for stage III of disease. Development of distant metastasis occurs in less than 10% in patients with stage I disease but increases up to 28% and 50% in patients with stages II and III rectal cancer, respectively.[7]
- Local pelvic recurrence of rectal cancer is also dependent on tumor and nodal stage. Local recurrence is less than or equal to 5% for patients with stage I rectal cancer but increases to 15% for stage II disease and 22% for stage III disease.[7] If a pelvic recurrence can be treated with a margin-negative surgical resection, 5-year survival can approach 40%. Often, this requires a pelvic exenteration which demands a multispecialty surgical approach.[8]

COMPLICATIONS

- Complications can occur in up to one-third of patients undergoing TME and coloanal anastomosis with 15% of patients experiencing major complications.[9]
- Rectal cancer patients who have received neoadjuvant chemoradiation and who undergo a coloanal anastomosis with a colonic conduit that depends on collateral blood flow have multiple risk factors for anastomotic leak. Fecal diversion with loop ileostomy after coloanal anastomosis reduces the clinical consequences of an anastomotic leak.[10,11]
- Most patients have defecatory dysfunction after removal of the rectum. In the native state, the rectum functions as a distensible organ to store stool until the patient initiates evacuation. Proctectomy patients loose this storage capacity and have more frequent bowel movements. They typically complain of a defecation pattern termed "low anterior syndrome," in which the patient senses a frequent defecation urge. Treatment includes fiber supplementation to bulk up the stool, use of Imodium or Lomotil to slow intestinal transit, and enemas to assist with evacuation. Patients with a severe decrease in quality of life may elect to undergo conversion to a permanent end colostomy.

REFERENCES

1. Muthusamy VR, Chang KJ. Optimal methods for staging rectal cancer. *Clin Cancer Res*. 2007;13:6877s-6884s.
2. van Gijn W, Marijnen CA, Nagtegaal ID, et al. Preoperative radiotherapy combined with total mesorectal excision for resectable rectal cancer: 12-year follow-up of the multicentre, randomised controlled TME trial. *Lancet Oncol*. 2011;12:575-582.

3. Kim CW, Kim JH, Yu CS, et al. Complications after sphincter-saving resection in rectal cancer patients according to whether chemoradiotherapy is performed before or after surgery. *Int J Radiat Oncol Biol Phys*. 2010;78:156-163.

4. Cipe G, Ergul N, Hasbahceci M, et al. Routine use of positron-emission tomography/computed tomography for staging of primary colorectal cancer: does it affect clinical management?. *World J Surg Oncol*. 2013;11:49.

5. Person B, Ifargan R, Lachter J, et al. The impact of preoperative stoma site marking on the incidence of complications, quality of life, and patient's independence. *Dis Colon Rectum*. 2012;55:783-787.

6. Schiessel R, Novi G, Holzer B, et al. Technique and long-term results of intersphincteric resection for low rectal cancer. *Dis Colon Rectum*. 2005;48:1858-1865.

7. Gunderson LL, Sargent DJ, Tepper JE, et al. Impact of T and N substage on survival and disease relapse in adjuvant rectal cancer: a pooled analysis. *Int J Radiat Oncol Biol Phys*. 2002;54:386-396.

8. Tanis PJ, Doeksen A, van Lanschot JJ. Intentionally curative treatment of locally recurrent rectal cancer: a systematic review. *Can J Surg*. 2013;56:135-144.

9. Bennis M, Parc Y, Lefevre JH, et al. Morbidity risk factors after low anterior resection with total mesorectal excision and coloanal anastomosis: a retrospective series of 483 patients. *Ann Surg*. 2012;255:504-510.

10. Huser N, Michalski CW, Erkan M, et al. Systematic review and meta-analysis of the role of defunctioning stoma in low rectal cancer surgery. *Ann Surg*. 2008;248:52-60.

11. Nurkin S, Kakarla VR, Ruiz DE, et al. The role of faecal diversion in low rectal cancer: a review of 1791 patients having rectal resection with anastomosis for cancer, with and without a proximal stoma. *Colorectal Dis*. 2013;15:e309-e316.

Chapter 30

Low Anterior Rectal Resection: Laparoscopic Technique

Antonio D'Urso, Jacques Marescaux, and Didier Mutter

DEFINITION

- A low anterior resection (LAR) combines total mesorectal excision (TME) with sphincter preservation and a colorectal or coloanal anastomosis.
- A complete mesorectal excision with an intact mesorectum including all regional lymph nodes significantly reduces locoregional recurrence. Preservation of pelvic innervation minimizes urinary and sexual sequelae after rectal resection.
- High or low transection of the inferior mesenteric artery (IMA) does not alter the rate of anastomotic leak, lymphatic nodal harvest, local recurrence rates, or 5-year survival rate.
- A ≥1 cm negative distal margin (distance from the lower pole of the tumor to the distal cut of the rectum) should be obtained.
- The circumferential margin remains an important independent prognostic factor in terms of recurrence and survival after optimal surgery with or without neoadjuvant chemoradiotherapy.

DIFFERENTIAL DIAGNOSIS

- **Middle** (6-10 cm from anal verge) **to low** (within 4-5 cm from anal verge) rectal tumors with ≥1 cm negative distal margin.
- All indications are discussed and validated in a multidisciplinary oncologic committee.
- Relative contraindications depend on surgeon experience, severe patient comorbidities, and tumor characteristics such as bulky lesions invading surrounding organs.

PATIENT HISTORY AND PHYSICAL FINDINGS

- A detailed family history that may suggest familial colorectal cancer syndromes (ie, Lynch syndrome) should be obtained.
- Genetic counseling should be proposed for patients younger than 40 years, for patients presenting with MSI + test associated with the absence of BRAF mutation, or for patients with families with 3 or more cases of colorectal cancer in first- or second-degree relatives, including 1 before the age of 50.
- An oncogeriatric counseling should be obtained in patients over 75 years of age with G8 score <14.
- A detailed history of symptoms and signs should include the following:
  - Presence of rectal pain and/or tenesmus
  - Presence of obstructive symptoms
  - Description of anorectal function, with any fecal incontinence or leakage documented preoperatively
  - Documentation of urinary and erectile function/dysfunction
- Physical examination should include the following:
  - Routine abdominal examination, noting any previous incisions
  - Digital rectal examination with assessment of sphincter function, the size, the mobility and the distance of the tumor from the anal margin and the puborectal muscle (upper pole of the anal canal)
  - Bilateral inguinal nodal examination
- **Rigid proctoscopy should complete the physical examination and is the key to a proper patient selection.**

- Proctoscopy should be standardized and well documented. It should:
  - Define correctly the distal extent of the lesion measured from the anal verge
  - Describe the exact position of the lesion in the lumen and the extent of the rectal circumference involved
  - Assess the presence or absence of fixation to perirectal structures
- Histological diagnosis should be confirmed.
- A complete colonoscopy with documentation of all polyps should be performed so the treatment plan can address synchronous pathology, as needed. If a preoperative colonoscopy is not feasible (ie, in obstructed patients), it should be performed within 3 to 6 months postoperatively.
- Evaluation of preoperative sphincter continence with an anal manometry should be considered in elderly patients or in patients with suboptimal sphincter function at clinical examination.

IMAGING AND OTHER DIAGNOSTIC STUDIES

Pelvic MRI

- Pelvic MRI should be routinely performed unless contraindicated to adequately stage the rectal cancer, to determine the potential need for neoadjuvant therapy, to verify the tumoral response after neo-adjuvant treatment, and to plan operative strategy. The MRI report should include the following elements:
  - The location of the lower pole of the tumor in relation to the anal margin, the upper border of the internal sphincter, the upper border of the puborectal muscle and the peritoneal reflection. For ultra-low tumors, it is important to determine if there is involvement of the levator ani muscles, puborectal muscle, and/or external/internal anal sphincter muscles.
  - Tumor T and N staging should be correctly reported.
  - The size, position of the tumor and its relation to the sacral space and surrounding organs, in case of high lesions the peritoneal reflection invasion.
  - Circumferential margin and potential fascia recti invasion.
  - The presence of suspicious mesorectal lymph nodes.

Computed Tomography

- A contrast-enhanced computed tomography (CT) of the chest, abdomen, and pelvis evaluates for potential metastases. In case of renal insufficiency, replaced by a noninjected thoracic scan combined with a liver MRI.
- Cancer should be staged according to the American Joint Committee on Cancer TNM system

Endorectal Ultrasound

Staging with endorectal ultrasound (ERUS) completes the workup to define the depth of invasion (with an accuracy for wall invasion of about 87.5%) and the potential invasion of the internal and external sphincters and/or the levator ani muscle and the lower rectum.

253

Positron Emission Tomography

- Positron emission tomography (PET-CT) is of particular interest for the evaluation of loco-regional lymph node involvement and to complete the investigations in case of doubt about the metastatic nature of a lesion.
- The preoperative carcinoembryonic antigen (CEA) level should be obtained.

SURGICAL MANAGEMENT

Preoperative Planning

- Informed consent is obtained preoperatively. The risks and benefits of the operation, potential complications, and eventual alternatives should be detailed.
- The patient has been informed of the necessity to perform a temporary stoma and even the risk to have a definitive colostomy.
- A clear explication about the risk of postoperative functional disorders and fecal incontinence and repercussion on lifestyle is essential.
- A detailed explication of the risk about the low anterior rectal resection syndrome (LARS) must be given.
- The possibility to conversion to an open procedure should be discussed.
- The stoma site is marked by a skin tattoo the evening before the intervention.
- We follow the Guidelines for Perioperative Care in Elective Colic and rectal/pelvic Surgery: Enhanced Recovery After Surgery (ERAS) Society Recommendations for perioperative optimization and bowel preparation as described elsewhere in this textbook.
- A dedicated ERAS nurse follows the patient from the preoperative counseling until the postoperative follow up.
- Appropriate intravenous antibiotics are administered within 1 hour of skin incision.

Equipment and Instrumentation

- 10-mm, 0° camera (30° camera is optional) with high-resolution monitors.
- Laparoscopic endoscopic scissors and a blunt tip, 5-mm energy device (10-mm in obese patients).
- Laparoscopic linear staplers.
- Three 10/12-mm trocars for the camera and stapler and suprapubic retraction, two 5-mm working trocars.
- A lone star self-retractor in case of coloanal anastomosis.

Positioning and Port Placement

Patient Setup

- Key elements for proper patient positioning include:
  - Supine position, with the right arm padded and tucked alongside the body. The left arm is left out for venous access. The legs are separated, in semiflexion, in Allen type stirrups to allow for easy abdominal and perineal access (**FIGURE 1A**).
  - **The thighs should be placed parallel to the ground to avoid conflict with the surgeon's arms/instruments.**
  - Adequate fastening to the table with padding in order to prevent neurovascular injuries to the extremities.
  - Deep vein thrombosis (DVT) prophylaxis using an intermittent pneumatic compression (IPC) device.
  - A body warmer device should be used to prevent patient hypothermia.
  - The patient is placed on a steep Trendelenburg position with the left side up to help retract bowel loops by means of gravity and enhance operative exposure.
  - The buttocks should be brought to the distal edge of the lower end of the table in order to allow for an easy access to the anal and perineal area.
  - An orogastric tube is inserted and removed at the end of the surgery.
  - A Foley catheter is inserted and left in place for 24 hours.

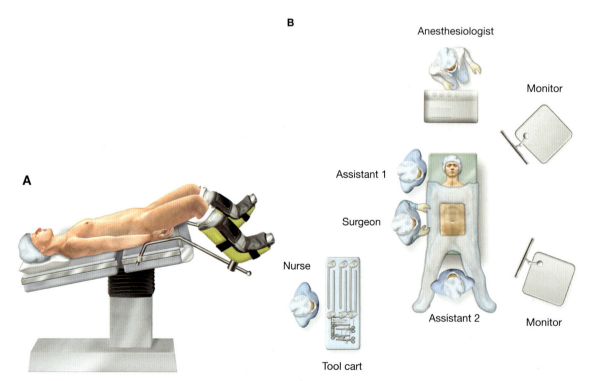

FIGURE 1 • Patient and Team position. **A,** Patient position. **B,** Team position and operative room setup.

Chapter 30 LOW ANTERIOR RECTAL RESECTION: LAPAROSCOPIC TECHNIQUE 255

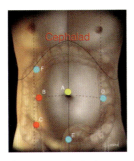

FIGURE 2 • Port placement: Optical port *(A)*. Working ports *(B and C)*. Retracting ports *(D and E)*. Additional retracting port *(F)*.

Team Positioning

- This procedure is performed with two assistants and a scrub nurse.
- Two instrument tables are used: one for the abdominal part and a second one for the perineal part of the operation in case a coloanal anastomosis is performed.
- The surgeon stands on the right flank of the patient, the first assistant lateral to the patient's right shoulder, and the second assistant between the patient's legs. The scrub nurse is placed to the right of the surgeon lateral to lower limbs (**FIGURE 1B**).
- If a coloanal anastomosis is performed the surgical team moves toward the perineal region.
- The monitors are placed in front of the operating team and at eye level to improve ergonomics.

- The light source, the insufflator, and the electronic generator are placed on the left side of the patient at the level of the leg in the instruments trolley.

Port Placement

- One 10/12-mm supraumbilical trocar (port A) is introduced using a mini-open technique. It will be used for the camera.
- Two other ports, a 5-mm port in the right flank (port B) and a 12-mm port in the right iliac fossa (port C), are used as operating ports.
- The fourth 5-mm port in the left flank at the level of the umbilicus is inserted through the rectus muscle (port D, 5 mm in diameter).
- The last 12-mm port introduced in the suprapubic area (port E) is used for pelvic retraction and for exposure of the root of the mesosigmoid.
- Port fixation in the wall should be perfect to prevent any risk of parietal injury and to prevent increased operative times due to a loss in abdominal pressure. One should not hesitate to fix ports to the skin.

Additional ports may be used in case of difficulty in exposure. In this case, a port will be positioned in the right hypochondrium (port F) to retract the ileocecal area. This is particularly useful in obese patients.

- Port placement is reported in **FIGURE 2**.

OPERATIVE STEPS

- Complete mobilization of the splenic flexure
- Transection of the IMA at its origin
- Left colon mobilization
- Total Mesorectal Excision (posterior, lateral, anterior dissection)
- Pelvic dissection
- Proximal and distal transection
- Anastomosis (colorectal or coloanal)
- See also ▶ Video 1.

LAPAROSCOPIC LOW ANTERIOR RESECTION

Exploration and Exposure

- The intervention begins with an exploration of the abdominal cavity to identify the presence of possible carcinomatosis and/or metastasis, and to verify potential unexpected extension to the surrounding organs.
- Once the feasibility is confirmed by laparoscopic exploration, the patient is placed in a Trendelenburg position with the table tilted to the right. The greater omentum is reflected over the transverse colon. The small bowel is moved to the patient's right side to obtain the visualization of the medial aspect of the rectosigmoid mesentery. The pelvis is exposed, and an evaluation of the length and quality of the sigmoid loop is performed.
- In women, exposure of the posterior pelvis and of the rectovaginal (Douglas) pouch can be obtained by direct or indirect suspension of the uterus by means of the T'Lift (VECTEC, France) tissue retraction device (**FIGURE 3A** and **B**) or suprapubic transparietal sutures (**FIGURE 4**).
- Visceral obesity (in male patients) is more incapacitating than subcutaneous obesity (in female patients). The use of retractors is very helpful.
- Tumor identification may be necessary especially for the determination of the lower transection; in this case, an intraoperative endoscopy is performed.

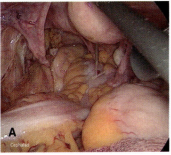 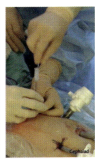 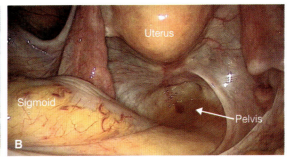

FIGURE 3 • T'Lift tissue retraction system. **A,** T'Lift tissue retraction system insertion with external view of the device. **B,** Pelvic exposure in women after bilateral uterine suspension with T'Lift tissue retraction system.

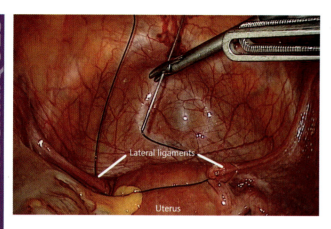

FIGURE 4 • Suprapubic suspension using transparietal sutures for uterine retraction.

OMENTAL DISSECTION AND SPLENIC FLEXURE MOBILIZATION

- The splenic flexure mobilization is performed as the initial step in order to have good length of colon for a tension-free anastomosis.
- The greater omentum is dissected at the level of the mild transverse colon. The assistant (located between the patient's legs) holds the omentum cranially with a 5-mm grasper while the transverse colon is pulled caudally by the grasper of the surgeon coming from the trocar in the right iliac fossa. Ligasure is placed in the 5-mm trocar on the right at the level of the umbilicus. The lesser sac is entered and the dissection of the transverse colon is performed from the right to left until the splenic flexure is reached.
- After this step, the transverse mesocolon is pulled cranially. The Treitz's ligament and the root of the transverse mesocolon are exposed. The inferior mesenteric vein (IMV) is grasped by the assistant with the grasper placed in the 5-mm trocar placed lateral to the umbilicus and the peritoneal sheet incised. The retroperitoneal space is dissected preserving the superior left hypogastric plexus and the prerenal fascia. The dissection is then continued laterally and toward the splenic flexure.
- The next step is the transection of the IMV: it is transected at the origin at the level of Treitz's ligament caudad to the inferior edge of the pancreas (**FIGURE 5**) with the LigaSure vessel-sealing device or in between clips.

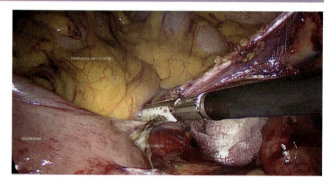

FIGURE 5 • The IMV is transected at its origin at the level of the Treitz's ligament underneath the inferior edge of the pancreas.

- Once this space created, the mesocolon is incised at the superior border of the pancreas at the left of the middle colic artery. A window is created and the lesser sac is entered. The mesocolic layer is now visible on its superior and inferior aspect. It is dissected with the Ligasure on the superior border of the pancreas until the splenic flexure is reached. A gauze can be placed at this level to join the dissection plane when completing the lateral dissection of the descending colon.
- The lateral attachments of the descending colon are dissected with the Ligasure. The left colic angle is freed from its lateral aspect, the eventual previous gauze placed is identified and removed, and the splenic flexure is now completely mobile.

VASCULAR ONCOLOGIC APPROACH

- The inferior mesenteric artery is dissected at its origin in order to perform an "en bloc" removal of all lymph nodes associated with the rectosigmoid junction (D3 resection). The inferior mesenteric artery (IMA) is exposed. The inferior mesenteric vein (IMV) is approached to prevent any venous overload related to the late ligation of the IMA.
- The posterior dissection created at the level of Treitz's ligament is continued toward the IMA origin.
- The sigmoid mesocolon is exposed, the posterior peritoneum is incised at the level of the promontory, and the left retroperitoneal space is entered, facilitated by the pneumodissection. The dissection is then continued in a cephalad direction reaching the previous dissection plane (**FIGURE 6**).
- Once the retroperitoneum is opened, dissection is initiated on the posterior aspect of the inferior mesenteric vascular sheath (ie, the superior rectal artery at this level). This step is facilitated by the anterior retraction on the mesocolon.
- Dissection is carried on always in contact with the posterior aspect of the vascular sheath of the IMA cranially until its origin on the aorta.
- An upward retraction on the sigmoid mesocolon and on the IMV expose the "T-shape" with the origin of the IMA (**FIGURE 7**).
- The IMA is skeletonized and the origin is identified thanks to the previous dissection (**FIGURE 8A** and **B**).

Chapter 30 LOW ANTERIOR RECTAL RESECTION: LAPAROSCOPIC TECHNIQUE   257

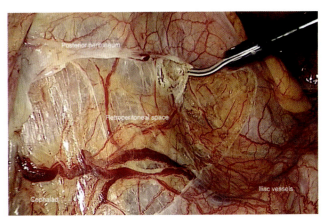

FIGURE 6 • The sigmoid mesocolon is exposed, the posterior peritoneum is incised at the level of the promontory, and the left retroperitoneal space entered.

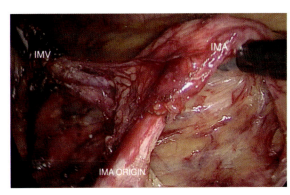

FIGURE 7 • A traction is performed on the sigmoid mesocolon and on the IMV in order to expose the "T-shape" that allows the identification of the origin of the IMA.

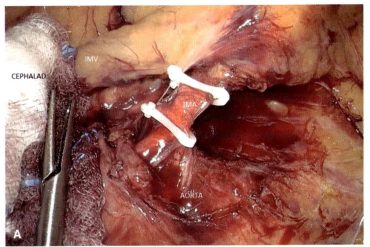

FIGURE 8 • IMA identification and dissection. A, Once the origin of the IMA has been identified, it is dissected and skeletonized 1 to 2 cm from the aorta. B, After a proper dissection, the IMA is transected.

- This technique preserves the sympathetic nerve plexuses, which run along the aorta on its anterior aspect.
- Once the origin of the IMA is correctly identified, the division is performed with the LigaSure vessel-sealing device. The stump of the IMA could be reinforced using an endoloop ligation or by placing clips.
- Once the IMA has been divided, the assistant, standing between the patient's legs, will grasp the artery using an atraumatic forceps introduced into the suprapubic port (port D) and apply anterior traction to ideally expose the dissection plane between the retroperitoneal space and the posterior aspect of the sigmoid mesocolon always remaining in contact with the posterior aspect of the artery.
- This type of dissection in contact with the artery helps to preserve the hypogastric nerve plexus, and notably the left sympathetic trunk of the neurovegetative system.

Mobilization of the Sigmoid Colon

- A medial to lateral mobilization of the mesocolon by opening the plane between Toldt's fascia anteriorly and Gerota's fascia posteriorly is performed (FIGURE 9). This mobilization

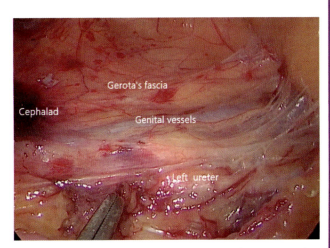

FIGURE 9 • Medial to lateral mobilization of the mesocolon. The retroperitoneal structures (gonadal vessels and left ureter) are correctly identified and preserved.

will help for the traction on the upper rectum allowing a perfect exposure of the anterior, posterior, and lateral aspects of the rectum.
- It is mandatory to identify the left ureter during this dissection. It is located between the aorta and the gonadal vessels, well protected by Gerota's fascia.
- The dissection is carried out laterally until the posterior aspect of the descending colon is reached laterally.
- Mobilization of the sigmoid colon is completed with a division of its lateral attachments to the abdominal wall (**FIGURE 10**).
- Caudally, the dissection is carried out toward the pelvic inlet. One should be cautious when in contact with the aorta as well as with the left iliac vessels where nerve rami of the superior hypogastric sympathetic plexus courses.

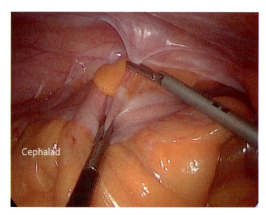

FIGURE 10 • Lateral dissection of left sigmoid colon attachments.

DISSECTION OF THE RECTUM ACCORDING TO THE PRINCIPLES OF THE TOTAL MESORECTAL EXCISION

- The principle of total mesorectal excision (TME) is respected.
- TME aims to eradicate the primary tumor and its lymphatic drainage by "en bloc" removal of the rectum and the mesorectum, along well-defined anatomical planes. A TME dissection proceeds under direct vision along the areolar tissue plane situated between the mesorectal fascia anteriorly and the presacral fascia posteriorly, the lateral pelvic fascia laterally, and Denonvilliers' fascia (rectovaginal space) anteriorly. A sharp dissection technique along these planes is associated with a higher probability of achieving a negative circumferential resection margin (CRM), a lower risk of bleeding from inadvertent tearing of the presacral veins, and a reduced risk of injuring the hypogastric nerves.
- A proper surgical intervention cannot be carried out without a detailed knowledge of the pelvic anatomy (**FIGURE 11**) and is essential to obtain a curative resection.

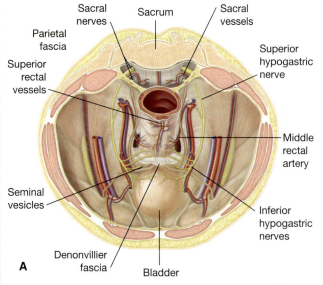

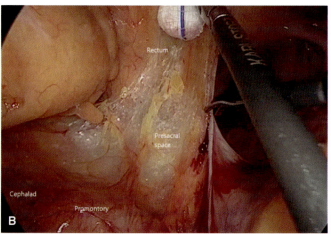

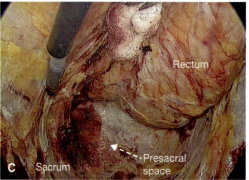

FIGURE 11 • Pelvic anatomy. **A,** Schematic description of pelvic anatomy. **B,** Presacral space opening and posterior rectal dissection. **C,** Surgical view of the holy plane between the presacral fascia and fascia propria of the rectum.

Chapter 30 LOW ANTERIOR RECTAL RESECTION: LAPAROSCOPIC TECHNIQUE   259

- In the case of a female patient, the suspension of the uterus facilitates the exposure and the dissection. If the patient had a previous hysterectomy, the dissection can be facilitated by the introduction of a vaginal bougie.

- The dissection is done in this order: posterior plane first, then the lateral dissection, starting with the right side facing the optic, the left side, and, finally the anterior dissection.

POSTERIOR DISSECTION OF THE RECTUM

- A cranial and anterior traction is exerted on the sigmoid rectal junction to expose the posterior aspect of the upper rectum.
- The presacral space (**FIGURE 11B** and **C**) is opened under the effect of traction and of pneumoperitoneum pressure. It is facilitated by the atraumatic anterior retraction of the posterior rectal wall exposing the space between the presacral fascia and the posterior aspect of the mesorectum, which is then dissected.

- Dissection should be continued toward the pelvic floor on the midline, until the presacral fascia fuses with the fascia propria (Waldeyer's fascia).
- The dissection is done in contact with but always outside the mesorectal fascia. The presacral space is avascular. There is little hemostasis to be done of a few small vessels which are coagulated and some branches of the hypogastric plexus for rectal use which are sectioned.
- The lateral pelvic fascia protects the main branches of the plexus along the pelvic side walls (**FIGURE 12A**).
- To complete the dissection, the recto-sacral ligament is transected at the level of the levators. This level will be completed after the end of the anterior dissection.

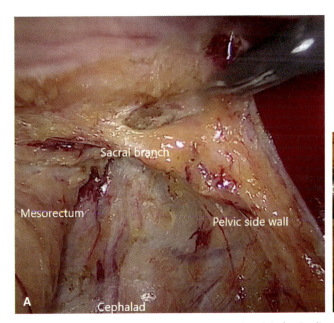

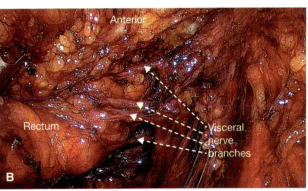

FIGURE 12 • Pelvic lateral dissection. **A**, Lateral pelvic fascia dissection and sacral branch dissection. **B**, The rectal branches of the inferior hypogastric plexus traverse along the so-called lateral rectal ligament. The lateral rectal ligament on the right side of the distal rectum has been skeletonized. The visceral nerve branches to the rectum and prostate originating from the lateral inferior hypogastric plexus trunk can be seen.

LATERAL DISSECTION OF THE RECTUM

- Lateral dissection is begun on the right side.
- The rectum is retracted cranially and medially to expose the lateral pelvic space.
- The right peritoneum is incised until seminal vesicles are reached (in male patients). Under the effect of pneumoperitoneum pressure and of medial retraction, parietalization of the inferior hypogastric plexus and especially of the sacral branches (3rd and 5th sacral nerves, parasympathetic nerves responsible for male erections) is carried out. Care is taken to avoid violating the parietal endopelvic fascia.

- Between three and five nerve branches can be observed crossing the space between the fascia and the rectum. These branches will be divided after skeletonization in order to preserve the trunks and prostatic branches as much as possible (**FIGURE 12B**).
- The LigaSure device allows a safe dissection.
- Middle rectal arteries are present in approximately 20% of patients and may be encountered during this dissection. These vessels can easily be taken using electrocautery, with Ligasure device or any other energy device.
- Once the right dissection is completed, the peritoneum is incised on the left side. The left-sided lateral dissection is

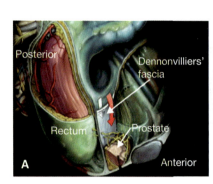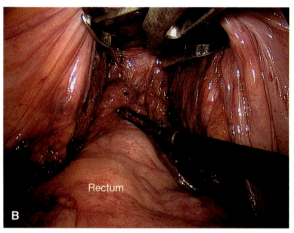

FIGURE 13 • Denonvilliers' fascia dissection. **A,** Schematic description of the anterior or posterior dissection of the Denonvilliers' fascia. **B,** Laparoscopic view of Denonvilliers' fascia adequately exposed by anterior retraction of the prostate.

performed in a similar fashion. The rectum is retracted cranially and toward the right side of the surgical for the left lateral dissection.
- During the deep lateral dissection, care must be taken to avoid an extensive dissection because the deepest areas seem superficial, especially as the pneumoperitoneum opens the space. Below the rectosacral ligament, which is not readily apparent in elderly patients, the curvature of the sacrum is in front of the view and care must be taken to dissect vertically along the levator muscles and not in the axis of the optic with the risk of transecting the rectococcygeal ligaments and expose the coccyx and presacral veins.

ANTERIOR DISSECTION OF THE RECTUM

- The last step of the rectal mobilization is the anterior dissection.
- The peritoneum is incised on the Douglas pouch on the relief of the seminal vesicles, 1 to 2 cm above the base of the Douglas pouch. The incision will join the previous lateral opening.
- In order to open and dissect the space between the anterior aspect of the rectum and Denonvilliers' aponeurosis, minimal cranial and posterior traction should be maintained on the rectum; Denonvilliers' aponeurosis should be retracted anteriorly.
- Retraction is usually easy to perform in female patients. In male patients, especially obese ones, this step is more difficult. Retraction is done using atraumatic graspers. Specific retractors developed by KARL STORZ (Endo-Retractors) exist in order to reproduce the technique used in open surgery with the St. Mark's retractor. It involves a three-directional retraction described by Heald's (3-D retraction), which ensures a safe dissection of the anterior aspect of the rectum.
- The plane of anterior dissection can be carried out either anterior or posterior to Denonvilliers' aponeurosis (**FIGURE 13A** and **B**). In advanced rectal cancer, it may be necessary to stay anterior to Denonvilliers' aponeurosis entering the latero prostatic space; in this case, the risk of injury of the neurovascular bundles of Walsh is much higher (impotence). Posterior tumors do not require Denonvilliers' fascia to be included in the specimen.
- The same problem can happen in female patients with the dissection of rectovaginal space.
- The dissection is carefully continued to the pelvic floor.
- The sacrorectal ligaments and the last attachments of the rectum are transected.

PELVIC DISSECTION, LOWER RECTUM DIVISION

- Sharp dissection in the avascular areolar plane is completed at the lower aspect of the mesorectum, 2 to 3 cm above the anorectal junction.
- The lower rectum should be completely dissected circumferentially and all the attachments are freed. Once the lower rectum is completely free, the level of rectal transection is confirmed with digital rectal or endoscopic examination.
- The rectum is then transected using a linear stapler introduced in the trocar placed in the right iliac fossa.
- We usually use an Endo-Gia with Tri-Staple technology (Medtronic), purple cartridge 30 mm or 45 mm.
- In difficult cases, the stapler can be introduced through the suprapubic port.
- Ideally, not more than two stapler applications should be applied to reduce the risk of anastomotic leak.
- Once the transection is performed, the staple line should be inspected and the rectal stump sealing tested by the injection of a Betadine solution.

Chapter 30 LOW ANTERIOR RECTAL RESECTION: LAPAROSCOPIC TECHNIQUE

PROXIMAL DIVISION, SPECIMEN EXTRACTION

- The suprapubic incision is enlarged without muscles division. A wound protector is placed (**FIGURE 14**).
- The specimen is exteriorized. The mesocolon is transected with the energy device (Ligasure). The proximal transection point of the colon is identified. A purse-string clamp is applied and the proximal colon is transected with scissors. The aspect and vascularization of proximal colon is verified. If available, the vascularization can be confirmed by fluorescence imaging injecting indocyanine green (ICG) (**FIGURE 15**).
- The anvil of a circular stapler is placed in the proximal colon and the purse-string is closed.
- The proximal colon with the anvil is then introduced in the abdominal cavity. The pneumoperitoneum is inflated. The anastomosis is performed under laparoscopic assistance using a Knight-Griffen technique with a circular stapler introduced transanally. It is important to verify the absence of tension on the descending colon to achieve a tension-free anastomosis. Before stapling, the absence of colon/mesocolon twisting should be verified. The anastomosis is performed. Two intact full-thickness doughnuts (colic and rectal) should be obtained and verified. The anastomosis is then tested with an air leak test or by means of an intraoperative endoscopy (**FIGURE 16**).
- After TME, the most widely used reconstructive technique is straight coloanal anastomosis. However, because the sigmoid colon is usually excised during surgery, which decreases the storage volume of stool, there is a common problem seriously influencing the life quality of patients, including increased tool frequency, urgency, and incontinence, which is termed as "anterior resection syndrome (ARS)." About 19% to 56% of patients would suffer from ARS. Thus, the demand for a technique with better functional outcomes made surgeons modify the straight anastomotic technique.

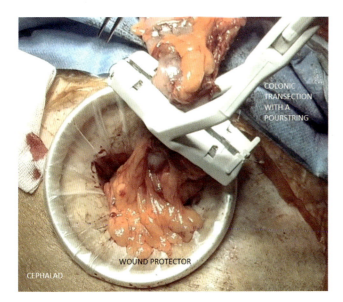

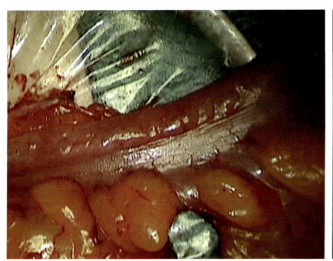

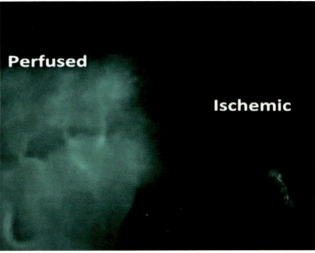

FIGURE 14 • External operative view: abdominal wall protection with a wound protector.

FIGURE 15 • Colonic perfusion evaluation by Fluorescence imaging.

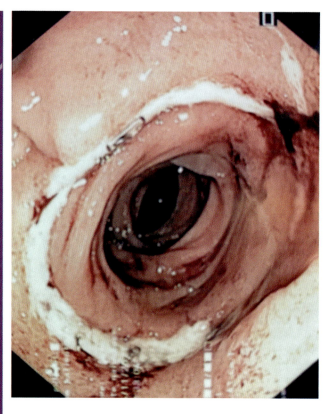

FIGURE 16 • Intraoperative endoscopy: inspection and testing of the anastomosis integrity.

ANASTOMOSIS TECHNIQUES

Knight-Griffen With Circular Stapler

- **Straight end to end colorectal anastomosis (FIGURE 17):** the anvil is introduced in a terminal fashion in the colonic opening and a purse string is performed to ensure the sealing.
- **Side to end colorectal anastomosis (FIGURE 18):** in case of very low anastomosis, the anvil is introduced in the colic lumen and comes out laterally at the level of the colic tenia in order to perform the side-to-end anastomosis. This is the first easy option in case of very low anastomosis representing an alternative to colonic J-pouch.
- **Colonic J-pouch (FIGURE 19):** in case of ultra-low anastomosis (colo-sus anal or colo-anal), a J-pouch can be performed. Colonic J-pouch was introduced by Lazorthes and

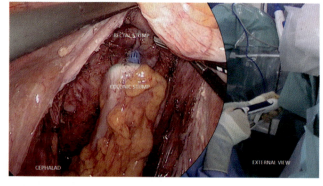

FIGURE 17 • Laparoscopic view of a straight-to-end colorectal anastomosis according to Knight and Griffen.

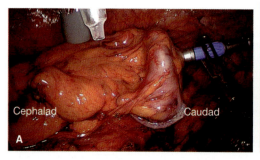
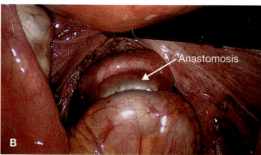

FIGURE 18 • Side to end colorectal anastomosis. **A**, The anvil of the circular stapler is placed laterally on the antimesenteric border of the colonic segment. **B**, Laparoscopic view of the intracorporeal side to end anastomosis, performed with a 28-mm EEA circular stapler.

Parc in 1986. Usually a 5 cm-long colonic segment was considered as the optimum size of the J-pouch but in some patients with a narrow pelvis or bulky mesentery, however, is not possible to perform it. The currently limited evidence suggests that colonic J-pouch and side-to-end anastomosis are comparable in terms of bowel functional outcomes, QoL, and surgical outcomes. Surgeons may choose either of the two techniques for anastomosis.

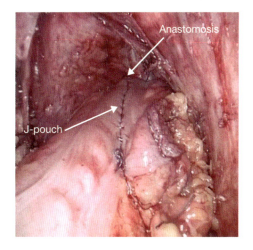

FIGURE 19 • Laparoscopic view of a colonic J-pouch colorectal anastomosis.

HAND-SEWN ANASTOMOSIS

- Hand-sewn anastomosis (**FIGURE 20**) is performed for ultra-low resections with or without intersphincteric resection. The descending colon is delivered into the pelvis and brought into position for a coloanal hand-sewn anastomosis. To pull down the colonic conduit, a laparoscopic grasper can be used or alternatively, tagging sutures can be placed into the proximal colon to guide the colonic conduit down. A self-retaining retractor is positioned to improve exposure and obtain adequate views of the anorectal stump wall. A one-layer (or two-layer) anastomosis is then fashioned using interrupted 3/0 resorbable sutures, as originally described by Sir Alan Parks. Each suture incorporates the mucosa of the anorectal cuff, a portion of the upper internal sphincter and full-thickness muscular layer of the colon.

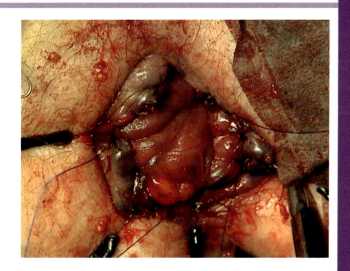

FIGURE 20 • Hand-sewn coloanal anastomosis.

PEARLS AND PITFALLS

Anatomy	■ Precise understanding of pelvic anatomy including fascia planes, autonomic nerves, pelvic floor anatomy, and muscular sphincter apparatus is critical in performing a proper LAR.
Preoperative	■ Accurate preoperative staging is crucial. ■ The distance between the inferior border of the tumor and the anorectal ring should be clearly determined and documented. ■ All rectal cancer cases should be discussed in a multidisciplinary team. ■ Multimodal therapy for rectal cancer is associated with a significant positive impact on long term functional and quality of life outcomes including risks for bowel, bladder, and sexual dysfunction and potential need for permanent colostomy.
Setup	■ Precise operating room (OR), patient, and team setup is critical to success.
Technique	■ A proper TME with sharp dissection along the visceral and parietal layers of the endovascular fascia facilitates margin-negative resection, reduces local recurrence, and limits nerve injury. ■ Medial to lateral dissection of the mesocolon is superior to a lateral to medial approach. ■ Splenic flexure mobilization is mandatory to perform a low colorectal anastomosis without tension and to reduce anastomotic leak rates. ■ TME principles must be observed at all times. ■ Pelvic dissection: ■ Posterior first ■ Lateral dissection/transection of the "lateral rectal ligaments": Avoid injury to autonomic trunks and genital nerve branches that would lead to autonomic dysfunction postoperatively
Perioperative care	■ Enhanced recovery program

POSTOPERATIVE CARE

- Postoperative care is driven by clinical pathways that include the following:
  - Pain control (score evaluation three times a day): 24 hours syringe pump (morphine 100 mg; Ketamine 50 mg; droperidol 5 mg). The transversus abdominis plane (TAP) nerve block greatly reduces the need for narcotics.
  - Deep vein thrombosis (DVT) prophylaxis with enoxaparin, starting within 6 hours of surgery and continued for 1 month postoperatively.
  - No additional antibiotics.
  - No nasogastric tube. Remove Foley catheter on postoperative day 1. Remove pelvic drains on postoperative day 2 or 3.
  - Early ambulation, normal diet, and aggressive pulmonary toilet.
  - Oral supplements three times a day during the first 3 POD.

OUTCOMES

- Recent multicenter trials show that laparoscopic total mesorectal excision is associated with more favorable short-term outcomes with no significant differences in terms of oncologic results as compared to open resection. Evaluation of adequate surgical resection, such as completeness of total mesorectal excision and negativity of circumferential and distal margins (CRM, DRM) associated with short- and long-term outcomes are similar when comparing laparoscopic surgery to open surgery for rectal cancer.
- TME with an intact mesorectum is critical to minimize locoregional treatment failures leading to a reduction in locoregional recurrence rates from 25% in the 1980s to under 4% today.

COMPLICATIONS

- Anastomotic leak
- Bleeding
- Surgical site infections
- Pelvic abscess
- Urinary/sexual dysfunction: It is important to preserve autonomic nerves intact

- Ureteral injury: critical to identify the left ureter prior to IMA transection
- DVT: lower risk with use of DVT prophylaxis
- Renal insufficiency in case of ileostomy high output

SUGGESTED READINGS

1. Cuna SA, Chesney TR, Ramjist JK, Shah PS, Kennedy ED, Baxter NN. Laparoscopic versus open resection for rectal cancer: a noninferiority meta-analysis of quality of surgical resection outcomes. *Ann Surg.* 2019;269(5):849-855.
2. Fleshman J, Branda ME, Sargent DJ, et al. Disease-free survival and local recurrence for laparoscopic resection compared with open resection of stage II to III rectal cancer: follow-up results of the ACOSOG Z6051 randomized controlled trial. *Ann Surg.* 2019;269(4):589-595.
3. Heald RJ, Husband EM, Ryall RD. The mesorectum in rectal cancer surgery the clue to pelvic recurrence? *Br J Surg.* 1982;69:613-616.
4. Hermanek P, Junginger T. The circumferential resection margin in rectal carcinoma surgery. *Tech Coloproctol.* 2005; 9(3): 193-199.
5. Kang SB, Park JW, Jeong SY, et al. Open versus laparoscopic surgery for mid or low rectal cancer after neoadjuvant chemoradiotherapy (COREAN trial): short-term outcomes of an open-label randomised controlled trial. *Lancet Oncol.* 2010;11(7):637-645.
6. Leonard D, Penninckx F, Fieuws S, et al. Factors predicting the quality of total mesorectal excision for rectal cancer. *Ann Surg.* 2010;252(6):982-988.
7. Martínez-Pérez A, Carra MC, Brunetti F, De'Angelis N. Pathologic outcomes of laparoscopic vs open mesorectal excision for rectal cancer: a systematic review and meta-analysis. *JAMA Surg.* 2017;152(4):e165665.
8. Penninckx F, Kartheuser A, Van de Stadt J, et al. Outcome following laparoscopic and open total mesorectal excision for rectal cancer. *Br J Surg.* 2013;100(10):1368-1375.
9. Stevenson ARL, Solomon MJ, Brown CSB, et al. Disease-free survival and local recurrence after laparoscopic- assisted resection or open resection for rectal cancer the Australasian laparoscopic cancer of the rectum randomized. *Clinical Trial.* 2019;269(4):596-602.
10. Stevenson AR, Solomon MJ, Lumley JW, et al. Effect of laparoscopic-assisted resection vs open resection on pathological outcomes in rectal cancer: the ALaCaRT randomized clinical trial. *JAMA.* 2015;314:1356-1363.
11. Tong G, Zhang G, Liu J, Zheng Z, Chen Y, Cui E. A meta-analysis of short-term outcome of laparoscopic surgery versus conventional open surgery on colorectal carcinoma. *Medicine (Baltim).* 2017;96(48):e8957.
12. van der Pas MH, Haglind E, Cuesta MA, et al. Laparoscopic versus open surgery for rectal cancer (COLOR II): short-term outcomes of a randomised, phase 3 trial. *Lancet Oncol.* 2013;14(3):210-218.

| Chapter | **31** | # Low Anterior Resection: Hand-Assisted Laparoscopic Surgery Technique |

Zhifei Sun and Matthew G. Mutch

DEFINITION

- Low anterior resection (LAR) is the full mobilization and resection of the rectum at the level of the levators, leaving behind only a short or no rectal stump.
- The hand-assisted laparoscopic surgery (HALS) technique uses a hand-assisted device that allows the surgeon to insert their hand into the peritoneal cavity while maintaining pneumoperitoneum. The location of the hand port is variable and is placed at the expected site of specimen extraction.
- HALS maintains all the short-term advantages of conventional laparoscopic surgery over open surgery.
- By reintroducing tactile feedback into the field, HALS results in higher laparoscopic usage rates, lower conversion rates, and shorter operative times, when compared to conventional laparoscopic surgery.

DIFFERENTIAL DIAGNOSIS

- The main indication for a HALS LAR is for the treatment of rectal cancer. Patients with diverticulitis with inflammation extending into the mesorectum may also require an LAR.

PATIENT HISTORY AND PHYSICAL FINDINGS

- A thorough history and a physical examination are necessary prior to initiation of therapy for patients with rectal cancers.
- It is important to identify the distance of the tumor from the anal verge. Digital rectal examination and rigid proctoscopy are used for this purpose and to determine whether the tumor is mobile, tethered, fixed, or involving the sphincter complex. These are important elements in determining whether the patient is a candidate for an LAR vs an abdominoperineal resection (APR). In addition, this may help determine the potential need for a multivisceral resection (pelvic exenteration) should the tumor be fixed to other pelvic organs on examination.
- Prior abdominal surgery is not a contraindication to HALS approach. If the patient has had prior surgery, an incision can be made at the site of the hand port, and if there are minimal adhesions, the hand port can be inserted. If the adhesions are prohibitive of the laparoscopic approach, the hand port incision can be extended into a full laparotomy incision for an open approach (described elsewhere in this textbook).

IMAGING AND OTHER DIAGNOSTIC STUDIES

- All patients with rectal cancer should have a complete colonoscopy prior to surgery. With the widespread use of neoadjuvant therapy, consider tattooing the lesion prior to initiating therapy. With a complete clinical response or significant downstaging, localization of the tumor can be difficult after neoadjuvant therapy.
- If the patient has an endoscopically obstructing lesion, a computed tomography (CT) colonography and a contrast enema study are acceptable alternatives to evaluate the proximal colon.
- Preoperative staging to rule out visceral and retroperitoneal lymph node metastases in the form of a CT scan of the chest and abdomen should be obtained.
- Preoperative staging of the primary tumor is paramount so the appropriate use of neoadjuvant therapy can be prescribed to help evaluate the need for an LAR vs an APR operation. This can be accomplished either by a rectal-protocol pelvic magnetic resonance imaging (MRI) or by a transrectal ultrasound. Both modalities provide greater accuracy than CT for assessing the depth of tumor invasion, the presence of regional nodal metastases, and the likelihood of a positive circumferential margin at the time of surgery. MRI provides superior evaluation of the circumferential resection margin as well as the potential need for a multivisceral resection (pelvic exenteration).
- Based on the preoperative T and N staging, the need for neoadjuvant therapy is determined. Typically, T3, T4, or N+ tumors receive neoadjuvant therapy, and the options include short-course radiation, long-course chemoradiation, or total neoadjuvant therapy with addition of chemotherapy. Surgical resection then occurs 6 to 8 weeks after completion of neoadjuvant therapy.

SURGICAL MANAGEMENT

Preoperative Planning

- Prior to the operating room, the patient should be marked for a possible diverting ileostomy. The patient needs to be assessed in the supine, sitting, and standing positions. The stoma should rest on the apex of skin fold and adequate distance from bony prominences, skin creases, and the waistline of their pants. The stoma should be brought through the rectus muscle to minimize the risk of developing a parastomal hernia.
- The use of ureteral stents at the time of surgery is left to the discretion of the surgeon.

Positioning

- The use of a mechanical bed that is able to place the patient in extreme gravity-assisted positions is necessary.
- There are many methods by which a patient can be secured to the bed. A beanbag, a nonslip pad, shoulder braces, or foam pads can be used for this purpose.
- The patient should be placed in a modified lithotomy position with Allen or Yellofin stirrups (**FIGURE 1**). This allows access between the legs to assist with mobilization of the left

265

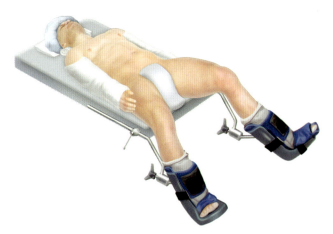

FIGURE 1 • Patient positioning. The patient is placed on a lithotomy position with the hips slightly flexed and the legs in Yellofin stirrups. The thighs are placed parallel to the ground to avoid interference with the surgeon's arms and instruments. The patient is secured to the table with tape applied over a towel across the chest. The arms are tucked to the sides. All pressure points are padded to avoid neurovascular injuries.

colon and to the perineum for the anastomosis. The thighs are placed parallel to the ground to avoid conflict with the surgeon's elbows during the surgery.

- Both arms are tucked to the patient's side with the thumbs facing up. This allows the surgeon, assistant, and camera driver plenty of room to maneuver during the case.
- A monitor should be placed off the patient's left shoulder during the mobilization of the left colon and splenic flexure. During the pelvic dissection, a monitor should be placed off the patient's left foot for the surgeon and another monitor should be placed off the patient's right foot for the assistant.

PORT PLACEMENT AND OPERATIVE TEAM SETUP

- There are several options for the position of the hand port:
  - The hand port can be placed through either a Pfannenstiel or a midline incision. The Pfannenstiel incision allows for greater space between the hand and instruments intracorporeally. It also has a lower incidence of incisional hernias and wound infections compared to the vertical midline incisions. It also allows for the direct visualization into the pelvis. The hand port can then be used to facilitate the rectal dissection, for division of the distal rectum, for the performance of the anastomosis, and to address any pelvic complications such as bleeding or anastomotic failure.
  - A vertical lower midline position for the hand port may be utilized if significant adhesions are anticipated or for patients with a BMI greater than 35. The incision can be conveniently extended to a full laparotomy if conversion to an open approach is needed.
  - The periumbilical position allows the surgeon to put their nondominant hand through the hand port.
  - A left lower quadrant (LLQ) position uses a muscle-splitting incision and allows for the right hand to be placed into the abdomen to facilitate the lateral and splenic flexure mobilizations of the left colon.
- For the purposes of this chapter, the suprapubic hand port position is discussed (**FIGURE 2**).
- The 5- or 12-mm camera port is placed in the supraumbilical position. The camera needs to be above the umbilicus, as the wound protector portion of the hand port

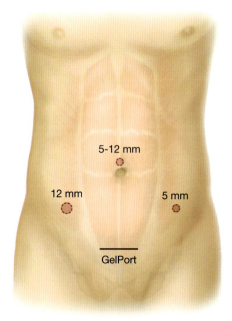

FIGURE 2 • Port placement. The GelPort is placed through a 5- to 6-cm Pfannenstiel incision. A 5- or 12-mm supraumbilical port is used for the camera. Two working ports, a 12-mm right lower quadrant port and a 5-mm left lower quadrant port, are inserted.

extends several centimeters beyond the edges of the incision.

- The primary laparoscopic working port (5-mm port) is placed in the right lower quadrant (RLQ), at an equal distance

between the hand port and the camera port and lateral to the rectus muscle.
- A 5-mm working port for the first assistant is placed in the LLQ. This will allow the assistant to help with the lateral and splenic flexure mobilization and the pelvic dissection. The lower the port is placed, the less time the assistant works in a reverse motion to the camera during the lateral and splenic flexure mobilization.
- The surgeon stands by the patient's right side with their right hand placed in the hand port. The camera operator stands to the left side of the surgeon. The assistant stands in between the patient's legs (**FIGURE 3**).

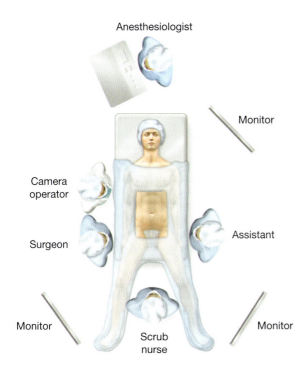

FIGURE 3 • Operating team setup. The surgeon stands by the patient' right side with their right hand placed in the hand port. The camera operator stands to the left side of the surgeon. The assistant stands by the patient's left side. The scrub nurse stands between the patient's legs. A monitor should be placed off the patient's left shoulder during the mobilization of the left colon and splenic flexure. During the pelvic dissection, a monitor should be placed off the patient's left foot for the surgeon and another should be placed off the patient's right foot for the assistant.

TRANSECTION OF THE INFERIOR MESENTERIC ARTERY

- The patient is placed in a steep Trendelenburg position and in an airplane position with the left side up to use gravity to place the small bowel in the right upper quadrant and the omentum in the upper abdomen to expose the transverse colon and splenic flexure. This helps to expose the inferior mesenteric artery (IMA) at its origin off the aorta and the inferior mesenteric vein (IMV) at the level of the ligament of Treitz.
- The surgeon's right hand is placed through the hand port and an energy source is placed through the RLQ working port.
- The retroperitoneum is accessed at the level of the sacral promontory. The superior hemorrhoidal artery is grasped and elevated (**FIGURE 4**). A wide incision is made in the peritoneum dorsal to this artery; the wider the incision, the more the artery can be elevated to obtain better exposure. Because of the curve of the pelvis at this point, the sigmoid mesentery curves up and away from the visual field. Therefore, the retroperitoneal plane is higher than expected, so the more mobile the arterial pedicle is, the easier it is to visualize the correct plane.
- Identification of the left ureter is necessary before the IMA can be ligated (**FIGURE 5**). The following text is a four-step algorithm to identify the left ureter.
    - Mobilization of the superior hemorrhoidal artery is as described earlier and the left ureter is identified.
    - At the level of the IMV, the IMV is grasped and elevated. The peritoneum is incised dorsal to the IMV and the retroperitoneum is accessed. The retroperitoneum is flat in this area and is often more easily accessed. Once in the correct plane, the dissection is carried in a caudad fashion to meet up with the initial plane under the superior hemorrhoidal artery.
    - If the left ureter is still not identified, the sigmoid and left colon is mobilized in a lateral to medial fashion.
    - Finally, the top of the hand port can be removed, and the left ureter can be located via an open fashion.
- After the left ureter is identified and swept into the retroperitoneum, the IMA can be isolated at its origin (**FIGURE 6**). The index finger elevates the superior rectal hemorrhoidal and the middle finger is used to sweep down the retroperitoneum along the course of the IMA. This motion continues until the bare area is exposed cephalad to the IMA and medial to the IMV.

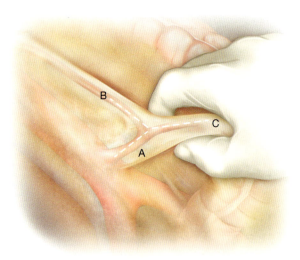

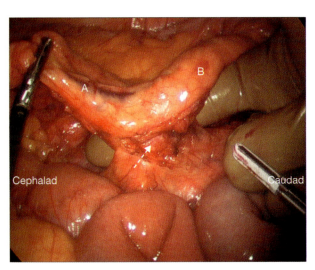

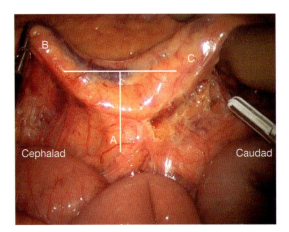

FIGURE 4 • Identification of inferior mesenteric artery (IMA) and its branches. Identify the "letter T" formed between the IMA (A) and its left colic artery (B) and superior hemorrhoidal artery (SHA) (C) terminal branches. The IMA takeoff is just cephalad from the aortic bifurcation. The thumb and index finger are lifting the SHA off the groove located anterior to the right common iliac artery.

FIGURE 6 • Circumferential dissection of the inferior mesenteric artery (IMA). After the left ureter has been identified, the IMA (arrow) is circumferentially dissected at its origin of the aorta. Again, the "letter T" formed between the IMA and its terminal branches, the left colic artery (A) and the superior hemorrhoidal artery (B), can be clearly identified.

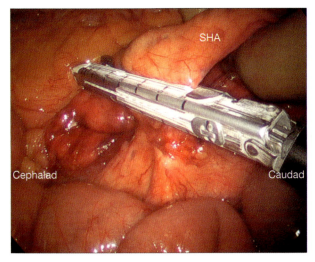

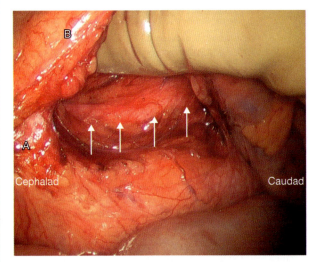

FIGURE 5 • Identification of the left ureter. After the inferior mesenteric artery (IMA) (A) and superior hemorrhoidal artery (B) have been lifted off the retroperitoneum, the left ureter (arrows) can be identified and preserved. Identification of the left ureter at this stage is critical in order to avoid injuring the ureter during the IMA transection.

FIGURE 7 • Transection of the inferior mesenteric artery (IMA). With the left ureter safely dissected away into the retroperitoneum, the IMA is transected with a linear vascular stapler at its origin of the aorta. The surgeon's hand is holding the superior hemorrhoidal artery (SHA) anteriorly.

- It is important to sweep down the retroperitoneal tissue in this area to help preserve the sympathetic plexus around the IMA. Once the IMA is safely isolated and the left ureter is clearly out of harm's way, the vascular pedicle can be ligated at its origin from the aorta with the surgeon's energy source of choice or with a linear stapler with a vascular cartridge (**FIGURE 7**).

TRANSECTION OF THE INFERIOR MESENTERIC VEIN

- The IMV courses parallel to the left colic artery. The previous IMA dissection plane is carried cephalad with Endo Shears and 5-mm energy device (sweeping the retroperitoneal tissues dorsally) until the left colic artery separates from the IMV as it courses toward the splenic flexure at the level of the ligament of Treitz.
- Now that the IMV is elevated off the retroperitoneum, it is isolated at the inferior border of the pancreas and near the ligament of Treitz (**FIGURE 8**). It can be isolated with the same technique used for the IMA: The index finger and the thumb elevate and create tension on the IMV and the middle finger and/or dissecting instrument sweeps the retroperitoneum dorsally along the course of the vein (**FIGURE 9**).
- A bare area is then created near the inferior border of the pancreas that allows the IMV to be safely isolated.
- Once isolated, the IMV can be safely transected with an energy device (**FIGURE 10**). The IMV should be transected cephalad to the left colic artery in order to preserve the marginal artery blood supply to the descending colon intact.

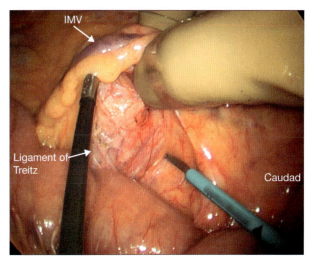

FIGURE 9 • Dissection of the inferior mesenteric vein (IMV). With the surgeon holding the IMV anteriorly, the retroperitoneal tissues are swept down (dorsally).

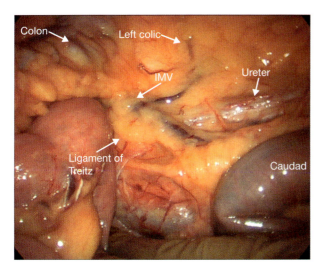

FIGURE 8 • Identification of the inferior mesenteric vein (IMV). The IMV can be identified at the root of the transverse/descending mesocolon at the level of the ligament of Treitz. At this level, the IMV has separated from the left colic artery (which courses away from the IMV and toward the splenic flexure of the colon) and from the left ureter.

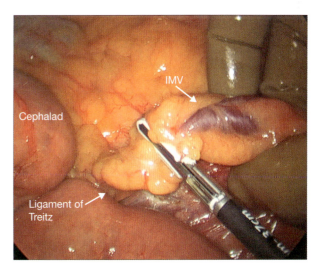

FIGURE 10 • Inferior mesenteric vein (IMV) transection. The IMV is transected with an energy device at the level of the IMV, cephalad of the left colic artery. This preserves the marginal artery of Drummond and ensures excellent blood supply to the descending colon segment for the anastomosis.

MOBILIZATION OF THE LEFT COLON

- The left colon mesentery is now dissected off the retroperitoneum using a medial to lateral dissection approach (**FIGURE 11**) all the way out to the lateral abdominal wall.
- The hand is placed palm down under the mesentery to elevate it as a fan-type retractor. The plane is dissected bluntly with an energy device from the sigmoid colon up to the splenic flexure. The further laterally and superiorly the dissection is carried, the easier the lateral dissection and splenic flexure mobilization will be later during the case. Care must be taken during mobilization near the inferior border of the pancreas, as it is very easy to carry the dissection deep to the pancreas.
- All that remains at this point are the lateral attachments. The hand is used to depress the sigmoid colon and lateral peritoneum is incised (**FIGURE 12A**). It is not uncommon for the hand to get in that way at this point, so it may be necessary to pass the energy source through the surgeon's fingers or the hand may be taken out and an instrument can be passed through the hand port to begin the dissection.
- Once the medial plane of dissection is accessed, the hand can be passed in the opening and the lateral attachments are elevated and exposed (**FIGURE 12B**). At this point, the surgeon uses a grasper for exposure and the first assistant uses the energy source through the LLQ port.

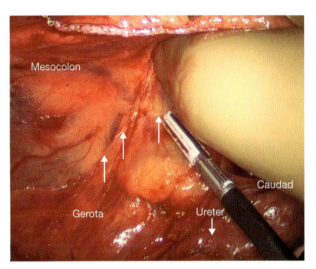

FIGURE 11 • Medial to lateral dissection. With the surgeon holding the mesocolon anteriorly (notice the stapled transected inferior mesenteric artery stump in between the surgeon's fingers), the retroperitoneal tissues are swept downward (dorsally) with an energy device. The dissection progresses along the transition of the two fat planes: mesocolon and Gerota (*arrows*).

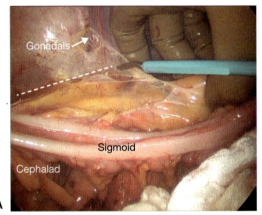
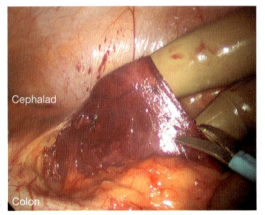

FIGURE 12 • Lateral mobilization of the sigmoid and descending colon. **A**, The white line of Toldt (*dotted line*) is transected with an energy device. **B**, The medial to lateral dissection plane is readily entered, greatly facilitating the lateral mobilization of the descending colon.

MOBILIZATION OF THE SPLENIC FLEXURE

- As the splenic flexure is reached, a transition to separate the omentum from the transverse colon must be made. The surgeon's hand reflects the colon downward and the grasper elevates the omentum in a vertical fashion. Only the peritoneum is divided moving along the transverse colon. Eventually, the lesser sac is entered.
- Once the peritoneum attaching the omentum to the transverse colon has been divided to the extent of the dissection, the next layer of attachments of the omentum and the transverse colon mesentery can be divided. The gastrocolic ligament is transected in this way medial to lateral until the splenic flexure is reached (**FIGURE 13**).
- Returning to the splenic flexure, the colon is grasped laterally with the hand and medially with a grasper. The colon is put on stretch and pulled down and medial to identify the next level of attachment between the splenic flexure of the colon and the diaphragm and spleen. The splenodiaphragmatic

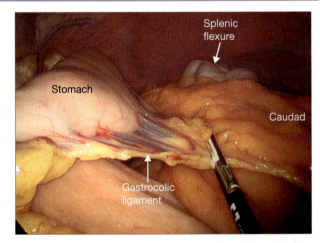

FIGURE 13 • Transection of the gastrocolic ligament. After entering the lesser sac (between the stomach and the transverse colon), the gastrocolic ligament is transected from medial to lateral (toward the splenic flexure of the colon) with an energy device.

and splenocolic ligaments are then transected with an energy device (**FIGURE 14**).
- All that remains are the posterior attachments to the inferior border of the pancreas. Division of these attachments to the midline allows for a full mobilization of the splenic flexure. This ensures adequate reach of the proximal colon for a tension-free anastomosis.

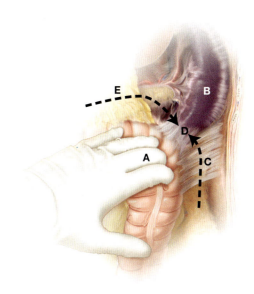

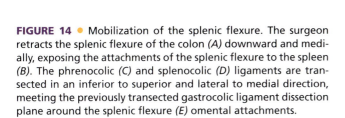

FIGURE 14 • Mobilization of the splenic flexure. The surgeon retracts the splenic flexure of the colon *(A)* downward and medially, exposing the attachments of the splenic flexure to the spleen *(B)*. The phrenocolic *(C)* and splenocolic *(D)* ligaments are transected in an inferior to superior and lateral to medial direction, meeting the previously transected gastrocolic ligament dissection plane around the splenic flexure *(E)* omental attachments.

THE PELVIC DISSECTION AND DISTAL RECTAL TRANSECTION

- The pelvic dissection can be performed with either the hand used as a retractor, straight laparoscopically, or open through the suprapubic hand port.
- Conceptually, the rectum and the mesorectum form a cylinder within the cylinder of the pelvis. This means the lines of dissection are circular and the ability to provide 360° exposure is necessary.
- The directions of retraction are anterior, posterior, medial, and lateral, with the goal being to make the plane of dissection perpendicular to the energy source. Avoid pulling the rectum and mesorectum out of the pelvis, as this does not optimize the exposure and space within the pelvis.
- The posterior dissection is performed first. The surgeon stands on the patient's right side with their right hand placed in the abdomen. With the thumb rotated medially and the palm up, the mesorectum is elevated and the presacral plane is entered (**FIGURE 15A**). Care is taken to identify and preserve the right and left hypogastric nerves.
- As the hand moves deeper into the pelvis, the fingertips are able to determine and expose the proper line of dissection. The mesorectum should be retracted anteriorly and not pulled out of the pelvis. The goal is to make the plane of dissection perpendicular to the energy source that is dividing the tissue.
- As the dissection proceeds on the right, posterior, and left, the hand subtly rotates the mesorectum to keep the plane of dissection perpendicular.

- Early on in the dissection, it is important to incise the peritoneum lateral to the rectum and mesorectum (Douglas pouch). The division should be carried all the way down to the peritoneal reflection. This helps to facilitate the lateral dissection and avoid carrying the lateral dissection too wide, minimizing the risk of injury to the parasympathetic nerves.
- The lateral dissection follows, with transection of the lateral rectal ligaments (**FIGURE 15B**).
- The posterior and lateral dissections are carried out down to the pelvic floor. All fat needs to be cleared off the levator muscles at the pelvic floor.
- The anterior peritoneal reflection is incised, with the hand retracting the uterus and cervix or prostate anteriorly. For the anterior dissection, the first assistant retracts the rectum posteriorly and rotates the direction of retraction as the dissection proceeds along Denonvilliers' fascia and behind the prostate/seminal vesicles in men (**FIGURE 15**) or the vagina in women. Once again, the assistant should avoid pulling the rectum out of the pelvis, as this does not optimize exposure and space within the narrow confines of the pelvis.
- For a tumor of the upper rectum, a tumor-specific mesorectal excision can be performed with a 5-cm distal margin. For a tumor of the mid to lower rectum, a total mesorectal excision should be performed.
- The rectum can then be stapled and divided with a linear stapler through the open hand port. This allows the rectum to be divided with a single firing of the stapler.

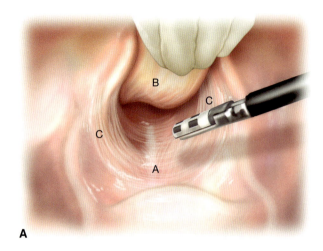
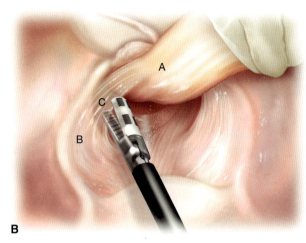
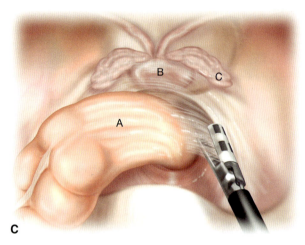

FIGURE 15 • Pelvic dissection. **A,** The posterior dissection is performed first, and it is carried in between the presacral fascia posteriorly *(A)*, the investing fascia of the mesorectum anteriorly *(B)*, and the endopelvic fascia laterally *(C)*. **B,** Transection of the lateral rectal ligaments follows. Dissection of the space between the rectum *(A)* and the lateral pelvic wall *(B)* anterior to the rectal ligament exposes the left lateral rectal ligament *(C)*, which can then be easily transected with the energy device. **C,** The anterior dissection is carried last. In men, the dissection is carried between the rectum posteriorly *(A)* and the prostate *(B)* and seminal vesicles *(C)* anteriorly.

EXTRACORPOREAL PROXIMAL TRANSECTION

- The rectum and colon can then be extracted through the hand port and the proximal site of division of the colon can be selected. For rectal cancer, the ligated IMA pedicle should be resected with the specimen to ensure an adequate lymph node harvest.
- The colon is divided proximally at the desired level between clamps. The specimen is now completely disconnected.
- Once the specimen is removed, it should be inspected and the quality of the mesorectal excision (complete, near complete, incomplete) should be noted and documented.

ANASTOMOSIS

- If an end-to-end anastomosis (EEA) will be constructed, a purse string is then created, and the EEA stapling anvil is placed in the open proximal colotomy. If a side-to-end anastomosis will be constructed, the EEA anvil is introduced through the open end of the descending colon and is exteriorized with the spear through an antimesenteric location in the descending colon approximately 5-cm proximal to the open end of the colon. The open end of the colon is then closed with a linear stapler.
- The type of reconstruction of the neorectum is left up to the discretion of the surgeon. Options include a colonic J-pouch, coloplasty, Baker-type anastomosis, and straight colorectal/coloanal anastomosis.

Chapter 31 LOW ANTERIOR RESECTION: HAND-ASSISTED LAPAROSCOPIC SURGERY TECHNIQUE 273

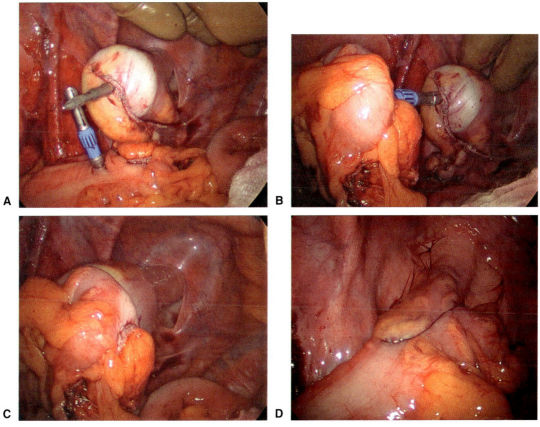

FIGURE 16 • An intracorporeal side-to-end colorectal anastomosis. **A,** The anvil of the end-to-end anastomosis (EEA) stapler is in antimesenteric location in the distal descending colon. The spear of the EEA stapler can be seen protruding through the rectal stump. **B,** The anvil and the spear of the EEA stapler have been mated. **C,** While the EEA stapler is fired, care is taken to avoid getting the bladder (or vagina) trapped in the stapler. **D,** The completed side-to-end colorectal anastomosis is tension-free and has excellent blood supply.

- Once the stapling cartridge is passed transanally to the top of the rectal stump, the spike is deployed and the anvil is reassembled. This can be performed either laparoscopically (**FIGURE 16A-D**) or open through the hand port. As the stapler is closed, ensure that the posterior wall of the vagina or the seminal vesicles is free from the stapler.
- The anastomosis should be assessed by inspecting the anastomotic doughnuts and by performing an air leak test (**FIGURE 17**) or endoscopic visualization of the anastomosis.
- A drain may be placed to drain whatever blood or fluid accumulates in the pelvis to minimize fibrosis of the neorectum.

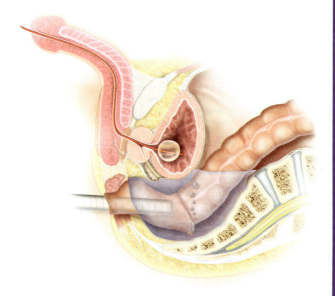

FIGURE 17 • Air leak test. The anastomosis is tested under water. The presence of air bubbles would indicate an anastomotic disruption and should trigger a revision of the anastomosis.

CLOSURE OF THE ABDOMEN

- All 12-mm port fascial sites should be closed. The 5-mm port fascial sites do not need to be closed. Skin incisions are closed with subcuticular closure.
- The hand port can be closed with either interrupted or running stitch of no. 1 polydioxanone suture.
- The indication for a diverting stoma is left at the discretion of the surgeon.

PEARLS AND PITFALLS

Indications	■ A complete history and review of preoperative staging is necessary to determine the need for neoadjuvant therapy. ■ The distance of the tumor to the anorectal ring needs to be clearly determined and documented. ■ T4 tumors, or those where there is concern for involvement of the circumferential margin, should not be approached laparoscopically.
Placement of the hand port	■ The suprapubic position offers many advantages such as access to the pelvis to help with the dissection, division of the rectum, performance of the anastomosis, or management of bleeding or anastomotic complications.
Accessing the retroperitoneum	■ Different options include a medial approach, either at the level of the sacral promontory or at the IMV by the ligament of Treitz. Alternatively, a lateral approach can be used.
Identification of the left ureter	■ A four-step technique was described earlier. Alternating the approach not only facilitates identification of the ureter, it also helps to complete other steps of the procedure.
Mobilization of the splenic flexure	■ Extensive medial to lateral mobilization facilities splenic flexure mobilization. ■ Be patient when entering the lesser sac. ■ Incise the peritoneum fusing the omentum to the transverse colon and dissect the omentum off the backside of the mesentery one layer at a time. ■ It is useful to alternate dissection between the lateral and medial aspects of the splenic flexure during this step.
Pelvic dissection	■ Creating space in the pelvis can be challenging. As a result, it is a natural reaction to pull the hand out of the pelvis; the exact opposite is necessary. The hand needs to be deeper in the pelvis; exposure is created by flexing the fingers and leaving the palm in place. ■ Small changes in the direction of tension are vital for increasing exposure and efficiency of the dissection.

POSTOPERATIVE CARE

- The patient can begin a liquid diet on the day of surgery. The diet can be advanced as tolerated. Solid food can be safely provided before the resumption of bowel function.
- A urinary catheter should remain in place for several days postoperatively to minimize the risk of urinary retention.
- Patients can begin ambulation as early as the day of surgery and by postoperative day 1; they are to be encouraged to spend more time out of bed than in bed.
- A protocol for multimodal pain control including acetaminophen, nonsteroidal anti-inflammatory drugs, and gabapentin should be established in order to reduce opioid usage, accelerate recovery, and improve patient satisfaction.
- Venous thromboembolism (VTE) prophylaxis is important due to several risk factors (cancer diagnosis, pelvic dissection, lithotomy positioning, etc) associated with this operation. Low molecular weight heparin (LMWH), subcutaneous heparin, or pneumatic compression boots are all acceptable methods. There are data supporting the use of LMWH for 21 days postoperatively to decrease the risk of VTEs.
- The drain can be removed on postoperative day 4 regardless of the volume of the output, unless it is draining urine, stool, or pus.

OUTCOMES

- Laparoscopic techniques for rectal resection have been shown to be safe and are associated with earlier return of bowel function, lower analgesic requirements, and shorter length of hospital stay.

- Three early trials of laparoscopic vs open resection of rectal cancer (The Conventional vs Laparoscopic-Assisted Surgery in Colorectal Cancer [CLASICC], COlorectal cancer Laparoscopic or Open Resection [COLOR II], and Comparison of Open vs laparoscopic surgery for mid or low REctal cancer After Neoadjuvant chemoradiotherapy [COREAN]) demonstrated similar 3-year local recurrence and 5-year disease-free survival rates. Lymph node harvest and margin positivity were also similar; however, there was a slightly higher circumferential margin positive rate for laparoscopy observed in the CLASICC trial (16% vs 14%).
- Two recent trials (ACOSOG Z6051 and Effect of Laparoscopic-Assisted Resection vs Open Resection on Pathological Outcomes in Rectal Cancer [ALaCaRT]) did not demonstrate noninferiority of laparoscopy with regards to a composite endpoint of pathologic outcomes; however, midterm oncologic outcomes were similar.
- When HALS is compared to conventional laparoscopic-assisted colectomy, multiple prospective randomized trials have demonstrated no difference in short-term outcomes including length of stay, return of bowel function, or pain scores. Furthermore, HALS has been shown to decrease the operative time for a left colectomy by 33 minutes and a total abdominal colectomy by 57 minutes and the risk of conversion over straight laparoscopy as well as to significantly decrease conversion rates. Oncologically, data show comparable lymph node harvest and margin status between HALS and straight laparoscopic proctectomy.

Chapter 31 **LOW ANTERIOR RESECTION: HAND-ASSISTED LAPAROSCOPIC SURGERY TECHNIQUE** **275**

- In order to optimize perioperative and oncologic outcomes, laparoscopic rectal cancer resections should be performed by experienced surgeons in well-resourced settings. Cases where there is concern for circumferential margin or history of obstruction/perforation should undergo an open approach.

COMPLICATIONS

- Bleeding
- Anastomotic leak
- Wound infection
- Pelvic abscess
- Ureteral injury
- Urinary and/or sexual dysfunction
- Incomplete mesorectal dissection
- VTE
- Incisional hernia

SUGGESTED READINGS

1. Fleshman J, Branda M, Sargent DJ, et al. Effect of laparoscopic-assisted resection vs open resection of stage II or III rectal cancer on pathologic outcomes: the ACOSOG Z6051 randomized clinical trial. *J Am Med Assoc.* 2015;314(13):1346-1355.
2. Guillou PJ, Quirke P, Thorpe H, et al. Short-term endpoints of conventional versus laparoscopic-assisted surgery in patients with colorectal cancer (MRC CLASICC trial): multicentre, randomised controlled trial. *Lancet.* 2005;365(9472):1718-1726.
3. Jayne DG, Guillou PJ, Thorpe H, et al. Randomized trial of laparoscopic-assisted resection of colorectal carcinoma: 3-year results of the UK MRC CLASICC Trial Group. *J Clin Oncol.* 2007;25(21):3061-3068.
4. Liu FL, Lin JJ, Ye F, et al. Hand-assisted laparoscopic surgery versus the open approach in curative resection of rectal cancer. *J Int Med Res.* 2010;38(3):916-922.
5. Marcello PW, Fleshman JW, Milsom JW, et al. Hand-assisted laparoscopic vs. laparoscopic colorectal surgery: a multicenter, prospective, randomized trial. *Dis Colon Rectum.* 2008;51(6):818-826.
6. Orcutt ST, Marshall CL, Balentine CJ, et al. Hand-assisted laparoscopy leads to efficient colorectal cancer surgery. *J Surg Res.* 2012;177(2):e53-e58.
7. Orcutt ST, Marshall CL, Robinson CN, et al. Minimally invasive surgery in colon cancer patients leads to improved short-term outcomes and excellent oncologic results. *Am J Surg.* 2011;202(5):528-531.
8. Pendlimari R, Holubar SD, Pattan-Arun J, et al. Hand-assisted laparoscopic colon and rectal cancer surgery: feasibility, short-term, and oncological outcomes. *Surgery.* 2010;148(2):378-385.
9. Stevenson AR, Solomon MJ, Lumley JW, et al. Effect of laparoscopic-assisted resection vs open resection on pathological outcomes in rectal cancer: the ALaCaRT randomized clinical trial. *J Am Med Assoc.* 2015;314(13):1356-1363.
10. Targarona EM, Gracia E, Garriga J, et al. Prospective randomized trial comparing conventional laparoscopic colectomy with hand-assisted laparoscopic colectomy: applicability, immediate clinical outcome, inflammatory response, and cost. *Surg Endosc.* 2002;16(2):234-239.
11. Trastulli S, Cirocchi R, Listorti C, et al. Laparoscopic vs open resection for rectal cancer: a meta-analysis of randomized clinical trials. *Colorectal Dis.* 2012;14(6):e277-e296.
12. van der Pas MH, Haglind E, Cuesta MA, et al. Laparoscopic versus open surgery for rectal cancer (COLOR II): short-term outcomes of a randomised, phase 3 trial. *Lancet Oncol.* 2013;14(3):210-218. doi:10.1016/S1470-2045(13)70016-0

Chapter 32

Low Anterior Rectal Resection: Robotic-Assisted Laparoscopic Technique

Perisa Ruhi-Williams, Mehraneh Dorna Jafari, and Alessio Pigazzi

DEFINITION

- Low anterior resection (LAR) is most commonly performed for patients with mid to low non–sphincter-invading rectal cancer. A simple surgical definition of LAR is full mobilization and division of the rectum below the level of the anterior reflection.
- LAR for rectal cancer involves an oncological resection of the rectum with removal of the inferior mesenteric and mesorectal lymph nodes. The resection of the rectum includes a total mesorectal excision (TME) to ensure a radical resection with adequate radial margins.[1] The goal is to achieve an R0 (negative margins) en bloc resection of the cancer with complete dissection of the lymph nodes contained within the mesorectum.
- Robotic-assisted laparoscopic LAR is a surgical technique that allows for a minimally invasive approach to TME. Robotic LAR can be performed via a totally robotic or laparoscopic/robotic hybrid techniques. Our preferred method is a hybrid approach involving a laparoscopic medial to lateral mobilization of the colon and of the splenic flexure followed by a robotic TME.

MINIMALLY INVASIVE VS OPEN RESECTION FOR RECTAL CANCER

- There have been multiple studies that have examined minimally invasive techniques (laparoscopic, robotic-assisted) vs open resection for rectal cancer.
  - The COREAN trial, a large randomized controlled trial (RCT), demonstrated that laparoscopic resection provides similar outcomes for 3-year disease-free survival as open resection in locally advanced rectal cancer after preoperative chemoradiation.[2] Overall survival and local recurrence rate also did not differ significantly between the two groups.
  - The COLOR II trial, another large RCT, demonstrated similar rates of locoregional recurrence and disease-free and overall survival between laparoscopic resection and open surgery.[3] Of note, in low rectal lesions (<5 cm from anal verge), circumferential resection margin positivity (CRM+) was significantly lower in the laparoscopic resection group than in the open resection group (9% vs 22%, respectively).
  - Robotic TME is comparable to laparoscopic TME in retrospective reviews of this technique. However, some studies report lower conversion rates to open surgery compared to conventional laparoscopy.[4-8] The ROLARR trial, a large, international, multicenter RCT, demonstrated there were no significant differences in the rates of conversion to open laparotomy for robotic-assisted laparoscopic surgery compared with conventional laparoscopic surgery (8.1% vs 12.2%, respectively).[9] This trial also demonstrated that there were no significant differences in CRM+ between the two groups (6.2% in the conventional laparoscopic group

and 5.1% in the robotic-assisted laparoscopic group). Additionally, no statistically significant differences were noted for multiple secondary outcomes including intraoperative complications, postoperative complications, 30-day mortality, bladder dysfunction, and sexual dysfunction.

PATIENT HISTORY AND PHYSICAL FINDINGS

- A full history and physical examination will allow the surgeon to determine if a sphincter-sparing operation is possible, whether a temporary ileostomy is likely, and will also aid in discussions regarding postoperative functional status.
- History elements elicited should include baseline functional status, bowel incontinence, sexual function, urinary function, and pain with defecation or tenesmus. Previous history of pelvic radiation and pelvic surgery should also be noted.
  - History of incontinence should prompt discussions regarding postoperative quality of life with a low anastomosis.
  - History of pain or tenesmus suggests involvement of the anal sphincter or a larger tumor. This will alter the course of treatment, and a sphincter-sparing operation may not be possible in this subgroup of patients.
- Physical examination should include a digital rectal examination (DRE), vaginal examination, flexible sigmoidoscopy, and a thorough abdominal examination.
  - DRE should assess tumor size, degree of fixation to rectal and pelvic wall, mobility, location (anterior/posterior/lateral), distance from the anorectal ring, and anterior extension into vagina/prostate.
  - Anal sphincter involvement can also be determined by DRE in the majority of patients. Maneuvers such as squeeze can determine involvement.
  - Anterior rectal tumors in female patients require a vaginal examination to rule out extension into the vagina.
  - Flexible sigmoidoscopy should be utilized for patients with rectal cancer. This is to measure distance from anal verge, location, and rule out obstruction. Rigid proctoscopy is another tool that can be utilized; however, numerous studies have demonstrated flexible sigmoidoscopy to be superior with respect to patient comfort, diagnostic value, and ease of performing biopsy and polypectomy.[10-12]
  - The abdominal examination should evaluate for liver metastasis. A bilateral groin examination should be performed to evaluate for potential inguinal lymphadenopathy.

IMAGING AND OTHER DIAGNOSTIC STUDIES

- The physical examination in conjunction with endoscopy and imaging modalities will aid in the preoperative surgical evaluation and staging. This preoperative workup will dictate the best surgical approach, the need for temporary diversion, and the need for neoadjuvant therapy.

Table 1: Sensitivity and Specificity of Pelvic Magnetic Resonance Imaging (MRI) and Endoscopic Ultrasound (EUS) in Determining T Stage in TNM Staging System

	T1 Sensitivity (%)	T1 Specificity (%)	T2 Sensitivity (%)	T2 Specificity (%)	T3 Sensitivity (%)	T3 Specificity (%)	T4 Sensitivity (%)	T4 Specificity (%)
MRI	58	97	62	81	80	74	71	97
EUS	88	98	81	96	96	091	95	98

- Colonoscopy must be performed in all patients with rectal cancer:
  - This will allow for assessment of tumor location and pathology.
  - It will also serve to rule out and possibly remove any synchronous colonic lesions.
  - A scope should be able to pass the mass in order to confirm there is no impending obstruction.
  - Malignant synchronous lesions have been reported in 2% to 8% of cases and benign synchronous polyps in 13% to 62% of cases.[13-15]
  - If a colonoscopy has already been done by another provider, it is our preference to perform a flexible sigmoidoscopy in all patients for documentation of the size, location, and distance of the tumor from the anal sphincter complex.
- The use of preoperative tattoos in rectal cancer patients should not be performed. The best assessment of the margin is obtained via frequent and thorough digital examinations, intraoperative flexible endoscopy, and adherence to the best TME surgery criteria.
- Accurate staging of rectal cancer should be able to determine the depth of invasion, presence of lymph node metastases, and resectability of locally advanced tumors.
  - Pelvic magnetic resonance imaging (MRI) should be used in diagnosis for all rectal cancers.
    - The MERCURY and MERCURY II trials demonstrate that high-resolution pelvic MRI is an essential tool for evaluating the mesorectal fascia and intersphincteric plane for tumor invasion for low rectal cancers.[16,17]
    - A recent meta-analysis included 35 studies evaluating diagnostic performance of MRI in the staging of rectal cancer and/or assessment of mesorectal fascia status. The pooled sensitivities and specificities of pretreatment MRI in diagnosing tumors for each stage can be seen in **TABLE 1**.[18]
  - Endoscopic ultrasound (EUS) is another imaging modality that may be used in the workup of rectal cancer and is particularly useful in early lesions. EUS has an overall 80% to 95% staging accuracy (**TABLE 1**).[19] When compared to MRI in staging of rectal cancer, EUS is superior at differentiating early T1 and T2 lesions as MRI provides limited visualization of the submucosa.[20]
    - The ability to visualize the layers of the bowel wall allows for accurate T staging (**FIGURE 1**).
    - Detection of lymph node metastasis is associated with 73% sensitivity and 76% specificity.[21]
  - Computed tomography (CT) scan of the chest, abdomen, and pelvis should be obtained for preoperative evaluation metastases as per the National Comprehensive Cancer Network (NCCN) guidelines.[22] It is associated with 40% to 86% accuracy in staging rectal cancers.[16,23,24]

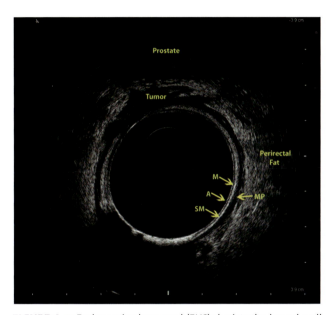

FIGURE 1 • Endoscopic ultrasound (EUS) depicts the bowel wall layers: *A* indicates balloon interface, *M* indicates mucosa/muscularis mucosa, *SM* indicates submucosa, and *MP* indicates muscularis propria. This patient has an anteriorly located tumor with invasion of the perirectal fat but no direct extension into the prostate (EUS T3).

- As per the NCCN guidelines, FDG-PET/CT should not replace contrast-enhanced CT or MRI. It should be reserved for cases of potentially surgically curable distant metastases.[22]

SURGICAL MANAGEMENT

Preoperative Planning

- Surgical decision is based on rectal cancer staging. As per the NCCN guidelines, neoadjuvant chemotherapy and radiation therapy (CRT) should be considered for all N+ positive tumors based on preoperative imaging.
- Neoadjuvant CRT has been shown to reduce the local recurrence rate and increase the chances of sphincter-sparing surgery in locally advanced rectal cancer.[22] A recent meta-analysis evaluated standard therapy consisting of chemoradiotherapy (CRT) followed by surgery and adjuvant chemotherapy compared to total neoadjuvant therapy (TNT) consisting of CRT plus neoadjuvant chemotherapy before surgery. TNT was associated with higher pathologic complete response (pooled prevalence 29.9% for the TNT group compared with 14.9% in the standard therapy group).[25] TNT is supported as an alternative treatment by the NCCN guidelines for locally advance rectal cancer.[9]

- The decision for preoperative therapy should stem from a multidisciplinary discussion among the surgeon, oncologist, radiation oncologist, and patient.
- An enterostomal therapist should be involved for counseling and for potential stomal marking prior to operation.
- In a 2019 publication to the Annals of Surgery in which the American College of Surgeons National Surgical Quality Improvement Program (ACS-NSQUIP) data were analyzed, combined mechanical bowel preparation and antibiotic bowel preparation was shown to significantly lower rates of surgical site infection (SSI), organ space infection, wound dehiscence, and anastomotic leak when compared to no bowel preparation in elective colorectal resections. The combined preparation also decreased SSI when compared to antibiotic bowel preparation alone.[26] As such, our institution's standard bowel preparation is two Dulcolax tablets, 510 gm of MiraLAX in 128 oz Gatorade, and neomycin and metronidazole 1 day before surgery.
- We also routinely allow patients to consume a low residue diet the night prior to surgery. A recently published randomized prospective trial demonstrated that patients who were allowed to consume a low residue diet the day prior to colonoscopy had superior bowel preparation quality to those who were restricted to a clear liquid diet.[27]
- A Foley catheter is placed in all patients after induction for bladder decompression.
- Prophylactic ceftriaxone and metronidazole are administered prior to induction of anesthesia. Prophylaxis with ertapenem is not routinely used as it may be associated with an increase in *Clostridium difficile* infection.[28]
- Sequential compression devices are placed in all patients. All patients also receive 5000 units of subcutaneous heparin preoperatively for venous thromboembolic prophylaxis. A 2016 RCT showed that bleeding complications were similar for patients undergoing major colorectal surgery who received preoperative vs postoperative chemical thromboprophylaxis.[29]

Positioning

- The patient is placed in a modified lithotomy position with attention placed to correct technique to minimize injury:
  - The patient is ideally placed on a large high-density viscoelastic foam mat to prevent sliding.
  - The patient is brought to the edge of the table and the legs are placed into Yellofin or Allen stirrups with the hips slightly flexed and abducted, the feet flat within the stirrups, and pressure avoided along the lateral aspects of the legs. The ankle, knee, and contralateral shoulder should be aligned.
  - A Velcro belt is strapped over the chest to prevent side-to-side sliding.
- The perineum is prepped if a transanal extraction and or hand-sewn anastomosis is anticipated.

TECHNIQUES

MEDIAL TO LATERAL DISSECTION OF COLON

Port Placement

- If performing the surgery totally robotically, ports are placed as follows:
  - Four robotic ports are placed along a diagonal line drawn from the right lower quadrant to the intersection of the left midclavicular line (MCL) and subcostal margin, each approximately 7 cm apart.
  - The port in the right lower quadrant is a 12-mm stapler port and may also be used as the stoma site.
- We prefer to perform a robotic-assisted laparoscopic procedure. Hybrid ports are placed as follows (**FIGURE 2**).
  - Pneumoperitoneum is established via a Veress needle at Palmer point (1-2 cm below the left costal border in the MCL).
  - The ports are triangulated and placed at a minimum of one handbreadth apart.

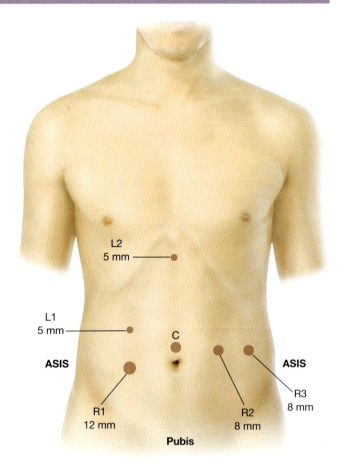

FIGURE 2 • Placement of hybrid ports. The camera (C) port is placed halfway between the xiphoid process and symphysis pubis. Three robotic (R) ports are placed as follows: R1 is a 12-mm trocar inserted in the midclavicular line (MCL) halfway in between C and the right anterior superior iliac spine. R2 is an 8-mm trocar inserted in the MCL to the left of C. R3 is an 8-mm trocar inserted 8 to 10 cm lateral to R2. Two laparoscopic-assisted (L) ports are placed as follows: L1 is a 5-mm trocar inserted in the MCL about 12 cm superior to R1. L2 is a 5-mm port inserted halfway between MCL and midline about 12 cm superior to L1.

Chapter 32 LOW ANTERIOR RECTAL RESECTION: ROBOTIC-ASSISTED LAPAROSCOPIC TECHNIQUE 279

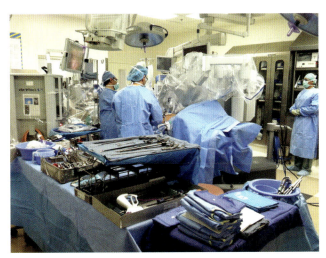

FIGURE 3 • Room setup with the robot docked from the left hip and surgeon and assistant surgeon on the right side of the patient.

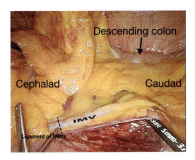

FIGURE 4 • The inferior mesenteric vein (IMV) is visualized lateral to the ligament of Treitz and is skeletonized. The IMV will then be transected just below the pancreas (*dotted line*).

- The camera (C) port is placed halfway between the xiphoid process and symphysis pubis.
- Three robotic (R) ports will be placed as follows:
  - R1 is a 12-mm trocar inserted in the MCL halfway in between C and the right anterior superior iliac spine. This port can be used for ileostomy placement at the end of the surgery.
  - R2 is an 8-mm trocar inserted in the MCL to the left of C.
  - R3 is an 8-mm trocar inserted 8 to 10 cm lateral to R2.
- Laparoscopic-assisted (L) ports (**FIGURE 2**):
  - L1 is a 5-mm trocar inserted in the MCL about 12 cm superior to R1.
  - L2 is a 5-mm port inserted halfway between MCL and midline about 12 cm superior to L1.
- Both surgeon and assistant stand on the right side of patient (**FIGURE 3**).
  - R1, L1, L2, and C ports are used during the laparoscopic section.

Transection of the Inferior Mesenteric Vein

- The peritoneal cavity is explored for evidence of metastatic disease.
- The patient is placed in a Trendelenburg position with the left side elevated.

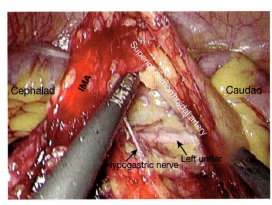

FIGURE 5 • The retroperitoneal plane dorsal to the superior hemorrhoidal artery is dissected. The inferior mesenteric artery (IMA) is identified and left ureter and hypogastric nerve are swept posteriorly.

- The small bowel is swept out of the pelvis. Nontraumatic bowel graspers are used to avoid injury.
- The dissection is begun at the inferior mesenteric vein (IMV), lateral to the ligament of Treitz (**FIGURE 4**).
- The IMV is identified and dissected from its attachments to the left mesocolon.
- The peritoneum is scored with monopolar electrocautery.
- Blunt dissection is used to skeletonize the vessel. Once this is achieved, the vessel is clipped and divided via vessel sealer device just below the pancreas. This can also be accomplished with an Endo GIA vascular stapler.
- Transection of the IMV will serve as a lengthening maneuver, which in turn will decrease tension on the anastomosis.

Transection of the Inferior Mesenteric Artery

- The sigmoid mesocolon is retracted toward the anterior abdominal wall, and the parietal peritoneum medial to the right common iliac artery at the sacral promontory is incised.
- Upward traction is maintained by the assistant and blunt dissection is used to enter the avascular retroperitoneal plane. This plane is developed under the superior hemorrhoidal artery (**FIGURE 5**).
- The left ureter and the hypogastric nerve are identified and swept posteriorly (**FIGURE 5**).
- This dissection is continued to the origin of the inferior mesenteric artery (IMA) at the aorta.
- The IMA is skeletonized using monopolar cautery. The junction of left colic artery and superior hemorrhoidal at the IMA can be visualized in a letter "T" configuration (**FIGURE 6A**).
- The IMA is clipped and divided at its origin from the aorta with a vessel sealer device (**FIGURE 6B**). This can also be accomplished via Endo GIA vascular stapler.
- The left colic artery is divided at its origin from the IMA (**FIGURE 6B**).
- Care is taken to avoid damage to the small nerve fibers of the preaortic sympathetic/superior hypogastric plexus.

Mobilization of the Left Colon and Splenic Flexure

- The assistant surgeon retracts the colon medially, and with a combination of cautery and blunt dissection, the lateral peritoneal reflections are dissected.

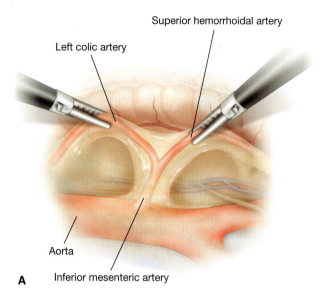
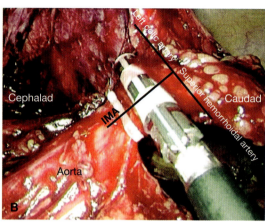

FIGURE 6 • **A,** The T configuration formed between the inferior mesenteric artery (IMA) *(A)* and its terminal branches, the left colic *(B)*, and the superior hemorrhoidal artery *(C)* is visualized. Notice the left ureter *(D)* dissected posteriorly in the retroperitoneum. **B,** The IMA is clipped and divided at its origin from the aorta with a vessel sealer device. The left colic artery will be transected at its origin from the IMA also with a vessel sealer device.

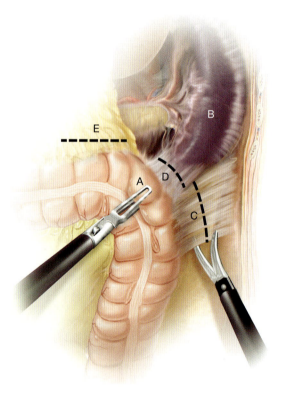

FIGURE 7 • Mobilization of the splenic flexure. The phrenocolic *(C)*, splenocolic *(D)*, and gastrocolic *(E)* ligaments are transected. *A,* splenic flexure of the colon; *B,* spleen.

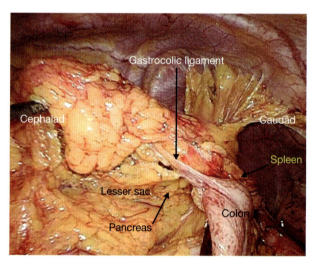

FIGURE 8 • Transection of the gastrocolic ligament allows for entry into the lesser sac during the splenic flexure mobilization. The dissection is carried to the base of the mesentery.

- The embryologic tissue plane between the descending colon mesentery and the retroperitoneum is entered. This bloodless areolar tissue plane is dissected toward the splenic flexure.
- The lateral dissection is continued cephalad by division of phrenocolic and splenocolic ligaments (**FIGURE 7**).
- The lesser sac is entered and the dissection is carried to the base of the mesentery (**FIGURE 8**).
- Care is taken to avoid injury to the tail of the pancreas in this location.
- The left and proximal transverse colon are now dissected free of their attachments allowing for greater length and decreased tension on the anastomosis.

ROBOTIC TOTAL MESORECTAL EXCISION

Robot Setup and Docking in Robotic-Assisted Laparoscopic Technique

- The patient is kept in a Trendelenburg position. A four-arm da Vinci robot is docked from a left hip approach (**FIGURES 3** and **9**). This will allow for easy access to the anus during the case.
- A 0° scope is inserted in port C.
- Robotic arms are docked as follows (**FIGURE 10**):
    - Arm 1 is docked in R1. A hook cautery or monopolar scissors will be inserted in R1.
    - Arm 2 is docked in R2. A bipolar grasper will be placed in R2.
    - Arm 3 is docked in R3. A "prograsper" will be placed in R3.
- The assistant surgeon will stay on the right side of the patient and will use L1 and L2 to assist in retraction and suction/irrigation.

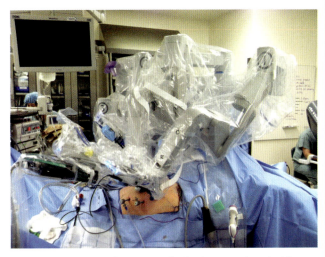

FIGURE 10 • Configuration of robotic arms after docking.

Robotic Total Mesorectal Excision

- The following principles should be adhered to during a robotic TME:
    - Minimal manipulation of the rectum
    - Identification of embryologic tissue planes
    - Oncologic resection with negative radial and distant margins without violation of the mesorectal envelope
- The surgeon at the robot's console will start dissection at the sacral promontory dorsal to the superior hemorrhoidal artery, following this plane distally over the promontory and into the presacral space.
- Arm 3 is used for retraction, whereas arms 1 and 2 develop a plane of dissection within the avascular presacral space between the presacral fascia, posteriorly, and the mesorectal fascia, anteriorly.
- Arm 2 of the robot (left hand of the surgeon) should avoid grasping the mesorectum for the strong robotic arm may tear the mesorectum, which would cause bleeding.
- Monopolar scissors are preferred for rapid development of the plane of dissection with minimal use of electrocautery.
- The pelvic dissection proceeds posteriorly first, then laterally, and then anteriorly.
    - Posterior exposure is achieved with the assistant retracting the sigmoid colon cephalad and anteriorly (**FIGURE 11**). Waldeyer fascia (rectosacral fascia) is entered distally at approximately the level of S3. This dissection is carried caudally to the level of levator muscles (**FIGURE 12**) (▶ Video 1).
    - Laterally, the hypogastric nerves are identified and preserved. The lateral dissection plane is carried anterior and medial to these nerves (**FIGURE 13A**). The nerve fibers are carefully dissected toward the pelvic sidewall (**FIGURE 13B**).
    - For the anterior pelvic dissection, exposure is achieved by the assistant retracting the rectum posteriorly and in a cephalad direction, as arm 3 anteriorly retracts the vagina (in females) or the prostate/seminal vesicles (in males). The Denonvilliers' fascia/pouch of Douglas

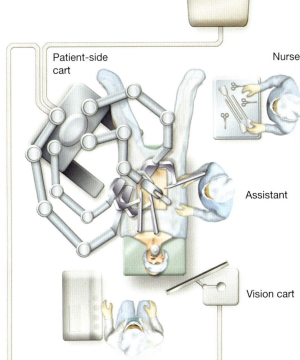

FIGURE 9 • The robot is docked from a left hip approach.

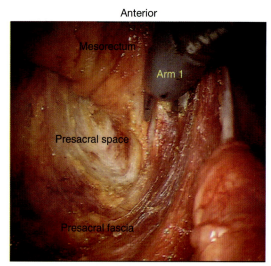

FIGURE 11 • The posterior pelvic dissection is carried out within the presacral space, staying between the presacral fascia, posteriorly, and the mesorectal fascia, anteriorly.

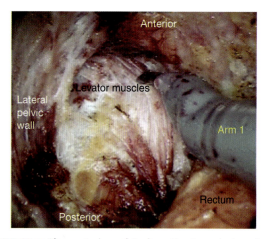

FIGURE 12 • The posterior pelvic dissection is carried caudally to the level of the levator muscles.

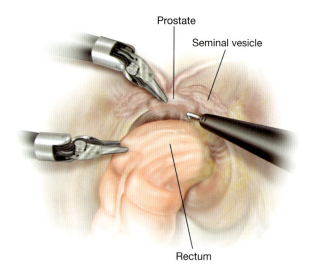

(rectovesical/rectovaginal pouch) is entered by incising the peritoneal reflection between the anterior wall of the rectum and the posterior wall of the vagina or the prostate/seminal vesicles (**FIGURE 14**) (▶ **Video 1**). In case of large anterior tumors, Denonvilliers' fascia is resected en bloc with the rectum.

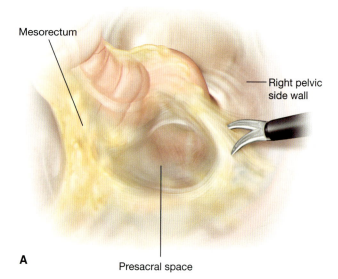

FIGURE 13 • Lateral dissection of the mesorectum off the right pelvic sidewall: transection of the right lateral rectal ligament (**A**). **B,** The hypogastric nerve can be seen posterolateral to the plane of the dissection.

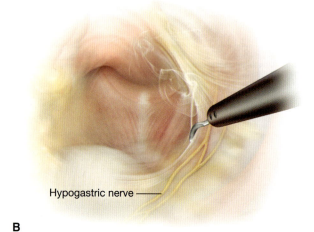

FIGURE 14 • Anterior pelvic dissection. Exposure is achieved by the assistant retracting the rectum posteriorly and in a cephalad direction, as arm 3 anteriorly retracts the prostate/seminal vesicles, respectively. The anterior plane of dissection is carried along Denonvilliers' fascia, between the rectum posteriorly and the prostate and seminal vesicles anteriorly.

DIVISION OF RECTUM AND CREATION OF ANASTOMOSIS

Division of Rectum

- DRE or flexible sigmoidoscopy under robotic vision is performed to establish the proper level of rectal division.
- In cases when the tumor is at least 2 to 3 cm from the anorectal ring, the distal rectum is transected with an articulating linear stapler.
    - An Endo GIA stapler is placed through the R1 port or in the lower assistant port (converted to a 12-mm port to accommodate the stapler).
    - The stapler is fired sequentially. Care is taken to avoid crossing staple lines during the sequential firing of stapler cartridges (**FIGURE 15**).
- For tumors that are less than 2 to 3 cm from the anorectal ring, an intersphincteric resection with hand-sewn coloanal anastomosis can be used (described elsewhere in this textbook).

Specimen Extraction

- Once the specimen is divided, the robot is undocked.
- The transected rectum and the contiguous sigmoid and descending colon are extracted through a 4- to 5-cm Pfannenstiel incision with a wound protector in place to protect the wound from potential oncologic contamination and soilage. The proximal transection is then performed with a linear stapler between the sigmoid and the descending colon. The specimen, including the rectum and sigmoid colon, is now completely disconnected and is sent to the pathologist for evaluation. The specimen should include the IMA pedicle and an intact mesorectum without any distal tapering (**FIGURE 16**).
- The anvil of a 29F end-to-end anastomosis (EEA) stapler is secured with a purse-string suture in the descending colon and the colon is returned into the abdomen. A colonic J pouch can be created at this point if preferred.

Creation of Anastomosis

- Once the colon is returned into the abdomen, an end-to-end stapled anastomosis with a circular EEA stapler is created laparoscopically (**FIGURE 17A** and **B**).
- A flexible sigmoidoscopy is then performed to assess the anastomosis integrity and to test for an air leak by filling the pelvis with saline and insufflating the rectum endoscopically. If there is an air leak, this indicates the presence of an anastomotic leak (**FIGURE 18**). In this situation, and at the discretion of the surgeon, the decision is made to either redo the anastomosis or reinforce it with sutures.
- A round Blake drain is routinely placed within the pelvis near the anastomosis.
- Anastomotic hypoperfusion may contribute to anastomotic leak, which in turn increases morbidity, mortality, and local recurrence rates. Fluorescence angiography may be used to assess intraoperative tissue perfusion during colorectal resection.[30]

Creation of Ileostomy

- A temporary diverting loop ileostomy is created based on surgeon preference and patient factors. However, it is generally recommended for low rectal anastomoses.

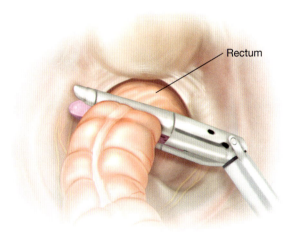

FIGURE 15 • The distal rectum is transected with an Endo GIA. The stapler is fired sequentially. Care is taken to avoid crossing staple lines during the sequential firing of stapler cartridges.

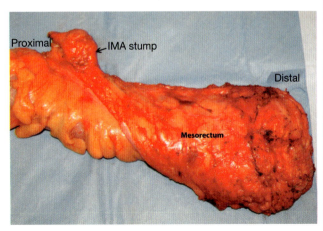

FIGURE 16 • The extracted specimen demonstrates the inferior mesenteric artery (IMA) pedicle and an intact mesorectal envelope without any distal tapering.

284   SECTION III   RECTAL RESECTIONS

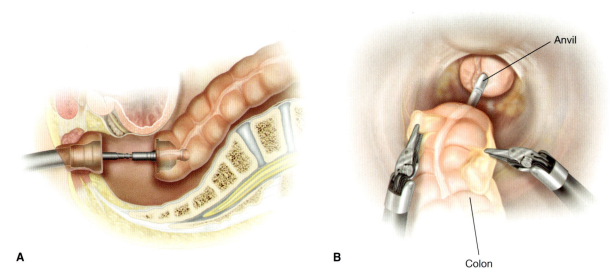

FIGURE 17 • **A** and **B,** Intracorporeal laparoscopic anastomosis. The descending colon is anastomosed to the rectal stump with a 29F end-to-end anastomosis circular stapler.

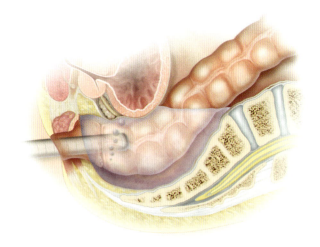

FIGURE 18 • Assessment of anastomotic integrity by sigmoidoscopy. The completed colorectal anastomosis is tested underwater. Air bubbles identified during insufflation of the anastomosis indicate an anastomotic leak.

PEARLS AND PITFALLS

Preoperative workup	▪ Obtain a complete and thorough history of urinary and bowel incontinence and sexual dysfunction. ▪ Perform your own endoscopy and verify the location of tumor.
Port placement	▪ Maintain triangulation. ▪ For narrower pelvic inlet, consider more medial robotic ports.
Division of IMA	▪ Visualize the T configuration to assure high ligation.
Robotic TME	▪ Avoid using arm 2 (surgeon's left hand) to grasp mesorectum. ▪ Dissection should be within the avascular plane of the presacral space. ▪ Avoid injury to hypogastric nerves laterally. ▪ Identify bilateral ureters prior to proceeding.
Division of rectum	▪ During repeated stapler firings, do *not* cross over previous transection points.
Anastomosis	▪ Visualize anastomosis via endoscope to assure good blood supply and integrity.

Chapter 32 LOW ANTERIOR RECTAL RESECTION: ROBOTIC-ASSISTED LAPAROSCOPIC TECHNIQUE

POSTOPERATIVE CARE

- The Foley catheter should be continued for 48 to 72 hours given the high likelihood of postoperative urinary retention after low pelvic surgery.
- The pelvic drain is discontinued prior to discharge.
- Stoma teaching is performed by the enterostomal nurse prior to discharge.

Enhanced Recovery Protocols

- We regularly use enhanced recovery after surgery (ERAS) protocols (described elsewhere in this textbook) at our institution following colorectal surgery, including minimization of intravenous fluid administration, early postoperative enteral feeding, and early mobilization. ERAS protocols have been shown to reduce morbidity and length of hospital stay for patients undergoing elective colorectal surgery.[31]

OUTCOMES

- Given improved surgical technique and adjuvant therapy, overall survival rates of rectal cancer have improvement over the recent decades.[32,33]
  - Overall 5-year survival for patients undergoing curative resection is 80% with 10% local recurrence rates.[34]

COMPLICATIONS

- Symptomatic anastomotic leaks after LAR have been reported to occur in 12% to 18% of patients with an associated risk of mortality of 15%.[34-39]
- Patients may complain of anorectal, sexual, and urinary dysfunction postoperatively. This may be due to dissection during surgery and/or secondary to pelvic radiation.
- LAR syndrome may occur and refers to a combination of symptoms including increased bowel frequency, fecal incontinence, and urgency.

REFERENCES

1. Heald RJ. The "Holy Plane" of rectal surgery. *J R Soc Med.* 1988;81(9):503-508.
2. Jeong SY, Park JW, Nam BH, et al. Open versus laparoscopic surgery for mid-rectal or low-rectal cancer after neoadjuvant chemoradiotherapy (COREAN trial): survival outcomes of an open-label, non-inferiority, randomised controlled trial. *Lancet Oncol.* 2014;15(7):767-774. doi:10.1016/S1470-2045(14)70205-0
3. Bonjer HJ, Deijen CL, Haglind E, Group CIS. A randomized trial of laparoscopic versus open surgery for rectal cancer. *N Engl J Med.* 2015;373(2):194. doi:10.1056/NEJMc1505367
4. deSouza AL, Prasad LM, Marecik SJ, et al. Total mesorectal excision for rectal cancer: the potential advantage of robotic assistance. *Dis Colon Rectum.* 2010;53(12):1611-1617. doi:10.1007/DCR.0b013e3181f22f1f
5. Koh DC, Tsang CB, Kim SH. A new application of the four-arm standard da Vinci® surgical system: totally robotic-assisted left-sided colon or rectal resection. *Surg Endosc.* 2011;25(6):1945-1952. doi:10.1007/s00464-010-1492-1
6. Baik SH, Kwon HY, Kim JS, et al. Robotic versus laparoscopic low anterior resection of rectal cancer: short-term outcome of a prospective comparative study. *Ann Surg Oncol.* 2009;16(6):1480-1487. doi:10.1245/s10434-009-0435-3
7. Pigazzi A, Ellenhorn JD, Ballantyne GH, Paz IB. Robotic-assisted laparoscopic low anterior resection with total mesorectal excision for rectal cancer. *Surg Endosc.* 2006;20(10):1521-1525. doi:10.1007/s00464-005-0855-5

8. Baek JH, McKenzie S, Garcia-Aguilar J, Pigazzi A. Oncologic outcomes of robotic-assisted total mesorectal excision for the treatment of rectal cancer. *Ann Surg.* 2010;251(5):882-886. doi:10.1097/SLA.0b013e3181c79114
9. Jayne D, Pigazzi A, Marshall H, et al. Effect of robotic-assisted vs conventional laparoscopic surgery on risk of conversion to open laparotomy among patients undergoing resection for rectal cancer: the ROLARR randomized clinical trial. *JAMA.* 2017;318(16):1569-1580. doi:10.1001/jama.2017.7219
10. Rao VS, Ahmad N, Al-Mukhtar A, Stojkovic S, Moore PJ, Ahmad SM. Comparison of rigid vs flexible sigmoidoscopy in detection of significant anorectal lesions. *Colorectal Dis.* 2005;7(1):61-64. doi:10.1111/j.1463-1318.2004.00701.x
11. Winnan G, Berci G, Panish J, Talbot TM, Overholt BF, McCallum RW. Superiority of the flexible to the rigid sigmoidoscope in routine proctosigmoidoscopy. *N Engl J Med.* 1980;302(18):1011-1012. doi:10.1056/NEJM198005013021806
12. Wilking N, Petrelli NJ, Herrera-Ornelas L, Walsh D, Mittelman A. A comparison of the 25-cm rigid proctosigmoidoscope with the 65-cm flexible endoscope in the screening of patients for colorectal carcinoma. *Cancer.* 1986;57(3):669-671. doi:10.1002/1097-0142(19860201)57:3<669::aid-cncr2820570345>3.0.co;2-w
13. Floyd CE, Stirling CT, Cohn I. Cancer of the colon, rectum and anus: review of 1,687 cases. *Ann Surg.* 1966;163(6):829-837. doi:10.1097/00000658-196606000-00003
14. Langevin JM, Nivatvongs S. The true incidence of synchronous cancer of the large bowel. A prospective study. *Am J Surg.* 1984;147(3):330-333. doi:10.1016/0002-9610(84)90161-2
15. Reilly JC, Rusin LC, Theuerkauf FJ. Colonoscopy: its role in cancer of the colon and rectum. *Dis Colon Rectum.* 1982;25(6):532-538. doi:10.1007/BF02564161
16. Brown G, Daniels IR. Preoperative staging of rectal cancer: the MERCURY research project. *Recent Results Cancer Res.* 2005;165:58-74. doi:10.1007/3-540-27449-9_8
17. Battersby NJ, How P, Moran B, et al. Prospective validation of a low rectal cancer magnetic resonance imaging staging system and development of a local recurrence risk stratification model: the MERCURY II study. *Ann Surg.* 2016;263(4):751-760. doi:10.1097/SLA.0000000000001193
18. Zhang G, Cai YZ, Xu GH. Diagnostic accuracy of MRI for assessment of T category and circumferential resection margin involvement in patients with rectal cancer: a meta-analysis. *Dis Colon Rectum.* 2016;59(8):789-799. doi:10.1097/DCR.0000000000000611
19. Puli SR, Bechtold ML, Reddy JB, Choudhary A, Antillon MR, Brugge WR. How good is endoscopic ultrasound in differentiating various T stages of rectal cancer? Meta-analysis and systematic review. *Ann Surg Oncol.* 2009;16(2):254-265. doi:10.1245/s10434-008-0231-5
20. Uberoi AS, Bhutani MS. Has the role of EUS in rectal cancer staging changed in the last decade?. *Endosc Ultrasound.* 2018;7(6):366-370. doi:10.4103/eus.eus_36_18
21. Puli SR, Reddy JB, Bechtold ML, Choudhary A, Antillon MR, Brugge WR. Accuracy of endoscopic ultrasound to diagnose nodal invasion by rectal cancers: a meta-analysis and systematic review. *Ann Surg Oncol.* 2009;16(5):1255-1265. doi:10.1245/s10434-009-0337-4
22. Network NCC. *Rectal Cancer (Version 1.2021).* 2021. https://www.nccn.org/professionals/physician_gls/pdf/rectal.pdf
23. Klessen C, Rogalla P, Taupitz M. Local staging of rectal cancer: the current role of MRI. *Eur Radiol.* 2007;17(2):379-389. doi:10.1007/s00330-006-0388-x
24. Martellucci J, Scheiterle M, Lorenzi B, et al. Accuracy of transrectal ultrasound after preoperative radiochemotherapy compared to computed tomography and magnetic resonance in locally advanced rectal cancer. *Int J Colorectal Dis.* 2012;27(7):967-973. doi:10.1007/s00384-012-1419-5
25. Kasi A, Abbasi S, Handa S, et al. Total neoadjuvant therapy vs standard therapy in locally advanced rectal cancer: a systematic review and meta-analysis. *JAMA Netw Open.* 2020;3(12):e2030097. doi:10.1001/jamanetworkopen.2020.30097

26. Klinger AL, Green H, Monlezun DJ, et al. The role of bowel preparation in colorectal surgery: results of the 2012-2015 ACS-NSQIP data. *Ann Surg.* 2019;269(4):671-677. doi:10.1097/SLA.0000000000002568

27. Samarasena JB, El Hage Chehade N, Abadir A, et al. Single-day low-residue diet prior to colonoscopy demonstrates improved bowel preparation quality and patient tolerance over clear liquid diet: a randomized, single-blinded, dual-center trial. *Dig Dis Sci.* 2021. doi:10.1007/s10620-021-07023-0

28. Itani KM, Wilson SE, Awad SS, Jensen EH, Finn TS, Abramson MA. Ertapenem versus cefotetan prophylaxis in elective colorectal surgery. *N Engl J Med.* 2006;355(25):2640-2651. doi:10.1056/NEJMoa054408

29. Zaghiyan KN, Sax HC, Miraflor E, et al. Timing of chemical thromboprophylaxis and deep vein thrombosis in major colorectal surgery: a randomized clinical trial. *Ann Surg.* 2016;264(4):632-639. doi:10.1097/SLA.0000000000001856

30. Jafari MD, Wexner SD, Martz JE, et al. Perfusion assessment in laparoscopic left-sided/anterior resection (PILLAR II): a multi-institutional study. *J Am Coll Surg.* 2015;220(1):82-92.e1. doi:10.1016/j.jamcollsurg.2014.09.015

31. Teeuwen PH, Bleichrodt RP, Strik C, et al. Enhanced recovery after surgery (ERAS) versus conventional postoperative care in colorectal surgery. *J Gastrointest Surg.* 2010;14(1):88-95. doi:10.1007/s11605-009-1037-x

32. Sauer R. Adjuvant and neoadjuvant radiotherapy and concurrent radiochemotherapy for rectal cancer. *Pathol Oncol Res.* 2002;8(1):7-17. doi:10.1007/BF03033695

33. Sauer R, Becker H, Hohenberger W, et al. Preoperative versus postoperative chemoradiotherapy for rectal cancer. *N Engl J Med.* 2004;351(17):1731-1740. doi:10.1056/NEJMoa040694

34. Enker WE, Merchant N, Cohen AM, et al. Safety and efficacy of low anterior resection for rectal cancer: 681 consecutive cases from a specialty service. *Ann Surg.* 1999;230(4):544-552; discussion 552-4. doi:10.1097/00000658-199910000-00010

35. Dehni N, Schlegel RD, Cunningham C, Guiguet M, Tiret E, Parc R. Influence of a defunctioning stoma on leakage rates after low colorectal anastomosis and colonic J pouch-anal anastomosis. *Br J Surg.* 1998;85(8):1114-1117. doi:10.1046/j.1365-2168.1998.00790.x

36. Law WL, Chu KW. Anterior resection for rectal cancer with mesorectal excision: a prospective evaluation of 622 patients. *Ann Surg.* 2004;240(2):260-268. doi:10.1097/01.sla.0000133185.23514.32

37. Matthiessen P, Hallböök O, Rutegård J, Simert G, Sjödahl R. Defunctioning stoma reduces symptomatic anastomotic leakage after low anterior resection of the rectum for cancer: a randomized multicenter trial. *Ann Surg.* 2007;246(2):207-214. doi:10.1097/SLA.0b013e3180603024

38. Montedori A, Cirocchi R, Farinella E, Sciannameo F, Abraha I. Covering ileo- or colostomy in anterior resection for rectal carcinoma. *Cochrane Database Syst Rev.* 2010(5):CD006878. doi:10.1002/14651858.CD006878.pub2

39. Karliczek A, Harlaar NJ, Zeebregts CJ, Wiggers T, Baas PC, van Dam GM. Surgeons lack predictive accuracy for anastomotic leakage in gastrointestinal surgery. *Int J Colorectal Dis.* 2009;24(5):569-576. doi:10.1007/s00384-009-0658-6

Chapter 33

Total Mesorectal Excision With Coloanal Anastomosis: Laparoscopic Technique

John H. Marks, Jane Yang, and Elsa B. Valsdottir

DEFINITION

- Total mesorectal excision with coloanal anastomosis via a transanal abdominal transanal proctosigmoidectomy is defined as the complete removal of the embryologic tissue block of the rectum, leaving the sphincter muscles intact and thus avoiding a permanent stoma. Neoadjuvant chemoradiotherapy is an essential component to successful sphincter preservation. The abdominal part of the procedure can be performed with laparoscopic technique.

DIFFERENTIAL DIAGNOSIS

- Several conditions, both benign and malignant, can have similar presentation to rectal cancer. These include adenomatous polyps, solitary rectal ulcer, radiation injury, carcinoid tumor, and squamous cell carcinoma. Hence, a tissue biopsy confirming the diagnosis of rectal cancer is imperative.

PATIENT HISTORY AND PHYSICAL FINDINGS

- Careful patient selection is crucial for successful sphincter preservation in rectal cancer. A detailed history and a physical examination are mandatory. Contraindications include inability to receive neoadjuvant chemoradiation therapy for distal rectal cancers, either because of comorbidities or previous radiation to the pelvis, previous radical surgery on rectum, distance of tumor from the dentate line, invasion of tumor into the sphincter muscles after completion of neoadjuvant chemoradiation therapy, and fecal incontinence on presentation.
- Detailed past medical history is obtained, emphasizing fecal continence, bowel habits, personal and family history of cancers and current medications and allergies, previous radiation to the pelvis, and previous abdominal surgeries.
- Prior radiation therapy for other cancers in the pelvis, such as cervical or prostate, is usually a contraindication. It is, however, helpful to review the previous records with regard to the dose and field treated and make decisions on individual basis.
- A detailed family history of cancers can help identify increased risk for other types of cancer as well as identify family members who are at an increased colon cancer risk. Recommendations should be given to first-degree relatives with regard to screening.
- Patient age, nodal status, and tumor size are not contraindications for sphincter preservation as long as the patient is a reasonable surgical candidate and negative margins (distally and circumferentially) can be obtained.
- Physical examination must include a thorough abdominal examination, including palpation of inguinal lymph nodes bilaterally. Most importantly, a careful digital rectal examination (DRE) and a rigid proctoscopy or flexible sigmoidoscopy are performed.

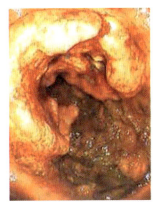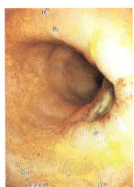

FIGURE 1 • Rectal cancer before (*left*) and after (*right*) neoadjuvant chemoradiation. This patient had a good response to treatment.

- During the DRE and proctoscopy, the location of the tumor (anterior, posterior, or lateral), distance from the anorectal ring, size, fixation, rectal circumference involvement, configuration, and ulceration of the tumor need to be documented. This is imperative in preoperative planning (determination of coloanal anastomosis vs abdominoperineal resection [APR]). It also allows for the assessment of response to neoadjuvant treatment later (**FIGURE 1**).

IMAGING AND OTHER DIAGNOSTIC STUDIES

- All patients require clinical and radiographic preoperative staging with regard to the primary rectal cancer, lymph node status, and potential metastatic spread.
- The most accurate way to determine size, length, and depth of the tumor invasion as well as any enlarged lymph nodes is with rectal protocol magnetic resonance imaging (MRI) or endoscopic rectal ultrasound (ERUS) (**FIGURE 2**).
- A computed tomography (CT) of the abdomen and chest should be obtained to evaluate for potential metastases to the retroperitoneum, liver, or lungs.
- Preoperative blood work should include a hemogram, blood chemistries, and a carcinoembryonic antigen (CEA) level.
- Full colonoscopy is needed to evaluate the entire colon for other pathology and synchronous malignant lesions or polyps.
- Histologic assessment with biopsy of the primary tumor is necessary and usually obtained at the time of colonoscopy.

SURGICAL MANAGEMENT

Preoperative Planning

- Neoadjuvant chemoradiotherapy is key to successful sphincter preservation. The radiation therapy is a high-dose, long-term treatment to maximize tumor downstaging. Preferred

287

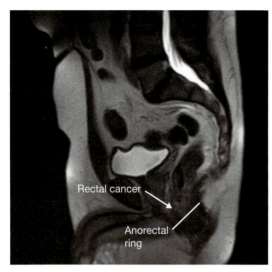

FIGURE 2 • Pre-neoadjuvant treatment MRI of a rectal cancer suitable for TATA.

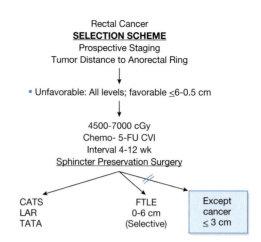

FIGURE 3 • Author's treatment algorithm for low rectal cancers (distal 3 cm of the true rectum). 5-FU, 5-fluorouracil; CATS, combined abdominal trans-sacral rectal resection; cGy, centiGray; CVI, continuous venous infusion; FTLE, full-thickness local excision; LAR, low anterior resection; TATA, transanal transabdominal rectal resection.

radiation dose is 5580 cGy, with 4500 cGy to the entire pelvis with a boost to the presacral area and tumor location, delivered over the course of 5 weeks. Concurrent chemotherapy based on 5-fluorouracil (5-FU) either orally or intravenously increases the sensitivity of the tissues to radiation, enhancing efficacy (**FIGURE 3**).

- Neoadjuvant chemoradiation apoptotic effect occurs only at cell division. Maximum cytotoxic effect is 8 to 12 weeks after completion of treatment. Extending the interval between completion of radiation therapy and surgery up to 8 to 12 weeks therefore gives the patient the fullest benefit of the treatment, maximizing downstaging and extending the options for sphincter preservation.
- Decision regarding sphincter preservation should be based on the status of the cancer *after* completion of chemoradiotherapy. All patients, except those whose cancers remain fixed at or below 3 cm from the anorectal ring level, are offered sphincter preservation.
- Accepting a distal margin of resection from the cancer as small as 5 mm is necessary for very low tumors. This does not adversely affect outcome. Dissection is started transanally to assure a known distal margin. This is particularly helpful in the postirradiated rectal cancer where there is often only a small scar left, making decisions as to where a stapler would be placed from above difficult.
- An intraoperative frozen section biopsy of the distal rectal margin is commonly needed to ensure that the patient is a candidate for a coloanal anastomosis vs an APR. Therefore, the final decision for sphincter preservation vs APR is made by the surgeon intraoperatively based on the intraoperative assessment of the distal margin.
- The patient should receive a bowel preparation the day before surgery.
- Perioperative antibiotics and deep vein thrombosis prophylaxis should be given.

Positioning

- The operation has both an abdominal part and a perineal part. The surgeon and the first assistant stand between the legs during the perineal part. For the abdominal part, which is performed laparoscopically, they stand at the patient's right side. It is important that the surgical team is free to move around the patient. The laparoscopic equipment and energy sources are positioned to patient's left (**FIGURE 4**).
- The patient is placed in the lithotomy position with the buttocks extending 2 cm over the padded table edge. Both arms are padded and tucked. The chest is taped to the table to further prevent slipping of the patient as the table is maneuvered. The Foley catheter is taped over the right thigh. The abdomen is prepped with Betadine and the perineum with povidone-iodine. In women, the vagina is prepped with povidone-iodine.

Chapter 33 TOTAL MESORECTAL EXCISION WITH COLOANAL ANASTOMOSIS: LAPAROSCOPIC TECHNIQUE   289

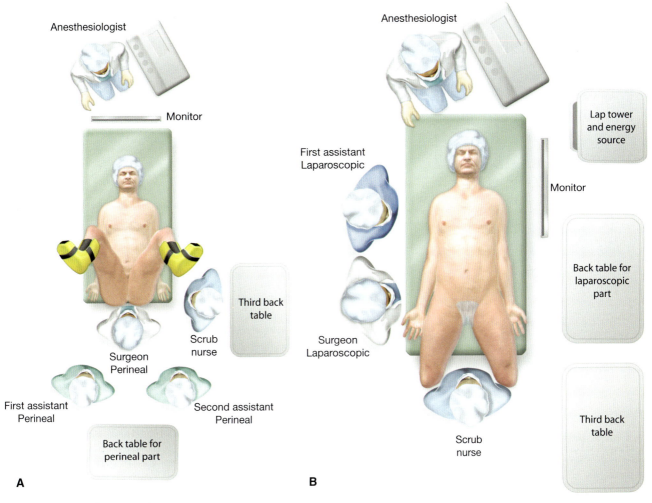

FIGURE 4 • A and B, Operating room setup.

TRANSANAL, INTERSPHINCTERIC RESECTION OF RECTUM

- Place a sponge soaked in povidone-iodine in the anal canal or irrigate it with povidone-iodine. In order to minimize the possibility of dislodging tumor cells, avoid digitalizing the canal after this.
- To allow visualization of the dentate line, Alice-Adair clamps are placed circumferentially around the anal canal to evert the anal tissue (FIGURE 5).
- The dentate line is incised circumferentially with electrocautery through the mucosa, thus defining the distal resection margin. This is a critical step to avoid radial tearing later in the dissection (FIGURE 6).
- The Metzenbaum scissors are spread posterolaterally and slightly off the midline, perpendicular to the axis of the anus, to enter into the plane between the transected upper half of the internal sphincter and the underlying puborectalis. This plane is developed circumferentially (FIGURE 7).

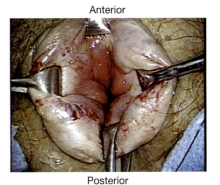

FIGURE 5 • To allow visualization of the dentate line, Alice-Adair clamps are placed circumferentially around the anal canal to evert the anal tissue.

- Alice-Adair clamps are applied to the transected distal portion of the rectum to facilitate retraction. One never applies more than four clamps at a time, as this is usually too bulky.

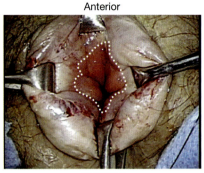

FIGURE 6 • Line of incision of the mucosa at the dentate line.

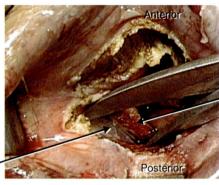

FIGURE 7 • The Metzenbaum scissors are spread slightly off the midline, perpendicular to the axis of the anus, to enter into the plane between the transected upper half of the internal sphincter and the underlying puborectalis. This defines the circumferential resection margin.

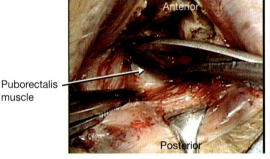

FIGURE 8 • The shiny, glistening white aspect of the puborectalis is identified using the scissors. Visualization of this white tissue is the key to ensuring that the dissection is carried out in the proper plane.

The shiny, glistening white aspect of the puborectalis is identified using the scissors. Visualization of this white tissue is the key to ensuring that the dissection is carried out in the proper plane (**FIGURE 8**). Placing a small Deaver retractor allows development of the plane between the rectum and the levator ani complex. Once the proper plane is entered, the dissection is essentially bloodless.

- The sharp dissection is brought around anteriorly (**FIGURE 9**). In women, a finger in the vagina allows palpation of the vaginal wall, and it is generally not a problem to avoid this structure. In men, one has to be careful when proceeding anteriorly to avoid taking the dissection anterior to the prostate. The length of dissection cephalad is up to the seminal vesicles in men and to the cervix in women. This dissection is carried circumferentially until the rectum is fully mobilized (**FIGURES 9** and **10**).

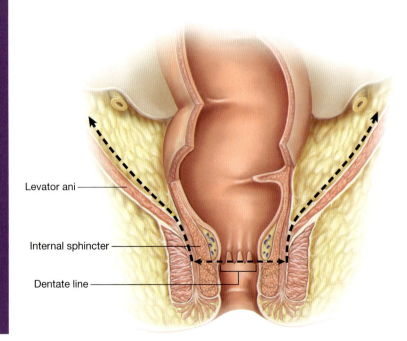

FIGURE 9 • The drawing shows the lines of pelvic dissection.

Chapter 33 **TOTAL MESORECTAL EXCISION WITH COLOANAL ANASTOMOSIS: LAPAROSCOPIC TECHNIQUE** 291

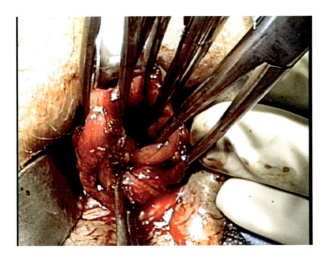

- The rectum is oversewn in a watertight fashion with a 0-Vicryl stitch, turning the edges inward to avoid potential spilling of feces or tumor cells during the abdominal part of the procedure. The pelvis is irrigated from below with saline; a sponge is placed through the anus with an occlusive dressing in the perineum.

FIGURE 10 • The distal rectum is fully mobilized.

ABDOMINAL LAPAROSCOPIC PROCTOSIGMOIDECTOMY

- The patient's knees are lowered from full lithotomy so that they are flat to the abdomen to avoid conflict with the surgeon's arms and instruments, allowing for laparoscopic access to the abdomen and, particularly, to the splenic flexure. The surgical team changes gowns and gloves. Five ports are placed as follows: (1) 5-mm port 20 cm above the pubic symphysis; (2) 12-mm port at the height of the umbilicus lateral to the rectus sheath; (3) 12-mm port in the right fossa, a hands width above the pubic tubercle; (4) 5-mm port suprapubically; and (5) 5-mm port in the left fossa (**FIGURE 11**).
- A careful exploration is carried out to rule out metastatic disease.
- The patient is placed in reverse Trendelenburg position of 5° with the right side down 18°. The monitor is placed above the patient's left shoulder. The surgeon and the assistant stand at the patient's right side (**FIGURE 4**).
- The first operative step is releasing the splenic flexure. The surgeon works with a bowel grasper in the left hand in port 2 and a LigaSure in the right hand in port 3. The 5-mm camera is in port 1. The gastrocolic ligament is identified and opened at the level of the middle epiploic perforating artery to enter the lesser sac. The gastrocolic ligament is divided laterally toward the lower pole of the spleen (**FIGURE 12**). Next, the lateral attachments of the flexure are taken down, using the epiploic to retract the colon medially. The splenocolic ligament is divided and the tail of the pancreas is identified. Finally, an incision is made in the peritoneal sheath of the mesentery of the transverse colon 1 cm below the inferior border of the pancreas (**FIGURE 13**). The avascular space between the fascia of Toldt and Gerota fascia is entered and the colonic mesentery is peeled off the Gerota fascia. The splenic flexure is now fully mobilized and the retroperitoneal structures are visualized (**FIGURE 14**).
- The second step is repositioning the small bowel to gain access to the pelvis and vasculature. The patient is placed in steep Trendelenburg position (18°); the right side remains down. The camera is changed to a 10-mm, 30° scope and

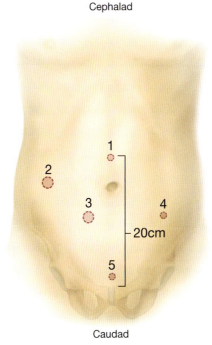

FIGURE 11 • Port placement for the abdominal (laparoscopic) phase of the operation. Five ports are placed as follows: (1) 5-mm port 20 cm above the pubic symphysis; (2) 12-mm port at the height of the umbilicus lateral to the rectus sheath; (3) 12-mm port in the right fossa, a hands width above the pubic tubercle; (4) 5-mm port suprapubically; and (5) 5-mm port in the left fossa.

moved to port number 2 and the surgeon's left hand to port number 1. The omentum is placed over the transverse colon; the small bowel is swept out of the pelvis and is placed in the right upper quadrant to expose the ligament of Treitz and the inferior mesenteric artery (IMA). The junction of the descending and sigmoid colon is marked with a suture to determine the level of transection to be performed later.

- The third step is a high ligation of the IMA. The right iliac artery and the left ureter are recognized. The peritoneum

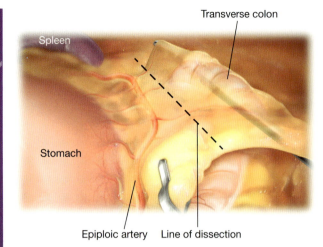

FIGURE 12 • The gastrocolic ligament is identified and opened at the level of the middle epiploic artery to enter the lesser sac. The gastrocolic ligament is divided laterally toward the lower pole of the spleen.

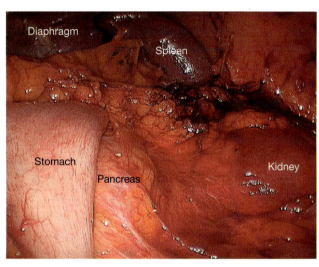

FIGURE 14 • Once the splenic flexure is fully mobilized and the colonic mesentery is peeled off Gerota fascia, the structures of the retroperitoneum can be visualized.

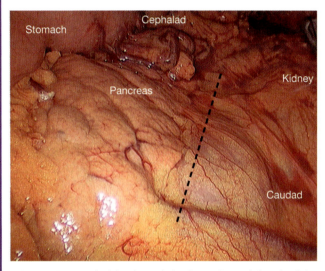

FIGURE 13 • An incision is made in the peritoneal sheath of the mesentery of the transverse colon 1 cm below the inferior border of the pancreas.

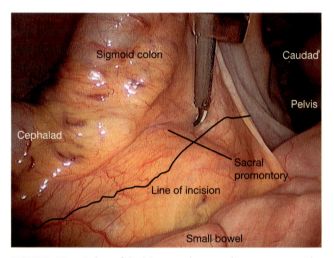

FIGURE 15 • Point of incision at the sacral promontory. The peritoneum is incised at the level of the promontorium of the sacrum and opened down to the right pararectal sulcus and cephalad along the aorta toward the ligament of Treitz.

is incised at the level of the promontorium of the sacrum and opened to the right pararectal sulcus distally and then cephalad along the aorta toward the ligament of Treitz (**FIGURE 15**). Blunt dissection is used to lift the mesentery of the proximal rectum off the retroperitoneum, revealing the left ureter (**FIGURE 16**). The nerves of the hypogastric plexus are the key to the dissection. They are identified and preserved intact under the IMA and gently pushed down toward the aorta. The base of the IMA is skeletonized circumferentially and the artery is divided with an energy device, clips, or endovascular stapler (**FIGURE 17**).

- The fourth step is the high ligation of the inferior mesenteric vein (IMV) (**FIGURE 18**). The IMV is dissected and divided at the

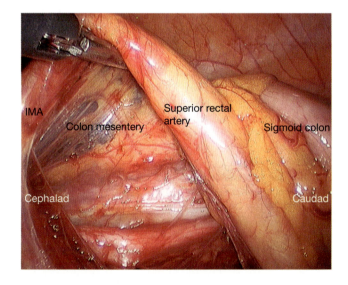

FIGURE 16 • Blunt dissection is used to lift the mesentery of the proximal rectum off the retroperitoneum, revealing the left ureter. IMA, inferior mesenteric artery.

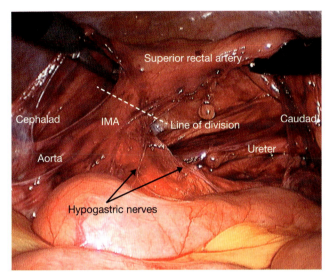

FIGURE 17 • The nerves of the hypogastric plexus are the key to the dissection. They are identified under the inferior mesenteric artery (IMA) and gently pushed down toward the aorta and preserved. The base of the IMA is skeletonized circumferentially and the artery is divided along the *dotted line*.

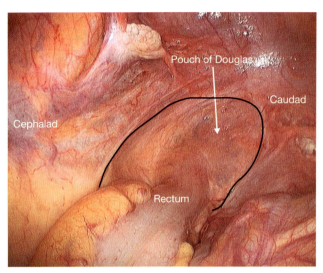

FIGURE 19 • The peritoneum of the rectum is incised to open the box circumferentially, going down the left and right pararectal sulcus and anteriorly across the pouch of Douglas.

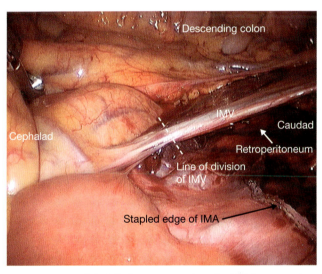

FIGURE 18 • High inferior mesenteric vein (IMV) transection. The IMV has been lifted up along with the mesentery of the descending colon and is transected (*dotted lines*) at the level of the ligament of Treitz. IMA, inferior mesenteric artery.

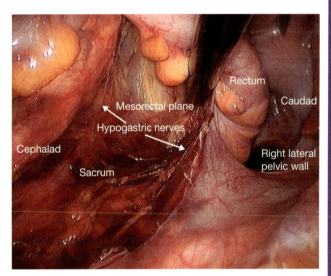

FIGURE 20 • The dissection around the rectum is carried posteriorly first.

level of the ligament of Treitz, where it dives under the duodenum to join the splenic vein. The remaining mesentery of the descending and sigmoid colon is then lifted off the Gerota fascia, completing the medial to lateral mobilization of the colon.
- The fifth step is the mobilization of the lateral attachments of the descending and sigmoid colon. This is relatively easy as the majority of the dissection has already been done in a medial to lateral fashion. Starting at the pelvic brim, the peritoneum in incised up to the previous mobilization of the splenic flexure and a connection made with the dissection from the medial side.
- The sixth step is the total mesorectal excision (TME) of the rectum. To accomplish this laparoscopically, a few key points

are made. First, the remaining peritoneum of the rectum is incised to "open the box" circumferentially, going down the left and right pararectal sulcus and anteriorly across the pouch of Douglas or the rectovesical fold (**FIGURE 19**). In anteriorly based lesions, this incision is a centimeter higher. The LigaSure is exchanged for Endo Shears with electrocautery attached to allow for finer dissection. The dissection is carried posteriorly along the mesorectal plane first (**FIGURE 20**), then brought around the right and the left sides (transection of the lateral rectal ligaments) (**FIGURE 21**), and is then finished anteriorly (**FIGURE 22**). This is repeated, alternating sides, as the dissection carries on deeper into the pelvis. To facilitate this, three-dimensional retraction is created by the surgeon retracting the rectum and assistants applying anterior and lateral retraction from the two 5-mm ports (**FIGURE 23**). The dissection is kept in the plane outside the mesorectal fascia, taking care not to taper the specimen and

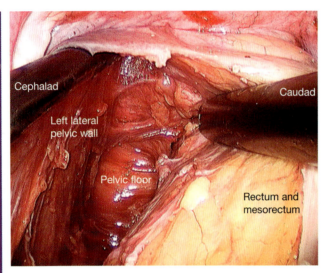

FIGURE 21 • The lateral dissection is brought around the left (shown here) and right sides.

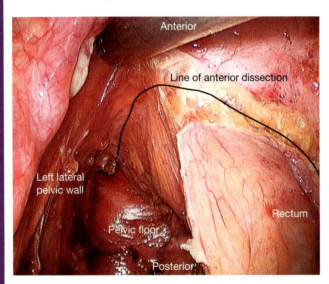

FIGURE 22 • The dissection around the rectum is finished anteriorly.

it is continued until it meets the previous perineal dissection from below. The sponge that was placed previously can be seen (**FIGURE 24**). The nerves are followed to direct the dissection in the proper plane.
- The rectum is delivered out the pelvis and the completeness of the dissection is checked as well as the hemostasis (**FIGURE 25**).

FIGURE 25 • The rectum is delivered out through the pelvis, and the completeness of the dissection and hemostasis are checked.

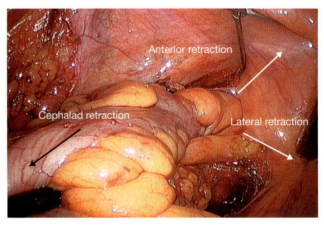

FIGURE 23 • To facilitate the dissection around the rectum, three-dimensional retraction is created by the surgeon retracting the rectum with the left hand and assistants applying retraction from the two 5-mm ports toward the sides and anteriorly.

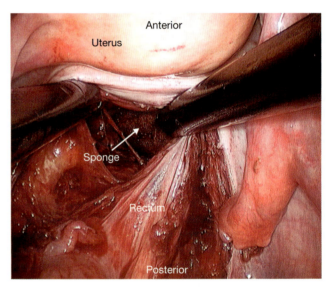

FIGURE 24 • The dissection is *continued* until it meets the previous perineal dissection from below and the sponge that was placed previously can be seen.

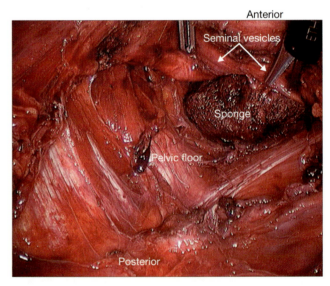

Chapter 33 TOTAL MESORECTAL EXCISION WITH COLOANAL ANASTOMOSIS: LAPAROSCOPIC TECHNIQUE   295

COLOANAL ANASTOMOSIS

- The surgeon moves back to the perineum. The patient's knees are raised again. The sponge and the perineal occlusive dressing are removed from the anus.
- The specimen is pulled through the anus carefully under direct laparoscopic visualization to assure orientation and is transected at the marking suture previously placed between the sigmoid and descending colon (**FIGURE 26**).
- The coloanal anastomosis is hand sewn. This can be direct, or a colonic pouch can be created if there is adequate length. Small Deaver retractors are used for exposure. Full-thickness bites are taken through the descending colon wall and the transected lower border of the internal sphincter, including the overlying anoderm. Four corner sutures are placed at 12, 3, 6, and 9 o'clock positions and left untied until one or two full-thickness bites have been placed between each corner suture (**FIGURE 27**).
- The anastomosis is either a direct coloanal, side-to-end or a colonic J-pouch, depending on the patient's body habitus and amount of fat (**FIGURE 28**).
- Digital examination is performed to ensure there are no gaps and the anastomosis is patent.

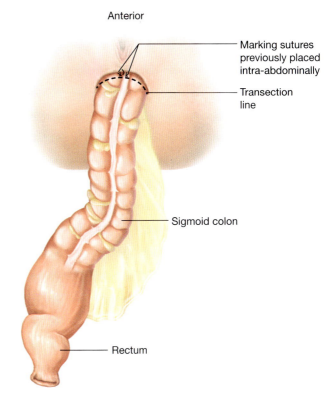

FIGURE 26 • The specimen is pulled through the anus carefully under direct laparoscopic visualization to assure orientation and is transected along the *dotted line* at the previously placed marking suture.

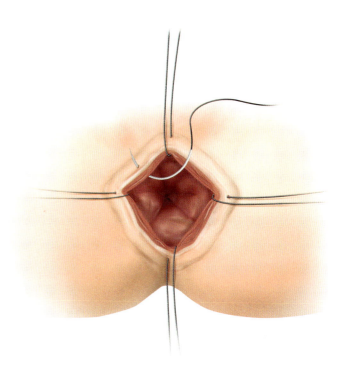

FIGURE 27 • The coloanal anastomosis is hand sewn. This can be direct or a colonic pouch can be created if there is adequate length. Small Deaver retractors are used for exposure. Full-thickness bites are taken through the descending colon wall and the transected lower border of the internal sphincter, including the overlying anoderm. Four corner sutures are placed at 12, 3, 6, and 9 o'clock positions and left untied until one or two full-thickness bites have been placed between each corner suture.

296 SECTION III RECTAL RESECTIONS

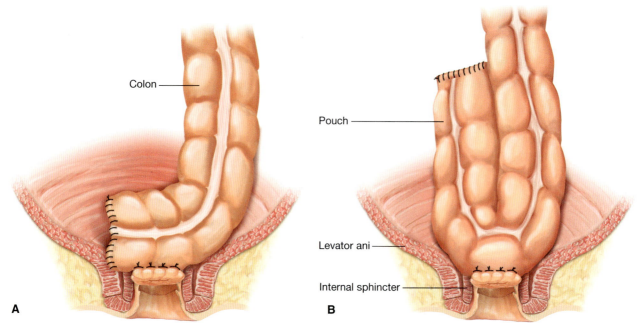

FIGURE 28 • The anastomosis is either a direct coloanal (A), a side-to-end, or a colonic J-pouch (B).

CREATION OF STOMA

- The last step is bringing out a loop of ileum in preparation for a diverting loop ileostomy. A locked bowel grasper is used to grasp the ileum about 20 cm proximal to the terminal ileum. This loop is brought out at the site of port 3 or at the infraumbilical fat fold.
- The abdominal part of the procedure is then concluded. The insufflation air is evacuated through the trocars. The fascia at the 12-mm port sites is closed with 0-Vicryl suture and all skin incisions with 4-0 Monocryl. Steri Strips and dressings are applied. Finally, the diverting loop ileostomy is matured; stoma plate and bag applied (FIGURE 29).

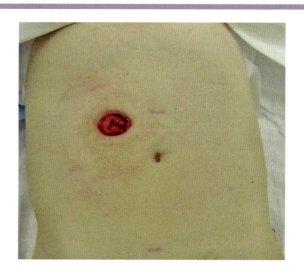

FIGURE 29 • The abdomen after all port sites has been closed and the diverting stoma has been matured.

PEARLS AND PITFALLS

Surgical decision-making	■ Decision on sphincter preservation based on *post* chemoradiation cancer characteristics
Patient selection	■ Patients whose cancer is not fixed to the levators in the distal third of the rectum after chemoradiation are offered sphincter preservation ■ Adequate baseline continence ■ Clinical staging and careful documentation of tumor location and size
Preoperative planning	■ Staging with MRI/ERUS, CT, physical examination ■ Full colonoscopy ■ Neoadjuvant chemoradiation therapy

Chapter 33 **TOTAL MESORECTAL EXCISION WITH COLOANAL ANASTOMOSIS: LAPAROSCOPIC TECHNIQUE** **297**

Intersphincteric dissection	▪ Incise mucosa at dentate line, marking distal margin ▪ Stay in the plane between the internal sphincter and the puborectalis sling—identified by the glistening white aspect of the puborectalis ▪ Carry the dissection cephalad to the cervix in women and to the seminal vesicles in men
Rectosigmoid resection	▪ Wide mobilization of the splenic flexure with freeing of the distal transverse mesocolon from the retroperitoneum ▪ Full medial to lateral mobilization of the left colon ▪ High transection of the IMA and the IMV ▪ TME resection of the rectum ▪ Avoid urethra or venturing anterior to the prostate in men
Anastomosis	▪ Maintain orientation when delivering specimen through the anus ▪ Full-thickness bites with interrupted sutures ▪ Can be colonic J-pouch, side-to-end, or end-to-end coloanal

POSTOPERATIVE CARE

▪ No nasogastric tube is needed. Oral diet with clear liquids is started immediately after surgery, and advanced as tolerated on the first postoperative day. Antibiotics are continued for 10 days postoperatively due to the poor vascularity of the radiated tissue and the ultralow anastomosis.

▪ The diverting stoma is closed at 3 months postoperatively, after flexible sigmoidoscopy, digital examination, and gastrograffin enema show that the anastomosis is intact. If the patient needs adjuvant chemotherapy, stoma closure is usually postponed until after completion of therapy.

▪ Close follow-up is mandatory for at least 5 years, with physical examination, flexible sigmoidoscopy, CT, and CEA measurements. Physical examination is performed every 3 months for 24 months, then every 4 months for 24 months, and then every 6 months for 12 months. Endoscopic evaluation (flexible sigmoidoscopy) is performed every 6 months for 24 months and then every 12 months for the next 3 years.

OUTCOMES

▪ Local recurrence is low and equivalent to best results after APR or 2.5% (at the author's institute) to 7.0%. The same holds for distant recurrence with metastasis (8% - 10%).

▪ Five-year survival for all patients undergoing sphincter preservation surgery for rectal cancer at the author's institution is 97%. Others have reported numbers from 71% to 82%.

▪ Sphincter preservation has been achieved in 90% of patients who have been considered for the procedure.

▪ Function is adequate in the majority of patients. In a survey among patients at the author's institute, more than half of patients report no or little inconvenience due to incontinence and 80% would not prefer to have kept their stoma.

COMPLICATIONS

▪ Infections
▪ Bleeding
▪ Anastomotic leak
▪ Ischemic neorectum
▪ Incontinence
▪ Rectal prolapse
▪ Bowel obstruction

SUGGESTED READING

1. Chamlou R, Parc Y, Simon T. Long-term results of intersphincteric resection for low rectal cancer. *Ann Surg.* 2007;246:916-922.
2. Habr-Gama A, Perez RO, Wynn G, et al. Complete clinical response after neoadjuvant chemoradiation therapy for distal rectal cancer: characterization of clinical and endoscopic findings for standardization. *Dis Colon Rectum.* 2010;53:1692-1698.
3. Laurent C, Paumet T, LeBlanc F, et al. Intersphincteric resection for low rectal cancer: laparoscopic versus open surgery approach. *Colorectal Dis.* 2012;14:35-41.
4. Marks GJ, Marks JH, Mohiuddin M, et al. Radical sphincter-preservation surgery with coloanal anastomosis following high-dose external irradiation for the very low lying rectal cancer. *Recent Results Cancer Res.* 1998;146:161-174.
5. Marks J, Mizrahi B, Dalane S, et al. Laparoscopic transanal abdominal transanal resection with sphincter preservation for rectal cancer in the distal 3 cm of the rectum after neoadjuvant therapy. *Surg Endosc.* 2010;24(11):2700-2707.
6. Marks JH, Frenkel JL, D'Andrea AP, et al. Maximizing rectal cancer results: TEM and TATA techniques to expand sphincter preservation. *Surg Oncol Clin N Am.* 2011;20:501-520.
7. Moore HG, Riedel E, Minsky BD, et al. Adequacy of 1 cm distal margin after restorative rectal cancer resection with sharp mesorectal excision and preoperative combined-modality therapy. *Ann Surg Oncol.* 2003;10:80-85.
8. Rullier E, Laurent C, Bretagnol F, et al. Sphincter-saving resection for all rectal carcinomas: the end of the 2 cm distal rule. *Ann Surg.* 2005;241:465-469.
9. Sauer R, Becker H, Hohenberger W, et al. Preoperative versus postoperative chemoradiotherapy for rectal cancer. *N Engl J Med.* 2004;351:1731-1740.
10. Swedish Rectal Cancer Trial. Improved survival with preoperative radiotherapy in resectable rectal cancer. *New Engl J Med.* 1997;336:980-987.

Chapter 34 | Abdominoperineal Resection: Open Technique

Curtis J. Wray and Stefanos G. Millas

DEFINITION

- The abdominoperineal resection (APR) refers to the operation for surgical treatment of distal rectal cancer. The APR, as originally described by Dr. Ernest Miles, involves the en bloc removal of the distal sigmoid colon, rectum, mesorectum, and anal canal. The operation uses both an abdominal and perineal approach.
- The APR requires a permanent end colostomy.

DIFFERENTIAL DIAGNOSIS

- This operation should be performed for those with a biopsy-proven diagnosis of malignancy (eg, rectal or anal cancer, anal melanoma).

PATIENT HISTORY AND PHYSICAL FINDINGS

- Patients may present with tenesmus, rectal bleeding, rectal pain, and/or obstructive symptoms. Iron deficiency anemia is common at presentation and should always prompt a full colonoscopy in adult patients. Asymptomatic patients are typically diagnosed during screening colonoscopy.
- A thorough history should be obtained to assess the patient's functional status and to ensure sufficient physiologic reserve to undergo a major abdominal operation.
- A detailed family history is necessary to identify risk of an inherited colon and rectal cancer syndrome as well as risk for metachronous colorectal cancer.
- Digital rectal examination and rigid proctosigmoidoscopy can be performed in the ambulatory office and provides a more accurate measurement of tumor distance from the anorectal ring when compared to a flexible sigmoidoscopy. It also allows for the evaluation of potential tumor fixation to the anal sphincter, pelvic side walls, sacrum, and/or urologic/gynecologic organs.

IMAGING AND OTHER DIAGNOSTIC STUDIES

- A complete colonoscopy is obtained to evaluate for potential synchronous lesions that may have to be addressed at the time of surgery.
- A computed tomography (CT) scan of the chest, abdomen, and pelvis with intravenous and oral contrast should be obtained to assess for the presence of metastatic disease and the extent of tumor involvement within the pelvis.
- A magnetic resonance imaging (MRI) of the pelvis with intravenous contrast, or endorectal ultrasound performed by a qualified endoscopist, should be obtained for local tumor staging that will guide neoadjuvant chemotherapy and radiation as per consensus guidelines.
- Laboratory blood work should include a complete blood count, serum electrolytes, liver function tests, and a carcinoembryonic antigen tumor marker level as a baseline measurement that will be the reference for future cancer surveillance.
  - Surgical decision is based on rectal cancer staging. As per consensus guidelines, neoadjuvant chemotherapy and radiation therapy (CRT) should be considered for all T4 and/or N+ positive tumors in the mid- or distal rectum based on preoperative imaging.
  - Neoadjuvant CRT has been shown to reduce the local recurrence rate and increase the chances of sphincter-sparing surgery in locally advanced rectal cancer.

SURGICAL MANAGEMENT

- Although controversial, a margin less than 2 cm between the tumor and the anorectal ring will typically require an APR to ensure adequate tumor clearance and a satisfactory functional outcome.
- The patient is placed in the lithotomy position and two surgical teams can work simultaneously. Alternatively, one team can perform both portions of the operation sequentially.

Preoperative Planning

- The patient should take a mechanical bowel preparation (GoLYTELY) the day before surgery.
- The best available evidence suggests that an oral antibiotic preparation reduces postoperative surgical site infections.
- The colostomy site should be marked preoperatively with the patient in a sitting and supine position to ensure skin folds and crevices do not interfere with the appliance. Ideally, this marking should be performed by a qualified enterostomal therapist (wound, ostomy, and continence nurse [WOCN]).
- The stoma is marked over the left rectus abdominus, typically below the level of the umbilicus, though it can be placed above the umbilicus to facilitate a large pannus or high belt line.
- Tumor fixation by rectal examination is unreliable in determining whether or not a low rectal tumor is resectable.
- Tumor fixation within the pelvis does not necessarily imply infiltration of tumor into surrounding structures.
- Inflammatory adhesions within the pelvis do not portend a worse prognosis with respect to local recurrence or overall mortality.
- Ultimately, the decision on whether to proceed with an APR is made at the time of laparotomy.

Positioning

- The patient is placed in a modified lithotomy position with Allen stirrups.
- The thighs are level with the abdomen as this allows efficient placement of a self-retaining retractor without creating excessive pressure between the retractor and the patient's thighs (**FIGURE 1**).
- The perineum is positioned flush with the edge of the operating room table.

Chapter 34 ABDOMINOPERINEAL RESECTION: OPEN TECHNIQUE   299

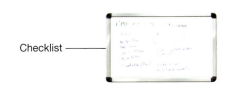
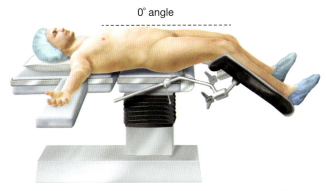

FIGURE 1 • Patient positioning on the operating table. Note the horizontal position of the thighs to ensure free movement of surgeon's arms and hands. The perineum is flush with the end of the table.

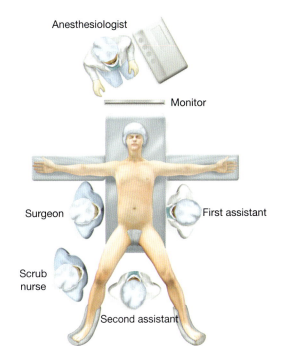

FIGURE 2 • Team setup. For the abdominal phase of the operation, the surgeon stands by the patient's right side with their assistant standing at the patient's left side. A second assistant, if available, stands in between the patient's legs. The scrub nurse stands by the surgeon's right side.

- The pelvis is supported with a folded sheet to lift the entire perineum and facilitate exposure during the perineal dissection.
- The arms are placed in a neutral position and supported with suitable armrests.
- The anus is closed with a purse-string monofilament suture (0-Prolene with circle taper 1 [CT-1] Ethicon needle, or equivalent) if there is relative certainty that an APR will be required for tumor clearance. In cases where a satisfactory distal margin for an anastomosis may be possible, the anus can be closed once the decision to proceed with an APR is made.
- For the abdominal phase of the operation, the surgeon stands by the patient's right side, with their assistant standing at the patient's left side. A second assistant, if available, stands in between the patient's legs. The scrub nurse stands at the surgeon's right side, by the patient's right leg (**FIGURE 2**). The surgeon and the first assistant will switch sides as necessary during the pelvic dissection.
- During the perineal phase, the surgeon and the first assistant will be situated in between the patient's legs, with the second assistant by the patient's right or left side.

EXPOSURE

- Exposure of the abdomen is obtained with a lower midline incision from the umbilicus to the pubic symphysis. A wound protector may be inserted to protect the wound from infectious and oncologic soilage (**FIGURE 3**).
- The abdomen should be fully explored for the presence of gross metastatic disease.
- Care should be taken to evaluate all peritoneal surfaces, the entire gastrointestinal tract, the omentum, and the liver.
- Any concerning lesions away from the primary tumor should be biopsied and evaluated by intraoperative cryosection.
- A self-retaining retractor is positioned to optimize exposure of the pelvis.
    - Two short Richardson attachments are used to retract the abdominal wall laterally, in a perpendicular orientation to the incision to avoid undue traction on the femoral nerves at the pelvic inlet (**FIGURE 4**).
    - A bladder blade is positioned at the inferior aspect of the incision to retract the bladder and uterus. A 2-0 silk,

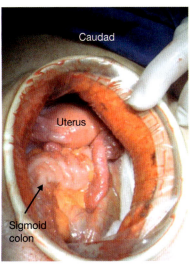

FIGURE 3 • Placement of a wound protector protects the wound from infectious and oncologic soilage.

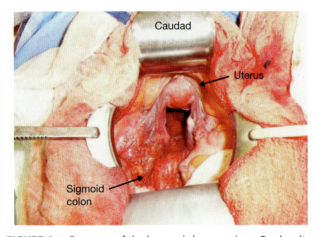

FIGURE 4 • Exposure of the lower abdomen using a Bookwalter retractor. Two short Richardson attachments are used to retract the abdominal wall laterally, in a perpendicular orientation to the incision, to avoid undue traction on the femoral nerves at the pelvic inlet. A bladder blade is positioned at the inferior aspect of the incision to retract the bladder and uterus. The small bowel is packed into the upper abdomen and held in place with a malleable retractor.

figure-of-eight suture through the fundus of the uterus can facilitate positioning the uterus behind the bladder blade.

- The patient is positioned in Trendelenburg position with the left side tilted upward to enhance operative exposure.
- The small bowel is packed into the upper abdomen; this maneuver is facilitated by not extending the incision beyond what is required to access the origin of the inferior mesenteric artery (IMA).
- A malleable retractor attachment for the Bookwalter and moistened laparotomy pads aid in keeping the small bowel out of the pelvis.

MOBILIZATION OF SIGMOID COLON AND TRANSECTION OF THE INFERIOR MESENTERIC ARTERY

- The lateral peritoneal attachments to the sigmoid colon are divided, exposing the plane between the sigmoid mesocolon and the retroperitoneum (**FIGURE 5**).
- Mobilization of the sigmoid mesocolon allows for exposure and preservation of the left ureter and gonadal vessels, which should always be identified prior to dividing the IMA at its origin (**FIGURE 6**).
- The left ureter courses over the left psoas and is located medial to the gonadal vessels; it travels over the left iliac artery at its bifurcation at the pelvic inlet.
- Direct exposure of the left psoas often indicates an incorrect dissection plane where the ureter and gonadal vessels are mobilized medially with the sigmoid mesocolon.
- The peritoneal reflection on the right side of the sigmoid mesocolon is incised to complete the dissection of the mesentery away from the retroperitoneum. Again, care must be taken to maintain the left ureter in its normal, anatomic position in the retroperitoneum.
- The origin of the IMA is identified at its origin off the aorta. The IMA is then ligated between Sarot clamps, incised, and doubly ligated with braided 2-0 suture (**FIGURE 7A** and **B**). An appropriate vessel-sealing energy device (LigaSure) or a stapler with a vascular load may also be used to ligate and divide the IMA. High IMA ligation allows for an excellent lymph node harvest.
- The colon is then transected proximally between the sigmoid and descending colon segments with a linear stapler. The intervening mesentery is ligated and divided between Sarot clamps and braided 2-0 ties or with an energy device.

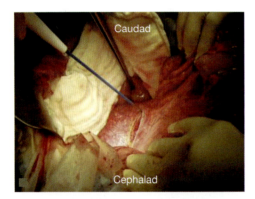

FIGURE 5 • Sigmoid colon mobilization. With the descending colon retracted medially, the lateral peritoneal attachments are transected with electrocautery along the left paracolic gutter.

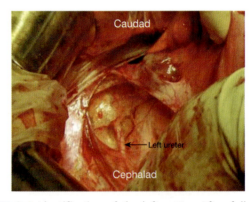

FIGURE 6 • Identification of the left ureter. After full mobilization of the descending colon, the left ureter is exposed in the retroperitoneum. The surgeon is retracting the descending colon medially.

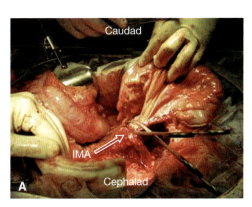
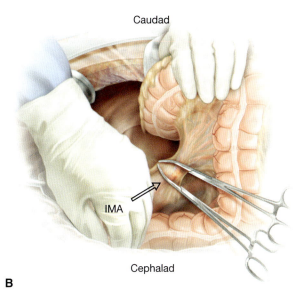

FIGURE 7 • **A** and **B,** Inferior mesenteric artery (IMA) division. The IMA is transected between clamps and will subsequently be ligated with heavy silk sutures.

MOBILIZATION OF THE RECTUM

- Once the sigmoid mesocolon is mobilized, dissection along the same anatomic plane between the mesentery and retroperitoneum is continued toward the pelvic inlet where the total mesorectal excision is initiated.
- The mesorectum is fully mobilized posteriorly using sharp dissection, typically with electrocautery. Care is taken not to injure the left and right hypogastric nerves posteriorly, as they can be intimately associated with the mesorectum (**FIGURE 8**).
- Dissection along the presacral plane is facilitated with anterior traction on the mesorectum provided by the St. Mark retractors (**FIGURE 9A** and **B**). A lighted St. Mark retractor can also provide good illumination during dissection in the distal pelvis.
- The presacral plane is an avascular tissue plane located between the presacral fascia, posteriorly, and the investing fascia of the mesorectum, anteriorly. As the dissection proceeds posteriorly, the curve of the sacrum and coccyx needs to be followed (**FIGURE 10**). It is imperative to avoid penetrating the presacral fascia, as inadvertent injury to the presacral venous plexus of the sacrum posteriorly can result in hemorrhage that can be very difficult to control. Division of the rectosacral facia (Waldeyer fascia) exposes the pelvic floor (levator ani).
- Once the rectum is fully mobilized posteriorly, the lateral mobilization can commence. This phase of the dissection is facilitated by the St. Mark retractors, and the dissection proceeds along the avascular mesorectal plane that was initiated posteriorly. The lateral rectal ligaments are transected with cautery or an energy device (**FIGURE 11**). Care must be taken to avoid penetrating the endopelvic fascia along the pelvic sidewalls to avoid injuring the hypogastric vein and its branches laterally which can result in severe bleeding. In the distal pelvis, penetrating the endopelvic fascia on the pelvic sidewalls can result in injury to the parasympathetic ganglia, which can result in autonomic pelvic organ dysfunction postoperatively.
- Pelvic dissection must be sharp at all times. It is important to avoid using blunt dissection. Special care must be taken to avoid inadvertent entry into the investing fascia of the mesorectum in order to avoid potential oncological contamination of the pelvis which can lead to rectal cancer recurrence in the pelvis. Also, care must be taken to injuring the ureters at the pelvic inlet, as it followed the lateral pelvic sidewalls toward the bladder trigone. The appropriate planes of dissection in the pelvis are properly exposed with sufficient traction.
- The anterior dissection is initiated with division of the rectovesical reflection in men and rectovaginal reflection in women. Mobilization is continued anterior to Denonvilliers' fascia, exposing the seminal vesicles in men (**FIGURE 11**) and the vagina in women.
- For posterior tumors in men, consideration can be given to dissecting posterior to Denonvilliers' fascia as this may lower the risk of injury to the nervi erigentes with concomitant sexual dysfunction.

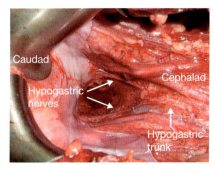

FIGURE 8 • View of the sympathetic plexus and the origin of the left and right hypogastric nerves.

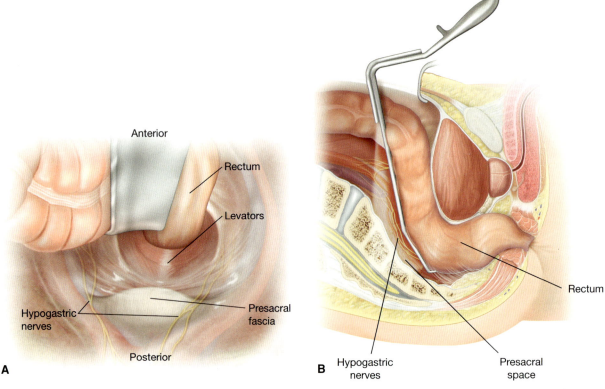

FIGURE 9 • Posterior pelvic exposure with the lighted St. Mark retractor. **A,** The rectum is retracted anteriorly, exposing the presacral space posteriorly. The hypogastric nerves are exposed and should be swept posteriorly and away from the mesorectum. This begins the superior and posterior portion of the total mesorectal excision. **B,** The presacral plane of dissection should be followed down to the levator ani muscles and the pelvic floor.

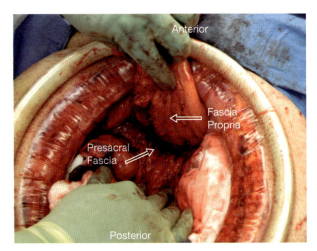

FIGURE 10 • The posterior plane of dissection proceeds in a semicircular fashion to release the posterolateral rectal attachments and to allow a better anterior retraction on the rectum. This allows *continued* exposure of the posterior plane of dissection down to the pelvic floor and prevents vascular and nerve injuries along the lateral pelvic walls. Mesorectum *(top arrow)*; presacral fascia *(bottom arrow)*.

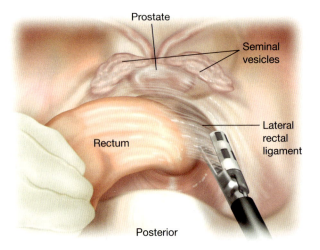

FIGURE 11 • Transection of the lateral rectal ligaments and anterior pelvic dissection. Posterolateral retraction of the rectum allows for good exposure of the lateral rectal ligament (the right one is shown here), which can then be transected with cautery or with an energy device. The anterior dissection will then proceed anterior to Denonvilliers' fascia, in the space between the rectum posteriorly, and the prostate and seminal vesicles anteriorly.

- The posterior, lateral, and anterior dissections are carried down to the level of the levator ani circumferentially.
- For distal tumors overlying the anal canal, creating a "waist" near the tumor when dividing the levator ani muscles has been associated with inadvertent bowel perforation, circumferential margin involvement, and local recurrence. An extended resection whereby the levator ani muscles are resected at their origin can improve the aforementioned oncologic parameters. An extended resection will likely require plastic surgery consultation to close the perineal wound with a vertical rectus abdominus myocutaneous (VRAM) flap.

DISSECTION OF THE PERINEUM

- This component of the operation can be performed concurrently with the abdominal dissection of the rectum.
- This technical description is applicable to a patient who has been placed in the lithotomy position and the legs are elevated in Allen stirrups. During the abdominal component of the operation, the Allen stirrups are lowered such that the thighs are level with the torso and abdomen, as this facilitates placement of the self-retaining retractor. For the perineal dissection, the Allen stirrups are elevated to fully expose the perineum. The self-retaining retractor should be repositioned if it places pressure on the thighs as they are elevated into position.
- The perineal surgeon should have a separate electrocautery with a dedicated grounding pad, and a separate suction, to allow the two operating teams to work independently. An instrument table should also be assembled for the perineal dissection, with the perineal instruments separated from those used in the abdomen and pelvis. The instrument set used is a typical major abdominal set, with the addition of two Gelpi retractors if they are not included.
- A monofilament suture (0-Prolene) is used to close the anus prior to initiating the dissection if it has not already been done. A large needle (CTX) is used to place two half-circle throws 1 cm lateral to the anal verge and the anus is closed by tying the suture (**FIGURE 12**). This helps prevent infectious and oncologic soilage of the perineal wound.
- Two Gelpi retractors are placed in an "X" configuration such that the anus and perianal skin are adequately exposed for the incision and subsequent dissection (**FIGURE 12**).
- A circular skin incision is placed around the anal verge to include all of the anoderm as well as a margin of perianal skin. The Gelpi retractors are repositioned inside of the skin

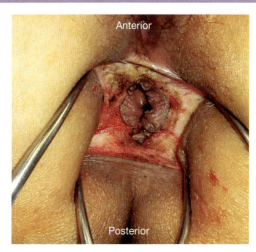

FIGURE 13 • Perineal dissection: lateral incision around the anal canal. The incision is carried through the skin and subcutaneous tissues.

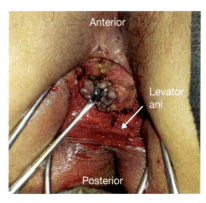

FIGURE 14 • Perineal dissection: dissection through the levator ani muscle complex.

incision to enhance exposure (**FIGURE 13**). A 3-cm margin (radius) around the closed anus is sufficient.
- Dissection should include the external sphincter muscle as the surgeon proceeds toward the levator ani (**FIGURE 14**). The lymphatic-bearing tissue surrounding the anal canal should be included with the specimen.
- The Gelpi retractors should be repositioned to maintain exposure. Handheld Richardson retractors can also be helpful and are held by the surgeon's assistant.
- As the external sphincter, perianal fat, and lymphatic tissue are mobilized, the coccyx should be palpated to ensure that dissection proceeds anterior to this structure. The surgeon in the abdominal field should place their hand posteriorly and serve as a guide for entry into the abdomen (**FIGURE 15**). A

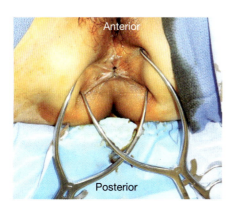

FIGURE 12 • Closure of the anus with a purse-string suture. This helps prevent infectious and oncologic soilage of the perineal wound.

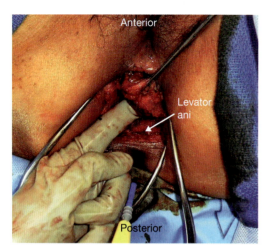

FIGURE 15 • Perineal dissection: posterior palpation of the coccyx during perineal dissection. The transection of the levators starts posteriorly, anterior to the coccyx. The index finger of the surgeon is placed into the pelvis and hooked on to top of the levator ani muscle, pulling it into the field. This allows for safe transection of the levator ani muscle with electrocautery.

- curved Mayo scissors is used to divide the anococcygeal ligament and levator ani muscle, which ultimately connects the abdominal and perineal dissections.
- The transection of the levator ani muscle starts posteriorly, anterior to the coccyx (**FIGURE 15**). The index finger of the surgeon is placed into the pelvis and hooked on to the top of the levator muscle, pulling it into the field. This allows for the safe transection of the levator ani muscle with electrocautery. The posterior and lateral component of the levator ani should be divided first, as the anterior dissection can be difficult, especially in anterior tumors.
- The surgeon's finger should then guide division of the perineal body anteriorly. In women, this component of the dissection is completed along the rectovaginal septum. In men, the surgeon should pay very close attention to the prostate gland anteriorly, as entry into the prostate can produce significant bleeding. Furthermore, if the dissection is too anterior, entry into the membranous urethra can occur. The appropriate

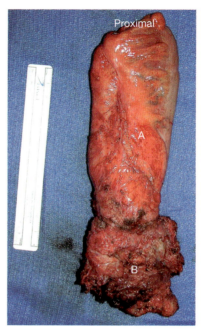

FIGURE 16 • Abdominoperineal resection specimen. The rectum should exhibit an intact mesorectum (A) with no distal "waisting" (B) in order to ensure excellent oncologic outcomes.

plane of dissection is anterior to Denonvilliers' fascia as the abdominal and perineal dissections are connected.
- The specimen, now completely disconnected proximally and distally, is then extracted through the perineal wound. The rectum should exhibit an intact mesorectum with no distal "waisting" (**FIGURE 16**) in order to ensure excellent oncologic outcomes.
- Anterior tumors in men can lead to loss of the normal plane between the rectum and prostate or even invasion into the prostate. In this case, removing the prostate en bloc with the rectum may be the best way to achieve a satisfactory oncologic margin.
- The pelvis is irrigated with saline and hemostasis achieved before the perineal wound is closed. Persistent bleeding from the remaining levator ani, the prostate, or vagina may be controlled with well-placed suture ligatures.

CLOSURE OF PERINEAL WOUND

- Once hemostasis is achieved, the levator ani are reapproximated with interrupted 0-Vicryl sutures. If the defect is large or insufficient levator ani muscle remains, consideration should be given to closure with a VRAM flap.
- The more superficial layers are sequentially closed with interrupted 2-0 Vicryl sutures and the skin can be reapproximated with interrupted 4-0 Monocryl sutures.
- A mobilized omental flap can be used to fill the pelvic cavity and help keep the small bowel in the upper abdomen. Closure of the peritoneum at the pelvic inlet can also facilitate keeping the small bowel in the upper abdomen.
- A closed suction drain is placed in the pelvis.

CREATION OF DESCENDING COLOSTOMY

- The site marked for the colostomy is identified. A Kocher clamp is used to lift the skin at the center of the mark and a circular skin incision is made approximately 2 cm in diameter.
- The subcutaneous fat is divided longitudinally, exposing the anterior rectus sheath, which is divided longitudinally as well. Removing a cylinder of subcutaneous fat is usually not necessary. The rectus abdominus is bluntly spread apart and the posterior rectus sheath is divided longitudinally.

Chapter 34 **ABDOMINOPERINEAL RESECTION: OPEN TECHNIQUE** **305**

Handheld Army-Navy retractors can facilitate exposure. The opening for the colostomy site should snugly accommodate two fingerbreadths.

- The descending colon should be sufficiently mobilized to allow a tension-free anastomosis between the colon and the skin. In patients with a thick layer of abdominal fat, additional length can be obtained by mobilizing the splenic flexure. If excessive tension at the skin persists, maturing the stoma as a loop-end can be the best option.

- The abdominal facia is closed in a standard manner.
- The staple line on the colon is removed with cautery and the stoma is matured to the dermis with interrupted 3-0 absorbable suture.
- Sterile dressings and a stoma appliance are placed such that the skin surrounding the stoma is completely protected with the wafer of the appliance.

PEARLS AND PITFALLS

Digital rectal examination and rigid proctoscopy	■ Should always be performed at the initial consultation as the lesion may decrease in size after neoadjuvant chemotherapy and/or chemoradiation.
Ureteral stent placement	■ Bulky pelvic tumors present a challenge and ureteral stents may assist in the identification of the ureters.
Pelvic dissection	■ Posterior first (along the presacral plane). Use sharp dissection (avoid blunt dissection) to prevent penetration through the investing fascia of the mesorectum and potential oncological contamination of the pelvis. ■ Lateral dissection and transection of the lateral rectal ligaments: Avoid injury to the autonomic trunks and genital nerve branches that can lead to autonomic dysfunction postoperatively. ■ Anterior dissection: Staying posterior to Denonvilliers' fascia reduces the incidence of injury to autonomic nerves near the prostate in posterior tumors. Bulky anterior lesions necessitate dissection anterior to Denonvilliers' fascia.
Perineal phase	■ Perform a circumferential dissection. Avoid "conization" of the specimen. The specimen should have an intact mesorectum without a "waist" effect distally.
Colostomy site	■ A location lateral to the rectus musculature increases the likelihood of peristomal hernia.
Perineal closure	■ Following neoadjuvant chemoradiation, a pedicled myocutaneous flap closure to the perineum warrants consideration in patients with extended resection or those at high risk for wound breakdown (ie, obese, diabetes, history of tobacco use).
Position in stirrups	■ Padded and positioned to avoid peroneal nerve injury.
Omental flap	■ Save the omentum, mobilize the omental pedicles, and place the omental flap into pelvic defect. This may prevent the small bowel from becoming entrapped in the new "potential" space created in the pelvis.

POSTOPERATIVE CARE

- Recent evidence has demonstrated that enhanced recovery after surgery (ERAS) pathways improve a number of important postoperative outcomes following colorectal surgery. Please refer to Chapter 52 for full details.

OUTCOMES

- Survival from rectal cancer after multimodality treatment is dependent on disease stage. Overall 5-year survival is approximately 90% for stage I, 74% to 65% for stage II, and 81% to 33% for stage III of disease. Development of distant metastasis occurs in less than 10% in patients with stage I disease but increases up to 28% and 50% in patients with stages II and III rectal cancers, respectively.
- Local pelvic recurrence of rectal cancer is also dependent on tumor and nodal stage. Local recurrence is 5% or less for patients with stage I rectal cancer but increases to 15% for stage II disease and 22% for stage III disease. If a pelvic

recurrence can be treated with a margin-negative surgical resection, 5-year survival can approach 40%. Often, this requires a pelvic exenteration, which demands a multispecialty surgical approach.

COMPLICATIONS

- Wound infections
- Incisional hernias
- Urinary/sexual dysfunction: important to preserve hypogastric nerves and parasympathetic ganglia intact
- Ureteral injury: critical to identify the left ureter prior to IMA transection
- Deep vein thrombosis (DVT): lower risk with use of adequate DVT prophylaxis
- Cardiac and pulmonary complications
- Pelvic abscess: reduced incidence with placement of an omental pedicle flap in the pelvis
- Perineal wound breakdown is a notorious problem, especially in high-risk patients

SUGGESTED READINGS

1. Lv L, Shao YF, Zhou YB. The enhanced recovery after surgery (ERAS) pathway for patients undergoing colorectal surgery: an update of meta-analysis of randomized controlled trials. *Int J Colorectal Dis.* 2012;27(12):1549-1554.
2. Nelson RL, Glenny AM, Song F. Antimicrobial prophylaxis for colorectal surgery. *Cochrane Database Syst Rev.* 2009;1:CD001181.
3. Ogilvie JW, Ricciardi R. Complications of perineal surgery. *Clin Colon Rectal Surg.* 2009;22(1):51-59.
4. Stelzner S, Koehler C, Stelzer J, et al. Extended abdominoperineal excision vs. standard abdominoperineal excision in rectal cancer—a systematic overview. *Int J Colorectal Dis.* 2011;26(10):1227-1240.
5. Turner GG, Pannett CA, Lloyd-Davies OV. Discussion on radical excision of carcinoma of the rectum with conservation of the sphincters. *Proc R Soc Med.* 1948;41(12):813-827.

Chapter 35

Abdominoperineal Resection: Laparoscopic Technique

Antonio D'Urso, Jacques Marescaux, and Didier Mutter

DEFINITION

- Abdominoperineal resection, or APR (once known as Miles operation), removes the distal colon, the entire rectum, with a total mesorectal excision (TME) with all regional lymph nodes, and the anus with the anal sphincter complex using both anterior abdominal and perineal approach, resulting in a permanent colostomy.
- The laparoscopic APR of the rectum described here is a totally laparoscopic procedure. Specimen removal is performed through a perineal excision without compromising the oncological principles of the surgical procedure.
- The definitive colostomy is extraperitoneal.
- Perineal closure could include advancement flap reconstruction.

Indications for Laparoscopic APR

- Rectal cancer: when unable to obtain a negative distal margin (less than 1 cm from the sphincter), and/or when there is external sphincter and/or levator ani muscle invasion, and/or in patients with poor sphincter function or severe comorbidities.
- Anal cancer: not responding to chemoradiotherapy or in the palliative setting.
- Inflammatory bowel disease (ie, Crohn disease with severe perianal disease).
- All indications are discussed and validated in a multidisciplinary oncologic committee.

PATIENT HISTORY AND PHYSICAL FINDINGS

Pretherapeutic Workup

- A detailed family history that may suggest familial colorectal cancer syndromes (ie, Lynch syndrome) should be obtained.
- Genetic counseling should be proposed for patients younger than 40 years, for patients presenting with MSI + test associated with the absence of BRAF mutation, or for patients with families with three or more cases of colorectal cancer in first- or second-degree relatives, including one before the age of 50.
- An oncogeriatric counseling should be obtained in patients older than 75 years with G8 score <14.

A Detailed History of Symptoms and Signs Should Include the Following

- Presence of rectal pain and/or tenesmus
- Presence of obstructive symptoms
- Description of anorectal function, with any fecal incontinence or leakage documented preoperatively
- Documentation of urinary and erectile function/dysfunction

Physical Examination Should Include the Following

- Routine abdominal examination, noting any previous incisions
- Digital rectal examination with assessment of sphincter function, the size, the mobility, and the distance of the tumor from the anal margin and the puborectal muscle (upper pole of the anal canal)
- Bilateral inguinal nodal examination

Rigid proctoscopy should complete the physical examination and is the key to a proper patient selection.
Proctoscopy should be standardized and well documented. It should:

- Define correctly the distal extent of the lesion measured from the anal verge
- Describe the exact position of the lesion in the lumen and the extent of the rectal circumference involved
- Assess the presence or absence of fixation to perirectal structures

The histological diagnosis should be confirmed.
A complete colonoscopy with documentation of all polyps should be performed so that the treatment plan can address synchronous pathology, as needed. If a preoperative colonoscopy is not feasible (ie, in obstructed patients), it should be performed within 3 to 6 months postoperatively.

IMAGING AND OTHER DIAGNOSTIC STUDIES

Pelvic MRI

Rectal protocol pelvic MRI should be routinely performed unless contraindicated to adequately stage the rectal cancer and to determine the need for neoadjuvant therapy and to plan operative strategy.

Computed Tomography

A contrast-enhanced computed tomography (CT) of the chest, abdomen, and pelvis evaluates for potential metastases. In case of renal insufficiency, it is replaced by a noninjected thoracic scan combined with a liver MRI.

- Cancer should be staged according to the American Joint Committee on Cancer TNM system.
  - Staging with endorectal ultrasound (ERUS) completes the workup to define the depth of invasion (with an accuracy for wall invasion of about 87.5%) and the potential invasion of the internal and external sphincters and/or the levator ani muscle and the lower rectum.
  - PET-CT (positron emission tomography) is recommended as part of an initial assessment for anal cancer. It is of particular interest for the evaluation of locoregional lymph node involvement. It can complete the investigations in case of doubt about the metastatic nature of a lesion for rectal adenocarcinoma.
- A preoperative carcinoembryonic antigen (CEA) level should be obtained.

SURGICAL MANAGEMENT

Preoperative Planning

- Informed consent is obtained preoperatively. The patient has been informed of the necessity to perform a definitive colostomy.
- The colostomy site is marked by a skin tattoo the evening before the intervention.
  - We follow the Guidelines for Perioperative Care in Elective Colic and rectal/pelvic Surgery: Enhanced Recovery After Surgery (ERAS) Society Recommendations for perioperative optimization and bowel preparation as described elsewhere in this textbook.
  - A dedicated ERAS nurse will follow the patient from the preoperative counseling through the postoperative follow up.
  - Appropriate intravenous antibiotics are administered within 1 hour of skin incision.

Equipment and Instrumentation

- 10 to 12 mm, 0° camera (30° camera is optional) with high-resolution monitors
- Laparoscopic endoscopic scissors and a blunt tip, 5-mm energy device (10-mm in obese patients)
- Laparoscopic linear staplers
- One 12-mm trocar for the stapler, 5 or 12 mm for suprapubic retraction, two 5-mm working trocars
- A lone star self-retaining retractor for the perianal phase of the operation

Positioning and Port Placement

Patient Setup

Correct patient positioning is a key step for a safe and successful operation.
Key elements of for proper patient positioning include:
- Supine position, with the right arm padded and tucked alongside the body. The left arm is left out for venous access. The legs are separated, in semiflexion, in Allen-type stirrups to allow for easy abdominal and perineal access (**FIGURE 1**)
- **The thighs should be placed parallel to the ground to avoid conflict with the surgeon's arms/instruments.**
- Adequate fastening to the table with padding in order to prevent neurovascular injuries to the extremities.
- Deep vein thrombosis (DVT) prophylaxis using an intermittent pneumatic compression (IPC) device.
- A body warmer device should be used to prevent patient hypothermia.
- The patient is placed on a steep Trendelenburg position with the left side up to help retract bowel loops by means of gravity and enhance operative exposure.
- The buttocks should be brought to the distal edge of the lower end of the table in order to allow for an easy access to the anal and perineal area.
- An orogastric tube is inserted and removed at the end of the surgery.
- A Foley catheter is inserted and left in place for 24 hours.

Team Positioning

- This procedure is performed with two assistants and a scrub nurse.
- Two instrument tables are used: one for the abdominal part and a second one for the perineal part of the operation.
- During the abdominal part of the procedure (**FIGURES 2** and **3**), the surgeon stands on the right flank of the patient, the first assistant lateral to the patient's right shoulder, and the second assistant between the patient's legs. The scrub nurse is placed to the right of the surgeon lateral to lower limbs.
- During the perineal part of the procedure, the entire team shifts toward the extremity of the table once the perineum has been exposed.
- The monitors are placed in front of the operating team and at eye level to improve ergonomics.
- The light source, the insufflator, and the electronic generator are placed on the left side of the patient at the level of the leg in the instruments trolley.

Port Placement

Ports are placed as follows (**FIGURE 4A** and **B**):
- One 10-/12-mm supraumbilical trocar (port A) is introduced using a mini-open technique. It will be used for the camera.

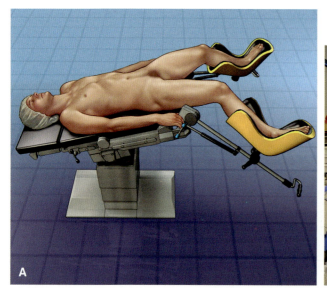 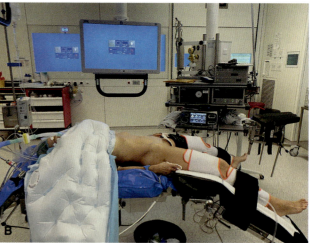

FIGURE 1 • **A**, Patient position. **B**, Patient setup.

Chapter 35 ABDOMINOPERINEAL RESECTION: LAPAROSCOPIC TECHNIQUE 309

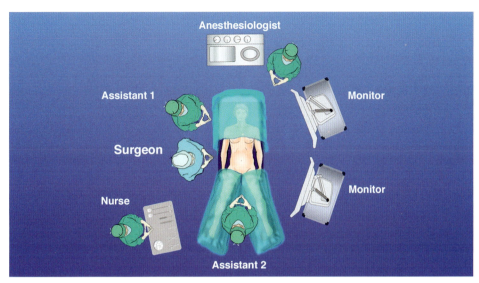

FIGURE 2 • Operative room setup.

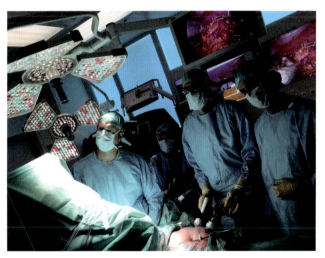

FIGURE 3 • Team position.

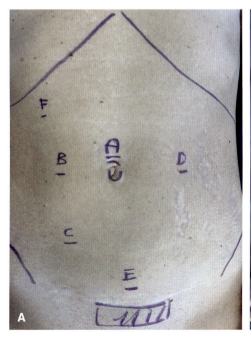
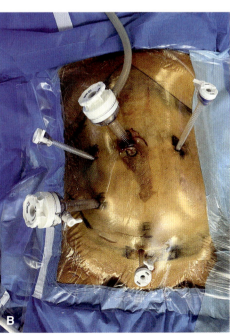

FIGURE 4 • Port placement. A, External view of the patient with positioning site: Optical port (A). Working ports (B, C). Retracting ports (D, E). Additional retracting port (F). B, External view of the patient with ports in place.

- Two ports, a 5-mm port in the right flank (port B) and a 12-mm port in the right iliac fossa (port C), are used as operating ports.
- The fourth port in the left flank at the level of the umbilicus is inserted through the rectus muscle (port D, 5 mm in diameter), preferably where the colostomy will be performed.
- The last port is introduced in the suprapubic area (port E, 12 mm in diameter), and is used for pelvic retraction and for exposure of the root of the mesosigmoid.
- Port fixation in the wall should be perfect in order to prevent any risk of parietal injury and to prevent increased operative times due to a loss in abdominal pressure. One should not hesitate to fix ports to the skin.
- Additional ports may be used in case of difficulty in exposure. In this case, a port will be positioned in the right hypochondrium (port F) to retract the ileocecal area. This is particularly useful in obese patients.

TECHNIQUE

- See Video 1.

LAPAROSCOPIC ABDOMINOPERINEAL RESECTION

Exploration and Exposure

- The intervention begins with an exploration of the abdominal cavity in order to identify the presence of possible carcinomatosis and metastasis. The evaluation of the length and quality of the sigmoid loop is performed in order to plan the type of mobilization of the left colon and rarely of the splenic flexure.
- The patient is the placed in a Trendelenburg position with the table tilted to the right.
- In women, exposure of the posterior pelvis and of the rectovaginal (Douglas) pouch can be obtained by direct or indirect suspension of the uterus by means of the T'Lift (VECTEC, France) tissue retraction device (**FIGURE 5A**) or suprapubic transparietal sutures (**FIGURE 5B**).
- Visceral obesity (in male patients) is more incapacitating than subcutaneous obesity (in female patients). The use of retractors is very helpful.
- The omentum and the transverse colon are retracted in a cephalad direction, and the small bowel is retracted toward the right side of the abdomen.

Primary Vascular Oncologic Approach to the Sigmoid Colon

- As for any oncologic surgical procedure, a primary vascular approach is performed.

- In rectal cancer, the inferior mesenteric vessels are dissected at their origin in order to perform an "en bloc" removal of all lymph nodes associated with the rectosigmoid junction (D3 resection). In the case of abdominoperineal resection, we prefer to dissect and preserve the left colic artery (LCA) to improve vascular supply for the future colostomy and because we do not need to lower the left colon for a lower anastomosis. Studies comparing ligation of the inferior mesenteric artery (IMA) at its origin or after the left superior colonic artery showed no statistically significant difference in survival between the two methods. These results suggest that the presence of invaded nodes at the origin of the IMA is associated with a tumor that has already spread along the aorta, and therefore beyond the aim of a curative removal.

The IMA is first exposed. The inferior mesenteric vein (IMV) is approached in order to prevent any venous overload related to the late ligation of the IMA.

The "Bottom-Up Technique"

The sigmoid mesocolon is exposed, the posterior peritoneum is incised at the level of the promontory and the left retroperitoneal space, facilitated by the pneumodissection is entered (**FIGURE 6**). The dissection is then continued in a cephalad direction up to the duodenojejunal junction (ligament of Treitz).

- Once the retroperitoneum is opened, dissection is initiated on the posterior aspect of the inferior mesenteric vascular

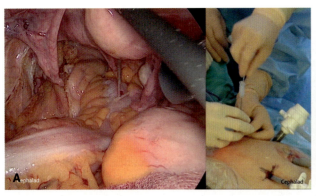
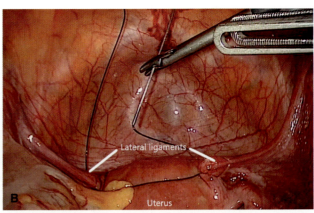

FIGURE 5 • Retraction system. **A,** T'Lift tissue retraction system passed through the round ligament. **B,** Transparietal suprapubic sutures for uterine suspension to enhance exposure.

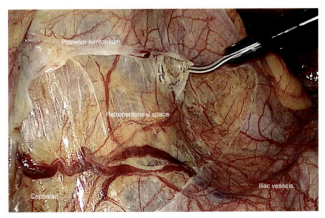

FIGURE 6 • Retroperitoneal incision at the level of the promontory and initiation of retroperitoneal dissection.

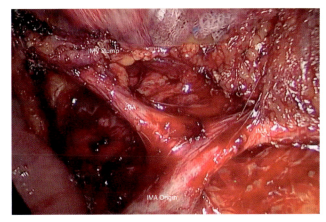

FIGURE 7 • Dissection of the IMA (at its origin and the left colic artery).

sheath (ie, the superior rectal artery at this level). This step is facilitated by the anterior traction on the mesocolon.
- Dissection is carried on always in contact with the posterior aspect of the vascular sheath of the IMA cranially until its origin on the aorta is reached.
- The IMA is skeletonized and the left colic artery and the terminal branch of the IMA are identified (**FIGURE 7**).
- This technique preserves the sympathetic nerve plexuses, which run along the aorta on its anterior aspect.

The "Top-Down" Technique

Sometimes, the identification of the origin of the IMA is not easy performing the dissection from the promontory. In this case, the retroperitoneal space is entered at the level of the ligament of Treitz facilitated by an upward traction on the IMV with the grasper placed in the 5-mm trocar placed lateral to the umbilicus and the peritoneal sheet incised (**FIGURE 8**). The retroperitoneal space is dissected preserving the superior left hypogastric plexus and the prerenal (Gerota) fascia. The dissection is then continued downwards toward the origin of the IMA thanks to the traction on the sigmoid mesocolon in order to expose the "T shape" created by the IMV and the IMA (**FIGURE 9A**).

- Once the IMA and the LCA are correctly identified, the superior rectal artery is divided with the LigaSure vessel-sealing device (**FIGURE 9B**). The stump of the IMA could be strengthened using ligation or placing clips.
- Once the superior rectal artery has been divided, the assistant standing between the patient's legs will grasp the artery using an atraumatic forceps introduced into the suprapubic port (port D) and apply anterior traction to ideally expose the dissection plane between the retroperitoneal space and the posterior aspect of the sigmoid mesocolon always in contact to the posterior aspect of the artery.
- This type of dissection in contact with the artery helps to preserve the nerve plexus, and notably the left sympathetic trunk of the neurovegetative system.
- The next step is the transection of the IMV: it can be transected at the level of the ligament of Treitz underneath the inferior edge of the pancreas (**FIGURE 10A**), or more distally when crossing the LCA (**FIGURE 10B**).
- The IMV is then transacted with the LigaSure vessel-sealing device or in between clips.

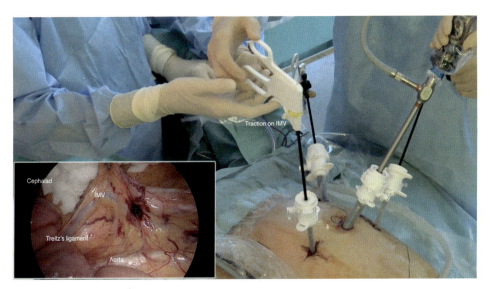

FIGURE 8 • Traction of the IMV at the level of the ligament of Treitz to access the retroperitoneal space in the top-down dissection technique toward the IMA.

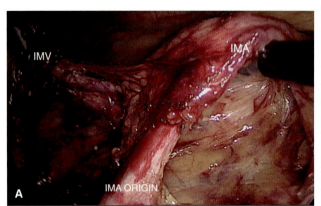
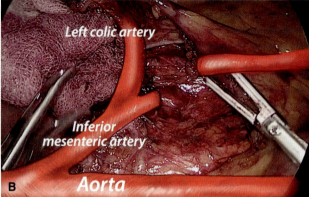

FIGURE 9 • **A,** Identification of the origin of the IMA thanks to the traction on the IMV and the mesosigmoid with the distal part of the IMA (T shape). **B,** Section of the superior rectal artery after correct identification of the IMA and its branches.

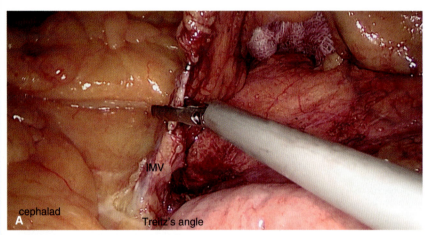

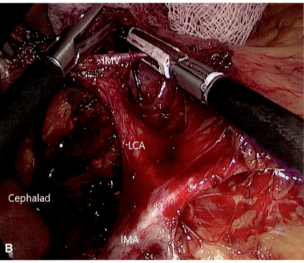

FIGURE 10 • Transection of the IMV **A,** Transection of the IMV performed at its origin at the Treitz's angle. **B,** Distal transection of the IMV when crossing the LCA.

MOBILIZATION AND DIVISION OF THE SIGMOID COLON

- A medial to lateral mobilization of the mesocolon by opening the plane between Toldt fascia anteriorly and Gerota fascia posteriorly is performed (**FIGURE 11**). This mobilization will help for the traction on the upper rectum allowing a perfect exposure of the anterior, posterior, and lateral aspects of the rectum.
- It is mandatory to identify the left ureter during this dissection. It is located between the aorta and the gonadal vessels, well protected by Gerota fascia.

Chapter 35 ABDOMINOPERINEAL RESECTION: LAPAROSCOPIC TECHNIQUE 313

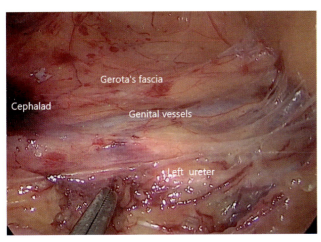

FIGURE 11 • Medial to lateral mobilization of the mesocolon. Gerota fascia is preserved intact. The left gonadal vessels and the left ureter are identified and preserved intact.

- The dissection is carried laterally until the posterior aspect of the descending colon is reached laterally.
- Mobilization of the sigmoid colon is completed with a division of its lateral attachments to the abdominal wall (**FIGURE 12**).
- The mesocolon is transected from the IMA transection site toward the sigmoid wall (**FIGURE 13A**). The sigmoid colon is transected at the level of the junction with the descending colon intracorporeally using an Endo GIA linear stapler (**FIGURE 13B**).
- Mobilization of the splenic flexure is not performed routinely in APR cases.
- Caudally, the dissection is carried toward the pelvic inlet. One should be cautious when in contact with the aorta as well as with the left iliac vessels where nerve rami of the superior hypogastric sympathetic plexus courses.

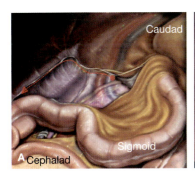
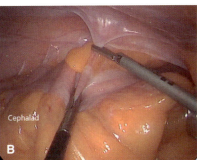

FIGURE 12 • **A,** Lateral mobilization of the sigmoid colon by dividing the lateral attachments to the abdominal wall. **B,** The previously dissected left ureter is again visualized.

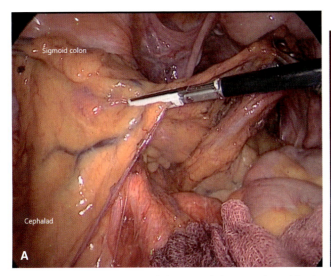
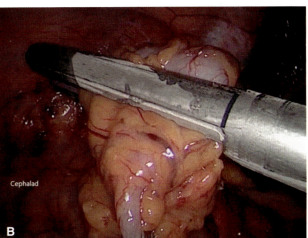

FIGURE 13 • **A,** Intracorporeal division of the mesosigmoid using the Ligasure device. **B,** Intracorporeal division of the proximal sigmoid colon with an Endo GIA linear stapler.

DISSECTION OF THE RECTUM ACCORDING TO THE PRINCIPLES OF THE TOTAL MESORECTAL EXCISION

- The principle of TME is respected.
- TME aims to eradicate the primary tumor and its lymphatic drainage by "en bloc" removal of the rectum and the mesorectum, along well-defined anatomical planes. A TME dissection proceeds under direct vision along the areolar tissue plane situated between the mesorectal fascia anteriorly and the presacral fascia posteriorly, the lateral pelvic fascia laterally, and Denonvilliers fascia (rectovaginal space) anteriorly. A sharp dissection along these planes is associated with a higher probability of achieving a negative circumferential resection margin (CRM), a lower risk of bleeding from inadvertent tearing of the presacral/hypogastric veins, and a reduced risk of injuring the hypogastric nerves.
- A proper surgical intervention is essential to obtain a curative resection and cannot be carried out without a detailed knowledge of this anatomy (**FIGURE 14A** and **B**).
- In an APR, the inferior limit of the dissection will depend on tumor's size and its distal location.
- The distal dissection is completed using a perineal approach as proposed by Miles.
- In the case of a female patient, the suspension of the uterus facilitates the exposure and the dissection. If the patient had a previous hysterectomy, the dissection can be facilitated by the introduction of a vaginal bougie.
- The dissection is done in this order: posterior dissection first, then lateral, starting with the right side, then the left side, and finally, the anterior dissection.

Posterior Dissection of the Rectum

- A cranial and anterior traction is exerted on the sigmoid rectal junction in order to expose the posterior aspect of the upper rectum.
- The presacral space (**FIGURE 14C**) is opened under the effect of traction and of pneumoperitoneum pressure. It is facilitated by the atraumatic anterior retraction of the posterior rectal wall exposing the space between the presacral fascia and the posterior aspect of the mesorectum, which is then dissected.
- Dissection should proceed toward the pelvic floor until the presacral fascia fuses with the fascia propria (Waldeyer fascia).
- During this dissection, left and right branches of the inferior hypogastric plexuses can be observed. The lateral pelvic fascia protects them along the pelvic side walls (**FIGURE 15A**).

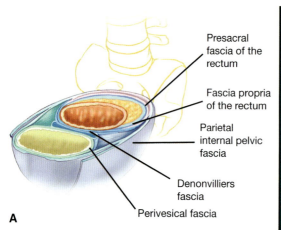
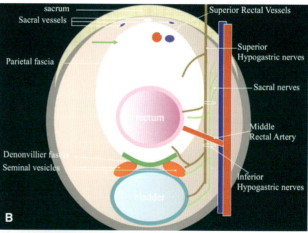
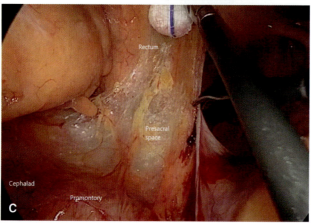

FIGURE 14 • **A,** Anatomy of pelvic fascias (in male patients). **B,** Pelvic anatomy with structures relationship. **C,** Posterior dissection of the rectum. Surgical view of the presacral "holy" plane.

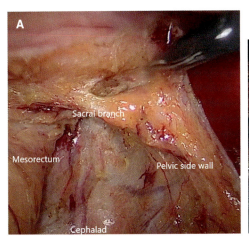
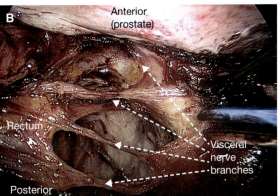

FIGURE 15 • Lateral dissection of the rectum. **A,** The rectal branches of the inferior hypogastric plexus traverse along the so-called lateral rectal ligament. **B,** The lateral rectal ligament on the right side of the distal rectum has been skeletonized. The visceral nerve branches to the rectum and prostate originating from the lateral inferior hypogastric plexus trunk can be seen.

Lateral Dissections of the Rectum

- Lateral dissection proceeds first on the right side.
- The rectum is retracted cranially and medially in order to expose the lateral pelvic space.
- The right peritoneum is incised until seminal vesicles are reached (in male patients). Under the effect of pneumoperitoneum pressure and of medial retraction, parietalization of the inferior hypogastric plexus and especially of the sacral branches (third and fifth sacral nerves, parasympathetic nerves responsible for male erections) is carried on. Care is taken to avoid violating the parietal endopelvic fascia.
- Between three and five nerve branches can be observed crossing the space between the fascia and the rectum (**FIGURE 15B**). These branches will be divided after skeletonization in order to preserve the trunks and prostatic branches as much as possible.
- The LigaSure device allows a safe dissection.
- Once the right dissection is completed the peritoneum is incised on the left side and the left sided lateral dissection is performed in a similar fashion. The rectum is retracted cranially and toward the right side of the surgical for the left lateral dissection.
    - During the deep lateral dissection, care must be taken to avoid an extensive dissection because the deepest areas seem superficial, especially as the pneumoperitoneum opens the space. Below the rectosacral ligament, which is not readily apparent in elderly patients, the curvature of the sacrum is in front of the view and care must be taken to dissect vertically along the levators muscles and not in the axis of the optic with the risk of transect the rectococcygeal ligaments and expose the coccyx and presacral veins.

Anterior Dissection of the Rectum

- The last step of the rectal mobilization is the anterior dissection. The Douglas pouch is opened (**FIGURE 16**).
- In order to open and dissect the space between the anterior aspect of the rectum and Denonvilliers aponeurosis, minimal cranial and posterior traction should be maintained on the rectum; Denonvilliers aponeurosis should be retracted anteriorly.
- Retraction is usually easy to perform in female patients. In male patients, especially obese ones, this step is more difficult. Retraction is done using atraumatic graspers. Specific retractors developed by KARL STORZ (Endo-Retractors) exist in order to reproduce the technique used in open surgery with the St. Mark's retractor. It involves a three-directional retraction described by Heald's (3-D retraction), which ensures a safe dissection of the anterior aspect of the rectum.
- The plane of anterior dissection can be carried either anterior or posterior to Denonvilliers aponeurosis (**FIGURE 17A** and **B**). In advanced rectal cancer, it may be necessary to stay anterior to Denonvilliers aponeurosis entering the latero prostatic space; in this case, the risk of genital nerve injury (impotence) is much higher.
- The same problem can happen in female patients with the dissection of rectovaginal space.

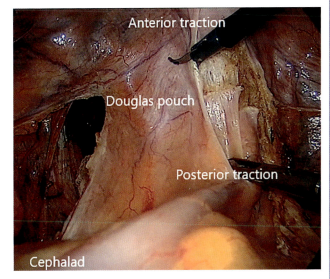

FIGURE 16 • Anterior dissection of the rectum. Douglas pouch incision.

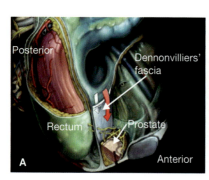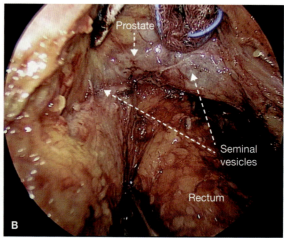

FIGURE 17 • Anterior dissection of the rectum. **A,** The dissection can be carried either anterior *(red arrow)* or posterior *(white arrow)* to Denonvilliers fascia. **B,** Surgical field after anterior dissection.

- It is important here to go as low as possible, especially anteriorly and laterally in men, and always down to the levators, as it may be difficult to complete the dissection of the lower part of the distal rectum during the perineal phase, even if the levators are largely resected.

- Before starting the perineal part of the operation, the colostomy is performed. An extraperitoneal colostomy, as described by Goligher, is performed in order to preserve as much as possible the quality of life of the patient reducing the risk of peristomal hernia and stomal prolapse when performing a definitive stoma.

EXTRAPERITONEAL COLOSTOMY TECHNIQUE

- The sigmoid colon is exposed and divided using the Endo GIA linear stapler after en bloc division of the mesocolon with the Ligasure device.
- The colostomy location is always determined and marked the day before the operation in order to avoid skin folds. Ideally, it should be placed in the left transrectal space at the level of the umbilicus.
   - A circular skin incision is performed and a patch of about 3 cm is removed (the size should be adapted if needed). The subcutaneous tissue is dissected until the aponeurosis of the rectus sheath is reached. A 3 cm-long cruciform incision of the aponeurosis is performed.
- A longitudinal rectus muscle splitting technique is used to expose the posterior leaflet of the rectus aponeurosis and is incised vertically to visualize the peritoneum, which is preserved.
- It is then necessary to detach the peritoneum from the posterior aspect of the rectus sheath aponeurosis, moving toward the left paracolic gutter and staying posteriorly to the aponeurosis of the transverse and oblique abdominis muscles.
- A tunnel is then created. It joins the intra-abdominal detachment of the left flank peritoneum performed during mobilization of the sigmoid and left colon.
- The tunnel can be created using a finger, a clamp, or with a bougie or even using an atraumatic retractor (**FIGURE 18A** and **B**).
- During this dissection, a permanent laparoscopic control helps to check the route and the width of the tunnel.
- The tunnel is widely dissected to allow the passage of the colon.
- In order to retrieve the colon, a clamp or a laparoscopic forceps is introduced into the tunnel. The colonic stump is grasped at the level of the staple line and taken out.
   - The colon should protrude 2 to 3 cm above the skin, checking whether there is no axial or lateral torsion in the preperitoneal tunnel. It has to remain spontaneous in this position (**FIGURE 19**). If the colonic stump retracts, it means that the colon has not been sufficiently mobilized and that there is a risk of stoma invagination.
   - The colostomy will be matured after closure of all wounds by opening the staple line and fixing the colonic serosa to the dermis with either interrupted or running sutures using a rapid resorption suturing material (Monocryl 3-0, Ethicon). Stitches transfix the dermal layer and extramucosal layer of the colon.

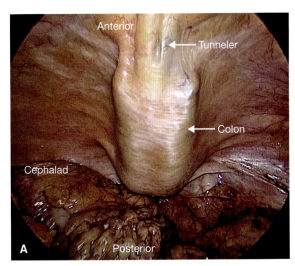 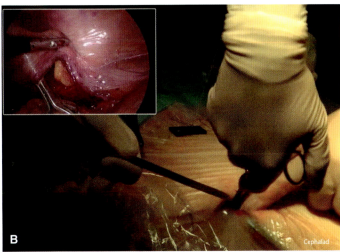

FIGURE 18 • Laparoscopic extraperitoneal end colostomy. **A,** Preperitoneal tunnelization with the H retractor. **B,** Preperitoneal tunnelization with a clamp.

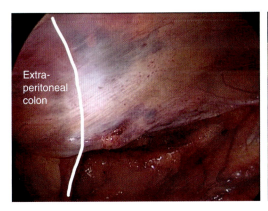 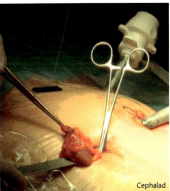

FIGURE 19 • Extraperitoneal colostomy, external view of the colostomy in correct position without retraction.

PERINEAL DISSECTION

- Once the perineal region has been perfectly exposed, the entire team is positioned opposite the perineum.
- The anal canal is closed by a purse-string suture. The skin incision is generally vertical and elliptical, away from the tumoral area in case of sphincteric invasion. It is possible to perform a circular incision 2 cm away from the closed anus (**FIGURE 20A**).
- The dissection can be performed using retraction on the purse string. The exposure can be facilitated by a retracting system (either a Gelpi retractor [**FIGURE 20B**] or the self-retaining Lina Sea Star [LineaMedical] retractor system) (**FIGURE 20C**) that is placed on the incision margins, dissection of deep structures is performed in a circular fashion first using the electrocautery and then using the LigaSure Atlas vessel-sealing device or ultrasonic scissors.
- During the posterior dissection, the subcutaneous cellular tissue is incised to the tip of the coccyx and to the presacral area to find the posterior pelvic plane previously dissected during the laparoscopic pelvic dissection phase. Laterally, the ischiorectal fossae fat is divided until the levator muscle is exposed.
- It is essential to maintain dissection along a vertical axis in order to prevent any conical route (conization).
- Anteriorly, the dissection is more subtle. The subcutaneous tissue and the anobulbar raphe are incised with the electrocautery. In male patients, it is recommended to stay dorsal to the urethra to avoid injuring or devascularizing it.
- More cranially, the dissection is carried dorsal to the prostate until reaching the anterior pelvic dissection plane.
- In female patients, the dissection is easier and it proceeds dorsal to the vagina.

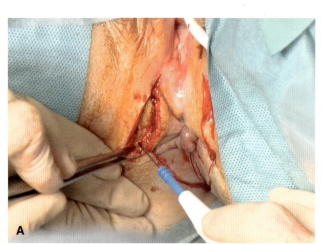
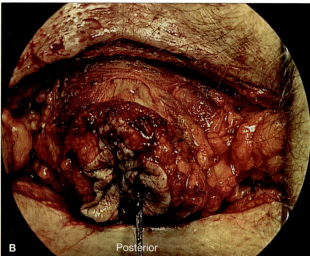
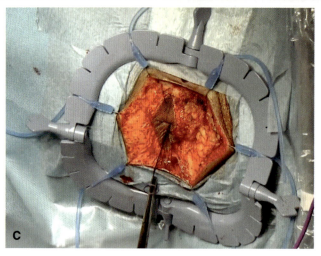

FIGURE 20 • Perineal dissection. **A,** Closure of anal canal with a purse-string and elliptical skin incision. **B,** Cylindrical dissection of the distal rectum is facilitated by the use of Gelpi retractors. **C,** Dissection facilitated with the application of a Lina Sea Star self-retractor.

DISSECTION OF THE PERINEAL RECTUM AND SPECIMEN EXTRACTION

We start with the posterior dissection first, entering the presacral dissection plane performed during the abdominal part.

- The closed stump of the anus is drawn forward and the anococcygeal raphe is transected with electrocautery. A finger is inserted into this space in front of the coccyx and into the presacral dissection plane dissected during the abdominal part. The opening is enlarged on each side as far as the posterior fibers of the posterior fibers of the levator muscles. The assistant pulls the anus to the right, exposing the right levator muscle. The operator's left index finger is introduced into the presacral space pulling the left levator into the field of view and then transects it with electrocautery close to its insertion on the pelvic sidewall. The same maneuver is performed on the right side but with the opposite hand index finger. The perineal opening is then sufficiently wide and the operator can use a long forceps to grasp the proximal colonic stump and evaginate the colonic stump behind the rectum to retract the specimen outside. At that moment, the distal rectum is held in place only by its anterior perineal attachments.
- The anterior dissection is tricky, as dissection too close to the rectum may result in a rectal opening and with potential soilage and oncological contamination, while a dissection too wide may result in a urethral injury.
- The closed anus is pulled outwards and posteriorly, putting tension on the anterior fibers of the levator muscles. In men, the anobulbar raphe is cut along the midline close to the bulb. There is a depression between the two medial edges of the anterior fibers of the levator, which represents the correct plane of cleavage.
- Dissection is continued on the posterior surface of the prostate until it reaches the anterior pelvic dissection plane of the abdominal phase. In women, the anovulvar raphe is sectioned on the midline in contact with the posterior wall of the vagina. The dissection is continued at its contact until the abdominal dissection plane is found.

Chapter 35 ABDOMINOPERINEAL RESECTION: LAPAROSCOPIC TECHNIQUE

- The specimen, including the sigmoid colon, the rectum, and anal canal, with an intact mesorectum without conization, can now be completely removed and sent to the pathology department for evaluation.

- Some authors suggest an extension of the lateral dissection, also called "extended APR," "extralevator abdominoperineal excision (ELAPE)," "cylindrical APR," or "Holm cylindrical abdominoperineal excision." This may be unnecessary, especially after radiochemotherapy.

PERINEAL CLOSURE, AND COLOSTOMY COMPLETION

- In order to obtain a good oncologic outcome, it is necessary to obtain a cylindrical specimen with an intact mesorectum and without a waist effect, removing the specimen along with the levator ani fixed to the anus (**FIGURE 21**).

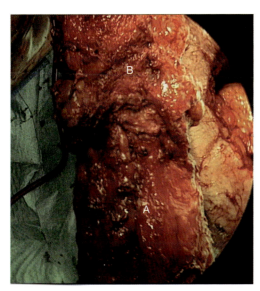

FIGURE 21 • Cylindrical specimen with an intact mesorectum *(A)* without a waist effect *(B)*.

- Complete hemostasis of the pelvis is then controlled through the perineal incision.
- One or two suction drains are placed (either 12-Fr Redon drain or 14-Fr Blake drain) in the presacral space.
- The deep cellular adipose plane is reapproximated using an absorbable suture. The perineal incision is then closed in layers (**FIGURE 22A**). In case of a wide dissection and resection by removing the vagina and the uterus or the prostate, closure of the perineal wound can be performed using a myocutaneous Taylor or Lotus flap (**FIGURE 22B**).
- An omental pedicle flap may be used to fill the pelvic space and to limit the risk of perineal hernia and urinary dysfunction due to a posterior falling of the urinary tract (**FIGURE 23**).
- It is better to perform the dissection for the omental pedicle flap at the beginning of the operation. The omentum is dissected off the greater curvature of the stomach with the Ligasure from the right to left by sectioning the right gastroepiploic pedicle and basing the flap on the left gastroepiploic pedicle.
- It will be descended into the left parietocolic gutter to the pelvis once the colostomy is ready or externalized.
- The extensive cylindrical rectal resection does not allow to reapproximate the muscular plane of the levator ani.
- The abdominal wound is closed in a standard fashion.
- The intervention is always completed with a final laparoscopic examination of the abdominal and pelvic cavity.

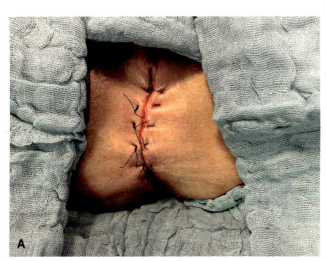
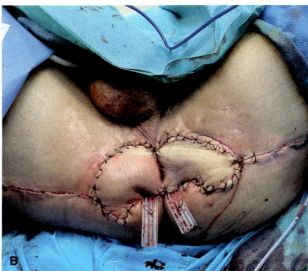

FIGURE 22 • Closures of the perineal defect. **A,** Simple suture. **B,** Perineal wound closure with a Lotus flap.

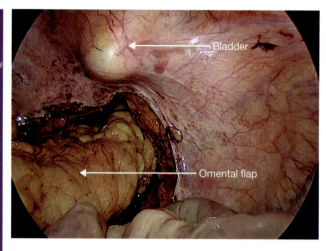

FIGURE 23 • An omental pedicle flap is used to obliterate the pelvic space after resection.

PEARLS AND PITFALLS

Anatomy and embryology	▪ Detailed knowledge of the pelvic fascial structures and tissue planes is essential.
Preoperative	▪ Adequate staging with colonoscopy and appropriate imaging is important in determining the need for an APR. ▪ A multidisciplinary team approach is essential.
Setup	▪ Precise operating room (OR), patient, and team setup is critical to success.
Technique	▪ Medial to lateral dissection of the mesocolon. ▪ TME dissection principles must be observed. ▪ Pelvic dissection: 　▪ Posterior first. 　▪ Lateral dissection/transection of the "lateral rectal ligaments": Avoid injury to autonomic trunks and genital nerve branches that would lead to autonomic pelvic dysfunction postoperatively. ▪ Perineal phase: Perform a circumferential dissection. ▪ Avoid "conization" of the specimen. ▪ The specimen should have an intact mesorectum without a "waist" effect distally. ▪ Subperitoneal colostomy to prevent stoma complications.
Perioperative care	▪ Enhanced recovery program.

POSTOPERATIVE CARE

- Postoperative care is driven by clinical pathways that include the following:
  - Pain control (score evaluation 3 times a day): 24-hour syringe pump (morphine 100 mg; Ketamine 50 mg; droperidol 5 mg). The transversus abdominis plane (TAP) nerve block greatly reduces the need for narcotics.
  - DVT prophylaxis with enoxaparin, starting within 6 hours of surgery and continued for 1 month postoperatively.
  - No additional antibiotics.
  - No nasogastric tube. Remove Foley catheter on postoperative day 1. Remove pelvic drains on postoperative day 2 or 3.
  - Early ambulation, normal diet, aggressive pulmonary toilet.
  - Oral supplements 3 times a day during the first 3 postoperative days.
  - Use soft pillow/jelly doughnut while seating.
  - Targeted discharge: postoperative day 3 or 4, 10 days in case of flap reconstruction

OUTCOMES

- Laparoscopic APR can promote patient recovery, overall outcome, and quality of life.
  - From an oncological standpoint, there is no difference in short-term outcomes between the laparoscopic and open approach. The long-term results of the limited number of trials conducted to date reported that the outcomes were similar between the two surgical groups' oncologic outcomes are at least comparable to those of open surgery.

Chapter 35 **ABDOMINOPERINEAL RESECTION: LAPAROSCOPIC TECHNIQUE** **321**

- TME with an intact mesorectum is critical to minimize locoregional treatment failures leading to a reduction in locoregional recurrence rates from 25% in the 1980s to under 4% today.

COMPLICATIONS

- Wound infections and hernias.
- Perineal wound infection/dehiscence and pelvic abscess incidence are reduced with the use of an omental pedicle flap to fill the pelvis.
- Urinary/sexual dysfunction: It is important to preserve autonomic nerves intact.
- Ureteral injury: critical to identify the left ureter prior to IMA transection.
- DVT: lower risk with use of DVT prophylaxis.

SUGGESTED READINGS

1. Bodin F, Dissaux C, Seigle-Murandi F, Dragomir S, Rohr S, Bruant-Rodier C. Posterior perineal reconstructions with "supra-fascial" lotus petal flaps. *J Plast Reconstr Aesthetic Surg.* 2015;68(1):e7-12.
2. Cuna SA, Chesney TR, Ramjist JK, Shah PS, Kennedy ED, Baxter NN. Laparoscopic versus open resection for rectal cancer: a noninferiority meta-analysis of quality of surgical resection outcomes. *Ann Surg.* 2019;269(5):849-855.
3. Fleshman J, Branda ME, Sargent DJ, et al. Disease-free survival and local recurrence for laparoscopic resection compared with open resection of stage II to III rectal cancer: follow-up results of the ACOSOG Z6051 randomized controlled trial. *Ann Surg.* 2019;269(4):589-595.
4. Goligher JC. Extraperitoneal colostomy or ileostomy. *Br J Surg.* 1958;46:97-103.
5. Heald RJ, Husband EM, Ryall RD. The mesorectum in rectal cancer surgery the clue to pelvic recurrence? *Br J Surg.* 1982;69:613-616.
6. Hermanek P, Junginger T. The circumferential resection margin in rectal carcinoma surgery. *Tech Coloproctol.* 2005;9(3):193-199; discussion 199-200.
7. Kroese LF, de Smet GHJ, Jeekel J, Kleinrensink GJ, Lange JF. Systematic review and meta-analysis of extraperitoneal versus transperitoneal colostomy for preventing parastomal hernia. *Dis Colon Rectum.* 2016;59(7):688-695.
8. Marr R, Birbeck K, Garvican J, et al. The modern abdominoperineal excision: the next challenge after total mesorectal excision. *Ann Surg.* 2005;242:74-82.
9. Stevenson AR, Solomon MJ, Lumley JW, et al. Effect of laparoscopic-assisted resection vs open resection on pathological outcomes in rectal cancer: the ALaCaRT randomized clinical trial. *JAMA.* 2015;314:1356-1363.
10. Tong G, Zhang G, Liu J, Zheng Z, Chen Y, Cui E. A meta-analysis of short-term outcome of laparoscopic surgery versus conventional open surgery on colorectal carcinoma. *Medicine (Baltim).* 2017;96(48):e8957.
11. West NP, Finan PJ, Anderin C, et al. Evidence of the oncologic superiority of cylindrical abdominoperineal excision for low rectal cancer. *J Clin Oncol.* 2008;26:3517-3522.

Chapter 36

Hand-Assisted Abdominoperineal Resection

Daniel Albo

DEFINITION

- An abdominoperineal resection, or APR, involves removal of the anus, the rectum, and part or all of the sigmoid colon along with the associated regional lymph nodes, through incisions made in the abdomen and perineum. The end of the remaining colon is brought out as an end colostomy.
- Hand-assisted laparoscopic surgery (HALS) is a minimally invasive surgical approach that uses conventional laparoscopic-assisted (LA) surgery techniques with the addition of a hand-assisted device (placed in the projected specimen extraction site) that allows for the introduction of a hand into the surgical field. HALS in colorectal surgery retains all of the same advantages of conventional LA surgery over open surgery, including less pain, faster recovery, lower incidence of wound complications, and reduction of cardiopulmonary complications, especially in the obese and in the elderly. Advantages of HALS over conventional LA colorectal surgery include the following:
  - Reintroduces tactile feedback into the field
  - Shorter learning curves; easier to teach and to learn
  - Shorter operative times
  - Lower conversion to open rates
  - Higher utilization rates of minimally invasive surgery

DIFFERENTIAL DIAGNOSIS

Indications for HALS APR include the following:

- Rectal cancer: when unable to obtain a negative distal margin and/or in patients with poor sphincter function or severe comorbidities
- Anal cancer: after failure of chemo/radiation therapy or in the palliative setting
- Inflammatory bowel disease (ie, Crohn with severe perianal disease)

PATIENT HISTORY AND PHYSICAL FINDINGS

- Most patients with rectal tumors generally present after an incidental finding during screening colonoscopy or with occult bleeding and anemia.
- A thorough history and physical examination should include:
  - Presence of rectal pain and/or tenesmus
  - Presence of obstructive symptoms
  - Description of anorectal function, with any fecal incontinence or leakage documented preoperatively
  - Documentation of urinary and erectile function/dysfunction
  - Previous history of pelvic radiation and pelvic surgery should also be noted
  - A detailed personal and family history of colorectal cancer, polyps, and/or other malignancies

- Physical examination should include:
  - Routine abdominal examination, noting any previous incisions
  - Digital rectal examination should assess tumor size, degree of fixation to anal sphincter, rectal and pelvic wall, mobility, location (anterior/posterior/lateral), distance from the anorectal ring, and anterior extension into vagina/prostate
  - Anterior rectal tumors in female patients require a vaginal examination to rule out extension into the vagina
  - Bilateral inguinal nodal examination
  - Rigid proctoscopy is arguably the most critical portion of the physical examination and is the key to proper patient selection of patients for an APR. Proctoscopy should be standardized and document at minimum:
    - The distal and proximal extent of the lesion measured from the anal verge and from the top of the anal sphincter
    - Exact position of the lesion and extent of the rectal circumference involved
    - Presence or absence of fixation to perirectal structures

IMAGING AND OTHER DIAGNOSTIC STUDIES

- A complete colonoscopy should be performed to rule out synchronous disease. Regardless of the primary location of the tumor, every patient should have a complete colonoscopy study whenever possible, since 2% to 9% of the patients may have synchronous tumors elsewhere in the colon and rectum.
- A colonic enema with double contrast may be used in patients in whom colonoscopy is not possible. Virtual colonoscopy (computed tomography [CT] colonography) is also an option for those that cannot undergo colonoscopy.
- A contrast-enhanced CT of the abdomen and pelvis is obtained to rule out adjacent organ involvement, to evaluate for extraluminal complications (eg, abscess, fistula), and to rule out metastatic disease in patients with cancer. A CT of the chest completes the metastatic workup.
- Preoperative should not be performed in rectal cancer patients. The best assessment of the margin is obtained via frequent and thorough digital examinations, intraoperative flexible endoscopy, and adherence to the best total mesorectal excision (TME) surgery criteria.
- Accurate staging of rectal cancer should be able to determine depth of invasion, presence of lymph node metastases, and resectability of locally advanced tumors.
- Pelvic magnetic resonance imaging (MRI) should be used in diagnosis for all rectal cancers.
- The MERCURY and MERCURY II trials demonstrate that high-resolution pelvic MRI is an essential tool for evaluating the mesorectal fascia and intersphincteric plane for tumor invasion for low rectal cancers.

Chapter 36 **HAND-ASSISTED ABDOMINOPERINEAL RESECTION** **323**

- Endoscopic ultrasound (EUS) is another imaging modality that may be used in the workup of rectal cancer and is particularly useful in early lesions. EUS has an overall 80% to 95% staging accuracy. When compared to MRI in staging of rectal cancer, EUS is superior at differentiating early T1 and T2 lesions as MRI provides limited visualization of the submucosa.
- Detection of lymph node metastasis is associated with 73% sensitivity and 76% specificity.
- A carcinoembryonic antigen (CEA) level is obtained in all cancer cases. The baseline preoperative result and postsurgical control must be obtained as an assessment for complete tumor resection. Absolute CEA presurgical value is an independent variable for survival.

SURGICAL MANAGEMENT

Preoperative Preparation

- We use an enhanced recovery after surgery (ERAS) clinical pathway (described elsewhere in this textbook) for the perioperative management of all of our colorectal surgery patients.
- A mechanical preoperative bowel preparation may be considered to facilitate the handling of the colon during laparoscopic surgery. Fleet enemas are prescribed to facilitate the performance of the anastomosis.
- All patients should receive preoperative prophylactic antibiotics, following published guidelines. We administer 1 to 2 g of ertapenem based on patient's BMI within 1 hour of surgical incision.
- Pharmacologic deep vein thrombosis (DVT) prophylaxis should be given to patients perioperatively, based on current recommendations and guidelines.
- Ultrasound-guided bilateral transversus abdominis plane block reduces the need for postoperative narcotics.

Equipment and Instrumentation

- We use a minimalistic approach to instrumentation, emphasizing a streamlined, efficient, and reproducible approach to our procedures. The entire operation is performed with essentially three instruments (a slotted grasper, am energy device, and a stapler) plus the camera. This approach minimizes clutter, makes the operation more efficient, and maximizes cost-efficiency.
- 5-mm, 30° scope with high-resolution monitors
- 5- and 12-mm clear ports with balloon tips. They hold ports in the abdomen during instrument exchanges, minimize dripping/condensation on the scope, and minimize intra-abdominal profile/fulcrum effect of the trocars during surgery
- A blunt tip, 5-mm, 37-cm long energy device
- A slotted laparoscopic grasper
- 60-mm linear roticulating laparoscopic staplers with vascular and tan cartridges
- We use the GelPort hand-assisted device due to its versatility and ease of use. This device allows for the introduction/removal of the hand without losing pneumoperitoneum and allows for insertion of multiple ports through the hand-assisted device if necessary. It also allows for the introduction of laparotomy pads into the field, which are very useful to retract bowel/omentum in obese patients and to clean up

the field and the scope during the procedure. It is imperative to mark every lap pad introduced into the abdomen on the operating room (OR) board and include them in the final counts to avoid inadvertently leaving a lap pad in the abdominal cavity after the procedure.
- We like to use a disposable three-instrument long pouch to place the energy device and slotted graspers during the procedure. This pouch is placed on the patient's left hip/thigh, in between the surgeon and the monitor. This pouch functions like a holster to facilitate an easy and intuitive handling of the two instruments used during the entire operation and allowing the surgeon's eyes to never leave the target in the monitor.

Patient Positioning and Surgical Team Setup

(FIGURE 1A)
- A preoperative briefing with the entire surgical team is conducted. Items discussed include patient identification, type of surgery, type of anesthesia, expected events during the surgery, the need for blood components, prophylactic antibiotic, surgical devices availability, and potential adverse events and their prevention.
- A dedicated, highly trained team in laparoscopic concepts is paramount. Critical members of this team concept are the scrub nurse, the circulating nurses, the assistants, and the anesthesia team members. I cannot emphasize enough the importance of a total team concept in accomplishing the highest level of performance during laparoscopic surgery.
- Proper patient position and OR setup is critical for successful performance of minimally invasive surgery.
- The patient is placed in a modified lithotomy position using Yellowfin stirrups with the heels firmly planted in the stirrups to avoid having the patient slide with gravity-assist maneuvers during the procedure.
- Pressure-bearing areas in the calf and lateral legs are padded to prevent DVTs and lateral peroneal nerve injury.
- The patient's toes, knee, and contralateral shoulders are aligned.
- The thighs are placed parallel to the ground to prevent conflict with the surgeon's arms.
- The patient's buttocks are placed at the edge of the table to allow for smoother introduction of the end-to-end anastomosis stapler at time of reconstruction. The coccyx should be readily palpable off the edge of the table.
- Both arms are tucked at the sides, with padding added to protect against neurovascular injuries.
- The patient is taped to the table across the chest over towels to avoid slipping. The shoulders are padded to avoid neurovascular injuries.
- All laparoscopic elements (CO_2 line, camera, light cord) exit through the right upper side. All energy device cords exit through the upper left side. This allows for a clutter-free working space for the operative team.

Team Positioning and Draping

(FIGURES 1B and 2)
- The patient is prepped with chlorhexidine and draped to facilitate easy access to the perineum.
- The surgeon stands at the patient's right lower side, with the assistant to their left side and the scrub nurse to their right side (**FIGURE 1B**).

324 SECTION III **RECTAL RESECTIONS**

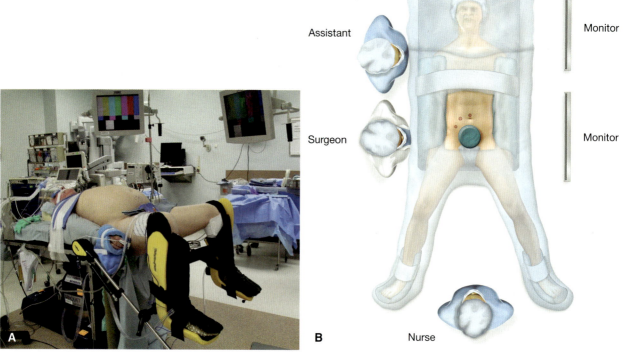

FIGURE 1 • **A,** Patient and operating room (OR) setup. The patient is placed in a modified lithotomy position with the thighs parallel to the floor and the arms tucked. The patient is secured to the OR bed using a chest tape-over-towel technique. **B,** Team, patient, and monitor setup. The patient is on a modified lithotomy position. The team, ports, targets, and monitors are aligned.

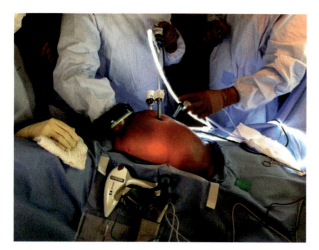

FIGURE 2 • Ports and instrumentation setup. The GelPort is placed through a Pfannenstiel incision. All ports are triangulated. Notice the energy devices placed in a pouch in front of the surgeon to minimize instrument transfer.

- There are four important principles that we follow for all laparoscopic cases: alignment, triangulation, a flat horizon, and gravity-assist.
- Alignment involves the placement of the team, ports, target lesion, and monitors in straight lines of vision.
- Triangulation involves the creation of an imaginary triangle, where the surgeon's hands/instruments/trocars are at the angles in the base of the triangle, and the target lesion is located at the apex of the triangle. The camera bisects this triangle and, in laparoscopic surgery, is always in front of the hands of the surgeon. This is in contrast to open surgery, where the surgeon's hands are in front of the eyes.
- The concept of horizon is a fundamental difference between laparoscopic and open surgery. In open surgery, the surgeon looks down into the field. In laparoscopic surgery, the surgeon looks to their front, introducing the concept of the horizon. It is imperative that the camera operator maintains a flat horizon in front of the operator to avoid disorientation. This is particularly important with the use of angled scopes (ie, a 30° scope).
- Extreme gravity-assist maneuvers are critically important in laparoscopic surgery to keep the bowel and omentum away from the operative field and to provide optimal exposure. To accomplish this while avoiding the patient sliding during the procedure, the patient needs to be secured to the table, so the table and the patient move as one. Padding on all pressure points is imperative to avoid neurovascular injuries to the extremities during the procedure.

- Two monitors are placed in front of the team at eye level and slighted tilted upward (to avoid ergonomic injury to the surgeon's lower neck/brachial plexus) on the patient's left side.

PORT PLACEMENT AND OPERATIVE FIELD SETUP (FIGURES 1 AND 2)

- Insert the GelPort through a 5- to 6-cm Pfannenstiel incision (**FIGURE 3**). One of the main advantages of HALS is that it uses the extraction site incision necessary in colorectal surgery procedures during the entire operation instead of just using it at the end of the procedure. This allows for the introduction of the surgeon's hand without losing pneumoperitoneum insufflation at various portions of the operation, reintroducing tactile feedback for the surgeon, making the operation much more efficient.
- The size of this incision in centimeters is usually 1 to ½ cm less than the surgeon's glove size. Make this incision as long as you need it to be comfortable during the operation; the size of the extraction size has no impact on any meaningful perioperative outcome.
- The Pfannenstiel incision (as opposed as vertical extraction site incisions) results in better cosmesis, lowers the incidence of wound infections and hernias, and allows for more working space between the hand and the instruments.
- Ports: Insert a 5-mm working port in the right upper quadrant (RUQ), a 12-mm working port in the right lower quadrant, and a 5-mm camera port above the umbilicus. These three ports are triangulated, with the camera port at the apex of the triangle. This setup avoids conflict between the working instruments and the camera and prevents disorientation (avoids "working on a mirror").

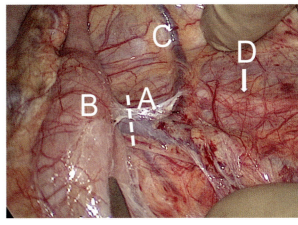

FIGURE 3 • Step 1: Key anatomy. *A*, Ligament of Treitz. *B*, inferior mesenteric vein (IMV). *C*, Left colic artery as it separates from the IMV and goes toward the splenic flexure of the colon. The left ureter *(D)* is located far from the IMV projected transection (dotted lines).

- A 5-mm accessory working port may be inserted at the planned colostomy site in the left lower quadrant. This port allows the surgeon to operate from the left side of the table (useful for the right-sided pelvic dissection, especially in males). It can also be valuable for the mobilization of the splenic flexure.

OPERATIVE STEPS

- All our operations are process-driven and highly standardized to maximize efficiency, quality, and cost-efficiency. We divide the operations in well-defined, sequential steps. Every step has a single strategic objective (it is the name of the step), a clear beginning and end, and a critical anatomy that is required to be identified.
- We believe that this stepwise approach makes it easier to teach and learn these complex operations. In fact, it is designed to strip down all complexity and to shorten the learning curve of the surgeon.
- Every step opens the planes of dissection that are necessary for the steps that will follow, flowing "downstream" and opening the planes of dissection sequentially always in front of the operator. This way, the only time that the surgeon encounters a virgin tissue plane is at the very beginning of the operation. We call this first step the point of entry.
- The ideal point of entry has three characteristics: it is easy to find, it has minimal to no anatomical variations, and it minimizes potential injury to other structures around it during its performance. In order to simplify our operations, we use only two potential points of entry for all our laparoscopic colorectal surgeries. For all resections to the left side of the middle colic vessels, we use the inferior mesenteric vein (IMV) as the point of entry.

- Our HALS APR operation consists of eight steps:
  1. Transection of the IMV
  2. Transection of the Inferior mesenteric artery (IMA)
  3. Medial to lateral dissection of the descending mesocolon
  4. Sigmoid colon mobilization off the pelvic inlet
  5. Descending colon mobilization
  6. Pelvic dissection
  7. Transection of the levator ani muscles
  8. Creation of colostomy and closure of abdominal wounds

Step 1: Transection of the IMV

- This is the critical "point of entry" in this operation. We favor it over starting dissection at the IMA level due to the IMV's constancy in location, the ease of its visualization by the ligament of Treitz, and the absence of structures that can be harmed around it (no iliac vessels, left ureter, or hypogastric nerve nearby). This will be the only time during the operation when a virgin tissue plane is entered. Every step will setup the following ones, opening the tissue planes sequentially.
- The patient is placed on a steep Trendelenburg position with the left side up. Using the right hand, move the small bowel into the RUQ and the transverse colon and omentum into the upper abdomen. If necessary, place a laparotomy pad to hold the bowel out of the field of view, especially in obese patients. This pad can also be used to dry up the field and

to clean the scope tip intracorporeally. Make sure that the circulating nurse notes the laparotomy pad in the abdomen on the white board.
- Identify the critical anatomy: IMV, ligament of Treitz, and left colic artery (**FIGURE 3**).
- If there are attachments between the duodenum/root of mesentery and mesocolon, transect them with laparoscopic scissors. This will allow for adequate exposure of midline structures.
- Pick up the IMV/left colic artery with the right hand. Dissect under the IMV/left colic artery and in front of Gerota fascia with endoscopic scissors or energy device, starting at the level of the ligament of Treitz and proceeding with the dissection caudally toward the IMA. The assistant provides upward countertraction with a grasper.
- Transect the IMV with the energy device (**FIGURE 4**) cephalad of left colic artery, which moves away from the IMV and toward the splenic flexure of the colon, with the 5-mm energy device, thus preserving intact the left-sided marginal arterial arcade and maintaining the blood supply to the descending colon segment.

Step 2: Transection of the Inferior Mesenteric Artery

- Identify the critical anatomy: The "letter T" formed between the IMA and its left colic and superior hemorrhoidal artery (SHA) terminal branches (**FIGURES 5** and **6A**).

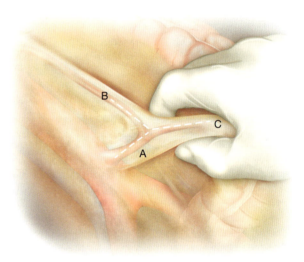

FIGURE 5 • Step 2: critical anatomy. Identify the "letter T" formed between the inferior mesenteric artery (IMA) *(A)* and its left colic artery *(B)* and superior hemorrhoidal artery (SHA) *(C)* terminal branches. The IMA takeoff is just cephalad from the aortic bifurcation (dotted lines). The thumb and index finger are lifting the SHA off the groove located anterior to the right common iliac artery.

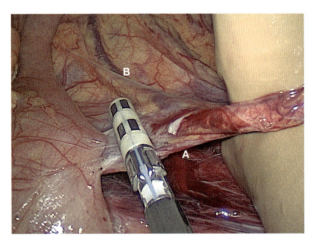

FIGURE 4 • Step 1: The surgeon holds the inferior mesenteric vein (IMV) *(A)* anteriorly with their right hand and transects it cephalad of the left colic artery *(B)* with a 5-mm energy device.

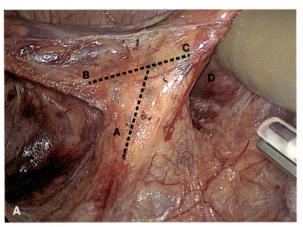
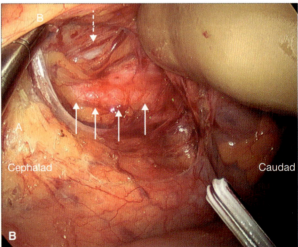

FIGURE 6 • **A,** The "letter T" dissected: inferior mesenteric artery (IMA) *(A)*, left colic artery *(B)*, superior hemorrhoidal artery (SHA) *(C)*. Notice the left ureter *(D)* in the retroperitoneum. **B,** Step 2: identification of the left ureter and gonadal vessels. After the IMA *(A)* and SHA *(B)* have been lifted off the retroperitoneum, the left ureter *(solid arrows)* can be identified and preserved intact. Identification of the left ureter at this stage is critical in order to avoid injuring it during the IMA transection. Distal to the takeoff of the IMA, the left gonadal vessels can be identified lateral to the left ureter *(dotted arrow)*.

Chapter 36 **HAND-ASSISTED ABDOMINOPERINEAL RESECTION** 327

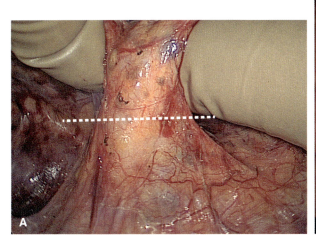
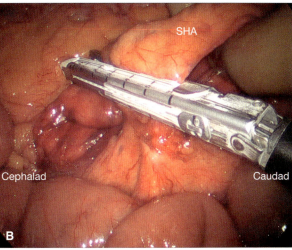

FIGURE 7 • **A,** The inferior mesenteric artery (IMA) is now completely encircled and will be transected at its origin (dotted line) with a stapler or energy device. **B,** Step 2: transection of the IMA. With the left ureter safely dissected away into the retroperitoneum, the IMA is transected with a linear vascular stapler at its origin of the aorta. The surgeon's hand is holding the superior hemorrhoidal artery (SHA) anteriorly.

- Using the hand, the aorta is identified and tracked down to the level of its bifurcation. The IMA will originate 1-2 cm proximal to this level.
- Using your thumb, palpate the groove between the left common iliac artery pulse and the SHA. Use your index finger to encircle the SHA and pick it up, turning it into an arch. The SHA fold is thicker than the inexperienced surgeon may think. A common mistake during this portion of the operation is to think that the SHA fold is too thick, wrongly thinking that you are instead under the left common iliac artery and the left ureter. This results in a too shallow dissection plane superficial to the SHA and, therefore, entering the wrong plane into the mesocolon, resulting in troublesome bleeding and disorienting the surgeon.
- Holding the SHA up with the right hand, dissect the plane along the palpable groove between the SHA and the left iliac artery using an energy device. After scoring the peritoneum under the SHA, use a 5-mm energy device to dissect (by gently pushing downward toward the retroperitoneum) along the avascular plane located between the meso descending colon, anteriorly, and the retroperitoneum, posteriorly. This avascular plane can be identified by the transition between the two distinctive fat planes.
- Preserve the sympathetic nerve trunk intact in the retroperitoneum. Identify the left ureter, located in front of the left iliac artery and psoas muscle and medial to the gonadal vessels, before transecting anything (**FIGURE 6B**). If you are directly on the psoas muscle, chances are that you left the left ureter attached to the dorsal surface of the mesocolon; bring it down into the retroperitoneum gently using blunt dissection with the energy device.
- If you cannot identify the ureter, try dissecting superior to inferior, starting from the IMV plane of dissection and moving caudally behind the IMA. If you still cannot find it, perform a lateral to medial mobilization of the sigmoid colon toward the midline. In this latter scenario, you will encounter the left gonadal vessels first, lateral to the left ureter.

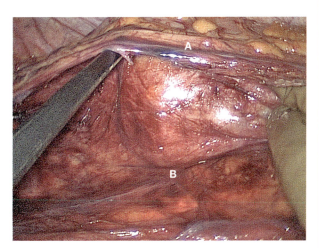

FIGURE 8 • Step 3: Medial to lateral dissection of the descending mesocolon. The surgeon's hand is holding the descending mesocolon and colon anteriorly *(A),* separating them from Gerota fascia and other retroperitoneal structures *(B).* The dissection proceeds along the transition between the two distinct fat planes.

- You can visualize the letter "T" formed between the IMA, the left colic artery, and the SHA (**FIGURE 6A**). Dissect with your thumb and index finger around and behind the IMA and transect the IMA at its origin (**FIGURE 7A**) with a vascular load stapler (**FIGURE 7B**). This ensures excellent lymph node harvest and great exposure for Step 3. The presence of the hand in the abdomen allows for a safe control of what could be serious bleeding from the IMA stump off the aorta should the staple line fail.

Step 3: Medial to Lateral Dissection of the Descending Mesocolon

- The surgeon's right hand and the assistant's grasper hold the descending mesocolon up, creating a working space between the mesocolon and the retroperitoneum (**FIGURE 8**). The

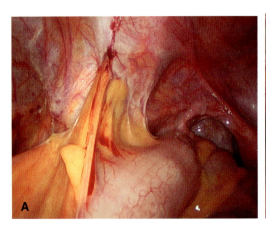
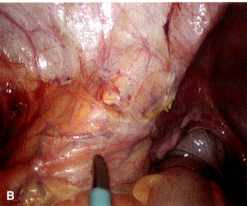

FIGURE 9 • Step 4. Panel **A**, Medial traction on the sigmoid exposes its lateral attachments to the pelvic inlet. Panel **B**, After the sigmoid mobilization is completed, the left ureter is visualized as it crosses over the left iliac artery.

plane between the mesocolon and Gerota fascia, readily identified by the transition between the two fat planes, is dissected bluntly in a downward direction toward the retroperitoneum with the 5-mm energy device.
- Dissect caudally toward the pelvic inlet; this will greatly facilitate performance of Steps 4 and 6. Dissect laterally until you reach the lateral abdominal wall; this will greatly facilitate performance of Step 5.

Step 4: Sigmoid Colon Mobilization Off the Pelvic Inlet

- The surgeon pulls the sigmoid colon medially, exposing the lateral sigmoid colon attachments (**FIGURE 9A**). Transect the attachments between the sigmoid and the pelvic inlet with laparoscopic scissors or energy device in your left hand, staying medially, close to the sigmoid and mesosigmoid, to avoid injuring the ureter/gonadal vessels.
- Dissect caudally until reaching the entrance to the left pelvic inlet.
- The left ureter and gonadal vessels, dissected in Step 3, should be visible (**FIGURE 9B**).

Step 5: Descending Colon Mobilization and Intracorporeal Proximal Transection

- The surgeon stands between the patient's legs. Retract the left colon medially with your hand to expose the white line of Toldt. The assistant holds the omentum/bowel out of way.
- Transect the white line of Toldt up to the splenic flexure using endoscopic scissors or energy device (**FIGURE 10**). You should readily enter the retroperitoneal dissection plane dissected during Step 2.
- Once the descending colon is properly mobilized, we perform an intracorporeal proximal transection. Using an energy device, divide the mesorectum, starting at the transected IMA stump and moving toward the junction of the sigmoid and descending colon. The marginal arcade is located adjacent to the bowel and is transected with the energy device.
- The colon is then transected between the descending and sigmoid colon with a laparoscopic stapler. The descending colon stump should be mobilized from its lateral attachments enough that a colostomy can be constructed later without tension.

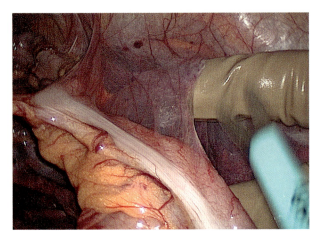

FIGURE 10 • Step 5: Transection of the lateral descending colon attachments. Notice that the hand has entered the retroperitoneal dissection plane previously dissected during Step 3.

- The proximal transection allows for an easier handling of the sigmoid/rectal stump during the performance of the pelvic dissection.

Step 6: Pelvic Dissection

- Once the sigmoid mesocolon is mobilized, dissection along the same anatomic plane between the mesentery and retroperitoneum is continued toward the pelvic inlet where the TME is initiated by entering the presacral space.
- The presacral plane is an avascular tissue plane located between the presacral fascia, posteriorly, and the investing fascia of the mesorectum, anteriorly.
- Start by following the dissection plane under the SHA, initiated during Step 2, over the promontory and into the presacral space. Dissect the presacral space using a 5-mm energy device staying between the presacral fascia, posteriorly, and the investing fascia of the mesorectum, anteriorly (**FIGURE 11A**). In the distal pelvis, Waldeyer fascia extends from the sacrum to the pubis, forming a suspensory hammock that supports the distal rectum as it angles anteriorly. Once you transect Waldeyer fascia with the 5-mm energy

Chapter 36 **HAND-ASSISTED ABDOMINOPERINEAL RESECTION** 329

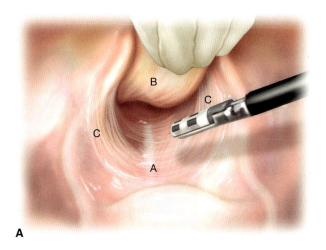
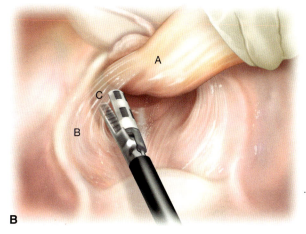
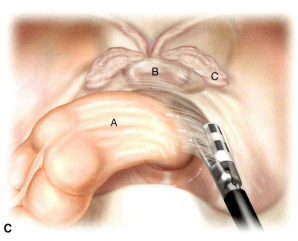

FIGURE 11 • Step 6: Pelvic dissection. Panel **A**, The posterior dissection is carried in between the presacral fascia posteriorly (A), the investing fascia of the mesorectum anteriorly (B), and the endopelvic fascia laterally (C). Panel **B**, Transection of the lateral rectal ligaments. Dissection of the space between the rectum (A) and the lateral pelvic wall (B) anterior to the rectal ligament exposes the left lateral rectal ligament (C), which can then be easily transected with the energy device. Panel **C**, The anterior dissection is carried (in men) between the rectum posteriorly (A) and the prostate (B) and seminal vesicles (C) anteriorly.

device, this posterior plane dissection changes direction in an anterior direction. It is important to make this turn to avoid injuring the most distal presacral veins. The posterior dissection is carried distally until the levator muscles are reached.

- Avoid penetrating the presacral fascia to avoid injuring the presacral veins, which could lead to severe bleeding that is difficult to control. It is critical to preserve the investing fascia of the mesorectum and the mesorectum intact to avoid oncological contamination of the pelvis.
- Once the rectum is fully mobilized posteriorly, the lateral mobilization can commence. Transect the lateral rectal ligaments between the rectum and the lateral pelvic wall (**FIGURE 11B**). There is a space in front of and behind the lateral rectal ligaments that can be easily dissected with the 5-mm energy device. In the distal pelvis, the lateral rectal ligaments have an anterior and a posterior leafs; they have to be transected separately to get adequate mobilization of the rectum of the pelvic floor. Care must be taken to avoid penetrating the endopelvic fascia along the pelvic sidewalls to avoid injuring the hypogastric vein and its branches laterally which can result in severe bleeding. In the distal pelvis, penetrating the endopelvic fascia on the pelvic sidewalls can result in injury to the parasympathetic ganglia, which can result in autonomic pelvic organ dysfunction postoperatively.

- From the right side of the table and using their right hand, the surgeon retracts the rectum to the right side, exposing the left lateral rectal ligament. The ligament is then transected with a 5-mm energy device.
- From the left side of the table and using their left hand, the surgeon retracts the rectum to the left side, exposing the right lateral rectal ligament. The ligament is then transected with a 5-mm energy device. Changing sides provides for a more ergonomic approach for the surgeon during the pelvic dissection.
- The posterior dissection is carried distally until the levator muscles are reached.
- Finally, the anterior dissection is carried out. For the anterior pelvic dissection, the assistant pulls the rectum up into the abdomen with a grasper. The surgeon holds the bladder (in males) or the uterus (in females) anteriorly using their right

hand and dissects between Denonvilliers fascia and the prostate/seminal vesicles (in males) (**FIGURE 11C**) or vagina (in females) with the 5-mm energy device. Continue with the circumferential dissection around the rectum until you can actually see the pelvic floor (levator ani muscle) (**FIGURE 12A**).
- At this point, you are ready for the intracorporeal proximal transection of the specimen. Transect the mesocolon between the sigmoid and left colic vessels with the 5-mm energy device. Start at the stapled IMA stump on the specimen side, and move up toward the colon wall, transecting the left colic artery (at its origin, off the IMA stump) and the marginal artery (close to the colon wall).
- Transect the colon intracorporeally using a 60-mm tan load linear stapler.

Step 7: Transection of the Levator Ani Muscle

There are two alternative techniques to accomplish this step.

Laparoscopic Anterior Circumferential Dissection

- We developed this approach to the levator muscle transection approach since it obviates the need for extensive open wound perineal dissection, thus greatly reducing perineal wound complications. Without the use of the hand for exposure, this technique is extremely difficult to accomplish.
- Very large tumors may impede proper visualization of the levator ani muscle, therefore necessitating a more conventional open transperineal approach.
- We first transect the posterior aspect of the levator ani with the 5-mm energy device, staying anterior to the coccyx followed by transection of the levator ani laterally until we reach the fat of the ischiorectal fossa (**FIGURE 12B**).
- We then perform a transection of the lateral levator ani muscles with the energy device.
- Finally, we perform the anterior transection of the levator ani muscles, staying posterior to the urethra (in males) or the distal vagina (in females).
- The rectum is now fully mobilized. By pulling up on the rectum, the anal canal comes up into the pelvis (**FIGURE 13A, B**). It is remarkable how far up into the pelvis the anal canal can be mobilized with this technique.
- While pulling up on the rectum with the left hand, the surgeon transects the specimen distal to the anal sphincter, using a 45-mm linear tan load stapler introduced through

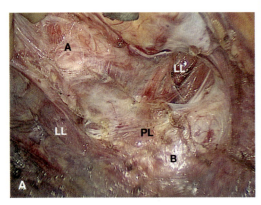 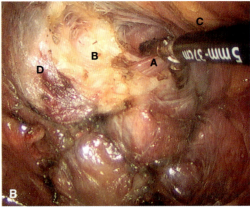

FIGURE 12 • Panel **A**, After completing the rectal mobilization, the levators are now fully exposed. A: Rectum. B: Coccyx. PL: Posterior levators. LL: Lateral levators. Panel **B**, Circumferential anterior transection of the levators. A: Transected lateral levators. B: Exposed ischiorectal fossa fat. C: Rectum. D: Lateral pelvic wall.

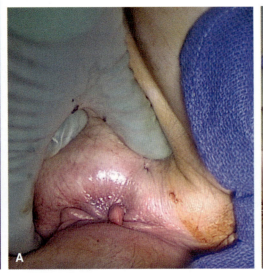 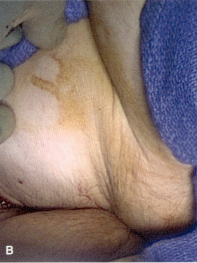

FIGURE 13 • The anus (**Panel A**) is pulled up into the pelvis and disappears from view (**Panel B**) when the anal canal is pulled up into the pelvis after circumferential anterior transection of the levators is completed.

Chapter 36 **HAND-ASSISTED ABDOMINOPERINEAL RESECTION** **331**

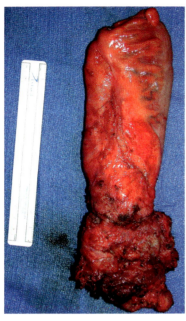

FIGURE 14 • APR specimen. Note the shinny surface of the intact mesorectum with no tapering.

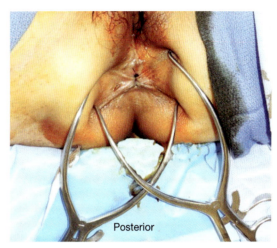

FIGURE 15 • Closure of the anus with purse-string suture. This helps prevent infectious and oncologic soilage of the perineal wound.

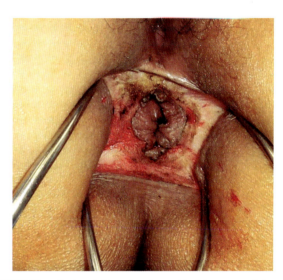

FIGURE 16 • Perineal dissection: lateral incision around the anal canal. The incision is carried through the skin and subcutaneous tissues.

- the RLQ port. We reticulate the stapler maximally and we fire the stapler on an anterior to posterior direction.
- The fully disconnected specimen is now extracted through the Pfannenstiel incision with the Alexis wound protector in place. It is paramount that the specimen has an intact mesorectum with no tapering down to the anal canal (**FIGURE 14**).

Open Transperineal Approach

- It is paramount to have completed the anterior pelvic dissection laparoscopically all the way down to the levator ani during Step 6.
- Key anatomic landmark: identify the coccyx posteriorly.
- Use headlight for illumination.
- This step of the operation can be performed concurrently with the abdominal dissection of the rectum by a second operative team.
- During the abdominal component of the operation, the Yellowfin stirrups are lowered such that the thighs are level with the torso and abdomen, as this facilitates placement of the self-retaining retractor. For the perineal dissection, the Yellowfin stirrups are elevated to fully expose the perineum. The self-retaining retractor should be repositioned if it places pressure on the thighs as they are elevated into position.
- The perineal surgeon should have a separate electrocautery with a dedicated grounding pad, and a separate suction, to allow the two operating teams to work independently. An instrument table should also be assembled for the perineal dissection, with the perineal instruments separated from those used in the abdomen and pelvis. The instrument set used is a typical major abdominal set, with the addition of two Gelpi retractors if they are not included.
- A monofilament suture (0-Prolene) is used to close the anus prior to initiating the dissection if it has not already been done. A large needle (CTX) is used to place two half-circle throws 1 cm lateral to the anal verge and the anus is closed by tying the suture (**FIGURE 15**). This helps prevent infectious and oncologic soilage of the perineal wound.
- Two Gelpi retractors are placed in an "X" configuration such that the anus and perianal skin are adequately exposed for the incision and subsequent dissection (**FIGURE 15**).
- A circular skin incision is placed around the anal verge to include all of the anoderm as well as a margin of perianal skin. The Gelpi retractors are repositioned inside of the skin incision to enhance exposure (**FIGURE 16**). A 3-cm margin (radius) around the closed anus is sufficient.
- Dissection should include the external sphincter muscle as the surgeon proceeds toward the levator ani (**FIGURE 17**). The lymphatic-bearing tissue surrounding the anal canal should be included with the specimen.
- The Gelpi retractors should be repositioned to maintain exposure. Handheld Richardson retractors can also be helpful and are held by the surgeon's assistant.

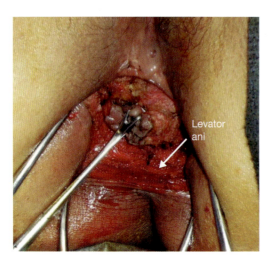
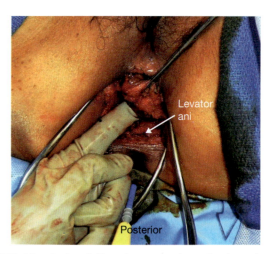

FIGURE 17 • Perineal dissection: dissection through levator muscle complex.

FIGURE 18 • Perineal dissection: posterior palpation of coccyx during perineal dissection. The transection of the levators starts posteriorly anterior to the coccyx. The index finger of the surgeon is placed into the pelvis and hooked on to top of the levator muscle, pulling it into the field. This allows for safe transection of the levator muscle with electrocautery.

- As the external sphincter, perianal fat, and lymphatic tissue are mobilized, the coccyx should be palpated to ensure that dissection proceeds anterior to this structure. The surgeon in the abdominal field should place their hand posteriorly and serve as a guide for the perineal surgeon's entry into the pelvis (**FIGURE 18**). A curved Mayo scissors is used to divide the anococcygeal ligament and levator ani muscle, which ultimately connects the abdominal and perineal dissections.
- The transection of the levator ani muscle starts posteriorly, anterior to the coccyx (**FIGURE 18**). The index finger of the surgeon is placed into the pelvis and hooked on to the top of the levator muscle, pulling it into the field. This allows for safe transection of the levator ani muscle with electrocautery. The posterior and lateral component of the levator ani should be divided first, as the anterior dissection can be difficult, especially in anterior tumors.
- The surgeon's finger should then guide division of the perineal body anteriorly. In women, this component of the dissection is completed along the rectovaginal septum. In men, the surgeon should pay very close attention to the prostate gland anteriorly, as entry into the prostate can produce significant bleeding. Furthermore, if the dissection is too anterior, entry into the membranous urethra can occur. The appropriate plane of dissection is anterior to Denonvilliers fascia as the abdominal and perineal dissections are connected.
- The specimen, now completely disconnected proximally and distally, is then extracted through the perineal wound. The rectum should exhibit an intact mesorectum with no distal "waisting" (**FIGURE 14**) in order to ensure excellent oncologic outcomes.
- Anterior tumors in men can lead to loss of the normal plane between the rectum and prostate or even invasion into the prostate. In this case, removing the prostate en bloc with the rectum may be the best way to achieve a satisfactory oncologic margin.
- The pelvis is irrigated with saline and hemostasis achieved before the perineal wound is closed. Persistent bleeding from the remaining levator ani, the prostate, or vagina may be controlled with well-placed suture ligatures.

CLOSURE OF PERINEAL WOUND

- Once hemostasis is achieved, the pelvis is copiously irrigated with warm normal saline solution (NSS) with antibiotic in the solution.
- The perineal wound is then closed in layers. If the defect is large or if preoperative radiation therapy was used, consideration should be given to closure with a myocutaneous flap.
- The more superficial layers are sequentially closed with interrupted 2-0 Vicryl sutures and the skin can be reapproximated with interrupted 4-0 Monocryl sutures.
- A mobilized omental flap can be used to fill the pelvic cavity and help keep the small bowel in the upper abdomen. Closure of the peritoneum at the pelvic inlet can also facilitate keeping the small bowel in the upper abdomen.
- A closed suction drain is placed in the pelvis.

CREATION OF DESCENDING COLOSTOMY

- The site marked for the colostomy is identified. A Kocher clamp is used to lift the skin at the center of the mark and a circular skin incision is made approximately 2 cm in diameter.
- The subcutaneous fat is divided longitudinally, exposing the anterior rectus sheath, which is divided longitudinally as well. Removing a cylinder of subcutaneous fat is usually not necessary. The rectus abdominus is bluntly spread apart and the posterior rectus sheath is divided longitudinally. Handheld Army-Navy retractors can facilitate exposure. The

opening for the colostomy site should snugly accommodate two fingerbreadths.

- The descending colon should be sufficiently mobilized to allow a tension-free anastomosis between the colon and the skin. In patients with a thick layer of abdominal fat, additional length can be obtained by mobilizing the splenic flexure. If excessive tension at the skin persists, maturing the stoma as a loop end can be the best option.
- After closure of all wounds, the staple line on the colon is removed with cautery and the stoma is matured to the dermis with interrupted 3-0 absorbable suture.
- Sterile dressings and a stoma appliance are placed such that the skin surrounding the stoma is completely protected with the wafer of the appliance.

Step 8: Closure of Abdominal Wounds

- The pelvis is irrigated again with warm NSS with antibiotic in the solution.
- We place a 19F round Blake through the RLQ port incision site and into the pelvis.
- The Pfannenstiel incision is closed using a running 2-0 Vicryl suture from the posterior rectus sheet and a running no. 1 polydioxanone (PDS) suture for the anterior rectus sheet. All skin incisions are closed with 4-0 PDS subcuticular sutures. Dermabond is applied to seal off all wounds.
- We retowel the field with clean towels and change gown and gloves, Bovie electrocautery, suction cannulas prior to wound closure in an effort to minimize wound infections.

PEARLS AND PITFALLS

Operative approach	A HALS approach improves minimally invasive surgery utilization, reduces conversions, and shortens OR times
	A standardized, stepwise approach leads to higher efficiency and quality
Positioning	- Gravity-assist maneuvers allow for good visualization and exposure - Secure the patient to the table, while protecting all pressure-baring areas - Make sure the heels are firmly planted on the stirrups to avoid patient sliding during the procedure - Make sure that all anesthesia lines and monitors are working appropriately after positioning the patient; there will be limited access to the arms during the procedure - Avoid unnecessary clutter of cables/lines; open the working space for the operating team
Port placement	- Align the surgeon, trocars, target, and monitor in straight lines - Triangulate all ports aiming to the target - Place the hand-access port in a Pfannenstiel location
	Use an accessory port in the left lower quadrant for the right-sided pelvic dissection
Setup	Proper patient, team, port, and instrumentation setup are critical
Operative technique	Point of entry: IMV at the ligament of Treitz
	Medial to lateral dissection step sets up all other steps
	Vascular dissection to visualize the "letter T" and high IMA ligation in malignancy; identify left ureter prior to IMA transection
	Pelvic dissection progression: first posterior, then lateral, and then anterior
	We prefer the anterior circumferential transection of the levators to prevent perineal wound complications
Pitfall: Dissecting anterior to the SHA	Solution: Identify "groove" between left common iliac artery and SHA and dissect in between the two vessels.
Pitfall: Floppy sigmoid difficult to handle	Use the back of the hand as a "shelf" to hold the sigmoid up while picking up the SHA with thumb and index finger

POSTOPERATIVE CARE

Postoperative care is driven by an ERAS clinical pathway (described elsewhere in this textbook) that includes the following:

- Multimodal analgesia
- DVT prophylaxis with enoxaparin
- No additional antibiotics. Judicious use of intravenous fluids

- No nasogastric tube. Remove
- Foley catheter on postoperative day 1
- Remove pelvic drain on postoperative days 2 to 3
- Early ambulation
- Diet ad lib
- Aggressive pulmonary toilette
- Use soft pillow/jelly donut while seating
- Targeted discharge: postoperative days 3 to 4

OUTCOMES

- HALS leads to improvements in short-term outcomes, including less pain, faster recovery, shorter hospital stay, and lower incidence of cardiac/pulmonary complications when compared to open surgery.
- When compared to conventional laparoscopy, HALS results in higher utilization rates of minimally invasive surgery, shorter learning curves, lower conversion rates, shorter operative times, and shorter hospital stays.
- For cancer resection, minimally invasive surgery oncologic outcomes are at least comparable to those of open surgery. TME with an intact mesorectum is critical to minimize locoregional treatment failures.

COMPLICATIONS

- Wound infections and hernias are markedly reduced with the use of a Pfannenstiel extraction site
- Perineal wound infection/dehiscence: this complication is virtually eliminated with the use of an anterior circumferential transection technique for the levators. Pelvic abscess are also markedly reduced
- Urinary/sexual dysfunction: important to preserve hypogastric nerves and parasympathetic ganglia intact
- Ureteral injury: critical to identify the left ureter prior to IMA transection
- DVT: low risk with use of DVT prophylaxis
- Cardiac and pulmonary complications: significantly reduced compared to the open surgery approach

SUGGESTED READING

1. Cima RR, Pattana-arun J, Larson DW, Dozois EJ, Wolff BG, Pemberton JH. Experience with 969 minimal access colectomies: the role of hand-assisted laparoscopy in expanding minimally invasive surgery for complex colectomies. *J Am Coll Surg.* 2008;206:946-952.
2. Jayne DG, Thorpe HC, Copeland J, Quirke P, Brown JM, Guillou PJ. Five-year follow-up of the Medical Research Counsel CLASICC trial of laparoscopically assisted versus open surgery for colorectal cancer. *Br J Surg.* 2010;97:1638-1645.
3. Marcello PW, Fleshman JW, Milsom JW, et al. Hand-assisted laparoscopic vs. laparoscopic colorectal surgery. A multicenter, prospective, randomized trial. *Dis Colon Rectum.* 2008;51:818-828.
4. Orcutt ST, Balentine CJ, Marshall CL, et al. Use of a Pfannenstiel incision in minimally invasive colorectal cancer surgery is associated with a lower risk of wound complications. *Tech Coloproctol.* 2012;16(2):127-132.
5. Orcutt ST, Marshall CL, Balentine CJ, et al. Hand-assisted laparoscopy leads to efficient colorectal cancer surgery. *J Surg Res.* 2012;177(2):e53-e58.
6. Orcutt ST, Marshall CL, Robinson CN, et al. Minimally invasive surgery in colon cancer patients leads to improved short-term outcomes and excellent oncologic results. *Am J Surg.* 2011;202(5):528-531.
7. Ozturk E, Kiran RP, Geisler DP, Hull TL, Vogel JD. Hand-assisted laparoscopic colectomy: benefits of laparoscopic colectomy at No extra cost. *J Am Coll Surg.* 2009;209:242-247.
8. Wilks JA, Balentine CJ, Berger DH, et al. Establishment of a minimally invasive program at a VAMC leads to improved care in colorectal cancer patients. *Am J Surg.* 2009;198(5):685-692.
9. Zhuang CL, Ye XZ, Zhang XD, Chen BC, Yu Z. Enhanced recovery after surgery program versus traditional care for colorectal surgery: a meta-analysis of randomized controlled trials. *Dis Colon Rectum.* 2013;56(5):667-678.

Chapter 37

Abdominoperineal Resection: Robotic-Assisted Laparoscopic Surgery Technique

Rodrigo Pedraza and Eric Mitchell Haas

DEFINITION

- Robotic-assisted laparoscopic abdominoperineal resection (APR) is a minimally invasive technique in which the rectum and anus are removed with the creation of a permanent end colostomy. The procedure is accomplished with the assistance of the da Vinci Surgical System (Intuitive Surgical Inc., Sunnyvale, CA) in a minimally invasive fashion.

PATIENT HISTORY AND PHYSICAL FINDINGS

- A thorough history and physical examination should include the following:
  - Presence of rectal pain and/or tenesmus
  - Presence of obstructive symptoms
  - Description of anorectal function, with any fecal incontinence or leakage documented preoperatively
  - Documentation of urinary and erectile function/dysfunction
  - A detailed personal and family history of colorectal cancer, polyps, and/or other malignancies
- Physical examination should include the following:
  - Routine abdominal examination, noting any previous incisions
  - Digital rectal examination with assessment of sphincter function, distal and proximal extent of the lesion measured from the anal verge, exact position of the lesion and extent of the rectal circumference involved, and the presence or absence of fixation to perirectal structures
  - Bilateral inguinal nodal examination
- Robotic-assisted laparoscopic APR is a safe and feasible approach.
- The most common indication is low rectal cancer in which the sphincter complex cannot be salvaged. Less commonly, APR is performed in those with persistent or recurrent squamous cell carcinoma of the anus following chemo/radiation therapy (ie, Nigro protocol).
- Other indications include severe inflammatory bowel disease (IBD) involving the rectum and recalcitrant to medical management.
- Low rectal cancer is typically diagnosed during screening colonoscopy or after presenting symptoms such as rectal bleeding, tenesmus, bowel obstruction, or pelvic pain.
- Patients presenting with residual or recurrent anal cancer and those with IBD with recalcitrant perianal disease have typically undergone thorough workup and extensive therapy for the disease prior to being considered candidates for APR.
- Absolute contraindications for robotic-assisted APR are those for any other major abdominal procedure, such as severe cardiovascular or hemodynamic compromise.

- Relative contraindications for robotic-assisted APR include those associated with the patient condition and surgeon experience.
  - Robotic-assisted laparoscopic procedures typically require steep patient positioning and result in prolonged operative times, especially early in the surgeon learning curve; thus, patient inability to tolerate a lengthy procedure may contraindicate the use of robotic-assisted APR.
  - History of prior abdominal surgery is not a contraindication but may additionally prolong the operative time for lysis of adhesions and proper exposure of tissue planes. We advocate performing laparoscopic lysis of adhesions prior to robotic docking so as to expedite the procedure.
  - Prior to offering challenging pelvic procedures such as robotic-assisted APR, we suggest the surgeon achieve competency with robotic surgery by performing several less demanding procedures such as rectopexy and/or left/sigmoid colectomy.

IMAGING AND OTHER DIAGNOSTIC STUDIES

- Appropriate imaging, endoscopic, and histopathologic evaluation is mandatory in all cases regardless of diagnosis.
- A full colonoscopy must be performed in all patients with rectal cancer. This allows for the assessment of tumor location and pathology. It also serves to rule out and possibly remove any synchronous colonic lesions. Malignant synchronous lesions have been reported in 2% to 8% of cases and benign synchronous polyps in 13% to 62% of cases.
- If a colonoscopy has already been done by another provider, consider performing either a rigid proctoscopy or a flexible sigmoidoscopy for accurate documentation of the size, location, and distance of the tumor from the anal sphincter complex.
- Patients with low rectal cancer requiring APR necessitate a full staging workup. Local tumor assessment and regional node involvement are optimally assessed with endoscopic ultrasound or rectal protocol magnetic resonance imaging (MRI). Distant metastases are evaluated with computed tomographic (CT) scan of the chest abdomen and pelvis.
- Following proper staging, the need for neoadjuvant chemoradiation is determined. Patients with T3 to T4 and/or N+ distal rectal cancer are offered neoadjuvant chemoradiation. Surgery is typically considered after 6 to 8 weeks following the last pelvic radiation session to allow for a full therapeutic radiation effect and to avoid operating in early inflammatory radiation tissue changes or late fibrosis; however, delayed intervention (8-12 weeks post completion of neoadjuvant therapy) has been recently suggested.
- For persistent or recurrent squamous cell carcinoma of the anus, APR is the rescue therapy of choice. These patients typically present after thorough imaging staging and following

335

conventional courses of chemoradiation with documented residual or recurrence disease.
- Most patients with recalcitrant perianal disease in the background of IBD present for the consideration of an APR after extensive imaging and endoscopic evaluation. It is imperative to endoscopically assess the disease to determine whether the APR should be accompanied with additional large or small bowel resection. Furthermore, the presence of additional fistulous tracts such as rectovaginal or rectovesical must be investigated during the preoperative planning.
- A carcinoembryonic antigen level is obtained preoperatively in cancer patients.

SURGICAL MANAGEMENT

Preoperative Planning

- Bowel preparation is typically achieved with preoperative enema. Full bowel preparation is performed selectively.
- In the operating room and under anesthesia, rigid proctosigmoidoscopy should be performed to affirm the surgical plan.
- The perineum is adequately prepped for the perineal portion of the procedure.
- Prophylactic antibiotics are administered according to the Surgical Care Improvement Project measures.

Positioning

- The patient is placed in a modified lithotomy position with moderate Trendelenburg position and with both arms tucked. All pressure points are padded to prevent neurovascular injuries to the extremities. The patient is secured with a wrapped technique using a 3-in tape at the level of the chest in such a fashion to prevent the patient from sliding but avoiding restriction of chest wall expansion (**FIGURE 1**). It is imperative to secure the patient firmly, as steep Trendelenburg position will be used later in the procedure before robotic docking.
- Optimal modified lithotomy position is crucial to ensure adequate perineal access while allowing appropriate robotic side docking (see the following text) to avoid external robotic arm conflict (**FIGURE 2**).

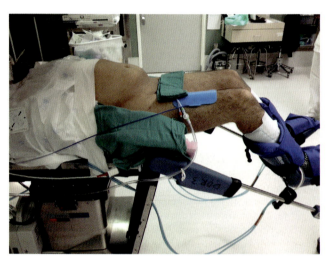

FIGURE 1 • Patient positioning. The patient is placed in a modified lithotomy position with moderate Trendelenburg and with both arms tucked. All pressure points are padded to prevent neurovascular injuries. The patient is secured with a wrap technique using a 3-in tape at the level of the chest in such a fashion to prevent movement but avoiding restriction of chest wall expansion.

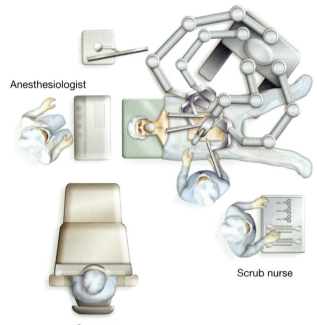

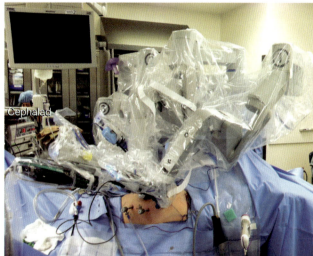

FIGURE 2 • Team and robot setup. The robot is docked on the left side of the patient's lower extremities in an acute angle. This configuration allows access to the perineum without undocking the robotic cart.

Chapter 37 ABDOMINOPERINEAL RESECTION: ROBOTIC-ASSISTED LAPAROSCOPIC SURGERY TECHNIQUE

INCISION, PORT PLACEMENT, AND INSTRUMENTS

- A total of five ports are used for robotic-assisted APR: two 12-mm ports for the robotic camera and assistant (the latter is for use with laparoscopic instruments) and three 8-mm ports for robotic instrumentation.
- The robotic camera port is placed in the periumbilical region and the assistant port in the right upper quadrant. The 8-mm instrument ports are placed in the right and left lower quadrants and in the left upper quadrant (**FIGURE 3**).
- The ports are placed approximately 8 cm apart to prevent conflict between the robotic arms and the camera.

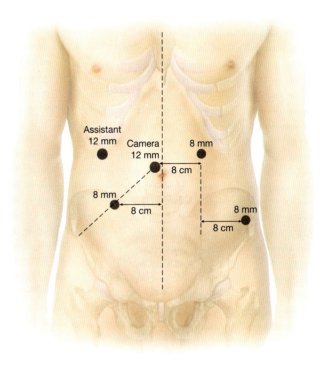

FIGURE 3 • Port placement. The camera arm is placed in the 12-mm port in the periumbilical region. The robotic arms 1, 2, and 3 are placed in the right lower, left upper, and left lower quadrants, respectively. A 12-mm port is placed in the right upper quadrant for the assistant to use with laparoscopic instruments. All ports are placed approximately 8 cm apart to avoid conflict between the robotic arms and the camera.

EXPLORATION AND ROBOTIC DOCKING

- The abdominal cavity is assessed, and, in oncologic cases, the presence of distant metastases is evaluated.
- Lysis of adhesions is performed laparoscopically, if needed.
- The patient is positioned in a steep Trendelenburg position with the left side elevated 15°. The small bowel and omentum are retracted out of the pelvis.
- The robot is docked on the left side of the patient's lower extremities in an acute angle (**FIGURE 2**). The camera arm is placed in the 12-mm port in the periumbilical region, whereas the robotic arms 1, 2, and 3 are placed in the right lower, left upper, and left lower quadrants, respectively (**FIGURE 3**).

ESTABLISHMENT OF THE PRESACRAL PLANE

- A medial to lateral approach is used with an incision of the peritoneum at the level of the sacral promontory. The avascular presacral plane is entered, which is confirmed by the identification of the areolar tissue (**FIGURE 4**). This plane is developed identifying the superior rectal artery and the left ureter (**FIGURE 5**). The vascular pedicle is isolated, identifying the inferior mesenteric artery, superior rectal artery, and the left colic artery (**FIGURE 5**).

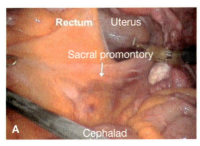
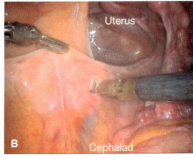

FIGURE 4 • Entering the presacral plane. A medial to lateral approach is used with an incision of the peritoneum at the level of the sacral promontory (*arrow*) (**A**). The avascular presacral plane is entered (**B**), which is confirmed by the identification of the areolar tissue (**C** and **D**).

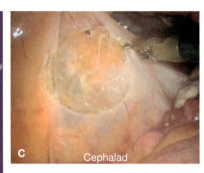
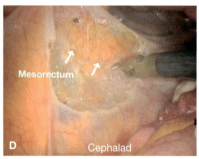

FIGURE 4 • Continued

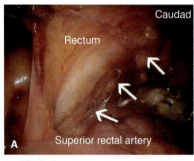
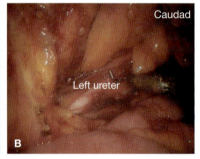
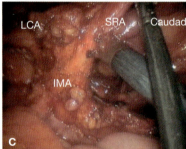
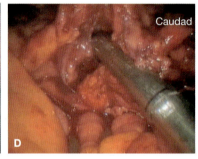

FIGURE 5 • Medial to lateral dissection. The anatomic landmarks, superior rectal artery (SRA) **(A)** and left ureter **(B)**, are identified prior to vascular pedicle isolation. The inferior mesenteric artery (IMA), left colic artery (LCA), and SRA are dissected and isolated **(C)**. The IMA is divided **(D)**.

VASCULAR DIVISION

- At this point, the inferior mesenteric artery is ligated at its origin from the aorta using a laparoscopic stapler, electrosurgical device, or clips (**FIGURE 5**).

MEDIAL TO LATERAL DISSECTION OF THE DESCENDING AND SIGMOID MESOCOLON

- Once the IMA is transected, the edge of the mesocolon is retracted upward. The plane between the mesocolon and Gerota fascia, readily identified by the transition between the two fat planes, is dissected with an energy device. The dissection is carried laterally until you reach the lateral abdominal wall and caudally toward the pelvic inlet. The left ureter and gonadal vessels are identified and preserved intact at all times.

LATERAL MOBILIZATION OF THE DESCENDING AND SIGMOID COLON

- The sigmoid and descending colon are retracted medially, exposing the lateral attachments. Transect the attachments with an energy device.

- The left ureter and gonadal vessels, previously dissected, should be readily visible.

Chapter 37 ABDOMINOPERINEAL RESECTION: ROBOTIC-ASSISTED LAPAROSCOPIC SURGERY TECHNIQUE

INTRACORPOREAL PROXIMAL TRANSECTION

- Once the descending colon is properly mobilized, we perform an intracorporeal proximal transection. Using an energy device, divide the mesorectum, starting at the transected IMA stump and moving toward the junction of the sigmoid and descending colon. The marginal arcade is located adjacent to the bowel and is transected with the energy device.

- The colon is then transected between the descending and sigmoid colon with a linear stapler. The descending colon stump should be mobilized from its lateral attachments enough that a colostomy can be constructed later without tension.
- The proximal transection allows for an easier handling of the sigmoid/rectal stump during the performance of the pelvic dissection.

MESORECTAL DISSECTION

- Attention is drawn to the pelvis for the mesorectal excision. The pelvic dissection proceeds posteriorly first, then laterally, and then anteriorly.
- First, the avascular presacral plane is entered for the posterior dissection. Arm 3 is used for retraction, whereas arms 1 and 2 develop a plane of dissection within the avascular presacral space between the presacral fascia, posteriorly, and the mesorectal fascia, anteriorly. Arm 2 of the robot (left hand of the surgeon) should avoid grasping the mesorectum, for the strong robotic arm may tear the mesorectum, which would cause bleeding.
- The fascia propria of the rectum is identified and preserved with sharp dissection using the robotic scissors or monopolar device. Dissection continues in the posterior mesorectal plane through the retrorectal (Waldeyer) fascia to the level of the anorectal junction (**FIGURE 6**).
- Avoid penetrating the presacral fascia to avoid injuries to the presacral veins, which could lead to severe bleeding that is difficult to control. It is imperative to preserve the mesorectal fascia and the mesorectum intact throughout the procedure to avoid potential oncological contamination of the pelvis.
- The lateral mesorectal dissection follows (**FIGURE 7**). The hypogastric nerve can be seen posterolateral to the plane of the dissection. It is important to preserve these nerves intact to avoid autonomic dysfunction postoperatively (**FIGURE 7**). Attention is first drawn to the right lateral pelvic attachments, which are divided starting at the level of the anterior peritoneal reflection and extending distally until reaching the levator ani muscle (**FIGURE 8**). The left lateral rectal ligament is then transected in a similar fashion (**FIGURE 9**).

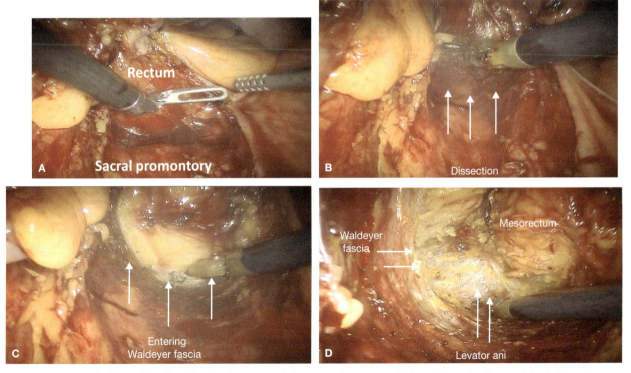

FIGURE 6 • Presacral plane dissection. **A,** Development of the avascular presacral plane. The robotic arm 3 (not shown) serves as retractor proximally, whereas robotic arm 2 countertracts the mesorectum anteriorly for dissection with robotic arm 1 (not shown). **B,** The dissection is carried out distally with the robotic arm 1 using monopolar energy or scissors. **C,** The plane is further developed and Waldeyer fascia is entered. **D,** The plane is completed distally to the level of the levator ani muscles.

340 SECTION III RECTAL RESECTIONS

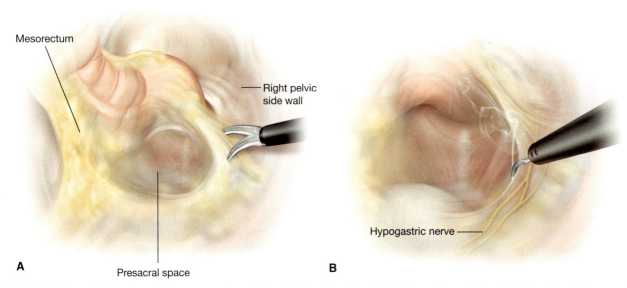

FIGURE 7 • Lateral dissection of the mesorectum off the right pelvic sidewall. **A,** Transection of the right lateral rectal ligament. **B,** The hypogastric nerve can be seen posterolateral to the plane of the dissection. It is important to preserve these nerves intact to avoid autonomic dysfunction postoperatively.

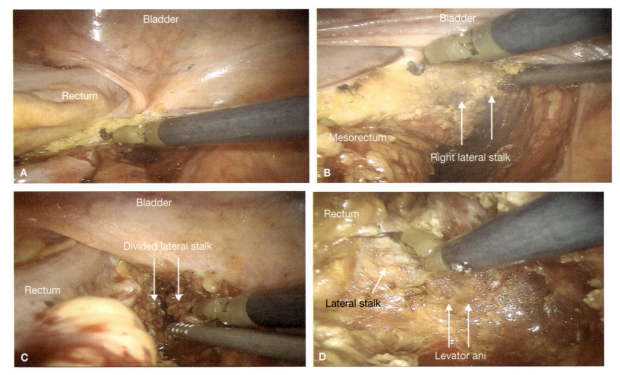

FIGURE 8 • Right lateral mesorectal dissection. The right lateral mesorectal dissection is initiated at the level of the cul-de-sac (**A**) and carried out distally taking down the right lateral stalk (**B** and **C**) and *continued* distally until reaching the levator ani muscle (**D**).

- Avoid penetrating the lateral endopelvic fascia to avoid venous injuries to the hypogastric vein and its branches, which could lead to severe bleeding that is difficult to control. In the distal pelvis, penetrating the lateral endopelvic fascia could also lead to injuries to the parasympathetic ganglia and its branches, resulting in potential autonomic pelvic organ dysfunction postoperatively.

- Lastly, the anterior mesorectal dissection is performed (**FIGURE 10**).
- For the anterior pelvic dissection, exposure is achieved by the assistant retracting the rectum posteriorly and in a cephalad direction, as arm 3 anteriorly retracts the vagina (in females) or the prostate/seminal vesicles (in males). The anterior dissection proceeds anterior to Denonvilliers fascia (**FIGURE 11**).

Chapter 37 ABDOMINOPERINEAL RESECTION: ROBOTIC-ASSISTED LAPAROSCOPIC SURGERY TECHNIQUE 341

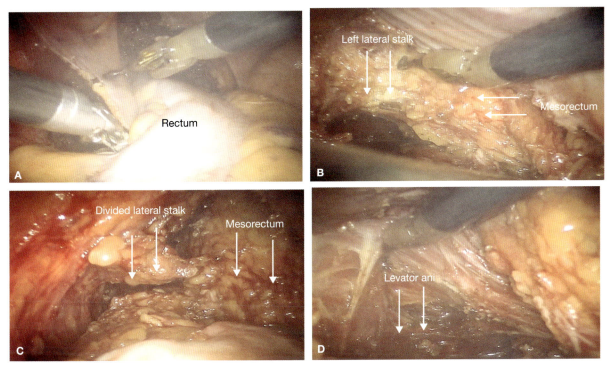

FIGURE 9 • Left lateral mesorectal dissection. The left lateral dissection is initiated **(A)** and carried out distally taking down the left lateral stalk **(B** and **C)** and *continued* up to the levator ani **(D)** in a similar fashion.

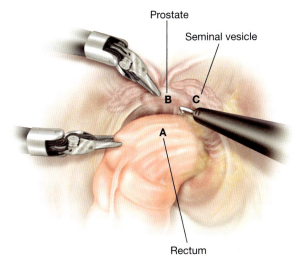

FIGURE 10 • Anterior pelvic dissection. Exposure is achieved by the assistant retracting the rectum *(A)* posteriorly and in a cephalad direction as arm 3 anteriorly retracts the prostate/seminal vesicles *(B, C)*, respectively. The anterior plane of dissection is carried along Denonvilliers fascia, between the rectum posteriorly *(A)* and the prostate *(B)* and seminal vesicles *(C)* anteriorly.

- In males, the Douglas pouch (rectovesical pouch) is entered by incising the peritoneal reflection between the anterior wall of the rectum and the prostate/seminal vesicles, taking care to avoid injury to the seminal vesicle and prostate (**FIGURE 11**).

- In the female patient, the anterior cul-de-sac is usually deeper, and the rectovaginal plane is readily established once entered.
- Following the anterior dissection, the lateral stalks of the rectum are further divided as necessary, achieving hemostasis with an electrosurgical device. Care is taken at this level to avoid excessive lateral dissection, which may result in injury to the pelvic nerve plexuses (this would lead to autonomic dysfunction postoperatively). It should be noted that, typically, brisk bleeding may occur if the wrong plane is entered (posteriorly, by injuring the presacral venous plexus, and laterally, by injuring the hypogastric veins or its tributaries).
- Once the planes have been divided, circumferential exposure of the levator complex is achieved. Thus, the robotic portion of the APR is carried out into the subcutaneous perineal tissue.
- In malignant cases, a cylindrical excision is then performed through the levator complex to ensure complete resection with proper radial margins. With the assistant retracting the rectum posteriorly and in a cephalad direction with a laparoscopic grasper and with the robotic arm 3 retracting the prostate/seminal vessels anteriorly, the levator ani muscle is exposed circumferentially around the distal rectum (**FIGURE 12A**). The levator ani is then circumferentially transected using monopolar electrocautery (**FIGURE 12B**).

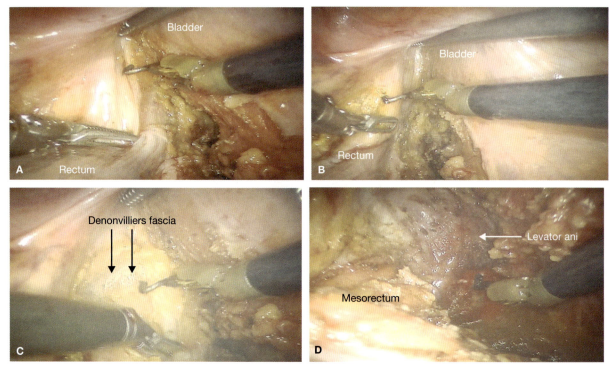

FIGURE 11 • Anterior mesorectal dissection. The peritoneum is incised at the peritoneal reflection (**A** and **B**) and the dissection is carried out distally entering Denonvilliers fascia (**C**) and continued inferiorly until complete anterior rectal mobilization is achieved and the levator ani muscle is encountered anteriorly (**D**).

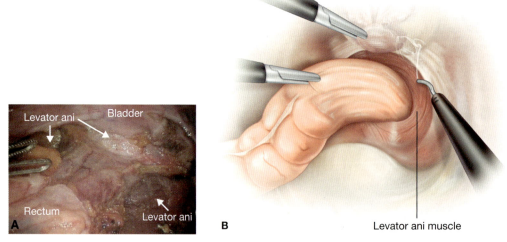

FIGURE 12 • Circumferential anterior transection of the levator ani. **A,** With the assistant retracting the rectum posteriorly and in a cephalad direction with a laparoscopic grasper and with the robotic arm 3 retracting the prostate/seminal vessels anteriorly, the levator ani muscle is exposed circumferentially around the distal rectum. **B,** The levator ani is then circumferentially transected using monopolar electrocautery.

PERINEAL PROCEDURE

- For malignant cases, a wide excision of the perineum circumferentially surrounding the anus is performed (**FIGURE 13A**).
- At this level, the incision is deepened to subcutaneous tissue and the planes achieved during the robotic portion of the procedure are reached (**FIGURE 13B**).
- The rectum and anus are extracted through the perineal wound.
- Appropriately performed cylindrical excision will result in a rectal specimen with an intact mesorectum and without an hourglass configuration in the final specimen (**FIGURE 14**).
- In cases involving benign disease, one should preserve levator ani to assist perineal closure and prevent perineal

Chapter 37 ABDOMINOPERINEAL RESECTION: ROBOTIC-ASSISTED LAPAROSCOPIC SURGERY TECHNIQUE 343

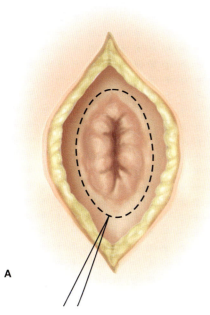
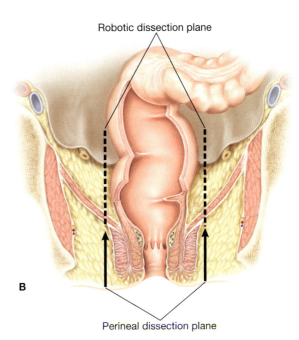

FIGURE 13 • The perineal portion of the procedure is performed in a conventional fashion, with an elliptical perianal incision **(A)**. The perineal plane reaches the robotic dissection plane in the subcutaneous level **(B)**.

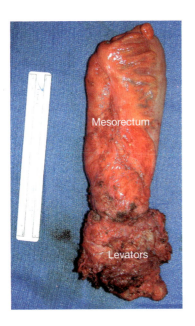

- hernias. Such a resection would result in an hourglass configuration.
- Myofascial rotational flaps should be considered for closing the large defect and/or in a radiated pelvic floor.
- For benign cases, a narrow excision should be performed to be able to close the levator ani and preserve as much pelvic floor function as possible. In these circumstances, consideration to an intersphincteric excision, in which the external sphincter complex and the levator ani are left intact, is given. These muscle and fascial layers can then be used for primary closure and myofascial flaps can be avoided.

FIGURE 14 • Abdominoperineal resection specimen. Note the shiny surface of the intact mesorectum with no distal tapering, avoiding an hourglass appearance on the specimen.

COLOSTOMY AND CLOSURE

- A circumferential incision in a predetermined size located on the left lower abdominal quadrant is performed through the rectus sheet for the creation of the colostomy.
- The subcutaneous tissue, fascia, and peritoneum are incised with a circumference of at least two fingerbreadths.
- The bowel proximal to the division is brought superficially to the abdominal wall and an end colostomy is performed in a conventional fashion. The colostomy is matured after wound closure.

- Before closure, the perineal incision is irrigated with normal saline and povidone-iodine.
- The perineal wound closure is initiated deep with imbrication of the levator ani (when preserved) with absorbable suture, typically 2-0 polyglactin 910 (Vicryl). The superficial perineal subcutaneous tissues are reapproximated with 3-0 Vicryl sutures. The skin is closed with interrupted 2-0 nylon sutures.
- Port sites are closed with subcuticular 4-0 polydioxanone sutures.

344 SECTION III **RECTAL RESECTIONS**

PEARLS AND PITFALLS

Indications	■ Low rectal cancer, anal cancer, recalcitrant IBD with anorectal involvement.
Preoperative evaluation	■ Colonoscopy, abdominal CT scan, pelvic MRI, and/or endorectal ultrasound. ■ Positron emission tomography scan selectively.
Port placement	■ Two 12-mm ports for camera and assistant in the right upper quadrant and periumbilical region, respectively. ■ Three 5-mm ports in the right lower, left upper, and left lower quadrants.
Technique—laparoscopic exploration	■ Abdominal exploration and lysis of adhesions are accomplished with conventional multiport laparoscopy.
Robotic docking	■ The robot is docked in the left side of the patient's legs at an acute angle.
Technique—robotic pelvic procedure	■ The posterior mesorectal dissection, along the presacral plane, is done first, followed by the lateral dissection, and then by the anterior dissection. ■ The levator ani muscles are incised circumferentially through an anterior approach; the dissection is continued to the subcutaneous perineal tissue. ■ The pelvic portion is started with a circumferential perianal incision and deepened to reach the robotically established planes. ■ The perineum is closed either primarily or using a myofascial flap. ■ An end sigmoid colostomy is performed in a conventional fashion.
Postoperative management	■ Optimal postoperative outcomes are accomplished with a fast-track perioperative protocol and an ostomy care program.

POSTOPERATIVE CARE

■ Patients following minimally invasive colorectal surgery are typically placed in an enhanced recovery pathway.

■ Return of oral intake is typically achieved with clear liquids 8 to 12 hours after the procedure and the diet is advanced as tolerated.

■ In contrast to purely abdominal procedures, for pelvic surgery the bladder catheter is not removed until postoperative day 2.

■ Ambulation is indicated to accelerate recovery.

■ Postoperative analgesia is accomplished with a combined modality involving intravenous acetaminophen, opioids, and nonsteroidal anti-inflammatory drugs. Alvimopan is used to eliminate the effects of opioids in the gastrointestinal tract. Additionally, patient-controlled analgesia is limited to 1 to 2 postoperative days.

■ Ostomy care is best achieved with a standardized protocol that includes preoperative and postoperative patient education and training. The program involves a multidisciplinary approach with patient and family, surgeon, and ostomy nurse.

OUTCOMES

■ Most patients following robotic-assisted colectomy managed with a fast-track perioperative protocol have a length of hospital stay of 4 days.

■ Longer hospital stay may be required to address complications.

■ Perineal wound complications are common; thus, close postoperative follow-up following APR is required.

■ Patients with malignancy should be placed on postoperative surveillance protocols.

COMPLICATIONS

■ Vascular injury with intraperitoneal bleeding
■ Ureteral injury
■ Sexual and/or urinary dysfunction secondary to autonomic nerve injury
■ Prolonged postoperative ileus
■ Abdominal wound complications (eg, hematoma, seroma, infection, and dehiscence)
■ Persistent perineal sinus
■ Intra-abdominal abscess
■ Perineal sepsis
■ Parastomal and perineal hernia formation

SUGGESTED READINGS

1. Bokhari MB, Patel CB, Ramos-Valadez DI, et al. Learning curve for robotic-assisted laparoscopic colorectal surgery. *Surg Endosc.* 2011;25:855-860.
2. Evans J, Tait D, Swift I, et al. Timing of surgery following preoperative therapy in rectal cancer: the need for a prospective randomized trial? *Dis Colon Rectum.* 2011;54:1251-1259.
3. Garcia-Aguilar J, Smith DD, Avila K, et al. Optimal timing of surgery after chemoradiation for advanced rectal cancer: preliminary results of a multicenter, nonrandomized phase II prospective trial. *Ann Surg.* 2011;254:97-102.
4. Patel CB, Ramos-Valadez DI, Haas EM. Robotic-assisted laparoscopic abdominoperineal resection for anal cancer: feasibility and technical considerations. *Int J Med Robot.* 2010;6:399-404.
5. Vlug MS, Wind J, Hollmann MW, et al. Laparoscopy in combination with fast track multimodal management is the best perioperative strategy in patients undergoing colonic surgery: a randomized clinical trial (LAFA-study). *Ann Surg.* 2011;254:868-875.

Chapter **38**

Restorative Proctocolectomy: Open Technique (Ileal Pouch-Anal Anastomosis)

Hasan T. Kirat and Feza H. Remzi

DEFINITION

- Restorative proctocolectomy with ileal pouch-anal anastomosis (RP/IPAA) is defined as removal of entire colon and rectum and construction of an anastomosis of ileal pouch to the anal canal using stapled or hand-sewn technique.

DIFFERENTIAL DIAGNOSIS

- When the patients with ulcerative colitis become refractory to medical therapy or steroid dependent, RP/IPAA has been the surgical choice.
- RP/IPAA can be performed with good functional results and quality of life, and low pouch failure for indeterminate colitis.
- Patients with Crohn disease have greater risk of pouch failure following RP/IPAA compared with those with ulcerative colitis.
- In patients with familial adenomatous polyposis, the risk of colorectal cancer is eliminated by performing RP/IPAA.

PATIENT HISTORY AND PHYSICAL FINDINGS

- A thorough history and physical examination should be obtained.
- In inflammatory bowel disease, it is important to note previous and/or concurrent use of steroids, immunomodulators, and nonsteroidal anti-inflammatory medications. Patients refractory to these medications are typically candidates for this procedure.
- Previous surgeries, particularly in patients with Crohn disease, need to be taken into consideration.
- Anal and urinary sphincter function needs to be evaluated. Patients with poor anal sphincter function may not be good candidates for RP/IPAA and may need a proctocolectomy with end ileostomy instead.
- A full nutritional assessment should be instituted.
- Significant cardiac and/or pulmonary comorbidities may prevent the patient to have this procedure.
- Family history of colorectal polyps, cancer, and/or inflammatory bowel disease should be elicited.

IMAGING AND OTHER DIAGNOSTIC STUDIES

- Preoperative colonoscopy is necessary.
- Diagnosis of ulcerative colitis and exclusion of Crohn disease by colonoscopic biopsy and by an experienced pathologist and/or with the assistance of other laboratory workup, such as Prometheus test, is necessary in order to establish the need for restorative proctocolectomy with ileoanal anastomosis.
- Colonoscopic evidence of terminal ileitis by biopsy may assist in the diagnosis of Crohn disease.

- Diagnosis of ulcerative colitis with proctitis and involvement of the anal canal by colonoscopy or rigid proctoscopy and biopsy may be necessary in order to establish the need for anal mucosectomy and hand-sewn ileal pouch anastomosis.
- Contrast-enhanced computed axial tomography (CAT) scan may help evaluate patients with cancer for locoregional extent of disease and metastases. CAT scan is also helpful in inflammatory bowel disease to evaluate for acute inflammatory processes (phlegmon, abscess, fistula, or obstruction).
- Endorectal ultrasound or rectal protocol magnetic resonance imaging (MRI) may assist with the staging of rectal carcinoma and identification of the anal sphincter muscle involvement. The latter would be a contraindication of a restorative proctocolectomy. It may also delineate the anatomy of the anal sphincter in case of previous obstetric trauma or episiotomies.
- Obtaining a Wexner fecal incontinence score preoperatively may assist with the diagnosis of fecal incontinence. Manometry studies may also be helpful in these patients. Preoperative fecal incontinence may lead to poor functional outcome following an ileoanal pouch anastomosis.
- Preoperative barium enema or small bowel follow-through contrast study may assist with the diagnosis of Crohn disease.

SURGICAL MANAGEMENT

Preoperative Planning

- The site for a diverting loop ileostomy is marked before surgery.
- A complete bowel preparation is recommended.
- Prophylaxis against deep venous thrombosis and prophylactic perioperative antibiotics should be administered.
- The rectum is washed out with normal saline in the operating room.

Positioning

- The procedure is performed with the patient in a Lloyd-Davies position (**FIGURE 1**).
- This position is defined as Trendelenburg position with legs apart.
- The thighs are level with the abdomen as this allows efficient placement of a self-retaining retractor without creating excessive pressure between the retractor and the patient's thighs.
- All pressure points are padded to avoid potential neurovascular injuries.
- The perineum is positioned flush with the edge of the operating room table for easy access during the perineal phase of the operation.

345

346   SECTION III RECTAL RESECTIONS

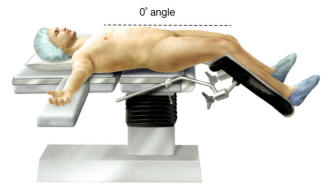

- The pelvis is supported with a folded sheet to lift the entire perineum and facilitate exposure during the perineal dissection.
- The arms are placed in a neutral position and supported with suitable armrests or tucked to the side.

FIGURE 1 • Patient positioning. The patient is placed on a Lloyd-Davies position, with the legs on stirrups. The thighs are positioned level with the abdomen, as this allows placement of a self-retaining retractor without creating excessive pressure between the retractor and the patient's thighs. The arms are tucked. All pressure points are padded to prevent neurovascular injuries.

TECHNIQUES

PLACEMENT OF INCISION

- A midline vertical incision is made.
- A suitable laparotomy retractor is inserted.

- After general inspection to see if there are any contraindications to performing RP/IPAA, the small bowel is packed with moist large swab packs into the upper abdominal cavity.

MOBILIZATION OF THE RIGHT COLON: PRESERVATION OF THE ILEOCOLIC VASCULAR PEDICLE

- The surgeon stands to the patient's left side. The patient is placed in a Trendelenburg position with the right side up to facilitate exposure.
- A full Cattell-Braasch maneuver is performed to mobilize the right colon of its retroperitoneal attachments.
- The cecum and ascending colon are freed from the peritoneal reflection by incising along the white line of Toldt (**FIGURE 2**). The terminal ileum is also freed from the retroperitoneum and mobilized by incising the peritoneum along the root of the mesentery.
- As the colon and terminal ileum are reflected anteriorly and medially, the right gonadal vessels and right ureter should be identified in the retroperitoneum and not mobilized anteriorly so as to avoid injury.
- The lateral dissection is carried sharply up and around the hepatic flexure in the avascular, embryologic plane between the mesocolon and the duodenum. The second and third portions of the duodenum are identified near the hepatic flexure, and injury to this structure must be avoided.
- The hepatocolic ligament is transected (**FIGURE 3**).
- Using an energy device, we hemostatically divide the ascending colon mesentery between the mesenteric vascular arcade and the colon wall (**FIGURE 4**) while protecting at all times the ileocolic vascular pedicle up to the mesenteric level of the ileocecal valve. This will allow excellent prograde blood supply to the pouch later on. Avoiding an ileocolic mesenteric bleeding or hematoma is crucial for preservation of the vascular supply to the ileal J-pouch.
- The mesenteric division extends from the midtransverse colon down to the mesenteric border of the terminal ileum at the selected site of proximal intestinal division—just proximal to the ileocecal valve.

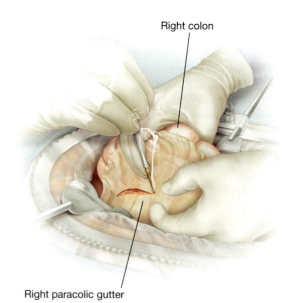

FIGURE 2 • Ascending colon mobilization. The surgeon retracts the ascending colon medially. Dissection proceeds along the right paracolic gutter.

Chapter 38 RESTORATIVE PROCTOCOLECTOMY: OPEN TECHNIQUE (ILEAL POUCH-ANAL ANASTOMOSIS) 347

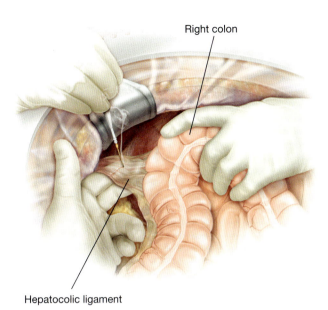

FIGURE 3 • Hepatic flexure mobilization. Gentle traction on the hepatic flexure of the colon exposes the hepatocolic ligament, which is then transected with electrocautery.

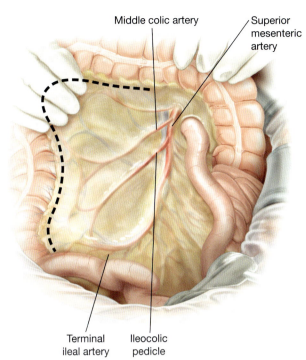

FIGURE 4 • Right colon vascular transection. Using an energy device, we hemostatically divide the ascending colon mesentery between the mesenteric vascular arcade and the colon wall (dotted line) while protecting at all times the ileocolic vascular pedicle up to the mesenteric level of the ileocecal valve. This will allow excellent prograde blood supply to the pouch later on.

TRANSVERSE COLON MOBILIZATION

- The gastrocolic ligament is exposed as the assistant retracts the greater omentum superiorly while the surgeon retracts the transverse colon anteroinferiorly.
- Diathermy is used to separate the greater omentum from the anterior leaf of the transverse mesocolon.
- Mobilization of the spleen needs to be approached from both sides to facilitate ease of mobilization of the splenic flexure (**FIGURE 5**). The patient is placed on a reverse Trendelenburg position with the left side up to allow the spleen to come down into the surgical field.
- Once the gastrocolic ligament has been completely transected, transection of the lateral peritoneal attachments (phrenocolic ligament) allows for lateral mobilization of the splenic flexure.
- At this point and from the right side of the table, the surgeon hooks the splenocolic ligament anteriorly with the right index finger, exposing the ligament adequately for the assistant to transect it using electrocautery. The splenocolic ligament is divided as close to the colon as feasible, avoiding undue traction on the spleen.

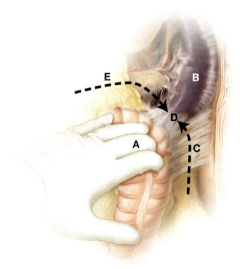

FIGURE 5 • Splenic flexure mobilization. The surgeon retracts the splenic flexure of the colon (A) downward and medially, exposing the attachments of the splenic flexure to the spleen (B). The phrenocolic (C) and splenocolic (D) ligaments are transected in an inferior-to-superior and lateral-to-medial direction. The gastrocolic ligament (E) is then transected in a medial-to-lateral direction, until both planes of dissection meet and the splenic flexure is fully mobilized.

DESCENDING COLON MOBILIZATION

- The surgeon stays on the right side of the table. The patient is placed in Trendelenburg position with the left side up.
- The descending colon is mobilized by medial traction and dissection along the left paracolic gutter using diathermy.
- The colon is mobilized from the retroperitoneum using a lateral-to-medial approach.
- Care is taken to identify, and avoid damage to, the left gonadal vessels and left ureter (**FIGURE 6**). In the lower abdomen, the left ureter is located medial to the gonadal vessels, close to the midline.

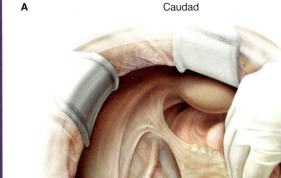
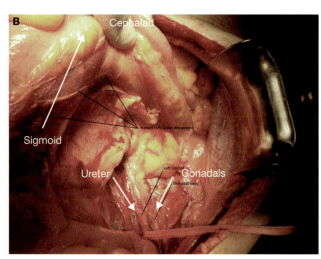

FIGURE 6 • Exposure of the left ureter. The illustration (**A**) shows the view of the operative field from cephalad to caudad direction. The operative picture (**B**) shows a caudad to cephalad view of the field. In the lower abdomen, as the descending and sigmoid mesocolon are separated from the retroperitoneum by the lateral-to-medial dissection, the left ureter is located medial to the gonadal vessels, close to the midline.

INFERIOR MESENTERIC ARTERY TRANSECTION

- With the assistant holding the proximal and distal sigmoid colon up, the root of the mesosigmoid colon is clearly visualized by the surgeon from the right side of the table. At the root of the mesentery, the arch of the superior hemorrhoidal vessels (SHVs) can be seen and palpated.
- Placing the index finger behind the SHV arch allows the surgeon to incise with electrocautery the right surface of the peritoneum just under the dorsal surface of the SHV.
- This plane of dissection along the dorsal aspect of the SHV is carried distally over the promontory (leading into the presacral space) and proximally, up to the origin of the inferior mesenteric artery (IMA). The IMA is dissected circumferentially at its origin from the aorta.
- The IMA is then ligated between Sarot clamps, incised, and doubly ligated with braided 2-0 suture (**FIGURE 7**).

Chapter 38 RESTORATIVE PROCTOCOLECTOMY: OPEN TECHNIQUE (ILEAL POUCH-ANAL ANASTOMOSIS)

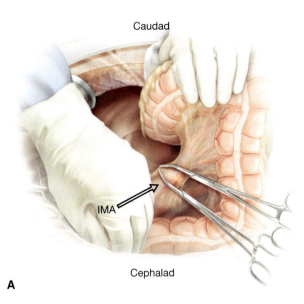
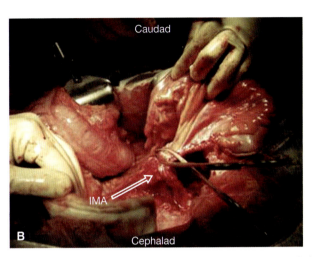

FIGURE 7 • IMA division. **A** and **B**, Illustration and operative picture. The IMA is transected between clamps and will subsequently be ligated with heavy silk sutures.

PROCTECTOMY

- The posterior pelvic dissection is performed first. Using a lighted St. Mark retractor for exposure, the presacral fascia is entered between the investing layer of fascia propria of the mesorectum and presacral fascia (**FIGURE 8**).
- The hypogastric nerves are identified at the pelvic rim and are preserved (**FIGURE 9**).
- The pelvic dissection is continued in the midline between Waldeyer fascia and the investing layer of the rectum to the level of the levator muscle. It is crucial not to violate the presacral fascia posteriorly where nervi erigentes and the lateral and presacral veins might be damaged.
- After the posterior dissection, a bilateral incision is made on the pelvic peritoneum and joined on the anterior rectal wall 1 cm above the peritoneal reflection. Dissection is then performed closer to the rectum to reduce the risk of nerve injury. The lateral ligaments are divided (**FIGURE 10**).
- The anterior dissection is done to the lower border of the prostate gland or lower one-third of the vagina (**FIGURE 10**). The Denonvilliers fascia is preserved in patients without a carcinoma. The rectum is completely mobilized.

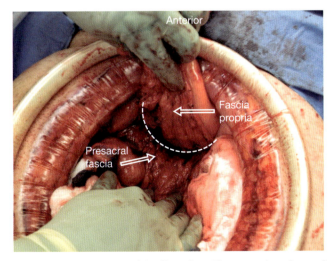

FIGURE 8 • Posterior pelvic dissection. The posterior plane of dissection *(dotted line)* proceeds in a semicircular fashion along the presacral space, located between the fascia propria of the rectum, anteriorly, and the presacral fascia, posteriorly. This allows continued exposure of the posterior plane of dissection down to the pelvic floor and prevents vascular and nerve injuries along the lateral pelvic walls.

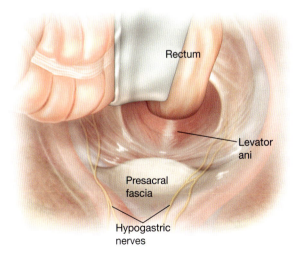

FIGURE 9 • Preservation of the hypogastric nerves. Using a lighted St. Mark retractor, the rectum is retracted anteriorly, exposing the presacral space posteriorly. The hypogastric nerves are exposed and should be swept posteriorly and away from the mesorectum. This begins the superior and posterior portion of the total mesorectal excision.

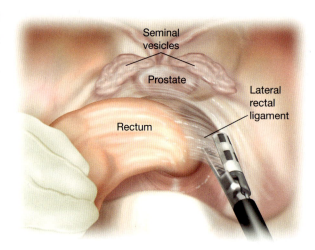

FIGURE 10 • Transection of the lateral rectal ligaments and anterior pelvic dissection. Posterolateral retraction of the rectum allows for good exposure of the lateral rectal ligament (the right lateral rectal ligament is shown here), which can then be transected with an energy device. The anterior dissection will then proceed between Denonvilliers fascia, posteriorly, and the prostate and seminal vesicles, anteriorly.

- A transanal digital evaluation with the tip of a finger is performed (**FIGURE 11**) to mark the level of distal rectal transection. The rectal transection is performed by a linear stapler

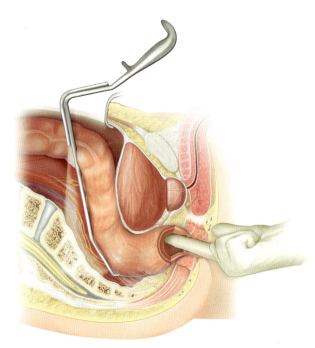

FIGURE 11 • A transanal digital evaluation with the tip of a finger is performed to mark the level of distal rectal transection.

for double-stapled IPAA or purse-string sutures for a single-stapled IPAA.

CREATION OF THE POUCH

- The pouch designs include J-, S-, or W-pouch (**FIGURE 12**). The J-pouch is the preferred technique because it is simpler to create. However, if there is an excessive tension in IPAA, an S-pouch can be created, because it usually reaches up to 4 cm further than the J-pouch.
- The J-pouch is created from the terminal 30 to 40 cm of small bowel, folded into two 15-cm or two 20-cm segments (**FIGURE 13**). A longitudinal 1.5-cm apical enterotomy is made. A side-to-side anastomosis of the two limbs of the ileum is done with 100-mm linear staplers, which is passed through apical enterotomy. After making sure that no small bowel mesentery is interposed between the anvil and the cartridge, the instrument is fired. A second stapler fire is required in the same way (**FIGURE 13A**).
- The end of the divided terminal ileum is closed by a linear stapler (**FIGURE 13B**) and usually reinforced by oversewing with 3-0 polyglycolic acid sutures.
- The pouch is filled with saline to confirm integrity of the anastomosis (**FIGURE 13C**). The staple lines are checked for hemostasis.

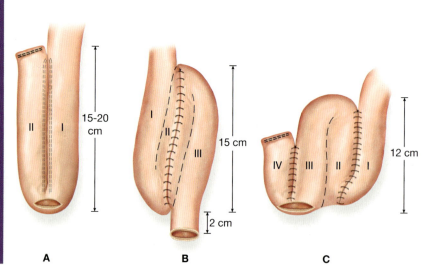

FIGURE 12 • Ileal pouch configurations. The potential pouch designs include a J-pouch (**A**), S-pouch (**B**), or W-pouch (**C**).

Chapter 38 RESTORATIVE PROCTOCOLECTOMY: OPEN TECHNIQUE (ILEAL POUCH-ANAL ANASTOMOSIS) 351

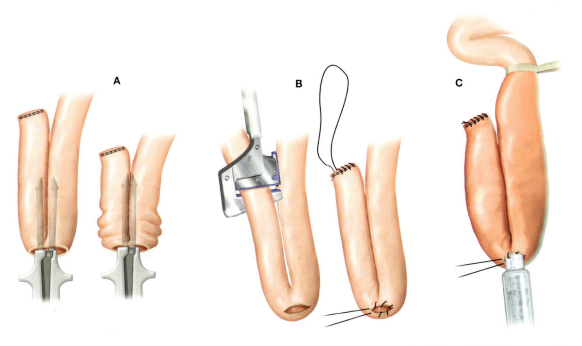

FIGURE 13 • Creation of a J-pouch. The J-pouch is created from the terminal 30 to 40 cm of small bowel, folded into two 15-cm or two 20-cm segments by creating a side-to-side anastomosis with two sequential 100-mm linear stapler loads introduced through an apical pouch incision **(A)**. The end of the divided terminal ileum is closed by a linear stapler and reinforced by oversewing with 3-0 polyglycolic acid sutures **(B)**. The pouch is then filled with saline to confirm integrity of the anastomosis **(C)**.

- The apical enterotomy is closed using a 0 polypropylene purse-string suture.
- An S-pouch is created using three limbs of 12 to 15 cm of terminal small bowel with a 2-cm exit conduit. The limbs are approximated by continuous seromuscular 3-0 polyglycolic acid sutures. An S-shaped enterotomy is made. Continuous or running all-coat sutures are applied to the two posterior anastomotic lines from within the pouch. Closure of the anterior wall is done with continuous seromuscular sutures. Lastly, interrupted 3-0 polyglycolic acid reinforcement sutures are applied.

THE POUCH DOES NOT REACH!

- The small bowel should be fully mobilized along the root of the mesentery up to the third portion of the duodenum so that the pouch reaches to the levator floor without tension.
- There may be difficulty with reach of the ileal pouch to the anal canal in obese patients or in patients who have had a previous small bowel resection.
- The reach can be estimated by grasping the ileal pouch at the apex and bringing it down to the pelvic floor.
- If the pouch does not reach, ligation and excision of the ileocolic artery and vein at their origin off the superior mesenteric artery (SMA) provides excellent pouch reach and allows for an anastomosis with no tension **(FIGURE 14A)**.
- If further mobilization is necessary, the peritoneal tissue to the right of the superior mesenteric vessels is excised with the use of translumination. In addition, transverse 1- to 2-cm peritoneal incisions over the superior mesenteric vessels border anteriorly and posteriorly can be done if needed **(FIGURE 14B)**.
- In a narrow pelvis, a bimanual maneuver can overcome the difficulty in reaching a bulky ileal pouch to the anal canal. A long Babcock clamp is passed transanally to grasp the apex of the pouch, and the surgeon's hand is passed behind the pouch to coax and ease the pouch and its exit conduit to the level of the levator floor **(FIGURE 15)**.

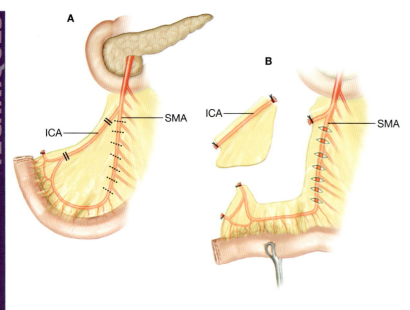

FIGURE 14 • **(A)** Pouch elongation. If the pouch does not reach, ligation and excision of the ileocolic artery and vein at their origin off the SMA provides excellent pouch reach and allows for an anastomosis with no tension **(B)**. If further pouch mobilization is necessary, the peritoneal tissue to the right of the superior mesenteric vessels is excised with the use of translumination. In addition, transverse 1- to 2-cm peritoneal stepladder incisions over the superior mesenteric vessels border anteriorly and posteriorly can be done if needed.

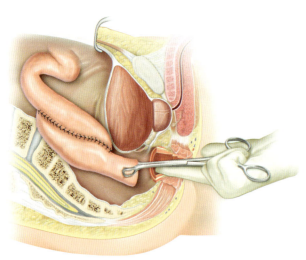

FIGURE 15 • Bimanual pouch delivery maneuver. A long Babcock clamp is passed transanally to grasp the apex of the pouch, and the surgeon's hand is passed behind the pouch to coax and ease the pouch to the level of the levator floor.

CREATION OF ILEAL POUCH-ANAL ANASTOMOSIS

Stapled Anastomosis

- IPAA can be created by either stapling or hand-sewn techniques. A stapled IPAA is constructed using either a double- or single-stapling technique.
- In the double-stapling technique (**FIGURE 16**), the distal anorectal stump is closed with a linear stapler. After the stapler is fired, the specimen is divided above the linear staple line. The linear staple line on the anorectum should rest at a level just below the superior border of the levator floor. Hence, the level of the planned IPAA should be determined and marked beforehand.
- A circular stapler with the anvil detached is inserted into the anus, and the pointed shaft/trocar is advanced just posterior to the linear staple line on the anorectum. This can be facilitated by putting the index finger into the anorectal area from the abdominal side and guiding the trocar just posterior to the linear staple line on the anorectum. The shaft of the circular staple line is then mated with the anvil shaft emerging from the ileal pouch. To prevent the twisting of mesentery, the small bowel is correctly oriented. The ends are approximated and anastomosis is completed. Both doughnuts are inspected for integrity. Care must be taken to avoid including the posterior vaginal wall and the anal sphincters within the anastomosis.
- Transanal insufflation with normal saline is performed to confirm that the anastomosis is intact.
- For a single-stapling anastomosis, a distal purse string is applied to the anorectal stump by hand with a 0 polypropylene suture. The surgical circular stapler is inserted transanally, the shaft is advanced completely, and the purse string is tightened. IPAA is then completed.

Chapter 38 RESTORATIVE PROCTOCOLECTOMY: OPEN TECHNIQUE (ILEAL POUCH-ANAL ANASTOMOSIS)   **353**

Hand-Sewn Anastomosis

- A hand-sewn IPAA is performed following mucosectomy of the anorectum (**FIGURE 17A**). The mucosa is stripped from the underlying sphincters starting at the dentate line to the level of the anorectal transsection. The anal verge is everted using sutures placed in four quadrants. An injection of 10- to 15-mL adrenalin solution (1:100,000) is used to raise the anorectal mucosa. A tube excision of anorectal mucosa is performed using cautery. Meticulous techniques are important to minimize risk of leaving islands of large bowel mucosa that are not amenable to surveillance.
- Excessive stretching of the anal canal may damage the anal sphincters; therefore, it should be avoided.
- 2-0 Polyglycolic acid sutures are placed radially at the dentate line, incorporating a small portion of internal anal sphincter. Stitches should not be taken too deeply anteriorly in female patients in order to prevent development of anastomotic-vaginal fistula.
- After the apex of the J-pouch or end of the exit conduit of the S-pouch is delivered to the anal verge using a Babcock clamp (**FIGURE 17B**), the previously placed sutures at the dentate line are serially placed through the full thickness of the ileum (**FIGURE 17C** and **D**).
- The retractor is then removed, and the sutures are tied.

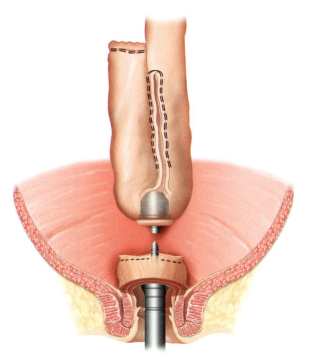

FIGURE 16 • J-pouch ileoanal anastomosis: double-stapled technique. An end-to-end stapled anastomosis is performed between the pouch and the anal canal.

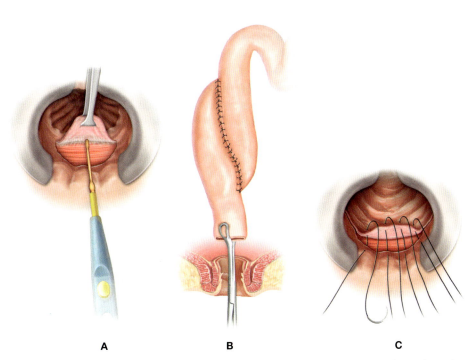

A   B   C

FIGURE 17 • J-pouch ileoanal anastomosis: hand-sewn technique. **A,** An anal mucosectomy is performed starting at the level of the dentate line. **B,** The apical opening of the J-pouch is delivered into the anal canal with a Babcock clamp. **C,** The anastomosis is constructed. **D,** This operative picture shows how the apical opening of the J-pouch is anchored to the anal canal. The previously placed four-quadrant distal sutures placed in the anal canal have now been placed full thickness through the open end of the J-pouch *(arrows)*. Placing full-thickness sutures in between these four quadrant sutures (along the *dotted lines*) will complete the anastomosis. A Lone Star retractor is used to enhance exposure.

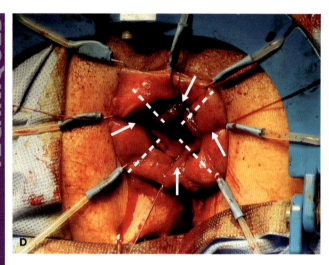

FIGURE 17 • Continued

CREATION OF DIVERTING STOMA AND CLOSURE

- A temporary diverting loop ileostomy is created in the right lower quadrant, 20 to 25 cm proximal to the pouch. In obese patients, if the ileal loop does not reach to the abdominal wall without tension, a divided end ileostomy may be preferred.
- A closed suction drain is placed into the presacral space.
- The incision is closed with running no. 1 polydioxanone (PDS) sutures. The skin incision is closed with staples.

PEARLS AND PITFALLS

Patient positioning	- Place the patient in a Lloyd-Davies position.
Incision	- Midline incision.
In severe fulminant colitis or toxic megacolon	- RP/IPAA should be performed in multistage: first, subtotal colectomy and end ileostomy, then completion proctectomy, IPAA, and loop ileostomy in 6 mo.
Creation of pouch	- J-pouch should be the preferred technique because of its simplicity. - S-pouch can be used if there is excessive tension.
The pouch does not reach	- Mobilize the small bowel to the third portion of the duodenum. - Transect and excise the ileocolic vessels at their origin from the SMA. - Stepladder incisions on the mesentery overlying the SMA.
IPAA	- The small bowel should be mobilized sufficiently so that it will reach to the levator floor without tension. - Stapled IPAA should be the preferred technique because it is associated with better outcomes.
Diverting stoma	- Reduces postoperative sepsis - In obese patients, if the ileal loop does not reach to the abdominal wall without tension, a divided end ileostomy may be preferred.

POSTOPERATIVE CARE

- Mean time to resuming a liquid diet is 3.8 days after surgery.
- The pelvic drain is left for 3 to 4 days or until the drainage is less than 50 mL a day.
- The mean length of hospital stay after RP/IPAA is 7.8 days.
- The diverting loop ileostomy is reversed in 6 weeks to 3 months, depending on the patient's performance and nutritional status, and only after a contrast study shows that the pouch and the anastomosis are intact.

OUTCOMES

- RP/IPAA is a good option for patients with ulcerative colitis, indeterminate colitis, and familial adenomatous polyposis and selected patients with Crohn disease.
- J is the preferred design of the ileal pouch.
- Stapled IPAA seems to be associated with significantly less complications and better functional outcomes and quality of life compared with a hand-sewn IPAA.
- Diverting ileostomy during RP/IPAA improves outcomes, especially sepsis.
- However, ileostomy may still be omitted in selected low-risk patients.
- Rate of pouch failure after RP/IPAA can be as low as 5% when it is performed at specialized centers.
- Patients who undergo RP/IPAA report good functional outcomes and quality of life after a long-term follow-up.

COMPLICATIONS

- Early complications: pelvic sepsis, anastomotic leak, hemorrhage, wound infection, small bowel obstruction, pouch fistula, stricture
- Late complications: small bowel obstruction, pelvic sepsis, pouch fistula, anastomotic leak, stricture, pouchitis, chronic pouchitis, pouch failure

SUGGESTED READINGS

1. Parks AG, Nicholls RJ. Proctocolectomy without ileostomy for ulcerative colitis. *Br Med J.* 1978;2(6130):85-88.
2. Fichera A, Silvestri MT, Hurst RD, et al. Laparoscopic restorative proctocolectomy with ileal pouch anal anastomosis: a comparative observational study on long-term functional results. *J Gastrointest Surg.* 2009;13(3):526-532.
3. Fazio VW, Kiran RP, Remzi FH, et al. Ileal pouch anal anastomosis; analysis of outcome and quality of life in 4035 patients. *Ann Surg.* 2013;257(4):679-685.
4. Kirat HT, Remzi FH, Kiran RP, et al. Comparison of outcomes after hand-sewn versus stapled ileal pouch-anal anastomosis in 3,109 patients. *Surgery.* 2009;146:723-729.
5. Weston-Petrides GK, Lovegrove RE, Tilney HS, et al. Comparison of outcomes after restorative proctocolectomy with or without defunctioning ileostomy. *Arch Surg.* 2008;143(4):406-412.

Chapter 39

Restorative Proctocolectomy: Single-Incision Laparoscopic Technique (Including Pouch Ileoanal Anastomosis)

Theodoros Voloyiannis

DEFINITION

- Single-incision laparoscopic restorative proctocolectomy, including pouch ileoanal anastomosis with temporary diverting loop ileostomy, is another application of the single-incision laparoscopic technique where a single multichannel laparoscopic port is used via a 2.5- to 3.5-cm total incision length.
- The procedure can be performed for benign or neoplastic diseases that require elective restorative proctocolectomy with a hand-sewn or stapled coloanal anastomosis including ileoanal pouch anastomosis such as ulcerative pancolitis, polyposis syndromes such as familial adenomatous polyposis or synchronous noninvasive rectal carcinoma, and colonic carcinomas and polyps after appropriate oncologic staging workup.
- A variation of this procedure may be applied for mid- or low rectal cancer with adequate oncologic distal rectal wall margin, preferably of at least 2 cm, for creation of an anastomosis. In these cases, a low anterior resection with stapled coloproctostomy or hand-sewn coloanal anastomosis and temporary loop ileostomy may be performed.
- A completion proctectomy, an ileoanal pouch anastomosis with temporary loop ileostomy after a total abdominal colectomy for ulcerative colitis, is another application of this technique.
- A new approach, the transabdominal-transanal single-port technique or transanal single-port total mesorectal excision (ta-TME) for completion of the total mesorectal excision with placement of a transanal single port, is discussed in this chapter.
- The goal is to keep the procedure simple, safe, and cost effective, with comparable outcomes to hand-assisted or multiport laparoscopic technique.
- Although single-incision laparoscopic surgery differs technically from conventional laparoscopic surgery, it follows the same steps and oncologic principles. However, it requires advanced laparoscopic skills.

PATIENT HISTORY AND PHYSICAL FINDINGS

- A detailed history and physical examination is essential preoperatively to determine if the patient is suitable for a laparoscopic approach. Rectal neoplasia after preoperative neoadjuvant chemoradiation or T4 rectal tumor extension to the sacrum, bladder trigone, prostate, posterior vaginal wall, or side pelvic wall with ureteral or major vessel involvement should be addressed preoperatively with appropriate staging workup. In these cases, laparotomy may be the best option,

or if the procedure can be accomplished laparoscopically, a hybrid approach with a single-port laparoscopic technique at the suprapubic area with subsequent conversion to a Pfannenstiel incision may be considered.

- Potential intraoperative consultation to other subspecialties, such as gynecology for addressing an incidental neoplastic adnexal pathology, urology for ureteral or bladder tumor involvement or other surgical service, may be necessary. It is the primary surgeon's responsibility to communicate with the consulting service regarding the feasibility of a single-incision laparoscopic approach in order to avoid a lengthy single-incision procedure that may lead to conversion to hand-assisted laparoscopy or to a laparotomy.
- A restorative proctocolectomy allows for extraction of the specimen via the single port or transanally, in case of a planned coloanal or ileoanal pouch hand-sewn anastomosis. A full-thickness rectal division is performed at the level of the dentate line. In case of underlying colonic or rectal neoplasia, the size of the tumor determines if it can be extracted without tension via the single-port wound protector. In general, tumors up to 7 cm can be extracted via a 5-cm maximum length single incision. The procedure can still be performed with elongation of the incision for extraction of larger tumors. In that case, the benefit of the single port is eliminated, with the exception of the avoidance of use of multiple laparoscopic ports. If the single port is placed via the new ileostomy site, then partial approximation of the fascia may be required prior to maturation of the ileostomy.
- A large palpable tumor preoperatively with fixation to the abdominal wall or other organs may be a contraindication to single-incision laparoscopy, although excision en bloc with soft tissue abdominal wall is still possible via a single incision in some cases.
- It is important to define the underlying pathology—benign vs malignant disease and the location of the lesion—preoperatively. Neoplasia may require formal lymphadenectomy with preferable high ligation of the involved vascular supply. This may not be necessary in benign conditions such as ulcerative colitis or polyposis syndromes without dysplasia or neoplasia.
- In case of a planned ileoanal pouch anastomosis, particular attention is paid to the preservation of the ileocolic vascular pedicle in order to maintain the vascular supply of the pouch. The ileal pouch can be fashioned extracorporeally, following extraction of the colon and rectum via the single-incision wound protector.
- Previous abdominal surgeries with extensive abdominal or pelvic adhesions may increase the operative time.

IMAGING AND OTHER DIAGNOSTIC STUDIES

- Preoperative colonoscopy is necessary to justify the planned restorative proctocolectomy.
- Diagnosis of ulcerative colitis and exclusion of Crohn's disease by colonoscopic biopsy and by an experienced pathologist and/or with the assistance of other laboratory workup, such as Prometheus test, are necessary in order to establish the need for restorative proctocolectomy with ileoanal anastomosis.
- Colonoscopic evidence of terminal ileitis by biopsy may assist in the diagnosis of Crohn's disease and avoidance of an ileoanal pouch formation.
- Diagnosis of ulcerative colitis with proctitis and involvement of the anal canal by colonoscopy or rigid proctoscopy and biopsy is necessary in order to establish the need for anal mucosectomy and hand-sewn ileal pouch anastomosis.
- Contrast-enhanced computed axial tomography (CAT) scan of the abdomen/pelvis assists the surgeon to decide on the feasibility of a single-incision laparoscopic approach. It also helps in identifying the exact location of large colonic or rectal neoplastic lesions, the potential involvement of adjacent organs or structures, and the potential presence of mesenteric adenopathy and/or metastases as well as inflammatory processes (phlegmon, abscess, fistula, or obstruction).
- Endorectal ultrasound or rectal protocol magnetic resonance imaging (MRI) may assist with the staging of rectal carcinoma and identification of the anal sphincter muscle involvement. The latter would be a contraindication of a restorative proctocolectomy and may also delineate the anatomy of the anal sphincter in case of previous obstetric trauma or episiotomies.
- Fecal incontinence—Wexner score preoperatively may assist with the diagnosis of fecal incontinence. Preoperative fecal incontinence may lead to poor functional outcome following an ileoanal pouch anastomosis.
- Preoperative barium enema or small bowel follow-through contrast study may assist with the diagnosis of Crohn's disease.
- The carcinoembryonic antigen (CEA) level is obtained in malignancies as a tumor marker.

SURGICAL MANAGEMENT

- Full bowel preparation is administered the day prior to surgery to reduce the weight and volume of the colon. This facilitates the laparoscopic handling of the colon and the extraction of the specimen via a small 3.5-cm single incision.
- Obtain preoperative medical or pulmonary cardiac clearance as necessary.
- Correct anemia, electrolyte imbalances, and malnutrition preoperatively as needed.
- Wean off preoperative steroids to preferably less than 20 mg prednisone per day, if possible.
- Give consideration to weight loss prior to surgery, especially in cases of chronic preoperative steroid usage. A short and thick ileal mesentery may preclude an ileoanal pouch anastomosis.
- Intravenous (IV) antibiotics are administered prior to skin incision.

Instrumentation

- A laparoscopic operating room (OR) table with steep tilting is used. Test maximum tilting prior to draping to assess patients' secure positioning on the table (**FIGURE 1**).
- Two laparoscopic high-definition screens, one on each side of the OR table, are used.
- We use a bariatric length, 10-mm 30° camera. If needed, we use a right-angle adaptor for fiberoptic attachment to the camera to avoid conflict of the fiberoptic cord with other laparoscopic instruments. Using camera heaters and a smoke evacuator channel can avoid the need for repeated camera cleansing, leading to a decrease in operative length.
- We use two bariatric length laparoscopic bowel graspers, laparoscopic scissors, and bariatric length laparoscopic 5- to 10-mm suction irrigation.
- We prefer to use a bariatric length laparoscopic energy device such as the 43-cm LigaSure 5-mm device. Energy devices that produce excessive moisture or fog may impair visibility.
- Laparoscopic Endoloop polydioxanone (PDS) for the ileocolic vascular pedicle.
- Staplers.
  - Linear GIA 100-mm, triple blue staple lines for the ileal pouch formation
  - A 28- to 29-mm circular stapler for a stapled ileoanal pouch anastomosis
  - A 60-mm Endo GIA for distal division of the rectum as indicated
- A second set of instruments is necessary for an extracorporeal anastomosis.

Patient Positioning

- The patient is placed on a modified lithotomy position on Allen stirrups with arms tucked (**FIGURE 1**). The patient is secured to the table, with foam pad placed under the patient's torso and with Velcro or broad tape placed across the chest. Rolled surgical towel is placed under the sacrum

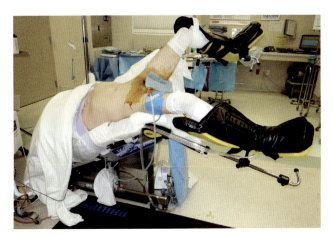

FIGURE 1 • Patient setup. The patient is secured to the table, with the arms tucked, a strap across the chest, and the legs on Yellofin stirrups. All pressure points are padded to avoid nerve and vascular injuries. The table tilt is tested prior to starting the case to ensure that the patient does not slide.

- to elevate the pelvis and assist with the coloanal or ileoanal anastomosis.
- A Foley catheter is inserted and taped over the right thigh in order to avoid urethral trauma with the OR table tilting.
- A bear hugger or other thermal device is applied to the chest and legs.
- A protecting foam pad is placed over the head to protect from injury with laparoscopic instrument positioning.
- We recommend using laparoscopic draping with side plastic bags or pockets to allow for bariatric instrument placement. All laparoscopic cords and energy device cords are brought out via the patient's upper chest.

DIAGNOSTIC LAPAROSCOPY—SINGLE MULTICHANNEL PORT TECHNIQUE

- A 2.5-cm circular incision is performed at the right lower quadrant (RLQ) premarked temporary ileostomy site. Alternatively, a 3.5-cm periumbilical vertical midline incision is performed. A wound protector is inserted, followed by attachment of the single-incision laparoscopic surgery (SILS) port (**FIGURE 2A** and **B**).
- Assemble all channels of the SILS port on the back table to avoid losing parts outside the sterile field. Insert the laparoscopic multichannel single port with a wound protector. Insufflate pneumoperitoneum carbon dioxide (CO_2) to 15 mm Hg of pressure.
- Perform a diagnostic laparoscopy. The surgical assistant/camera holder and the surgeon stand by the patient's right side when addressing the left colon, sigmoid, or rectum and by the patient's left side when addressing the right colon. For the transverse colon mobilization, either side may be suitable or the surgeon may be positioned between the patient's legs. Tilt the OR table to a steep Trendelenburg position and airplane it to the left or right for maximum exposure.
- Minimize excursion/cluster effect around hands and camera between the surgical assistant and operating surgeon with adherence to the principle that the surgeon should position their assisting (nondominant hand) instrument's distal tip (used for grasping, retracting, or suctioning) as close as possible to their operating (dominant hand) instrument's (ie, energy device) tip. This distance should be about 3 to 4 cm between the two instruments' tips. For example, hold the ileocolic vascular pedicle just above the site of the division site rather than holing the cecum itself, which is far more distant from the pedicle. This technique allows achieving a wide angle between the two instruments outside the abdomen as they exit and cross via the single port, thus minimizing instrument conflict effect between the surgeon's hands.
- The assistant/camera holder will avoid conflict with the surgeon's instruments outside the abdomen by holding the camera as far as possible from the surgeon's hands and by using the camera's 30° angulation for side view as well as the zoom-in option (**FIGURE 2B**).
- Minimize the need for frequent laparoscopic instrument exchange, such as exchanging of graspers with monopolar laparoscopic scissors. Instead, consider using multiuse energy devices that provide dissection and sealing-cutting capabilities, thus allowing constant progress in the operating field and significant time saving.
- The surgeon and the assistant can either switch sides during the various steps of the procedure or just rotate the single port clockwise or counterclockwise while the instruments stay in the abdomen under direct visualization with the camera, thus achieving different camera angles, better exposure, and better visualization.
- The OR table can also be tilted accordingly during the various steps of the procedure to increase the exposure and prevent instrument conflict.

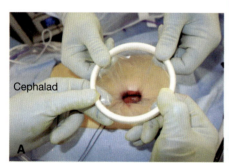 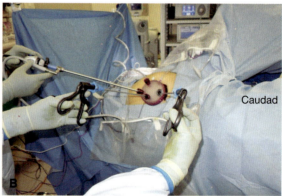

FIGURE 2 • SILS port placement and configuration. **A,** A wound protector is inserted in the RLQ at the diverting loop ileostomy site. **B,** A multiport channel with four working ports, insufflation port, and a smoke evacuator port is used. The port is assembled on a side table prior to insertion in the patient. The assistant/camera holder will avoid conflict with the surgeon's instruments outside the abdomen by holding the camera as far as possible from the surgeon's hands.

MOBILIZATION OF THE RIGHT COLON: PRESERVATION OF THE ILEOCOLIC VASCULAR PEDICLE

- The patient is positioned in a steep Trendelenburg position with the OR table tilted maximally toward the patient's left side. The surgeon is standing on patient's lower left side using a grasper in the nondominant hand and the energy device on the dominant hand. The camera holder stands cephalad to the surgeon.
- If the omentum is adherent medially to the hepatic flexure or the ascending colon itself, we start the procedure with the dissection of the omentum off the colon. We may perform omentectomy by including the omentum with the transverse colectomy.
- Dissect the terminal ileal retroperitoneal attachments and mobilize it toward the midline (FIGURE 3), exposing the origin of the superior mesenteric artery and the third and fourth portions of the duodenum. Morbidly obese patients require a generous terminal ileal medial mobilization to allow for a tension-free ileoanal pouch anastomosis.
- Proceeding from a caudad to cephalad direction, dissect the ascending colon mesentery off its retroperitoneal attachments without entering Gerota's fascia and preserving the right gonadal vessels and the right ureter intact. Dissect the ascending colon mesentery off the second and third portions of the duodenum in an atraumatic fashion.
- Using an energy device, we hemostatically divide the ascending colon mesenteric vascular arcade while protecting the ileocolic vascular pedicle up to the mesenteric level of the ileocecal valve (FIGURE 4). This is critical to ensure a good blood supply to the pouch. Avoiding an ileocolic mesenteric bleeding or hematoma is crucial for preservation of the vascular supply to the ileal J-pouch.
- Divide with the energy device the ascending colon mesentery flush to the ileocolic vascular pedicle (staying close to the colonic wall), up to the mesenteric border of the terminal ileum at the selected site of proximal intestinal division, just proximal to the ileocecal valve.
- Proceed with laparoscopic division of the incidental right colonic artery/vein if present.
- Mobilize the ascending colon medially by transecting the white line of Toldt.

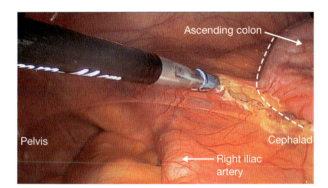

FIGURE 3 • Mobilization of the ileum and ascending colon. The mobilization starts by transecting the ileocecal retroperitoneal attachments (*dotted line*). The dissection will then proceed on a caudad to cephalad direction, eventually exposing the origin of the superior mesenteric artery and the third portion of the duodenum.

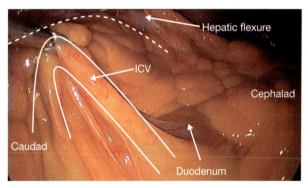

FIGURE 4 • Preservation of the ileocolic vessels (ICVs). During the dissection of the right colon, it is critical to divide the mesentery close to the colonic wall (*dotted line*), preserving the ICVs (here seen crossing over the third portion of the duodenum) intact. This will ensure excellent blood supply to the pouch.

MOBILIZATION OF THE TRANSVERSE COLON

- The surgeon stands in between the patient's leg. Place the patient on Trendelenburg and keep the OR table tilted to the left for the proximal transverse colon mobilization or to the right for the distal transverse colon and the splenic flexure mobilization. Alternatively, we may place the patient on reverse Trendelenburg for exposure and the assistant may use a laparoscopic grasper to assist with the retraction—"tenting"—of the transverse colon.
- Enter the lesser sac via the antimesenteric border of the proximal transverse colon and perform a hepatic flexure mobilization by dividing the hepatocolic ligament with the energy device (FIGURE 5).

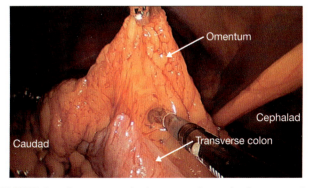

FIGURE 5 • Entrance to the lesser sac. Enter the lesser sac via the antimesenteric border of the proximal transverse colon and perform a formal hepatic flexure mobilization using the energy device.

- Divide the gastrocolic ligament adjacent to the mesenteric border of the transverse colon while preventing inadvertent injury of the gastroepiploic arcade.
- The omentum may be included with the transverse colon into the specimen.
- Dissect the root of the hepatic flexure and proximal transverse colon mesentery and identify the origin of the middle colic artery and vein. Using an energy device, divide the middle colic vascular pedicle at the root of the mesocolon while holding the stump with a grasper to avoid retraction or residual bleeding (**FIGURE 6**).
- Place hemostatic clips or Endoloop PDS at the divided stump to secure the hemostasis. There is no need to use an Endo GIA stapler, unless severe atherosclerosis or vessels larger than 7 mm in size are present, which preclude usage of an energy device.
- Complete the dissection of the root of the distal transverse mesocolon off the retroperitoneum, pancreas, and fourth portion of the duodenum with the energy device.

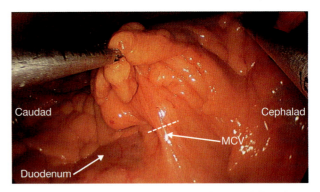

FIGURE 6 • Identification and division of the middle colic vascular pedicle. With the transverse colon tented up with two graspers, the middle colic vessels (MCVs) can be identified at the intersection of the root of the mesotransverse colon and the third portion of the duodenum. After dissection, the middle colic vessels will be transected (*dotted line*) with an energy device.

SPLENIC FLEXURE MOBILIZATION, LEFT COLECTOMY, AND SIGMOID COLECTOMY

- The surgeon stands on the patient's right side and caudally to the assistant, with the OR table tilted to the right.
- Start the dissection of the root of the sigmoid mesocolon off the retroperitoneal attachments by dissecting dorsal to the superior hemorrhoidal vessels (**FIGURE 7A**). Identify and preserve the left ureter (**FIGURE 7B**), gonadal vessels, and hypogastric nerves intact.

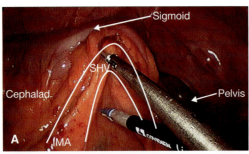

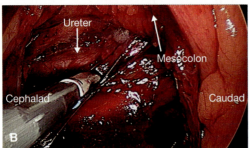

FIGURE 7 • Dissection of the IMA and the superior hemorrhoidal vessels (SHVs). **A,** The dissection starts at the root of the sigmoid mesentery, dorsal to the SHV. **B,** The retroperitoneal structures, including the left ureter, are swept down (dorsally) with the energy device, separating them for the mesocolon.

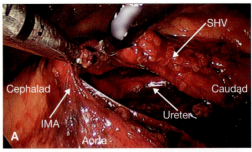

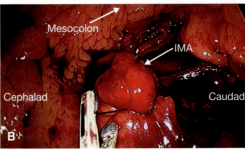

FIGURE 8 • IMA transection. **A,** With the left ureter safe in the retroperitoneum, a high IMA transection is performed off the aorta with the energy device. **B,** The IMA stump is secured with an Endoloop.

- Skeletonize the origin of the inferior mesenteric artery (IMA). Perform a high IMA transection (**FIGURE 8A** and **B**) as described earlier for the middle colic vascular pedicle.
- Perform a medial to lateral mobilization of the descending colon mesentery off the retroperitoneal attachments by sweeping the retroperitoneal tissues down (dorsally) with an energy device (**FIGURE 9**). This dissection is carried laterally to the lateral abdominal wall, superiorly separating the tail of the pancreas from the splenic flexure of the colon, and inferiorly to the pelvic inlet. This dissection greatly facilitates the lateral mobilization of the descending colon and the splenic flexure mobilization.

Chapter 39 RESTORATIVE PROCTOCOLECTOMY: SINGLE-INCISION LAPAROSCOPIC TECHNIQUE **361**

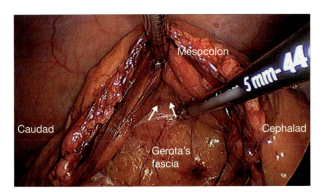

FIGURE 9 • Medial to lateral mobilization of the descending colon. The descending mesocolon is separated from Gerota fascia and other retroperitoneal structures. The dissection proceeds laterally until reaching the lateral abdominal wall. The dissection proceeds at the transition between the two distinctive fat planes (*arrows*).

- Divide the inferior mesenteric vein and the left colic artery by the ligament of Treitz with the energy device.
- Perform a lateral mobilization of the descending and sigmoid colon by transecting the white line of Toldt. The medial to lateral dissection plane is readily entered.
- Mobilize the splenic flexure of the colon by dividing the gastrocolic, splenocolic, and phrenocolic ligaments using an energy device. Care is taken to avoid injury to the pancreatic tail and to the spleen (**FIGURE 10**).

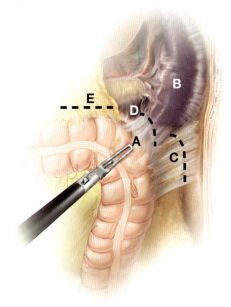

FIGURE 10 • Mobilization of the splenic flexure. The splenic flexure (*A*) is separated off the spleen (*B*) by transecting the phrenocolic (*C*), the splenocolic (*D*), and the gastrocolic (*E*) ligaments using an energy device.

PROCTECTOMY AND TOTAL MESORECTAL EXCISION

- The surgeon stands on the patient's right side and cephalad to the assistant; the OR table is tilted to the right. The RLQ single port site allows for excellent exposure during the total mesorectal excision.
- Start with the posterior mobilization of the rectum by dissecting the presacral avascular plane. The dissection proceeds caudally in this plane to the level of the levator muscles while preserving the hypogastric nerves (**FIGURE 11**). Avoid penetrating the presacral fascia in order to avoid potentially serious bleeding from the presacral venous plexus.
- The lateral mobilization of the rectum is then performed by dissecting the lateral rectal attachments and dividing the lateral ligaments with the energy device. Care is taken to avoid penetrating the endopelvic fascia at the lateral pelvic walls, which could result in severe bleeding from injury to the hypogastric vein and its branches (**FIGURE 12**).
- At this point, mobilize the rectum anteriorly. Include into the specimen the anterior (Denonvilliers') fascia for mid- to low anterior rectal carcinoma while completing the dissection caudally to the levator muscles. Care is taken to avoid injury to the nervi erigentes, bladder, trigone, seminal vesicles, prostatic capsule, and urethra in males or the uterus and posterior vagina in females (**FIGURE 13**).
- The superior hemorrhoidal pedicle is divided with the energy device at the chosen distal rectal division site if a stapled coloproctostomy is planned.

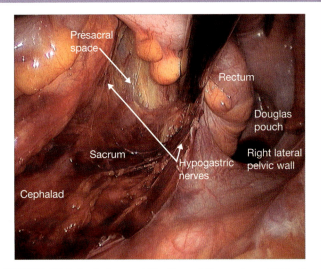

FIGURE 11 • Posterior mobilization of the rectum. With the assistant retracting the rectum anteriorly, the presacral space is dissected with the energy device. The dissection proceeds caudally to the level of the levator muscles while preserving the hypogastric nerves. Avoid penetrating the presacral fascia in order to avoid potentially serious bleeding from the presacral venous plexus.

- The perineum may be pushed manually into the pelvis by the assistant surgeon. This maneuver may add another critical 2 cm to the distal rectal resection margin caudally.
- Intraoperative identification of the distal rectal resection site, either with preoperative anterior rectal wall tattoo

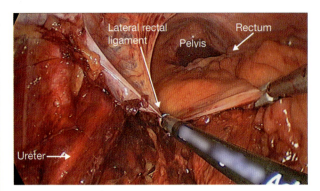

FIGURE 12 • Lateral mobilization of the rectum. The lateral rectal ligaments (the left one is shown here) are transected with the energy device. Care is taken to avoid violating the endopelvic fascia along the lateral pelvic walls, which could lead to injury to the ureters and, more distally, the hypogastric vein and its branches. The latter could result in serious bleeding that is difficult to control.

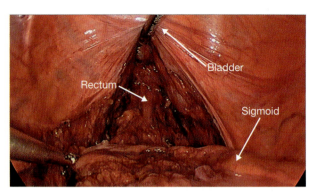

FIGURE 13 • Anterior mobilization of the rectum. The dissection proceeds anterior to Denonvilliers' fascia, separating the rectum from the bladder, and more distally, from the seminal vesicles and prostate in men (shown here) or the vagina in females.

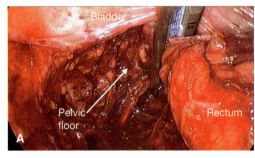
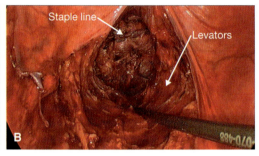

FIGURE 14 • Distal rectal transection. **A,** When a stapled coloanal anastomosis is planned, the distal rectum is stapled from an anterior to posterior direction above the dentate line. This technique avoids the need for multiple stapler fires, reducing anastomotic leak rates. **B,** After resection of the rectum, the staple line can be seen in the distal pelvis at the level of the pelvic floor.

placement 2 cm distal to the carcinoma or with intraoperative proctoscopy, is necessary. Preoperative tattooing is particularly helpful in cancer patients who had a complete response to neoadjuvant therapy.
- In case of a distal rectal division at the level of the dentate line with the intention of a stapled coloproctostomy, an Endo GIA laparoscopic stapler is used either via the single port site at the RLQ or by placing a suprapubic 12-mm port and stapling the rectum vertically via that site.
- A vertical stapling of the rectum via a suprapubic port (**FIGURE 14A** and **B**), especially in males or patients with narrow pelvis, may prevent from usage of multiple overlapping Endo GIA loads for the rectal division, which lowers anastomotic leak rates. The suprapubic port may be used for placement of the low pelvic Jackson-Pratt drain at the end of the case.
- If a hand-sewn anastomosis is planned, then the dissection is carried to the levator muscle/dentate line with care to obtain an adequate negative radial mesorectal margin.

TRANSANAL SINGLE-PORT TOTAL MESORECTAL EXCISION: THE NARROW PELVIS

- The surgeon is now seated between the patient's legs, with the patient on Trendelenburg position. A back table with instruments for the perineal portion of the procedure is used.
- The surgeon may use a Mayo tray placed on their knees and a headlight.
- In case of a planned hand-sewn coloanal or ileoanal pouch anastomosis, a Lone Star retractor may be placed in the anus for exposure.
- In case of neoplasia, the rectum proximally to the dentate line is obliterated with a mucosal 0-Vicryl or 2-0 PDS purse-string suture (**FIGURE 15**). A full-thickness division of the rectum at the level of the dentate line is performed with electrocautery, with care not to injure the internal sphincter muscle (**FIGURE 16**).
- If the pelvic total mesorectal excision is adequate caudally, then the rectum is freed up and the colon and rectum may be extracted either via the RLQ abdominal single port site with the wound protector in place (**FIGURE 17**) or via the anus. The specimen is divided at the level of the terminal ileum/ileocecal valve with a linear stapler.
- If the rectum is still adherent in the inner pelvis secondary to a narrow/deep pelvis precluding further laparoscopic dissection transabdominally, then a Transanal Minimally Invasive Surgery (TAMIS) laparoscopic single port is inserted in the anus after placement of the purse-string rectal lumen

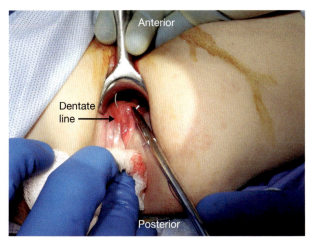

FIGURE 15 • Transanal single-port total mesorectal excision. In case of neoplasia, the rectum proximal to the dentate line is obliterated with a mucosal 0-Vicryl or 2-0 PDS purse-string suture.

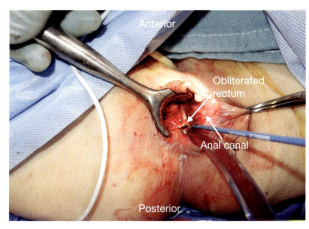

FIGURE 16 • Transanal single-port total mesorectal excision. A full-thickness division of the rectum at the level of the dentate line is performed with electrocautery. In this picture, the dissection is proceeding right lateral to the obliterated distal rectum and the distal rectal wall.

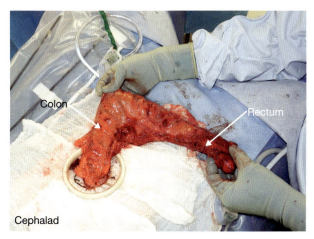

FIGURE 17 • Extracorporeal mobilization of the specimen. The colon and rectum may be extracted via the RLQ abdominal single port site with the wound protector in place.

obliteration and the division of the rectum at the dentate line is completed (**FIGURE 18A** and **B**). This allows for excellent visualization in the distal narrow pelvis.

- Pneumoperitoneum CO_2 to 15 mm Hg is insufflated via the transabdominal and pneumopelvis via the transanal single port; two insufflators are needed.
- Using the transanal single port, a 30° 5-mm laparoscopic camera, a 5-mm laparoscopic grasper, and the same laparoscopic energy device (**FIGURE 19**), we proceed with the completion of the total mesorectal division with a circumferential caudal to cephalad direction. The endpoint of the dissection

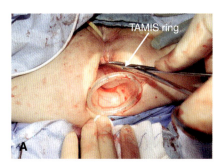

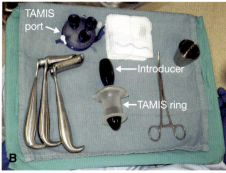

FIGURE 18 • Transanal single-port total mesorectal excision: transanal insertion of the TAMIS port. **A**, The TAMIS ring is introduced first, followed by application of the TAMIS port. **B**, The multichannel TAMIS port is assembled on a side table prior to insertion into the anus.

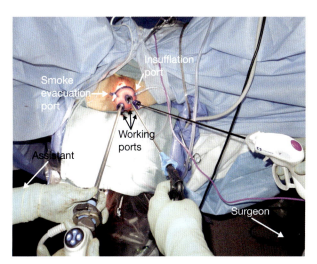

FIGURE 19 • Transanal single-port total mesorectal excision. The surgeon operates with an energy device and a grasper while the assistant operates the camera.

is accomplished by meeting the transabdominal distal dissection site in the inner pelvis (**FIGURE 20**).
- Upon completion of the transanal single port dissection, the specimen is extracted as described earlier. If the specimen is too thick, then elongate the circular incision superiorly using an Army-Navy to "hook" under the fascia protecting the wound protector from perforation. Use a no. 11 scalpel in a sawing move or electrocautery to elongate the incision; extract the specimen, divide it at the terminal ileum, and send it to pathology.
- The transanal single port is removed and an anal canal mucosectomy may be performed as indicated (such as in ulcerative colitis with involvement of the anoderm) by elevating the anoderm with a submucosal injection of Marcaine with epinephrine and performing a sharp excision anal mucosectomy with scalpel or scissors.

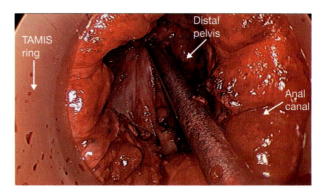

FIGURE 20 • Transanal single-port total mesorectal excision. The dissection is carried through the TAMIS port into the distal pelvis until the distal dissection planes from the transabdominal phase of the operation are reached.

ILEOANAL POUCH FORMATION AND J-POUCH ILEOANAL ANASTOMOSIS

- Following division of the terminal ileum at the level of the ileocecal valve with a linear GIA blue load stapler, the ileal pouch is fashioned.
- Place wet lap sponges around the abdominal wound protector and use a second towel for the instruments used for creation of the pouch formation in order to avoid fecal contamination to the laparoscopic surgical drapes.
- Fold the distal 30 cm of terminal ileum in the shape of the letter "J"; a pouch length of 15 cm is usually adequate (**FIGURE 21**). Use a linear GIA stapler 100-mm blue load (double line) or 75-mm blue (triple line) or, if already opened and used, the Endo GIA laparoscopic triple line 60-mm stapler (blue load for Ethicon or tan load for Covidien staplers) to create the pouch.
- Insert the stapler via the antimesenteric border of the terminal ileum at the tip of the J-pouch and fire the loads (usually two loads with the 100-mm linear stapler) in an antimesenteric side-to-side fashion. Inspect the inside of the pouch for bleeding.
- If a stapled anastomosis is planned, place a 28- to 29-mm circular stapler anvil into the tip of the pouch and secure it with a 3-0 Prolene purse string.
- Reintroduce the pouch into the abdomen and place it into the inner pelvis with the pouch mesentery facing posteriorly. Reinsufflate the pneumoperitoneum via the abdominal single port and perform a circular stapled ileal pouch-anal anastomosis (**FIGURE 22A** and **B**). Two intact doughnuts should be obtained.
- Test the integrity of the anastomosis by insufflating the pouch under saline immersion. If a major anastomotic leak is noted, 2-0 Vicryl or 2-0 PDS sutures maybe placed transanally using a Hill Ferguson or a Sims Parks retractor. The air leak test may be repeated as discussed earlier to confirm resolution of the leak.
- If a hand-sewn anastomosis is planned, then place a purse string to close the tip of the pouch in order to prevent soilage

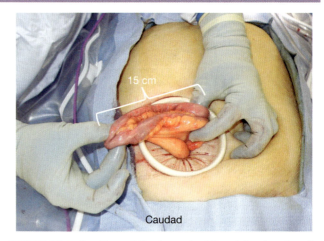

FIGURE 21 • Creation of the J-pouch. After delivering the distal 30 cm of terminal ileum through the SILS port site (with the wound protector in place), the ileum is folded in the shape of the letter "J." The J-pouch will then be created with a 100-mm stapler (usually two loads are needed) inserted via the antimesenteric border of the terminal ileum at the tip of the J-pouch.

in the pelvis. Place the pouch into the inner pelvis with the pouch mesentery facing posteriorly toward the sacrum. The pouch should reach to outside of the anal canal (**FIGURE 23**). Perform a hand-sewn ileoanal pouch anastomosis using the Lone Star retractor for exposure (a 2-0 Quill double ended may be used alternatively) using 2-0 Vicryl or 2-0 PDS in interrupted full-thickness fashion, incorporating the internal sphincter muscle and the anoderm at the level of the dentate line (**FIGURE 24**).
- A Surgicel hemostatic agent may be placed into the anus following completion of the anastomosis.
- A 19-Fr Jackson-Pratt circular drain, placed posteriorly to the pouch with the tip superiorly to the anastomosis, is brought via the suprapubic port site and is placed on bulb suction.

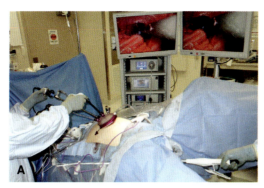
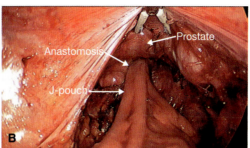

FIGURE 22 • Creation of the stapled J-pouch ileoanal anastomosis. **A,** After reintroducing the J-pouch with the anvil in its tip into the abdomen, the pneumoperitoneum is reinsufflated. With an experienced assistant introducing the 28-mm end-to-end anastomosis (EEA) stapler transanally and the scrub nurse holding the camera, the surgeon mates the anvil to the stapler's opened torch intracorporeally, as seen in the OR monitors. **B,** After firing the stapler, the anastomosis is now completed. The J-pouch, its mesentery (posteriorly located along the sacrum), and the tension-free anastomosis can be seen here.

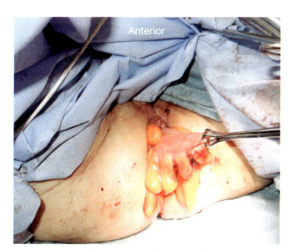
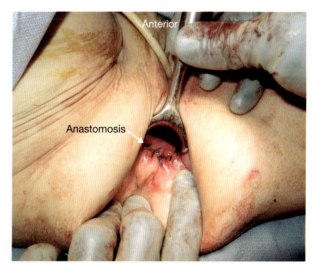

FIGURE 23 • Hand-sewn J-pouch ileoanal anastomosis. The pouch should reach to outside of the anal canal.

FIGURE 24 • Hand-sewn J-pouch ileoanal anastomosis. The completed anastomosis is seen here.

ILEOANAL POUCH ANASTOMOSIS: THE POUCH WILL NOT REACH!

- Perform mesenteric J-pouch serosal dissections.
- Perform mesenteric pouch "windows" by dividing the afferent or efferent mesenteric vessels. Consider the risk for pouch ischemia-necrosis.
- Perform mesenteric ileal serosal dissections laparoscopically up to the origin of the superior mesenteric artery.

DIVERTING LOOP ILEOSTOMY

- Remove the abdominal wound protector and bring a loop of terminal ileum proximal to the afferent limb of the pouch.
- It is advised to place an antiadhesive sheet posterior to the ileostomy fascia edges.
- Mature the loop ileostomy with the proximal limb in a Brooke's fashion and the distal limb as a mucous fistula (**FIGURE 25**) and place an ileostomy appliance.
- The patient has no wound for approximation.

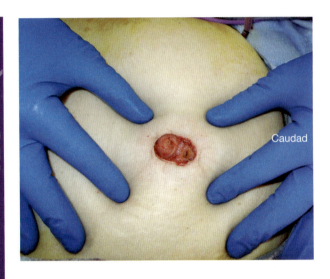

FIGURE 25 • The abdomen after the completed SILS restorative proctocolectomy with J-pouch ileoanal anastomosis and protective temporary diverting loop ileostomy. The temporary ileostomy is constructed at the SILS port site.

PEARLS AND PITFALLS

Preoperative workup	■ Correct identification of the underlying pathology allows for careful selection of the laparoscopic single-incision restorative proctocolectomy technique.
Patient positioning, laparoscopic instruments, surgeon assistant position	■ Securing the patient's position, OR table tilting, single port rotation, and usage of instruments and camera with bariatric length are necessary for a laparoscopic single-incision surgery. Surgeon should change their position in relation to the assistant several times during the procedure in order to achieve adequate exposure and visualization.
Laparoscopic instrument tissue handling	■ The tips of the assisting and dominant laparoscopic instruments are positioned as close as possible to each other in the surgical field in order to avoid hand conflict outside the abdomen.
Insertion of the SILS port	■ May use the new temporary loop ileostomy site at the RLQ. Alternatively, an umbilical or suprapubic site may be chosen.
Will the pouch reach?	■ Preoperative evaluation is essential. Intraoperative laparoscopic single port evaluation and surgical approach may be challenging.
Difficult dissection in the distal narrow pelvis	■ Consider the ta-TME technique.
Distal rectal division	■ Divide the rectum on an anterior to posterior direction with a linear reticulating stapler inserted via the suprapubic port. Use this port site to bring a Jackson-Pratt pelvic drain out at the end of the case.

POSTOPERATIVE CARE

- A fast-track postoperative laparoscopic pathway is initiated.
- The orogastric tube is discontinued in the OR upon completion of the procedure.
- IV acetaminophen alvimopan and opioid patient-controlled anesthesia (PCA) is used as per surgeon's preference the day of surgery, with the goal of discontinuing the PCA within 36 hours and adding IV or oral nonsteroidal antiinflammatory drugs (NSAIDs), such as ketorolac, and transition to oral analgesics.
- Ice chips/water diet is introduced the day of surgery with the goal to advance to clear liquids within 24 hours and to regular high-fiber diet within 48 hours postoperatively.
- The Foley catheter is kept until the third postoperative day secondary to the risk for urinary retention from the pelvic surgery/hypogastric nerve manipulation.
- Perioperative antibiotics, pharmacologic venous thromboembolism protocol, incentive spirometry, and early ambulation are initiated the day of surgery.
- Wound care need is minimal. If the umbilicus is used for the single port entry, umbilical skin edges are tucked with Vaseline/Adaptic gauze and cotton, which is removed in 48 to 72 hours. If the ileostomy site is used for single port entry, there is no abdominal wound.
- Surgicel is removed from the anus after 24 hours and the anastomosis is inspected for bleeding.

Chapter 39 **RESTORATIVE PROCTOCOLECTOMY: SINGLE-INCISION LAPAROSCOPIC TECHNIQUE** 367

- The patient usually can be safely discharged home within 72 hours when passage of flatus/succus is documented from the ileostomy and a regular diet is tolerated by at least two consecutive meals and there are no other adverse postoperative findings.
- No weight lifting of more than 20 lb is recommended for 4 to 6 weeks postoperatively in order to avoid incisional hernia.

OUTCOMES

- Single-port laparoscopic restorative proctocolectomy is considered to be an equally safe and cost-effective technique with excellent cosmesis, similar morbidity and operative time, possible less postoperative pain and faster return to full activities, possible shorter hospital stay, and comparable oncologic outcomes when performed for neoplastic diseases to conventional hand-assisted or multiport laparoscopic approach.
- It is achieved with equipment that the hospital already has available and requires no additional training for the operative room personnel.
- It is feasible by surgeons who perform advanced laparoscopy.
- It does require one assistant who has advanced laparoscopic skills for camera handling.
- The laparoscopic single-incision restorative proctocolectomy technique may therefore contribute to decreased total hospital cost.

COMPLICATIONS

- The procedure has similar morbidity and mortality and comparable rates for conversion to laparotomy with conventional laparoscopy.
- The single-incision laparoscopic technique for restorative proctocolectomy has the option for conversion to multiport or hand-assisted laparoscopy.
- Mobilizing/elongating the small intestinal mesentery for an ileoanal anastomosis may be challenging laparoscopically.

- The ileal pouch may not reach the perineum. In these cases, an end ileostomy is needed.
- It may require a longer operative time during the learning curve of the surgeon; this can complicate an already challenging procedure.
- Elongating the ileostomy site single port incision for specimen extraction with fascial reapproximation prior to the ostomy maturation may increase the incidence of parastomal hernia rate.
- It is intrinsically a one-operating surgeon technique with less involvement of the assistant surgeon and a potential impact on resident education during the learning curve period.

SUGGESTED READING

1. Geisler DP, Kirat HT, Remzi FH. Single-port laparoscopic total proctocolectomy with ileal pouch-anal anastomosis: initial operative experience. *Surg Endosc.* 2011;25(7):2175-2178. doi:10.1007/s00464-010-1518-8
2. Costedio MM, Remzi FH. Single-port laparoscopic colectomy. *Tech Coloproctol.* 2013;17(suppl 1):S29-S34. doi:10.1007/s10151-012-0935-1
3. Paranjape C, Ojo OJ, Carne D, et al. Single-incision laparoscopic total colectomy. *J Soc Laparoendosc Surg.* 2012;16(1):27-32. doi:10.4293/108680812X13291597715826
4. Leblanc F, Makhija R, Champagne BJ, et al. Single incision laparoscopic total colectomy and proctocolectomy for benign disease: initial experience. *Colorectal Dis.* 2011;13(11):1290-1293. doi:10.1111/j.1463-1318.2010.02448.x
5. Wexner SD, Berho M. Transanal TAMIS total mesorectal excision (TME)—a work in progress. *Tech Coloproctol.* 2014;18(5):423-425. doi:10.1007/s10151-014-1141-0.
6. Atallah S, Martin-Perez B, Albert M, et al. Transanal minimally invasive surgery for total mesorectal excision (TAMIS-TME): results and experience with the first 20 patients undergoing curative-intent rectal cancer surgery at a single institution. *Tech Coloproctol.* 2014;18(5):473-480. doi:10.1007/s10151-013-1095-7
7. Atallah S. Transanal minimally invasive surgery for total mesorectal excision. *Minim Invasive Ther Allied Technol.* 2014;23(1):10-16. doi:10.3109/13645706.2013.833118

Chapter 40

Restorative Proctocolectomy: Hand-Assisted Laparoscopic Surgery Ileal Pouch-Anal Anastomosis

Robert R. Cima

DEFINITION

- An ileal pouch-anal anastomosis (IPAA) is a restorative procedure used when the entire colon and rectum needs to be removed and the patient wishes to avoid a permanent ileostomy. The two most common indications for IPAA are chronic ulcerative colitis (CUC) and familial adenomatous polyposis syndrome. Although the procedure is basically the same, the frequency and indications for surgery are different, and for the purposes of this chapter, the focus will be on the surgical treatment of CUC.[1]
- IPAA involves removal of the entire colon and rectum followed by construction of an ileal reservoir most commonly in a "J shape" that is anastomosed to the anal canal by either a stapled or handsewn technique.
- This maintains the normal route of defecation, although the frequency and consistency of the stool is different than normal bowel function.

DIFFERENTIAL DIAGNOSIS

- Primarily, CUC needs to be distinguished from Crohn colitis. This is particularly important, because a restorative IPAA is not recommended in Crohn disease patients.
- Other acute colitis syndromes (ie, toxic bacterial colitis, cytomegalovirus [CMV] colitis, ischemic colitis) can mimic CUC. Thus, a thorough workup to differentiate between CUC and other disease processes needs to be considered prior to surgery.
- A detailed review of the patient's disease course including past endoscopic findings, prior imaging studies, and any history of perianal disease needs to be evaluated. Any history of small bowel inflammation or perianal abscesses, fistulas, or fissures is highly suggestive of underlying Crohn disease.
- In patients with an established history of CUC presenting with an acute worsening of their symptoms, it is important to rule out an infectious cause such as *Clostridium difficile* or CMV colitis as the *cause* of their disease exacerbation.

PATIENT HISTORY AND PHYSICAL FINDINGS

- CUC is characterized by recurrent episodes of bloody diarrhea associated with urgency and tenesmus.
- Approximately 15% of patients will present initially with fulminant disease, characterized by high-volume bloody diarrhea, severe abdominal distension and pain, fever, and systemic signs of illness. In severe situations, the patient might have peritonitis as the result of colonic perforation or hemodynamic compromise from volume depletion and systemic inflammation.
- More commonly, the CUC patient with medically refractory disease will not have any characteristic physical findings. However, prolonged disease activity can be associated with poor overall nutritional status and significant weight loss.

IMAGING AND OTHER DIAGNOSTIC STUDIES

- Computed tomography (CT) enterography is the most commonly used imaging study in CUC patients (**FIGURE 1**). The use of intravenous (IV) contrast is essential to highlight intestinal inflammation and helps identify any evidence of small bowel inflammation, which is highly suggestive of Crohn disease.
- In active CUC, the CT will demonstrate inflammatory changes around the involved colon with thickening of the colonic wall. This inflammation usually starts in the rectum and extends proximally into the colon for a varying distance.
- Endoscopic imaging of the colon is essential (**FIGURE 2**). It should demonstrate continuous inflammation from the rectum for a variable distance, extending proximally into the colon. Evidence of discontinuous mucosal inflammation is worrisome for an underlying diagnosis of Crohn disease.

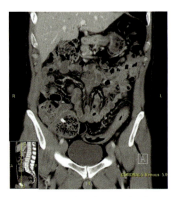

FIGURE 1 • CT enterography (coronal view, venous phase). Severely inflamed distal colon in a chronic ulcerative colitis patient with normal appearing small bowel.

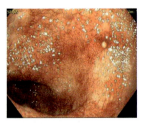

FIGURE 2 • Colonoscopy shows diffuse severe inflammation and friable mucosa, with a loss of the vascular appearance of the colon, erythema, hemorrhage, and inflammatory pseudopolyps.

SURGICAL MANAGEMENT

- Frequently, an IPAA for the treatment of CUC is performed in stages, depending on the patient's overall health at the time of surgery or the indications for surgery.
- The primary indications for surgery are toxic or fulminant disease activity, medically refractory disease, and/or evidence of dysplasia/malignancy.
- In an emergency situation, or in an ill patient on multiple immunosuppressive medications, the first operation is a subtotal colectomy with an end ileostomy.
- Once the patient recovers their health, a completion proctectomy with IPAA and diverting ileostomy may be performed. At the last operation (the third stage), the ileostomy is reversed.
- In outpatients with mild disease that are coming to surgery, the total proctocolectomy with IPAA and diverting loop ileostomy may be performed at a single operation.
- In some institutions, the diverting loop ileostomy may be routinely omitted, depending on a number of patient- and procedure-specific factors. However, the majority of centers recommend use of a temporary diversion.

PATIENT PREPARATION PRIOR TO SURGERY

- After a detailed discussion regarding the risks, alternatives, benefits, and expected outcomes from the IPAA, the patient should see a certified wound, ostomy, and continence nurse (WOCN) for preoperative education and appropriate site marking for a temporary diverting loop ileostomy. Many patients are provided with a mechanical bowel preparation with oral antibiotics. This is an optional step as there are mixed data as to the necessity of such preparation. An alternative approach would be to perform a tap water enema the morning of surgery to clear the distal colon and rectum. All patients are provided with antimicrobial soap (Hibiclens) to shower with the night prior to surgery and the morning of surgery.

PATIENT INDUCTION AND POSITIONING

- Prior to the induction of anesthesia, the patient is given 5000 units of heparin subcutaneously and sequential compression devices are placed on the lower extremities. The patient is positioned supine on the operating table lying on an upper body gel pad to minimize movement during operating room position changes. Once induction of anesthesia is complete, an orogastric tube is placed. An indwelling urinary catheter is placed using sterile technique.
- Once all necessary IV access is secured, the patient is repositioned in a modified lithotomy position (**FIGURE 3**). The heels are firmly planted on the stirrups to avoid pressure along the calves and the lateral peroneal nerves. The thighs are placed parallel to the ground to avoid conflict with the surgeon's arms and instruments during the procedure.
- Both arms are wrapped in gel pads and the patient's right arm is placed next to their side and secured in position by positioning of an acrylic toboggan. The left arm is placed on an arm board positioned straight outward (**FIGURE 3**). Alternatively, both arms may be placed at the patient's side, but this will impede access to the arms during the procedure in case the anesthesia team needs to intervene. A chest strap is applied to minimize the risk of the patient shifting on the operating table during frequent position changes during the procedure. A forced air warming device is placed on the chest and over the left arm is positioned outward.
- The abdominal wall skin is prepared with a chlorhexidine–alcohol mixture after the perineum has been scrubbed and painted with a Betadine–iodine skin preparation kit. The patient is then draped in a fashion that allows access to the entire abdomen and perineum (**FIGURE 4A**).
- Video monitors should be placed directly off of the patient's left and right shoulders. If a monitor is available on a boom, it can be positioned over the patient's head, which facilitates the dissection in the midportion of the patient's upper abdomen. The scrub nurse should have their instruments positioned over the patient's chest and head and they should stand on the patient's left side above the outward-positioned left arm (**FIGURE 4B**). The surgeon will stand between the patient's legs for the hand-assisted laparoscopic mobilization and resection of the abdominal colon. The first assistant/camera operator will initially stand on the patient's right side (**FIGURE 5**).
- Prior to incision, Surgical Care Improvement Project (SCIP)–compliant antibiotics are administered and documented. A procedural pause is performed, confirming the patient identity, procedure, position, antibiotic administration, allergies, and special equipment needs.

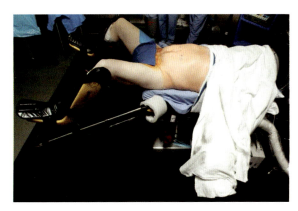

FIGURE 3 • Patient positioning. The patient is on a modified lithotomy position with the thighs parallel to the ground to avoid conflict with the surgeon's elbows and instruments. The left arm is placed laterally on an arm board for access by the anesthesia team during the operation. The patient is strapped to the Yellofin stirrups and taped to the table across the chest to avoid sliding during the procedure.

SECTION III RECTAL RESECTIONS

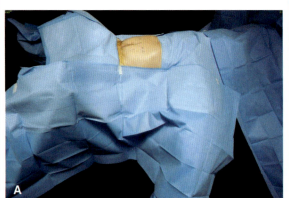
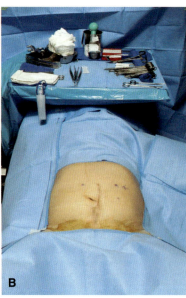

FIGURE 4 • **A,** Field setup. The patient is draped in a fashion that allows access to the entire abdomen and perineum. **B,** Field setup. The scrub nurse sets their or her instruments positioned over the patient's chest and head.

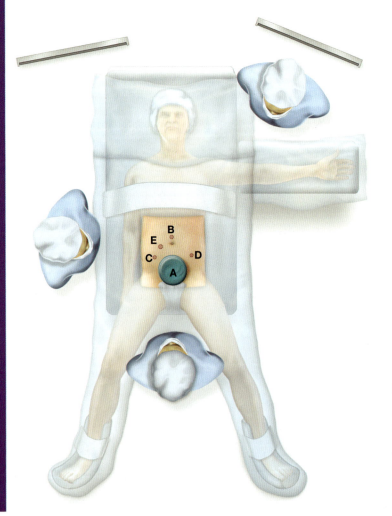

FIGURE 5 • Team and monitors setup. The surgeon stands between the patient's legs for the hand-assisted laparoscopic mobilization and resection of the abdominal colon. The first assistant/camera operator stands on the patient's right side. The scrub nurse stands on the patient's left side above the outward-positioned left arm. The monitors are positioned above the right and left shoulders. *A,* Gelport; *B,* 5 mm camera; *C* and *D,* 5 mm working; and *E,* the marking for the planned stoma location.

INCISION AND TROCAR PLACEMENT

- A midline incision is marked on the patient's abdomen from the pubis to the xiphoid process in case emergent entry into the abdomen is required. In men, our preferred incision for the hand port is a 7-cm lower midline incision starting 1.5 cm above the pubic bone. In women, we prefer a 7-cm Pfannenstiel incision centered on the midline 1.5 cm above the pubis. If a prior midline or Pfannenstiel incision exists, we will use that incision.[2,3]
- The hand-port incision is made and the abdomen is entered under direct vision. With the surgeon's hand in the abdomen through the primary incision, a small 5-mm incision is made in the upper aspect of the umbilicus and a nonbladed 5-mm trocar is guided into the abdomen with the surgeon's hand protecting the abdomen content from inadvertent injury. Next, the hand access device is placed in the lower abdominal incision and pneumoperitoneum is established.
- Under laparoscopic visualization, a 5-mm nonbladed trocar is placed in the left lower abdomen and another in the right lower abdomen. Usually, the best location is 2 to 2.5 cm medial and 1 cm inferior to the superior iliac crest (**FIGURE 6**).

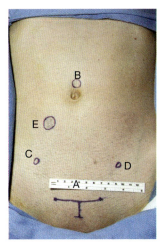

FIGURE 6 • Port placement. The hand port will be placed through a 7-cm Pfannenstiel incision *(A)*. Three 5-mm ports are placed for the camera (supraumbilical, *B*) and instruments (right and left lower abdomen, *C, D*). The diverting ileostomy site *(E)* is marked in the right lower quadrant.

MOBILIZATION OF THE LEFT COLON

- The patient is placed in steep Trendelenburg position with left side up. The surgeon stands between the legs and the camera operator is on the patient's right side. A 5-mm camera is placed through the supraumbilical trocar. The surgeon places their left arm through the hand-port device and uses the left lower quadrant trocar for their dissecting scissors (**FIGURE 7**). The surgeon uses their hand to push the small bowel into the right lower quadrant and to lift the omentum into the upper abdomen. The left colon is then grasped and pulled medially and anteriorly. The camera is used to look over the surgeon's hand into the left abdomen.
- The surgeon starts dissecting from the mid- to lower sigmoid and works upward toward the splenic flexure while maintaining medial retraction of the left colon. The dissecting scissors attached to monopolar cautery are used to incise the peritoneal lining about 1 cm lateral to the edge of the colon (**FIGURE 8**). A common mistake is to incise too far laterally from the colon in what appears to be a "natural" plane. The surgeon should move in a cephalad direction along the entire left colon in a continuous fashion upward toward the spleen while maintaining medial traction (**FIGURE 9**).

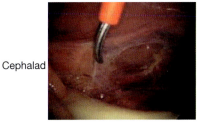

Cephalad — Caudad

FIGURE 8 • Mobilization of the left colon. The lateral peritoneal attachments are incised about 1 cm lateral to the edge of the colon while the surgeon's hand retracts the colon medially.

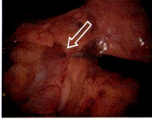

FIGURE 9 • Mobilization of the left colon. The lateral dissection is *continued* in a cephalad direction until reaching the splenic flexure (*arrow*).

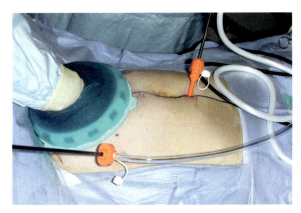

FIGURE 7 • Finalized setup. The surgeon stands between the patient's legs with their left hand in the abdomen and their right hand controls the dissecting scissors for the mobilization of the left colon. The assistant operates the camera from the right side of the table.

- The mesentery of the left colon is then dissected off the retroperitoneum (anterior to Gerota fascia) in a lateral to medial direction. Care is taken to identify the left ureter and gonadal vessels, which should be preserved intact in the retroperitoneum.

SPLENIC FLEXURE MOBILIZATION AND MESENTERY DIVISION

- Once the left colon mesentery is mobilized medially toward the lateral border of the aorta, the patient is placed in steep reverse Trendelenburg position. The surgeon retracts the upper left colon medially to see the back portion of the splenic flexure as it attaches to Gerota fascia. Using the dissecting scissors attached to monopolar cautery, the phrenocolic is divided as the surgeon retracts the flexure medially and downward toward the right lower quadrant (**FIGURE 10**).
- To further free up the splenic flexure of the colon, the gastrocolic ligament, exposed by retracting the omentum in a cephalad direction with the left hand (**FIGURE 11**), is transected at the midline, entering the lesser sac (**FIGURE 12**). The gastrocolic ligament is then transected from medial to lateral, toward the splenic flexure of the colon, until the previous dissection plane around the flexure is encountered (**FIGURE 12**). At this point, the splenocolic ligament is easily visualized and transected (**FIGURE 13**).
- Once the splenic flexure is fully mobilized, a 5-mm vessel-sealing device is placed through the left lower quadrant port,

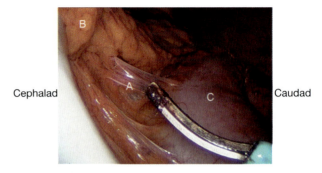

FIGURE 11 • Exposure of the gastrocolic ligament. The surgeon exposes the gastrocolic ligament (A) by retracting the omentum (B) in a cephalad direction with their left hand while the assistant retracts the transverse colon (C) in a caudad direction.

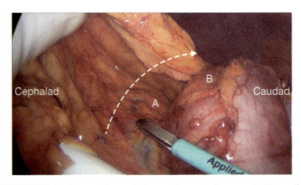

FIGURE 12 • Transection of the gastrocolic ligament allows for entrance into the lesser sac, exposing the tail of the pancreas (A). While holding the omentum in a cephalad direction, the gastrocolic ligament is transected in a medial to lateral direction (arrow) toward the splenic flexure of the colon (B), until the precious dissection plane is encountered and the splenic flexure of the colon is fully mobilized.

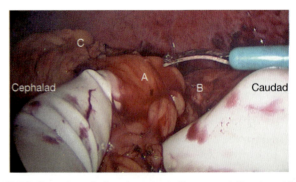

FIGURE 13 • Completing the splenic flexure mobilization. After the superior to inferior and the medial to lateral dissection planes meet around the splenic flexure of the colon, the splenocolic ligament (A) is easily exposed between the colon (B) and the spleen (C) and is transected.

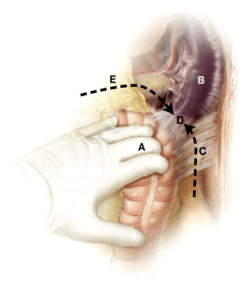

FIGURE 10 • Mobilization of the splenic flexure. The surgeon retracts the splenic flexure of the colon (A) downward and medially, exposing the attachments of the flexure to the spleen (B). The phrenocolic (C) and splenocolic (D) ligaments are transected in an inferior to superior and lateral to medial direction. The gastrocolic ligament (E) is transected in a medial to lateral direction, until both planes of dissection meet and the splenic flexure is fully mobilized.

replacing the scissors, and the transverse colon mesentery is divided. Once the flexure mesentery is divided, the left colon mesentery and what remains of the gastrocolic ligament are divided (**FIGURE 14**) while working toward the hepatic flexure. To ensure that the small bowel mesentery is not divided, the surgeon's hand is used to control the colon mesentery while pushing the small bowel mesentery away below the hand.

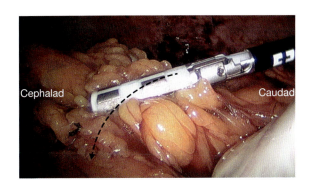

FIGURE 14 • After the splenic flexure has been mobilized, the transverse colon mesentery is divided, proceeding from the splenic toward the hepatic flexure (*arrow*), with an energy device.

HEPATIC FLEXURE AND RIGHT COLON MOBILIZATION

- Once the dissection of the transverse colon mesentery has proceeded past the midline of the abdomen, the camera assistant moves to the patient's left side. The patient is kept in reverse Trendelenburg but is placed with the right side up. The surgeon places their left hand through the hand access device and uses the dissecting scissors attached to monopolar cautery through the right lower quadrant port. The surgeon's left hand is used to retract the hepatic flexure downward and toward the left lower quadrant (**FIGURE 15**), exposing the hepatocolic ligament. This ligament is transected with scissors. Once incised, the surgeon's index finger is placed under the lateral peritoneal attachments of the right colon and the dissection is started downward along the lateral edge of the right colon (**FIGURE 16**). All the while, the surgeon is placing firm and constant traction on the colon toward the left lower quadrant. This action literally peels the right colon and its mesentery off of the retroperitoneum.
- The dissection is carefully continued medially toward the duodenum. The filmy attachments of the colon mesentery are divided off of the anterior wall of the duodenum, the head of the pancreas, and Gerota fascia (**FIGURE 17**).
- Once the right colon mesentery is completely mobilized, the 5-mm vessel-sealing device is placed through the right lower quadrant trocar and the hepatic flexure mesentery is divided, progressing from right to left. To facilitate this dissection, the surgeon's left hand grabs the transverse mesentery from where the previous mesenteric division was performed. The surgeon places their fingers behind the mesentery while the thumb is anterior to the mesentery. The fingertips are near the hepatic flexure mesentery and these are used to facilitate the movement of the vessel-sealing device as it traverses the mesentery from right to left, eventually completing the division of the transverse colon mesentery.
- Once the hepatic flexure and transverse colon mesentery are divided, the entire colon and distal small bowel can be exteriorized through the hand access port site with the wound protector in place (**FIGURE 18**). The right colon mesentery is divided under direct vision close to the colon wall, thus preventing any

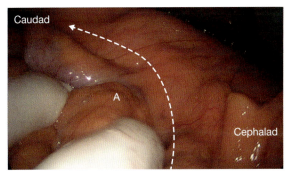

FIGURE 16 • While retracting the hepatic flexure of the colon (*A*) with the hand, the hepatocolic ligament and the lateral peritoneal attachments of the right colon are transected in the direction shown (*arrow*).

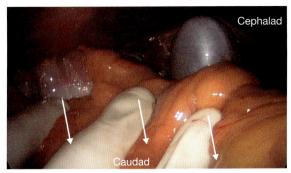

FIGURE 15 • The surgeon pulls the hepatic flexure of the colon downward and toward the left lower quadrant of the abdomen (*arrows*).

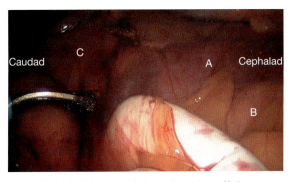

FIGURE 17 • Mobilization of the right colon off the retroperitoneum. The right mesocolon is dissected off the duodenum (*A*), head of the pancreas (*B*), and Gerota fascia (*C*).

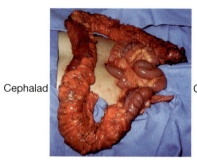

FIGURE 18 • Extracorporeal delivery of the colon and terminal ileum.

injury to the ileocolic vessel and the right-sided marginal arterial arcade. This is critical to ensure good antegrade blood supply to the J-pouch to be constructed later.

- The terminal ileum is divided using a linear stapling device about 1 to 2 cm proximal to the ileal–cecal valve. The distal sigmoid colon is divided with a stapling device. The abdominal colon is sent to pathology to confirm the diagnosis of ulcerative colitis.
- To facilitate pouch placement in the pelvis, the small bowel mesentery needs to be mobilized off of the retroperitoneum. Once the abdominal colon is removed, the small bowel is returned to the abdomen and the pneumoperitoneum is reestablished. The surgeon with their left hand in the abdomen places their hand under the small bowel mesentery and pushes it up and to the left upper quadrant. Using the dissecting scissor from the right lower quadrant trocar, the mesentery is dissected off of the retroperitoneum and duodenum. If needed, this dissection can be carried out up over the pancreas to the origin of the superior mesenteric vessels.

OPEN PROCTECTOMY THROUGH THE HAND ACCESS DEVICE

- The patient is leveled from a right to left perspective and then placed in steep Trendelenburg position. The surgeons then moves to the patient's right side, the first assistant is on the left side, and the second assistant goes between the patient's legs. The small bowel is packed off into the upper abdomen. The hand access device is maintained in the incision as a wound protector. The distal sigmoid colon is exteriorized through the hand access device and used as a "handle" to initiate the dissection into the pelvis. The superior rectal vessels are divided and the presacral space is entered posteriorly.
- The dissection is carried out into the posterior deep pelvis facilitated by the use of two long, narrow, specially designed St. Mark retractors, one lighted and the other not lighted (**FIGURE 19**). Both retractors are used through the hand access device so that no hands are placed through the device that would obstruct the view into the pelvis.
- The posterior pelvic dissection is carried first, along the presacral space between the presacral fascia, posteriorly, and the investing fascia of the mesorectum, anteriorly (**FIGURE 20**). The lateral rectal ligaments are transected with an energy device.
- The pelvic dissection is then carried anteriorly in a circumferential fashion around the rectum. The Douglas pouch is incised open with cautery. The plane of dissection anteriorly is carried in between Denonvilliers fascia (along the anterior wall of the rectum), posteriorly, and the prostate/seminal vesicles (in males, **FIGURE 21**) or the vagina (in females), anteriorly. The pelvic floor (with the levator muscles) is identified (**FIGURE 21**).
- Once the pelvic floor is reached, a transverse stapling device is placed through the hand access device and around the low rectum at the level of the pelvic floor (**FIGURE 22**). Before the stapler is fired, a digital rectal examination is performed to ensure that the device will be dividing the rectum at the top of the anal canal. Once the device is fired, the rectum is removed and a check of hemostasis in the pelvis is made.

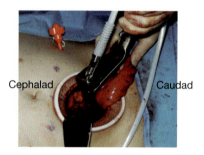

FIGURE 19 • Rectal dissection through the hand access device using two narrow, double bent St. Mark's retractor (one lighted).

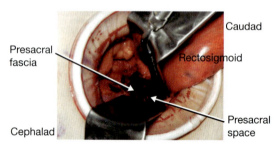

FIGURE 20 • The posterior pelvic dissection is carried along the presacral space between the presacral fascia, posteriorly, and the investing fascia of the mesorectum, anteriorly.

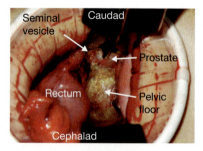

FIGURE 21 • The pelvic dissection is then carried anteriorly in a circumferential fashion around the rectum. The pelvic floor (with the levator muscles) is identified. The seminal vesicles and the prostate can be seen anteriorly.

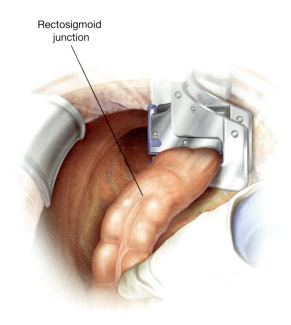

FIGURE 22 • Once the pelvic floor is reached, a transverse stapling device is placed through the hand access device and around the low rectum at the level of the pelvic floor.

J-POUCH CONSTRUCTION AND POUCH-ANAL ANASTOMOSIS

- Once the rectum is removed, the small bowel is exteriorized through the hand access device. The last 25 to 30 cm of the terminal ileum is folded into a "J" shape and the apex of the fold is opened anteriorly to allow placement of a linear stapler (**FIGURE 23**). The common wall between the two limbs of the J is divided with the linear stapler. To make an adequate-sized pouch (approximately 15 cm in length), many sequential firings of the linear stapler are usually required. Before the stapler is fired, care must be taken to ensure that the small bowel mesentery of the pouch is not trapped by the stapler in between the limbs of the pouch.

- Through the same opening that the linear stapler was placed, a monofilament suture is placed as a purse string and the anvil of a circular stapling device is secured to the apex of the J-pouch (**FIGURE 24**). The end of the J staple line and the anterior pouch staple lines are oversewn with 3-0 suture to reinforce the staple lines.
- An end-to-end stapled anastomosis is performed between the pouch and the anal canal (**FIGURE 25**). The mesentery of the pouch should be placed posteriorly against the sacrum. In a woman, prior to the firing of the circular stapler, great care must be taken to ensure that the vagina is not trapped into the circular stapling device. A diagnostic rigid proctoscopy is performed through the anus after the pelvis has been filled with saline to check for any evidence of an air leak from the pouch (**FIGURE 26**).
- Two 19-Fr closed bulb suction drains are placed behind the pouch and brought out at the lower abdominal trocar sites. These are secured to the skin with monofilament suture.

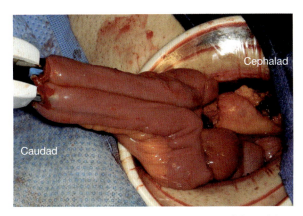

FIGURE 23 • Creation of the J-pouch. The small bowel is exteriorized through the hand access device. The last 25 to 30 cm of the terminal ileum is folded into a J shape and the apex of the fold is opened anteriorly to allow placement of a linear stapler. The common wall between the two limbs of the J is divided with the linear stapler.

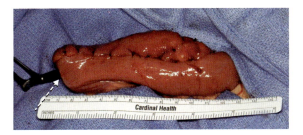

FIGURE 24 • Creation of the J-pouch. Through the same opening that the linear stapler was placed, a monofilament suture is placed as a purse string and the anvil of a circular stapling device is secured to the apex of the J-pouch (*arrow*). The pouch is approximately 15 cm long.

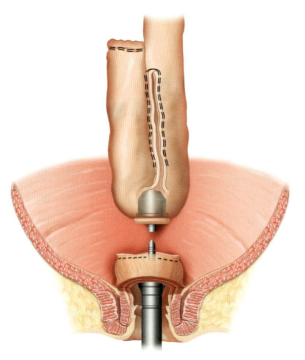

FIGURE 25 • An end-to-end stapled anastomosis is performed between the pouch and the anal canal.

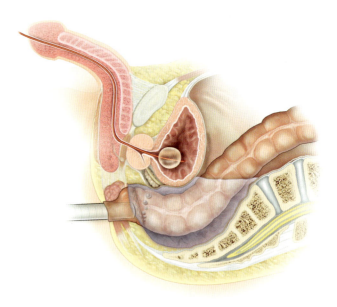

FIGURE 26 • A diagnostic rigid proctoscopy is performed through the anus after the pelvis has been filled with saline to check for any evidence of an air leak from the pouch.

TEMPORARY DIVERTING LOOP ILEOSTOMY CONSTRUCTION

- Prior to surgery, the patient should have been counseled by a WOCN and site marked for a temporary ileostomy. At the marked site in the right lower quadrant, a diverting loop ileostomy is constructed. Usually, the loop should be 20 to 30 cm proximal to the J-pouch. To facilitate ileostomy reversal in the future, the bowel can be wrapped in an adhesion barrier material, which should also be placed in the abdomen under the site of the stoma to minimize adhesions.
- The hand access device/wound protector is removed and the incision is closed in the standard fashion. The 5-mm camera trocar site is closed at the skin level with a monofilament suture.

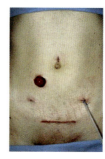

FIGURE 27 • The end result after a HALS-IPAA.

- The loop ileostomy is matured, with the proximal limb matured in a Brooke's fashion. The distal limb is matured as a mucous fistula (**FIGURE 27**).

PEARLS AND PITFALLS

Indication	■ In cases of acute disease or indeterminate colitis, proceeding to a subtotal colectomy as the initial operation is preferred to allow thorough pathologic review of the specimen and withdrawal of the medications to unmask potential Crohn disease.
Conduct of the abdominal portion	■ It is best to start with the left colon and the splenic mobilization first as this will determine if you can use a hand-assisted laparoscopic surgery (HALS) approach.
Creation of the J-pouch	■ Preservation of the right-sided marginal arterial arcade is critical to ensure good blood supply to the pouch. ■ Separation of the pouch mesentery from the retroperitoneum allows for adequate pouch length to reach the pelvic floor. ■ Place the pouch mesentery along the presacral space posteriorly.
Conduct of the pelvic portion	■ Avoid placing the surgeon's hands into the pelvis as this will completely obstruct the view through the hand access device.

POSTOPERATIVE CARE

- We use an enhanced recovery pathway approach to the postoperative care in our patients. They are started on a regular ileostomy diet upon arrival to the ward.
- IV fluids are kept to a minimum (<40 mL per hour) the night of surgery. All IV fluids are discontinued the morning after surgery.
- The urinary catheter is removed at 8 AM the morning after surgery.
- The two drains are removed the morning of the second day after surgery.

OUTCOMES

- The functional outcomes of IPAA over the last few decades in numerous institutional experiences have been quite comparable. Most patients report six to eight bowel movements in a 24-hour period, with one of those occurring at night.
- Depending on the patient's age and gender, about 20% to 30% will experience minor leakage of stool, particularly at night.
- The majority of patients will experience one or more episodes of pouchitis, with approximately 20% having chronic pouchitis, which requires treatment.
- IPAA patient's quality of life is usually significantly improved relative to their presurgery health state.
- Finally, IPAA is a durable operation with over 90% of patients having a well-functioning pouch at 20 years after surgery.

COMPLICATIONS

- The most concerning complication is a pouch leak or pelvic sepsis. Unexplained tachycardia, lower abdominal pain, and low back/pelvic pain are worrisome signs for a pouch leak. Early operative intervention with pelvic irrigation/washout and drain placement is the procedure of choice. Later presentation with fever, pelvic pain, and urinary symptoms warrant abdominal imaging with a CT scan and percutaneous drain placement.[4]
- Prior to ileostomy reversal, usually 2 to 3 months after the pouch surgery, a contrast enema is obtained to evaluate for a possible anastomotic leak or narrowing. If a small anastomotic sinus is observed, closure should be delayed for another 2 to 3 months and a repeat contrast study obtained. Commonly, the sinus will close. However, if it persists, an examination under anesthesia is required in an attempt to open the sinus or to curette the tract to promote healing.

REFERENCES

1. Cima RR, Pemberton JH. Surgical indications and procedures in ulcerative colitis. *Curr Treat Options Gastroenterol*. 2004;7:181-190.
2. Nakajima K, Nezu R, Ito T, et al. Hand-assisted laparoscopic restorative proctocolectomy for ulcerative colitis: the optimization of instrumentation toward standardization. *Surg Today*. 2010;40:840-844.
3. Bordeianou L, Hodin R. Total proctocolectomy with ileoanal J-pouch reconstruction utilizing the hand-assisted laparoscopic approach. *J Gastrointest Surg*. 2009;13:2314-2320.
4. Cima RR, Pendlimari R, Holubar SD, et al. Utility and short-term outcomes of hand-assisted laparoscopic colorectal surgery: a single-institution experience in 1103 patients. *Dis Colon Rectum*. 2011;54:1076-1081.

Chapter 41: Pelvic Exenteration

Cherry E. Koh and Michael J. Solomon

DEFINITION

- Pelvic exenteration, also known as extended radical resection, is a form of radical surgery first described for the treatment of locally advanced cervical cancer, which was adopted for locally advanced colorectal cancer shortly thereafter. Currently, locally advanced primary rectal cancers (LARCs) and locally recurrent rectal cancers (LRRCs) are among the more common indications for pelvic exenteration.
- The fundamental surgical principle of pelvic exenteration is complete en bloc removal of all viscera or structures contiguously involved by tumor with a clear resection margin (R0 resection). Therefore, depending on the location of the tumor, different types of exenteration will be required, which may include en bloc cystoprostatectomy, vaginectomy, radical hysterectomy, or even sacrectomy. The same surgical principles may be applied to other locally advanced pelvic cancers, including uterine, bladder, and prostate cancers and sarcomas.
- Different classifications have evolved to describe the different types of recurrence and exenteration, although of note, there is no universally accepted terminology.
- Although lengthy anatomical discussion is beyond the scope of this chapter, a brief discussion is necessary to facilitate understanding of the key concepts and principles of surgery.

- Anatomically, the pelvis can be divided into four compartments: the anterior, central, posterior, and lateral compartments (**FIGURE 1**). Each compartment overlaps at the margins, but the axis of each compartment is centered on a different structure. The urethra, the tip of the coccyx, the third sacral vertebra, and the ischial spine form the axis of the anterior, central, posterior, and lateral compartments, respectively.
- For clarity, exenteration is best classified as complete exenteration or partial exenteration. Complete exenteration is defined as complete removal of all compartments of the pelvis with or without en bloc bony resection, whereas a partial exenteration is defined as the removal of at least three compartments of the pelvis, with or without en bloc bony resection. Within partial exenteration, there are many subtypes of exenterations that often involve surgery on parts of different compartments (**FIGURE 2A** and **B**).
- As a general principle, the resection margin for a compartment will involve excision of the soft tissue at its attachment to the bone or en bloc excision of the involved bone (eg, en bloc sacrectomy, excision of ischial spine or of pubic ramus). Attempting to obtain a soft tissue margin within a compartment will invariably result in a very high rate of highly involved margins. **FIGURE 2A** and **B** illustrate the potential dissection planes depending on the location of the tumor.
- In addition to consideration of the compartments of the pelvis, the "height" of the tumor is also important to determine resectability (if there is high sacral involvement), the extent of perineal resection and reconstruction required, as well as whether or not intestinal continuity can be restored.

PATIENT HISTORY AND PHYSICAL FINDINGS

- Patients with LARC are usually symptomatic. Patients with LRRC may be symptomatic or asymptomatic (see below), although most patients are symptomatic.
- Symptoms experienced by the patient reflect the location of the cancer. Common symptoms include pain, rectal bleeding, altered bowel habits, and tenesmus. Pain may be the result of direct nerve (sacral nerve roots and sciatic nerve), muscle (levator, piriformis, and obturator internus), or bony (sacral) infiltration or the result of referred pain, usually to the buttock or hamstring.
- As the tumor gets larger, mass effect may ensue with ureteric or bowel obstruction. Advanced cancers of the pelvis may also present with malignant fistulae between the small or large bowel and an adjacent viscera such as the vagina or bladder. Occasionally, patients may present with an offensive fungating tumor or lymphedema of the lower limb because of venous compression.
- Asymptomatic local recurrences may be detected on routine follow-up with elevated carcinoembryonic antigen (CEA), surveillance computed tomography (CT), or colonoscopy. Asymptomatic anastomotic recurrence following low rectal

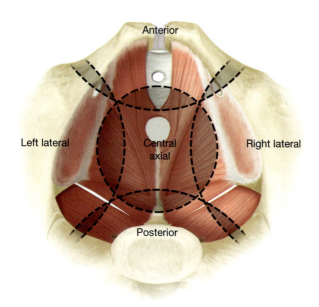

FIGURE 1 • The compartments of the pelvis are shown in this diagram. The pelvis can be divided into the anterior, central, posterior, and lateral compartments, which are centered on the urethra, the tip of the coccyx, the third sacral vertebra, and the ischial spines, respectively. A complete pelvic exenteration is one where all viscera are removed and involves surgery in all five compartments of the pelvis with or without bony resection, whereas a partial exenteration is one which involves removal of at least three compartments of the pelvis with or without bony resection.

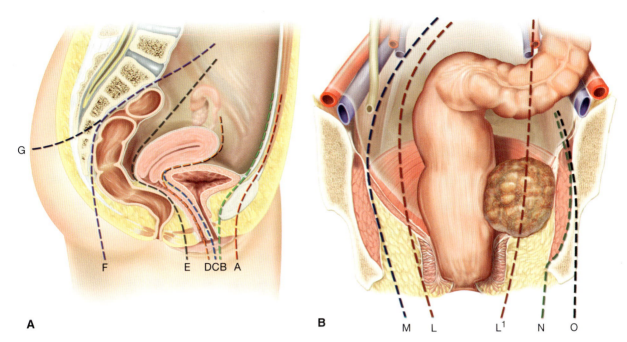

FIGURE 2 • **A,** This is the sagittal section of a female pelvis. *Planes A and B* are the dissection planes for complete or partial exenterations involving the anterior compartment with and without en bloc pubic excision, respectively. *Planes C and D* are dissection planes for partial exenteration involving the central compartment with total or subtotal vaginectomy and posterior vaginectomy, respectively. Note that *planes C and D* do not exist in men. *Planes E and F* are the anterior and posterior total mesorectal excision planes, respectively, whereas *plane G* is the plane for en bloc sacrectomy. **B,** Coronal section of the pelvis. There are four possible lateral dissection planes. *Plane L* represents the total mesorectal excision plane and is the lateral plane for a partial exenteration not involving the lateral compartment. *Plane M* represents the extravascular plane, which is a plane lateral to the iliac vasculature but medial to obturator internus. *Plane N* involves excision of the entire lateral compartment including obturator internus, whereas *plane O* includes en bloc bony resection such as the ischial spine or ischial tuberosity. The right-hand side of **FIGURE 2B** shows a tumor that involves the lateral compartment. Dissection in the lateral mesorectal plane depicted by *plane L1* will invariably result in an involved surgical margin. In order to achieve R0 resection margins, dissection should follow *plane N*.

- resection may be readily palpable with digital rectal examination or be visible on rigid sigmoidoscopy.
- As pain frequently accompanies LARC or LRRC, clinical assessment may require an examination under anesthesia, which will also permit biopsies and other investigations to be undertaken concurrently such as a completion colonoscopy or cystoscopy where ureteric stents may also be inserted at the same time if necessary.
- In patients with a previous abdominoperineal excision, clinical findings are often limited.
- A general assessment for obvious systemic metastasis such as hepatomegaly or inguinal lymphadenopathy should also be performed to rule out the presence of metastatic disease.

IMAGING AND OTHER DIAGNOSTIC STUDIES

- CT scan of the chest, abdomen, and pelvis is a useful first step to rule out systemic metastasis. In general, CT scans do not provide adequate soft tissue delineation in the pelvis to permit accurate staging of LARC for decision making on neoadjuvant therapy. In patients with potential LRRC, CT scans are limited in their ability to distinguish between postsurgical fibrosis and tumor recurrence.
- Positron emission tomography (PET) scans complement CT scans in detecting the presence of metastatic disease (**FIGURE 3A** and **B**). By detecting metabolically active tissue, it

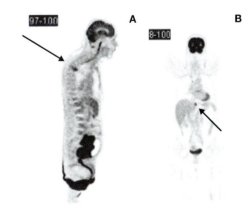

FIGURE 3 • **A,** PET scan of a patient with locally advanced rectosigmoid cancer referred for pelvic exenteration. PET scan was consistent with metastatic disease *(arrow)*. **B,** PET scan of a patient with an anastomotic recurrence after a previous sigmoidectomy who presented with an asymptomatic recurrence manifesting with an elevated CEA. The patient was being considered for pelvic exenteration. PET scan showed a small liver metastasis otherwise undetected on CT scan *(arrow)*.

has the advantage of being able to distinguish between postoperative fibrosis and metabolically active local recurrence. PET in LARC or LRRC has been shown to alter clinical decision making by 20% to 40% by detecting occult metastatic disease.

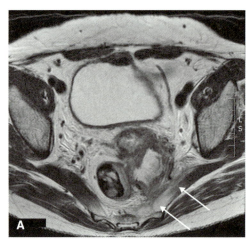 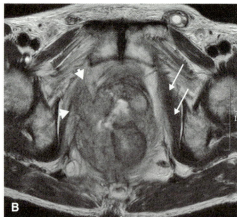

FIGURE 4 • **A,** MRI of the pelvis showing locally advanced cervical cancer. The cancer is seen to the left of the rectum and is invading the left piriformis muscle *(arrows)*. This patient has pain in the left S2-S3 nerve root territory consistent with sacral plexus infiltration. **B,** MRI of the pelvis of a patient with a large LRRC abutting the left obturator internus muscles *(arrows)* and directly infiltrating the right obturator internus muscle *(arrowheads)*.

- Magnetic resonance imaging (MRI) is currently the gold standard to determine the local extent of tumor, to assess resectability, and to determine the potential need of neoadjuvant (for LARC) therapy (**FIGURE 4A** and **B**). The accuracy of MRI in confirming anterior compartment, pelvic sidewall, and sacral involvement ranges between 60% and 100%. The major limitation of MRI with LRRC resides in its inability to accurately diagnose pelvic sidewall involvement.
- Tissue diagnosis, although easily obtained in LARC, is a contentious issue in patients with LRRC when the lesion may be inaccessible luminally and a biopsy would necessitate a percutaneous route that could lead to tract seeding. However, without tissue diagnosis, patients in whom the final pathology report shows no recurrence of cancer may have been subjected to an unnecessary major operation with significant morbidity. It is our practice to accept a diagnosis of LRRC when there is a positive PET scan provided that there is corroborative history, MRI findings, and elevated CEA level.
- CEA level is helpful for ongoing disease surveillance in patients with LARC. The sensitivity of CEA for detecting recurrent disease is low but the specificity is 85%.
- A complete colonoscopy is performed to obtain tissue diagnosis and to rule out synchronous colon cancer prior to embarking on a major resection.
- CT or magnetic resonance angiography may be useful to ensure the patency of inferior epigastric arteries if a rectus abdominis myocutaneous flap is being considered for perineal reconstruction in a patient who previously had or currently has stoma(s). They may also help to determine if a vascular surgeon may be needed if there is major arterial involvement of the common iliac or external iliac vessels.
- Cystoscopy can help diagnose bladder involvement and may allow ureteric stenting to relieve ureteric obstruction and prevent impending renal failure.

SURGICAL MANAGEMENT

Preoperative Planning

- All patients should be discussed preoperatively at a multidisciplinary team meeting to determine resectability and operative strategy.
- Patients who are radiotherapy naive should be considered for preoperative long-course chemoradiation prior to pelvic exenteration.
- A detailed informed consent is obtained. Because studies have shown that patients often underestimate the magnitude of the procedure, we encourage family members to participate in the discussions and we schedule at least two separate consultations.
- A preoperative review by the cancer coordinator and psycho-oncologist is obtained. Furthermore, as most patients will require the creation of at least one, if not two, stoma, it is essential that the patient receive stomal education prior to the procedure.
- Bowel preparation is usually necessary for patients without an existing colostomy.

Positioning

- Depending on the location and the extent of the cancer, the patient may require surgery from the abdominal and the perineal compartments. In patients in whom a high sacrectomy is required, repositioning in a prone position after completion of the abdominal and perineal components of the operation is also necessary.
- Patients are placed in a modified Lloyd-Davies position directly on a gel mat with both arms tucked by their sides and protecting all pressure areas (**FIGURE 5**). In patients who require major perineal resections, the buttocks should be elevated with a rolled towel and overhang the end of the operating bed by up to 5 cm to permit access into the natal cleft if needed.
- To avoid muscle compartment syndrome, the legs should not be elevated more than 30° during the abdominal phase and only elevated for the perineal phase.

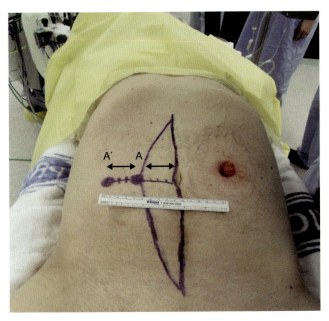

FIGURE 5 • The patient is positioned in modified Lloyd-Davies position with both arms tucked by their sides. The previous midline scar is marked. In this patient, a high sacrectomy and rectus abdominis myocutaneous is planned. The rectus abdominis myocutaneous flap is to be harvested from the patient's right where there has not been a previous stoma, and this has also been marked out with the ileal conduit site being lateralized to A′ by the same distance as that between the midline and the first stoma site A.

- Patients will require an arterial line, a central line, and a large-bore intravenous cannula. These lines need to be well secured prior to be being tucked away by the patient's sides.
- Patients should also receive prophylactic antibiotics, subcutaneous heparin, mechanical venous thromboprophylaxis in the form of graduated compression stockings and calf compressors.
- An indwelling Foley catheter is inserted. The anterior thigh is prepped and draped if a vascular graft using the great or common saphenous veins needs to be harvested. The vagina should also be included in the preparation.
- A purse-string suture at the anal verge is used to prevent fecal spillage during the procedure.
- Prior midline incisions or scars should be marked so that the same incision can be used. In patients in whom a rectus abdominis myocutaneous flap is planned, this should also be premarked prior to prepping and draping (**FIGURE 5**). The colostomy is prepped and covered with a swab, which is then held in place by an impervious adhesive plastic dressing.
- Insertion of bilateral ureteric stents is not routinely done in all cases.

ABDOMINAL PHASE

- We start with a meticulous adhesiolysis to mobilize all small bowel loops from the pelvis. Avoiding enterotomies in pelvic small bowel loops that may have been damaged by previous radiotherapy is important to prevent a postoperative enterocutaneous fistula.
- The abdominal cavity is inspected for peritoneal carcinomatosis or unresectable metastatic liver disease not identified during preoperative staging. Presence of either usually precludes curative resection and is likely to alter the surgical plan.
- Pelvic small bowel loops invaded by cancer should be resected en bloc using linear staplers. The remaining small bowel loops are packed into the upper abdomen using moist sponges held in a fixed table retractor such as the Omni-Tract.
- If the colon is still intact, it should be mobilized along its anatomic planes. Reflection of the sigmoid and descending colon on its mesentery medially will expose the left ureter. Identification of the ureter is important to avoid inadvertent ureteral injury.
- For a LARC, a high ligation of the inferior mesenteric artery is performed. The colon is divided at a point of convenience that remains well vascularized. The proximal divided colon can then be packed into the upper abdomen, isolating the pelvis from the abdominal contents.
- The appendix is prophylactically removed in patients who require a conduit as dense adhesions and mesh closure of the abdomen would make a future appendectomy difficult.

Lateral Compartment Dissection

- There are four possible planes of dissection in the lateral compartment (**FIGURE 2B**). Plane L is the conventional total mesorectal excision plane that is familiar to all colorectal surgeons. This plane is used for partial exenterations not involving the lateral compartment or in small anastomotic recurrence that only requires a reoperative anterior resection.
- For dissections in plane M, N, or O, the procedure begins with identification and mobilization of the ureters with a cuff of connective tissue to preserve their blood supply (**FIGURE 6**). Both ureters are mobilized as distal as possible into the pelvis. If en bloc cystectomy is planned, the ureters are divided without compromising resection margins and to provide adequate ureteric length for urinary reconstruction with an ileal or colonic conduit. Ureters should be anastomosed to the conduit out of the field of prior radiotherapy when possible. Even if en bloc cystectomy is not required, mobilizing the ureters along their entire length allows them to be mobilized off the pelvic sidewall such that the next layer of structures under the ureter (the common, external, and internal iliac arteries) can be accessed (**FIGURE 7**).

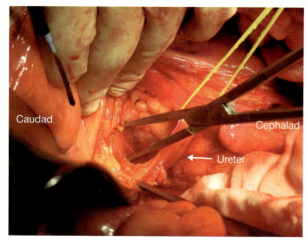

FIGURE 6 • Mobilization of the right ureter with a cuff of connective tissue around the ureter so as to preserve its blood supply. We use yellow vessel loops for ureters (blue for veins and red for arteries). Ureterolysis is performed with the operator dissecting using right-angle forceps and the assistant dividing tissue between the forceps using diathermy.

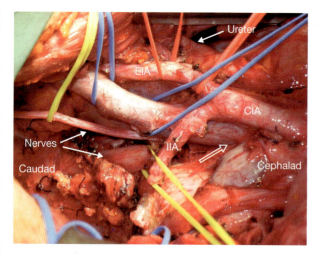

FIGURE 7 • Right pelvic sidewall. The ureter has been fully mobilized and divided and is placed in the right iliac fossa away from the pelvic sidewall while further dissection of the right pelvic side wall continues *(top arrow)*. Pelvic lymphadenectomy has been performed from the bifurcation of the aorta and the common iliac artery (CIA). This exposes the common iliac vessels and the confluence between the external and internal iliac vessels *(block arrow)*. The right external iliac artery (EIA) is held in red vessel loops, and the right internal iliac artery (IIA) has been ligated and divided. The external iliac and common iliac veins are held in blue vessel loops with the internal iliac vein ligated and divided. The two yellow vessel loops demonstrate two nerves. The smaller nerve is the obturator nerve, and the larger nerve is the lumbosacral trunk *(left sided arrows)*. Note the "layered" arrangement of the pelvic sidewall where the iliac arterial system lies superficial to the iliac venous system, which in turn lies superficial to the lumbosacral trunk. Note that, after ligation and division of the internal iliac artery or vein, the external iliac artery and vein can then be "floated off" the pelvic sidewall.

- Other than an early anastomotic recurrence, complete pelvic lymphadenectomy, starting at the level of the aortic bifurcation, is routinely performed for most other LRRCs. **FIGURE 7** also demonstrates the appearances of the iliac vasculature after complete pelvic lymphadenectomy.
- Dissecting in *plane M* will require ligation and excision of the internal iliac vasculature so as to get into and to remain in the extravascular plane. Even if formal excision of the internal iliac vasculature is not required, in situ ligation of the internal iliac artery and vein can be helpful to provide vascular control to limit blood loss as the dissection continues, especially if sacrectomy is planned. In LRRC, previous total mesorectal excision and radiotherapy usually cause tissue fibrosis and obliterate tissue planes making dissection difficult. Even if extravascular dissection is not necessary, the plane is typically virginal and may be comparatively easier to dissect.
- To get into plane M, after ureterolysis is performed, the internal iliac artery is dissected. When an adequate segment of internal iliac artery has been mobilized, it can be suture ligated and divided.
- Continued mobilization of the common iliac and external iliac arteries, which do not have any branches within the pelvis, will allow the common and external iliac arteries to be "floated" out of the operative field using two vessel loops held apart to prevent acute kinking of the artery. This exposes the next layer of structures—the common, external, and internal iliac veins. The combination of ligation of the internal iliac venous system and lymphadenectomy will result in progressive exposure of the sacral nerve roots on the piriformis muscle (**FIGURE 8**).
- Next, the internal iliac vein can then be ligated and excised en bloc together with the specimen, allowing the operator to get progressively more lateral within the lateral

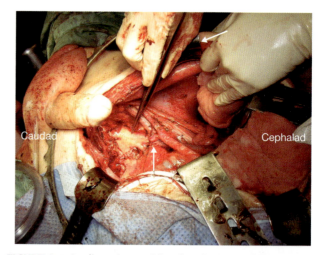

FIGURE 8 • By dissecting and ligating the internal iliac vasculature and performing a lymphadenectomy, the lumbosacral trunks and the sacral plexus (S1, S2, and S3 nerve roots) are displayed. The internal iliac artery and internal iliac vein stumps are seen *(arrows)*. The DeBakey forceps points to the S1 and S2 sacral plexus nerve roots. (S3 has been divided.)

compartment. Variable venous anatomy and tributaries coupled with thin-walled veins make dissection of the venous system particularly challenging. Once the internal iliac vein is ligated, the external iliac vein and distal common iliac vein can be similarly mobilized (as with the common and external iliac arteries) to allow these veins to be floated out of the pelvis providing access to the deeper structures—the lumbosacral trunk (**FIGURE 7**). The lumbosacral trunk is derived from L4 and L5 nerve roots and joins the sacral plexus on the piriformis muscle to form the sciatic nerve, which exits the pelvis by coursing posterior to the ischial spine via the greater sciatic notch.

- Identification of the lumbosacral trunk is an important step as this ensures the nerve is preserved for lower limb function and serves as an anatomic gatekeeper that helps guide the operator to the obturator internus muscle and ischial spine.
- Continued lateral dissection staying within the extravascular plane (*plane M*) will stay medial to the obturator internus muscle within the lateral compartment. While dissecting in *plane M*, numerous small branches and tributaries of the internal iliac vessels will be encountered that will need to be individually ligated to ensure hemostasis is secure. Continued dissection within *plane M* will lead to the origin of the levator ani, which can then be divided to enter the perineal compartment (**FIGURE 2B**).
- For complete excision of the lateral compartment (*plane N*), the lumbosacral trunk is traced distally to the obturator internus muscle and ischial spine. The entire obturator internus muscle can be excised by detaching it at its origin from the medial aspect of the pelvis (pubic bone) using diathermy. The ischial spine may also be excised en bloc to gain wider exposure. To do this, a large curved right-angle forceps is passed from the posterior to anterior around ischial spine (**FIGURE 9A**). The free end of a Gigli saw is pulled through. Using a malleable retractor to protect the sciatic nerve, which is immediately deep to the ischial spine, the Gigli saw may be used to saw off the spine at its origin from the remainder

of ischium (**FIGURE 9B**). The combination of dividing the ischial spine and the obturator internus exposes the entire pregluteal, pelvic course of the sciatic nerve (**FIGURE 8**) and releases the sacrospinous ligament exposing the sacrotuberous ligament.

- For wider excision of the medial wall of the ischium or of the ischial tuberosity (**FIGURE 2B**, *plane O*), the origin of the obturator internus is mobilized as described earlier. The perineal surgeon commences perineal dissection to gain wide exposure of the perineal aspect of inferior pubic ramus, leading to ischial tuberosity. Soft tissue attachments (origin of adductor magnus and semimembranosus muscles) are mobilized from the inferolateral aspect of ischial tuberosity, which then allows the ischial tuberosity to be excised using either an electric or Gigli saw while protecting the sciatic nerve using a malleable retractor. In some cases, the ischium can be removed through an abdominolithotomy approach.

Anterior Compartment Dissection

- The anterior plane of dissection for complete exenteration or partial exenteration involving the anterior compartment is depicted by *planes A* and *B* in **FIGURE 2A**.
- To dissect *plane B*, the peritoneum overlying the bladder is incised to enter the retropubic space of Retzius (**FIGURE 10A**). This incision continues laterally to open the endopelvic fascia. This is largely a bloodless plane, although anterolaterally, the superior vesical pedicle, vas deferens in a male patient, and the inferior vesicle pedicle will be encountered, which will require suture ligation. Laterally, the obturator neurovascular bundle will be seen and obturator lymphadenectomy is also performed with preservation of the obturator nerve.
- Anteriorly, the dorsal venous complex is the next to be encountered, which will require suture ligation (**FIGURE 10B**). Division of the dorsal venous complex will allow the bladder to be reflected more posteriorly.
- In the male patient, the prostate will be encountered next (**FIGURE 10C**). Further mobilization of the prostate from

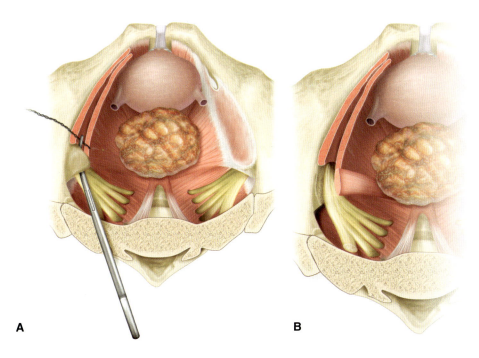

FIGURE 9 • **A,** Curved large right-angle forceps passed around ischial spine in preparation to its excision. The end of a Gigli saw is grasped and pulled through. The sciatic nerve under the saw is protected by a malleable retractor while the ischial spine is being divided. **B,** View of the pelvic sidewall after ischial spine has been excised. This exposes the entire intrapelvic course of the sciatic nerve.

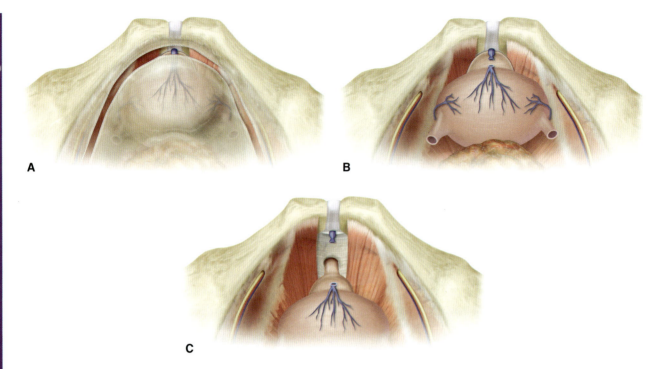

FIGURE 10 • **A,** Anterior dissection plane for complete exenteration or partial exenteration involving the anterior compartment. This step involves incising the peritoneum over the bladder anteriorly. This enters the space of Retzius and is largely bloodless. However, the superior and inferior vesical pedicles and vas deferens (in men) will need to be ligated and divided. Laterally, the endopelvic fascia is also released. **B,** The dorsal venous complex has been ligated, which allows the bladder to be mobilized further. In males, this exposes the prostate. **C,** Continued mobilization of the anterior plane exposes the urethra as it exits the prostate. The presence of urethra can be confirmed by palpating the indwelling urinary catheter.

the pelvic floor will lead to the urethra as it exits the prostate and traverses the urogenital diaphragm to become the penile urethra (**FIGURE 10C**). Presence of the urethra can be confirmed by palpation of the indwelling urinary catheter.

- The urethra is first partially incised to allow the catheter to be completely divided and removed before completely transecting the urethra and suture ligating the distal end of urethra. This completes the abdominal dissection in *plane B*.
- If restoring intestinal continuity is not possible, the perineal surgeon then begins dissection from the perineum to join the abdominal dissection similar to an abdominoperineal excision. In LRRC, if the tumor invades the prostate or membranous urethra (eg, after previous abdominoperineal excision), then the urethra can be transected more distally from the perineal approach often with a cuff of pubic bone (see the following text).
- Dissection in *plane A* involves the first step in anterior plane mobilization, which is incision of the peritoneum overlying the bladder to enter the retropubic space of Retzius immediately deep to pubic symphysis and superior pubic rami. This incision is extended laterally to incise the endopelvic fascia. Mobilization of the bladder and ligation of the superior and inferior vesical vessels and the vas deferens (in the male patient) as described earlier are also carried out, but ligation of the dorsal venous complex is not performed.
- In order to perform en bloc pubic excision, the pubic symphysis and pubic ramus will need to be defined and widely exposed both from the abdominal as well as perineal compartments. Thus, once the abdominal surgeon enters the

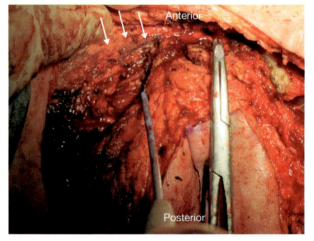

FIGURE 11 • Perineal dissection with wide exposure of the pubic symphysis, inferior pubic ramus, and ischial tuberosity in preparation for en bloc pubic bone excision. The inferior pubic ramus bony edge is illustrated by the *arrows*.

retropubic space of Retzius, the perineal surgeon commences perineal dissection working toward defining the pubic symphysis, inferior pubic ramus up to the ischial tuberosity widely (**FIGURE 11**).

- The anterior levator plane is not excised but is also defined widely. The origins of the adductor and gracilis muscles as well as the obturator fascia deep to the adductors are divided to expose the anteroinferior surface of the inferior pubic

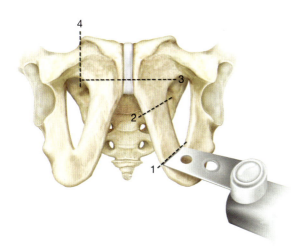

FIGURE 12 • Diagram of the bony pelvis with *lines 1* to *4* demonstrating possible excision planes. Dividing pubic bones between *lines 1* and *2* will resect the inferior pubic ramus; between *lines 2* and *3* will cause central partial pubic excision; between *lines 2* and *4* bilaterally will result in central pubic excision.

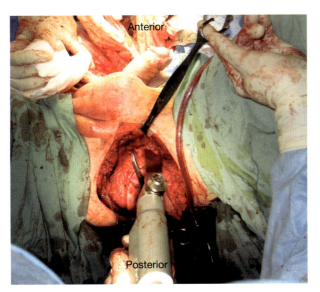

FIGURE 13 • A handheld oscillating saw being used to divide the inferior pubic ramus.

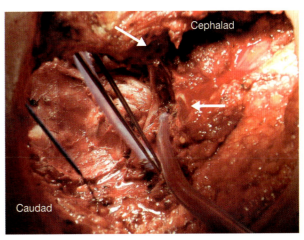

FIGURE 14 • This patient has had en bloc excision of the left inferior pubic ramus. The picture demonstrates an oblique caudal to cephalad view into the pelvis. The divided ends of the pubic ramus can be seen in the photo *(block arrows)*.

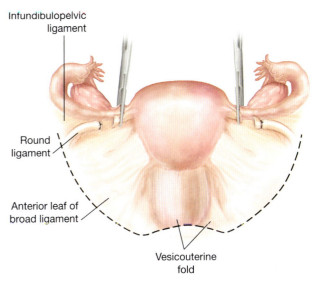

FIGURE 15 • Uterine dissection. Two Kocher forceps grasp the uterus by the uterine cornu so as to provide retraction. The base of the broad ligament is incised as shown. The round ligament is also ligated and divided.

ramus. Depending on the site of tumor involvement, different extent of bony resections can be performed ranging from unilateral or bilateral pubic ramus excision (**FIGURE 12**, lines 1 and 2), partial pubic symphysis excision (**FIGURE 12**, lines 2 and 3), or central pubic excision (**FIGURE 12**, line 2 and 4) using either a Gigli saw or a handheld electric saw (**FIGURES 13** and **14**).

- Internal fixation following pubic symphysis excision is generally not required even when it has been completely excised. Mesh reconstruction using polypropylene mesh to the cut ends of all four pubic rami and flap closure is usually all that is required.
- *Plane C* is the anterior dissection plane for a partial exenteration not involving the anterior compartment. Dissecting in this plane is dissecting in the vesicovaginal plane for en bloc radical hysterectomy and bilateral salpingo-oophorectomy.

- The procedure begins by grasping each uterine cornu for retraction (**FIGURE 15**). Gonadal vessels are ligated at the level of pelvic brim, and the broad ligament is incised with ligation of the round ligament. The peritoneum between the uterus and bladder is incised (**FIGURE 15**) to permit placement of a lipped St. Mark retractor to maintain retraction of the bladder anteriorly.
- Bilateral ureterolysis should be performed in order to mobilize the ureters from the lateral aspects of lower uterus and cervix to prevent inadvertent injury.
- Whether or not an en bloc hysterectomy is required depends on whether or not the uterus is involved more proximally.
- Whether a total vaginectomy or subtotal vaginectomy is required depends on the location of the cancer. When only posterior vaginectomy is required, dissection is carried out in *plane D*. Using a swab-on stick or a vaginal retractor is useful

so that the operator is able to confidently incise the posterior wall of vagina without damaging the anterior wall.
- Vaginal reconstruction can be achieved using the skin paddle from a rectus abdominis myocutaneous flap to reconstruct the posterior and lateral walls of vagina.
- Note that *planes C* and *D* do not exist in men.

Posterior Compartment Dissection

- *Plane E* is the anterior dissection plane for a partial exenteration involving the central and posterior compartments or the posterior dissection plane for a partial exenteration involving the central and anterior compartments. This is also a plane familiar to all colorectal surgeons and is the anterior mesorectal plane.
- Dissection proceeds in the usual manner using a total mesorectal excision technique with an assistant retracting the uterus and/or the bladder forward using a lipped St. Mark retractor while the operator provides backward and downward countertraction on the rectum.
- This dissection continues to the pelvic floor. If a low rectal anastomosis is to be fashioned, the rectum is stapled at the level of the pelvic floor, but if an anastomosis is inappropriate, then an abdominoperineal excision can be performed with the abdominal surgeon guiding the perineal surgeon about the point of entry into the pelvis.
- *Plane F* is the surgical plane for a complete exenteration or partial exenteration without sacral involvement. Rectal mobilization begins by incising the peritoneum over the left or right mesorectal fold. This plane, which is usually bloodless, is dissected using sharp dissection. Retrograde dissection in this plane joins the mesocolic plane and allows the inferior mesenteric artery to be ligated if this is not ligated yet. With an assistant providing traction on the rectum and retracting the rectum forward using a St. Mark retractor, the surgeon can continue to dissect in this bloodless plane until the coccyx is reached, where Waldeyer fascia is incised in order to mobilize the rectum down to the pelvic floor.
- When an en bloc sacrectomy is necessary, plane G is the suggested plane of dissection. Depending on the level of sacrectomy (high vs low), a different surgical approach is needed. Furthermore, sacral resection is usually the last step in the procedure after completion of abdominal (anterior, lateral dissections) and perineal phases.
- A low sacrectomy involving S3, S4, and S5 can usually be performed with the patient in modified Lloyd-Davies position via an abdominolithotomy approach, whereas a high sacrectomy (excision of S1 or S2) generally requires a prone approach.
- Surgery begins as described earlier with the abdominal phase of dissection. Lateral compartment dissection with vascular ligation and exposure of the lumbosacral trunk so as to preserve lower limb function is performed. The ischial spine may also need to be excised laterally.
- Dissection in the appropriate anterior plane is performed and posterior dissection stops about 2 cm above the site where the tumor is adherent to the sacrum. Overlying S3, S4, and S5 in the midline is the anterior longitudinal ligament, which is often abnormally thickened in patients with LRRC as a result of previous radiotherapy and surgery. Lateral to this at S3 level is piriformis medially and sacral nerve roots laterally. These may also need to be disconnected depending on the level of sacral resection.

- Perineal dissection should also be completed before attempting en bloc distal sacrectomy (see "Perineal Phase"). To perform abdominal sacrectomy, the perineal surgeon will have to extend the posterior dissection to first get to the coccyx. Once the coccyx is defined, the perineal surgeon continues dissection immediately posterior to the coccyx mobilizing the posterior aspect of the coccyx and sacrum from surrounding attachments of gluteus maximus and ligamentous attachments.
- By tunneling to the appropriate level of sacral excision, a malleable retractor or osteotome can then be inserted to protect the natal cleft tissue as the abdominal surgeon performs sacrectomy using a 20-mm osteotome and mallet (**FIGURE 16**). Once all bony attachments are divided, the specimen can then be delivered from the perineal wound.
- Where a high sacrectomy (excision of S1 and S2) is necessary, abdominal and anterior compartment perineal phases of the operation have to be completed before the patient is turned prone for posterior compartment excision. This includes completion of all aspects of abdominal and perineal procedures such as visceral reconstruction, drain placement, abdominal wound closure and temporary perineal wound closure, harvest of rectus abdominis flap, as well as formation of a colostomy.
- To ensure the appropriate sacral segments are excised from a prone approach, an orthopedic pin or staple is secured into the sacrum about 1 to 2 cm above the desired point of transection (11 × 15 mm, Smith & Nephew fixation staple). The position of this stapler is checked with an intraoperative x-ray to confirm the point of transection (**FIGURE 17A**) when commencing the prone approach.
- It is also useful to leave both lumbosacral trunks marked with a yellow vessel loop and to have a suture to orientate a rectus abdominis myocutaneous flap to avoid flap malrotation. Abdominal sponges may also be left just anterior to the sacrum to prevent small bowel from coming into contact with the anterior aspect of sacrum, which may be inadvertently injured as the sacrus is being transected from the prone approach.

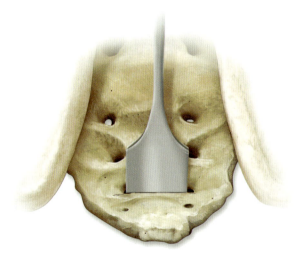

FIGURE 16 • Diagram showing how low sacrectomy is performed by using an osteotome and a mallet.

Chapter 41 PELVIC EXENTERATION

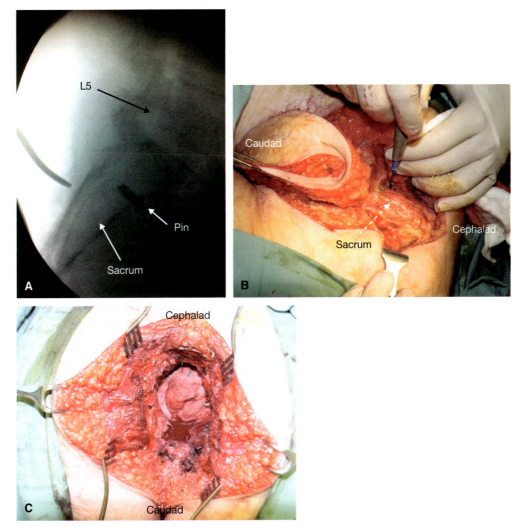

FIGURE 17 • **A,** A pin is placed in the sacrum to mark the intended level of sacral transection for high sacrectomy. Posterior dissection usually stops about 1 to 2 cm above the site of tumor adherence. An intraoperative x-ray is then performed to confirm the site of intended sacral transection from a prone approach. **B,** Intraoperative photo of prone sacrectomy. The sacrum is being defined by detaching the attachments of gluteus maximus. **C,** Intraoperative photo showing the result after transecting sacrum and the specimen has been retrieved. The sponge placed abdominally to protect small bowel loops from being damaged by the saw used to transect sacrum. This diagram also demonstrates the defect after completing a high sacrectomy.

- Prone approach to high sacrectomy is usually performed in collaboration with orthopedic surgeons or neurosurgeons and begins with a longitudinal incision in the natal cleft that extends from the posterior aspect of the perineal incision.
- The incision is deepened until the sacrum is reached. Attachments of gluteus maximus are released bilaterally so as to provide access to the sacrum (**FIGURE 17B**). Deep to gluteus maximus are the sacrococcygeal, sacroiliac, and the sacrotuberous ligaments, which are also released. Dividing these soft tissue attachments frees the lateral borders of the sacrum. Deep to the sacrotuberous ligament is the sacrospinous ligament, which is divided exposing the underlying piriformis muscles. Immediately deep to piriformis are the sacral nerve roots. It is imperative that the operator remains close to the lateral border of the sacrum to avoid any injury to these nerve roots.

- The level of transection is confirmed by a cross-table x-ray to check the position of the pelvic staple placed above the tumor (**FIGURE 17A**). This enables the sacrum to be transected with the staple in situ so as to ensure adequate bony margins.
- Once the level is determined, the sacral crest between the median and intermediate sacral crest is resected to expose the dural sac, which is ligated to prevent ongoing leakage of cerebrospinal fluid.
- Sacrectomy is then completed by using a handheld oscillating saw. The specimen is removed, exposing the abdominal pack protecting small bowel loops (**FIGURE 17C**). Hemostasis is secured; bone wax may be necessary to stop bleeding from exposed cancellous sacrum. The vessel loops around lumbosacral trunks should be intact and need to be removed. The preinserted abdominal drain needs to be repositioned, and the preorientated rectus abdominis flap can then be retrieved and secured in place.

388 SECTION III **RECTAL RESECTIONS**

Perineal Phase

- The perineal phase is carried out with the patient in wide lithotomy position. This phase is usually only commenced when abdominal dissection is near completion.
- The extent of perineal excision required depends on the location of the cancer. The wider the perineal excision, the more likely the patient is to require closure using a pedicled myocutaneous flap to avoid tension closure, which will only predispose to perineal wound breakdown and prolonged healing due to previous irradiation.
- An elliptical skin incision is made. Using the Lone Star retractor, the incision is deepened into the ischiorectal fossa fat. Depending on the planned dissection plane from the abdominal compartment, the incision is deepened to approximate the dissection plane from the abdominal compartment. Wide excision of levator muscle is usually performed even if the amount of perineal skin excised does not have to be excessive.
- When en bloc distal sacrectomy is required, the perineal surgeon continues dissecting immediately posterior to the coccyx to the proposed level of sacrectomy, detaching gluteus maximus from the lateral and posterior aspects of the coccyx and lower sacrum. A malleable retractor blade or second osteotome is then placed into the space to protect the natal cleft soft tissue, which the abdominal surgeon divides the sacrum using an osteotome and mallet.
- When a proximal sacrectomy is required, the perineal wound is temporarily closed so that the patient can be turned prone for the posterior dissection.

Urinary Reconstruction

- When an en bloc cystectomy is required, reconstruction using ileal or colonic conduit is usually performed. The decision for an ileal or colonic conduit is surgeon dependent, and although ileal conduits are usually preferable in the urologic literature, in patients with LRRC where pelvic small bowel loops may have been previously irradiated, isolating a segment of ileum may be associated with increased risk of postoperative complications including anastomotic leak from the ureteroileal anastomosis and the ileoileal anastomosis.
- A colonic conduit is usually out of the radiation field, and a study from our institution found a higher leak rate with ileal conduits as opposed to colonic conduits. Furthermore, to minimize the risk of ileoileal anastomotic leaks, the segment of ileum isolated should be such that the subsequent ileoileal anastomosis is at least 10 to 15 cm away from the ileocecal valve so that it is away from the back pressure exerted by the valve.
- The use of orthotopic neobladder reconstruction is popular within the gynecologic oncology literature, but few, if any, are considering the technique in LARC or LRRC.
- When en bloc partial cystectomy is required, double-layered suture repair of the bladder in conjunction with leaving the indwelling urinary catheter in situ for a minimum of 7 days with a check cystography prior to catheter removal is usually sufficient.
- When a segment of ureter is involved unilaterally, depending on the extent of ureteric excision and preexisting renal function in the kidney involved, the options are to consider a ureteric reimplantation with a psoas hitch, reimplanting the resected ureter to the contralateral ureter, or if

renal preserving options are not available, a nephrectomy. Anastomosing the resected ureter to the contralateral ureter is avoided where possible as any anastomotic problem or surgical complication can have repercussions on both kidneys instead of one.
- To perform ureteric reimplantation and psoas hitch, the bladder has to be adequately mobilized bilaterally. Once the bladder is mobilized, a transverse cystostomy is performed. By inserting a finger through the cystostomy, an assessment is made to determine the best position for the ureter to be anastomosed to the bladder without excessive tension. A separate small cystostomy is created, and the ureter is pulled through and anastomosed to the bladder using fine absorbable sutures over a ureteric stent. Reinforcing sutures are placed between the bladder and the psoas tendon to avoid traction injury on the newly created ureterovesical anastomosis. The cystostomy is then closed longitudinally in two layers, completing the reconstruction.

Intestinal Reconstruction

- When an ileal conduit is fashioned and when a segment of small bowel is resected en bloc with the main specimen, intestinal continuity needs to be restored, using either a hand-sewn or stapled anastomosis.
- Most patients with LRRC will require an end colostomy.
- Patients with LARC or selected patients with early anastomotic recurrences may be suitable for a colorectal anastomosis provided there are no other contraindications for the anastomosis. Even if a colorectal anastomosis is performed, in view of the complex surgery and previous irradiation, these patients should be at least temporarily defunctionalized with a proximal stoma.

Abdominal and Perineal Closure and Reconstruction

- In patients in whom a wide perineal excision, high sacrectomy, or complete pelvic exenteration has been performed, consideration needs to be given to flap reconstruction. Although our preference is for rectus abdominis myocutaneous flap, other perforator flaps based on the inferior gluteal artery perforator (I-GAP) or anterior thigh flaps may be necessary when the rectus abdominis is not available due to previous stomas.
- Rectus abdominis on the side where there are no prior stomas is preferable. In our practice, a vertical elliptical skin paddle (used for simplicity and ease of abdominal skin closure) with a maximum diameter of 5 cm is harvested (**FIGURE 5**) with the underlying anterior sheath and rectus abdominis muscle but leaving the posterior sheath intact. We avoid excessively wide skin paddles as this may introduce donor site morbidity with difficult abdominal skin closure and tension on stomas.
- The flap can then be rotated into the pelvis after harvesting. There are two possible ways of rotating the flap. The first is to rotate the flap with the pedicle acting as a pivot and the second is to roll the flap downward like a "Swiss roll."
- After harvesting the flap, it is important to raise skin flaps either on the ipsilateral side alone or bilaterally (if there are no existing stomas) prior to fashioning stomas. Broad-based skin flaps are raised on the external oblique with hemostasis of perforators as they penetrate the anterior abdominal wall to supply the overlying skin.

- Prior to abdominal and perineal wound closure, a thorough lavage of the abdomen, pelvis, and perineal wound is carried out. Hemostasis is checked to ensure there is no active bleeding. Minor oozing is not uncommon but should be controlled with electrocautery, clips, or sutures where possible. Ongoing oozing may require topical hemostatic agents such as Gelfoam, Surgicel, or Nu-knit. At least one large-bore drain is placed in the pelvis, making sure that it drains the most dependent part of the pelvis.
- The myocutaneous flap is usually secured in the perineum using a combination of absorbable dermal and nonabsorbable skin sutures.
- When myocutaneous flaps are not required, the perineal wound is closed in layers. Owing to wide excision of levator ani, muscle closure is generally not possible and closure is generally that of subcutaneous fat and skin using a braided suture such as Vicryl.
- There has been an increasing interest in prophylactic mesh repairs of the perineal wound to prevent subsequent perineal hernias. Currently, the safest and cost-effective method remains unclear, with some authors reporting the use of flaps and others the use of biologic mesh. Considering the high prevalence of postoperative pelvic septic complications and low prevalence of perineal hernias in our practice, we have not found prophylactic perineal mesh repair beneficial.
- Abdominal closure when a rectus abdominis flap is not required is relatively straightforward using mass closure with either a no. 1 polydioxanone (PDS) suture or nylon suture. However, when a rectus abdominis flap has been harvested, the abdominal wall will require mesh reconstruction to prevent a future incisional hernia. In these patients, closure of the posterior sheath on the ipsilateral side of harvest to full thickness of the abdominal wall on the contralateral side is performed using no. 1 PDS suture. It is important to remain mindful of the inferior aspect of the midline laparotomy wound where closure should be loose to prevent strangulating the arterial supply or impeding venous drainage of the flap particularly when edema sets in after surgery.
- An onlay mesh repair using polypropylene mesh is then carried out to reinforce the abdominal wall, securing it to the linea semilunaris laterally and the linea alba in the midline wound using 2.0 Prolene suture (**FIGURE 18**). A drain is also placed to prevent wound seromas.
- Abdominal skin closure is performed using a combination of skin staples and nonabsorbable interrupted vertical mattress sutures.

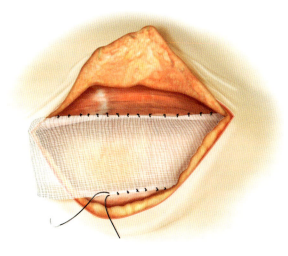

FIGURE 18 • Abdominal wall reconstruction using polypropylene mesh.

PEARLS AND PITFALLS

Intraoperative surgical management	■ Meticulous adhesiolysis to avoid inadvertent enterotomies will prevent future complications. A trial of dissection is permissible, but if the tissue is very adherent, consideration should be given to en bloc excision of that structure to avoid an involved surgical margin.
Lateral compartment dissection	■ The pelvic sidewall is organized in a "layered" structure. The layers are the ureter, the iliac arteries, the iliac veins, the lumbosacral trunk, and pelvic sidewall muscles.
Meticulous venous dissection	■ Although highly variable, there is an underlying pattern to venous drainage. ■ Usually, there is at least one spinal, gluteal, and visceral tributary entering the main trunk of internal iliac vein at each level. ■ Dissection of each tributary such that there is an adequate cuff before ligation of each tributary is advisable to prevent ties from slipping due to a short cuff. ■ Suture ligation is preferred over clips as it is not unusual for clips to slip or be inadvertently dislodged. ■ When suture ligation fails to control bleeding, adjacent muscle tissue can be used as a pledget and provides additional bulk for providing direct pressure for hemostasis.
Visceral reconstruction	■ In patients with LRRC, heavily irradiated small bowel loops are poor candidates for ureteroileal or ileoileal anastomosis. In these patients, a colonic conduit may be considered as the colon is typically beyond the irradiation field. ■ Mixed colostomies (combined urine and stool stomas) are not routinely advised.

Perineal reconstruction	■ Most recurrences do not require wide perineal excision. However, in patients with wide perineal excision and/or with a sacrectomy, a rectus abdominis myocutaneous flap reconstruction provides well-vascularized tissue in the pelvis to fill the "dead space" and to additional skin paddle to facilitate tension-free skin closure. ■ Alternatively, a pedicled omental flap is also very useful to fill the space within the pelvis to prevent infected fluid collections.
Postoperative management	■ Prolonged ileus is common. Early commencement of total parenteral nutrition should be considered. ■ In view of high complication rates, a high index of clinical suspicion is required for early recognition and treatment to prevent further morbidity.

POSTOPERATIVE CARE

- All exenteration patients are routinely admitted to an intensive care unit for postoperative care. The patient is often left intubated overnight.
- Aggressive fluid and blood product replacement and correction of coagulopathy is often required after a complete exenteration with en bloc sacral resection.
- Prolonged ileus is common; early initiation of total parenteral nutrition is recommended.
- Mechanical venous thromboprophylaxis is vital.
- Patients who have had a flap reconstruction are usually required to rest in bed for the first 5 to 7 days after surgery. It is important that these patients are turned regularly to minimize pressure on their flaps. Flap observations should also be performed regularly to ensure the flap remains well perfused.
- In patients with a urinary conduit, it is imperative to ensure that the patient is well hydrated to maintain a good urine output. Regular drain fluid creatinine check (1-2 days) also helps to detect urinary leaks early so that intervention can be readily instituted to avoid further morbidity.
- Septic complications are also particularly common in this group of patients; thus, it is common to continue prophylactic antibiotics for 5 days after surgery. Most causes of sepsis originate from urinary sepsis, infected abdominal or pelvic collections, and hospital-acquired pneumonia. Early mobilization and chest physiotherapy are helpful.
- Infected pelvic collections are common and are usually diagnosed on CT performed for persistent fevers with no obvious source. One of the challenges with interpreting CT scans after such surgery is distinguishing between infected and noninfected fluid collections as postoperative fluid collections are also very common. Postoperative inflammatory changes also take a longer time to dissipate; hence, interpretation of the CT by an experienced radiologist in conjunction with the surgeon is helpful. Keeping an abdominal drain in situ for a longer period of time may allow the drain to be rewired for abdominal drain replacement as opposed to a transgluteal approach for drain insertion, which is usually uncomfortable.
- In patients who have undergone a high sacrectomy, early documentation of neurologic deficit in lower limbs is helpful before swelling of nerves. Neuropathic pain in this group of patients is common, and early input from the acute and chronic pain teams with early consideration for gabapentin may be helpful to facilitate pain management.

- Most patients will require ongoing input from dietitians, stomal therapists, and psycho-oncologists. Furthermore, most patients will require a period of inpatient rehabilitation at a rehabilitation center. Thus, early involvement of all allied health specialists is important. As follow-up plans are often complex, clear written instructions and contact persons should be provided.

OUTCOMES

- The main aim of surgery is to achieve a clear resection margin (R0) as this is the single most important predictor of long-term survival.
- R0 rates within the literature vary between 38% and 85%. In as much as R0 is the most important surgical outcome, R0 is by no means an accurate reflection of a recurrent cancer unit's experience and performance because, as alluded to early in the chapter, different units have different resectability criteria. Without an understanding of the types of exenterations offered, units performing only limited exenterations on patients with good prognostic features may be seen to outperform higher-volume and more established units.
- Pelvic sidewall recurrence was traditionally considered a formidable challenge because of the difficult dissection, risk of major bleeding, and concerns for involved surgical resection margins, and, therefore, often considered incurable. However, with improved surgical techniques, pelvic sidewall as a site of recurrence is no longer considered a contraindication for surgery, and provided clear margins can be obtained, comparable survival with recurrence at other sites can be achieved.
- Quality of life in patients following pelvic exenteration is an area that remains understudied. Although much remains unknown, it is known that quality of life following exenteration is comparable with that of patients after total mesorectal excision for primary rectal cancer.

COMPLICATIONS

- Reported mortality rates range between 0.3% and 8%, although larger series in recent years have tended to report mortality rates of less than 1%.
- Published complication rates range from 21% to 72%, with major complication rates within the contemporary literature originating from high-volume centers at about 25%.
- Common complications published are listed in **TABLE 1**.

Table 1: Complications From Pelvic Exenteration

Septic complications
- Urinary tract infection
- Wound infection
- Pneumonia
- Deep-seated intra-abdominal/pelvic collections
- Osteomyelitis

Gastrointestinal complications
- Prolonged ileus
- Small bowel obstruction
- Enterocutaneous fistula
- Anastomotic leak
- Colovaginal fistula

Cardiorespiratory complications
- Atrial fibrillation or other cardiac arrhythmias
- Myocardial infarction
- Pulmonary embolism (deep venous thrombosis)

Wound complications
- Wound dehiscence
- Persistent perineal sinus
- Perineal flap necrosis
- Infected prosthetic mesh
- Hematomas

Urologic
- Urinary retention
- Urologic leak
- Colovesical fistula

Neurologic
- Sciatic nerve palsy

Stomal complications
- Stomal dehiscence
- Ischemia

SUGGESTED READINGS

1. Austin K, Solomon M. Pelvic exenteration with en bloc iliac resection for lateral wall involvement. *Dis Colon Rectum.* 2009;52(7):1223-1233.
2. Austin K, Young J, Solomon M. Quality of life of survivors after pelvic exenteration for rectal cancer. *Dis Colon Rectum.* 2010;53(8):1121-1126.
3. Heriot AG, Byrne CM, Lee P, et al. Extended radical resection: the choice for locally recurrent rectal cancer. *Dis Colon Rectum.* 2008;51:284-291.
4. Koda K, Tobe T, Takiguchi N, et al. Pelvic exenteration for advanced colorectal cancer with reconstruction of urinary and sphincter functions. *Br J Surg.* 2002;89(10):1286-1289.
5. Milne T, Solomon M, Lee P, et al. Assessing the impact of a sacral resection on morbidity and survival after extended radical surgery for locally recurrent rectal cancer. *Ann Surg.* 2013;258(6):1007-1013.
6. Nielsen MB, Rasmussen PC, Lindegaard JC, et al. A 10-year experience of total pelvic exenteration for primary advanced and locally recurrent rectal cancer based on a prospective database. *Colorectal Dis.* 2012;14(9):1076-1083.
7. Pawlik TM, Skibber J, Rodriguez-Bigas MA. Educational review. Pelvic exenteration for advanced pelvic malignancies. *Ann Surg Oncol.* 2006;13(5):612-623.
8. Solomon MJ. Re-exenteration for recurrent rectal cancer. *Dis Colon Rectum.* 2013;56(1):4-5.
9. Teixeira SC, Ferenschild FT, Solomon MJ, et al. Urological leaks after pelvic exenterations comparing formation of colonic and ileal conduits. *Eur J Surg Oncol.* 2011;38(4):361-366.
10. Young JM, Badgery-Parker T, Masya LM, et al. Quality of life and other patient-reported outcomes following exenteration for pelvic malignancy. *Br J Surg.* 2014;101(3):277-287.
11. Zoucas E, Frederiksen S, Lydrup ML, et al. Pelvic exenteration for advanced and recurrent malignancy. *World J Surg.* 2010;34(9):2177-2184.

Chapter 42

Transanal Excision of Rectal Tumors: Open Technique

Angel M. Charles, Barry W. Feig, and Ryan M. Thomas

DEFINITION

- Transanal excision (TAE) of rectal tumors refers to the complete resection of a benign or malignant neoplasm of the distal rectum such that negative surgical resection margins are achieved while avoiding the morbidity of transabdominal resection procedures.[1]

PATIENT HISTORY AND PHYSICAL FINDINGS

- A full history must be performed with special focus on any changes in bowel habits including stool caliber, the presence of melena or hematochezia, personal or family history of colorectal cancer, and the use of any antiplatelet or anticoagulant medications in preparation for surgical excision.
- A thorough physical examination must be performed with special focus on digital rectal examination including information on rectal tone, location of the rectal tumor and degree of circumferential rectal wall involvement, distance of the tumor from the anal verge, and mobility/fixation of the tumor to surrounding structures. These physical factors of the mass are critical to determine the feasibility of resection as the criteria for resection demands that the lesion:
  - Be within 8 cm of the anal verge to be able to reach the lesion transanally. Distal rectal lesions may be more amendable to TAE than transanal minimally invasive surgery (TAMIS; Chapter 43) or transanal endoscopic microsurgery (TEM).[2,3]
  - Must be mobile and not fixed to surrounding structures.
  - Must involve less than 30% of the circumference of the rectal wall on endoscopic evaluation, as resection of lesions encompassing >30% of the circumference risks narrowing the rectal lumen after excision is performed.
  - Favorable histopathologic features: <3 cm in size; T1 only; grade 1 or 2 (well to moderately differentiated); no lymphatic, venous, or perineural invasion; and ability to obtain negative margins of resection.[1]
  - Full-thickness excision (all four rectal layers) must be feasible.[1]
  - Often, patients are referred for TAE of a rectal tumor after having undergone endoscopic evaluation that diagnosed a malignant mass, indeterminate pathology, or a benign mass not amenable to endoscopic resection.
- Differential diagnosis for a rectal mass includes:
  - Benign polyp
  - Hemorrhoidal disease
  - Infectious (abscess)
  - Arteriovenous malformation
  - Malignancy.[1]

IMAGING AND OTHER DIAGNOSTIC STUDIES

- Endoscopy and endoscopic rectal ultrasound (ERUS) for malignant lesions play a critical role in the management of mid- to low-rectal lesions in patients who may be candidates for TAE. Endoscopy defines the anatomy of the lesion and special attention should be made to the anatomic location, as this will affect surgical positioning. The tumor diameter, location from the anal verge, degree of circumferential involvement, and depth of invasion and nodal involvement are noted as they dictate the appropriateness of TAE as well.
- Assuming that a malignant lesion is technically resectable via a transanal approach, one must ensure that the lesion is a T1 stage and without nodal involvement. The transanal approach for rectal tumors has garnered support because of the decreased morbidity compared with a transabdominal approach, but lymph node metastasis has been reported in 10% to 18% of T1 lesions.[4,5]
- A retrospective study of 282 patients undergoing either transanal local excision or radical resection of T1 rectal cancers from 1985 to 2004 revealed a local recurrence of 13.2% and 2.7%, respectively ($p = .001$). A similar study of 2124 patients showed local recurrence of 12.5% and 6.9% for patients who underwent local excision and radical resection, respectively ($p = .003$).[6,7]
- Imaging is integral in the preoperative planning for TAE of rectal tumors in selected patients. In the case of malignancy, staging imaging should include the following:
  - A chest x-ray and computed tomography (CT) of the abdomen and pelvis to assess for metastatic disease.
  - Critical to the determination of the local resectability of a rectal lesion is the assessment of the T stage and N stage of the tumor. The accuracy of determining the depth of invasion by CT scan, magnetic resonance imaging (MRI), and ERUS is 73%, 82%, and 87%, respectively. Nodal metastases are accurately assessed by CT scan, MRI, and ERUS in 66%, 74%, and 74% of cases, respectively. The use of endorectal coils during MRI has been found to be equivalent to ERUS for T stage determination but superior in terms of nodal status.[8,9]
  - In a 2004 meta-analysis, EUS and MRI have similar sensitivity and specificity when evaluating lymph nodes (sensitivity 67% and 66%, and specificity 78% and 76%, respectively), whereas CT had lower sensitivity and specificity for lymph node involvement (55% and 74%, respectively); therefore, CT is not recommended for rectal staging.[1,10]
  - ERUS is unable to visualize high or bulky lesions and is operator-dependent. Therefore, ERUS is recommended if MRI is contraindicated in these patients (ie, patient has a pacemaker that is not MRI-compatible).

Chapter 42 TRANSANAL EXCISION OF RECTAL TUMORS: OPEN TECHNIQUE 393

- Any biopsies that are performed of the rectal tumor prior to definitive excision should be re-reviewed to confirm the tumor depth of invasion, differentiation, and the presence of lymphovascular invasion (LVI) or perineural invasion (PNI).
- Established pathologic criteria for TAE of a malignant lesion include T1 lesions, no evidence of LVI or PNI, moderately to well-differentiated tumors, or an endoscopically removed polyp with indeterminate pathology.[11]

SURGICAL MANAGEMENT

Preoperative Planning

- Not all patients are candidates for TAE of rectal tumors and many factors may prove to be a contraindication to such treatment. The surgeon must consider physiologic, anatomic, and pathologic factors to determine if a patient is an appropriate candidate for TAE (**TABLE 1**).
- Physiologic factors and patient desires may make TAE a viable option, namely, in patients who physiologically cannot tolerate an extensive transabdominal resection or have a short life expectancy because of metastatic disease yet have a bleeding tumor in need of palliation. In addition, some patients may not desire an abdominoperineal resection and resultant permanent colostomy or the possibility of sexual and/or urinary dysfunction. Given appropriate physical and pathologic criteria, these patients may be appropriate candidates for TAE as well.
- In most cases, patients should be instructed to discontinue anticoagulation and antiplatelet medications 7 to 10 days prior to the planned procedure if medically feasible.
- A formal bowel preparation is unnecessary other than an enema the evening prior to the procedure to evacuate the rectal vault.

Patient Positioning

- Positioning of the patient depends on the anatomic location of the rectal tumor to be excised, which should be determined on preoperative physical examination and endoscopy. Patients with a rectal tumor along the posterior rectal wall should be positioned in high lithotomy such that their coccyx can be easily palpated (**FIGURE 1A**). In contrast, patients with lesions located along the anterior rectal wall should be placed in the prone jackknife position (**FIGURE 1B**).
- For patients placed in the prone position, heavy tape should be applied to the buttocks so that they can be retracted laterally and secured to the operating room table. Benzoin or Mastisol ointment applied to the skin prior to application of the tape assists in preventing the tape from slipping during the procedure.
- Once in position with pressure points appropriately padded, a digital rectal examination is performed to confirm tumor location and the rectum is irrigated with saline until all solid material has been removed. The perineum is then prepped with Betadine and appropriately draped.
- A pudendal and perineal nerve block with local anesthesia should be considered once the patient is prepped and draped, which will aid in relaxation and postoperative pain control.

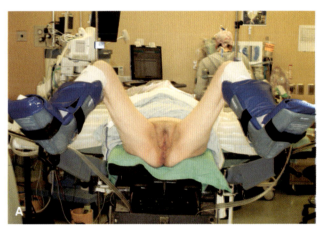

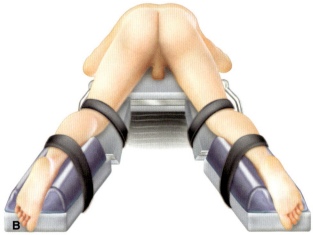

FIGURE 1 • **A,** Patient positioning. For posterior lesions, the patient is placed on a high lithotomy position. It is important that the coccyx can be palpated, which ensures that they are low enough on the bed and adequate exposure to the lesion can be obtained. **B,** Prone position: ideal for patients with anteriorly located lesions. The arms are resting without straining on arm boards. The lower extremities are resting on a split-table configuration. The patient is firmly secured to the table position changes during the procedure. All pressure points are padded to prevent nerve and/or vascular injuries.

Table 1: Criteria for Transanal Excision of Rectal Tumors

Patient factors	Anatomic factors	Pathologic factors
• Comorbidities that preclude transabdominal resection • Short life expectancy in need of surgical palliation • Refusal of abdominoperineal resection and resultant permanent colostomy	• Lesion ≤8 cm from the anal verge • Lesion involves ≤30% of rectal circumference • Lesion ≤3 cm in diameter • Mobile and not fixed to underlying tissue • Negative margins achievable depending on pathology of primary lesion (0.3-1 cm)	• Moderately or well-differentiated tumor • T1 tumor • No lymphovascular or perineural invasion • Indeterminate pathology on polypectomy • No evidence of lymphadenopathy on preoperative imaging

EXPOSURE OF THE LESION

- Because of the limited working area, exposure is key to safe TAE with adequate margins.
- A high-intensity headlight aids in the visualization, and a long, narrow suction apparatus is helpful for both smoke evacuation and fluid removal.
- The goal of exposure for TAE is to bring the lesion closer to the anus and avoid retractors that tend to push the lesion away. There are several methods and instruments that are available to achieve this goal.
- A Lone Star retractor (CooperSurgical; Trumbull, CT) may be used to help evert the anus and gain better exposure. Alternatively, a series of nylon sutures placed circumferentially in a simple fashion from the internal sphincter to the thigh can achieve a similar result. The use of these techniques is particularly helpful for posterior lesions when the patient is in the lithotomy position.
- For men in the lithotomy position, it may be helpful to secure the scrotum to the inner thigh with a 2-0 silk or other similar suture to remove it from the operative field. This is not necessary in the prone jackknife position as gravity provides the necessary retraction.
- A Parks anal self-retaining retractor, with the option of the additional center blade, is then placed in the anus to provide exposure, with an assistant using an appropriately sized lighted Hill–Ferguson retractor for additional exposure (**FIGURE 2**). A variety of other self-retaining and handheld retractors may be considered depending on the patient's anatomy or surgeon preference.

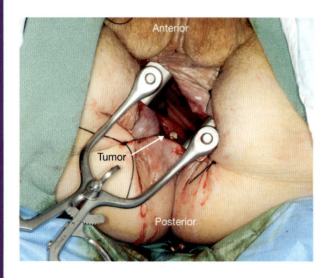

FIGURE 2 • Exposure of the lesion. A self-retaining retractor, such as the Parks retractor, is placed into the anus and rectum and gently opened. A Lone Star retractor or a series of 2-0 nylon sutures placed around the periphery of the anus can be used to evert the anal canal and bring the lesion closer to the field prior to placing the Parks retractor. This is especially useful in obese individuals or for lesions that are at the maximum extent of reach (8-10 cm from the anal verge).

DEFINING THE SURGICAL MARGIN

- Once the lesion has been identified, electrocautery is used to score the mucosa circumferentially around the mass. This step is critical to define the appropriate margin: 1 cm for malignant lesions and at least 0.3 cm for benign lesions or those with indeterminate pathology on preoperative pathologic evaluation (**FIGURE 3**).

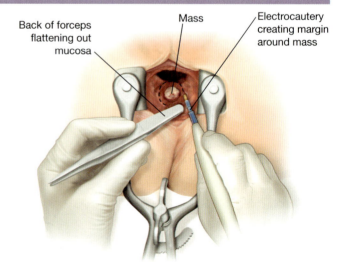

FIGURE 3 • Defining the surgical margin. Once adequate exposure is obtained, electrocautery is used to mark out the surgical margin: 1 cm for malignant lesions and 0.3 cm for benign lesions or those of indeterminate pathology. Because mucosal folds can obscure the true margin and lead to a margin that is lesser or greater than intended, using the back of a DeBakey forceps or a handheld retractor such as the Hill–Ferguson retractor can help flatten the mucosal folds so an appropriate margin can be defined.

- It is important to flatten the surrounding mucosa with the use of the Hill–Ferguson retractor or a flat right-angle (Haney) retractor as the margin is being scored. The back end of DeBakey forceps is especially useful for this purpose as well (**FIGURE 3**). Failure to flatten the mucosa may result in a margin that is far greater or lesser than the intended margin because of mucosal folding.

PLACEMENT OF RETRACTION AND ORIENTATION SUTURES

- For proximal lesions or in patients where visualization is less optimal, a 2-0 Vicryl with a UR-6 needle retraction (stay) suture can be placed at the apex of the surgical specimen outside of the scored margin, tied into place, and used to bring the lesion closer to the operator, if necessary, during resection (**FIGURE 4A**).

- Next, sutures should be placed within the outlined margin to serve as orientation sutures once the specimen has been removed. A short proximal suture with one suture end cut and a long left lateral suture leaving both suture ends long avoids confusion and will ensure proper orientation of the specimen should additional margins need to be removed (**FIGURE 4B**).

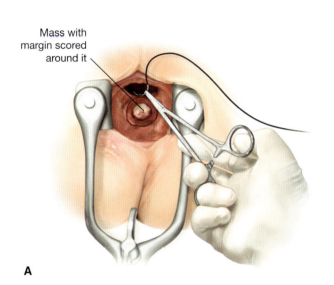
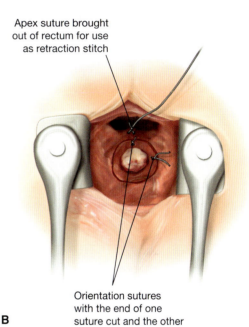

FIGURE 4 • Placement of retraction and orientation sutures. **A,** Just outside of the most proximal extent of the surgical margin, a 2-0 Vicryl suture is placed and tied. The suture is left long and is brought out of the rectum and secured to the surgical drapes. This suture can be used during the excision for retraction and to help bring the lesion closer to the operator. **B,** Sutures of different lengths are then placed within the surgical margin that will serve as orientation sutures. As an example, a single short suture may be used for the proximal margin and a long suture for the left lateral margin. These sutures should be placed early in the case to maintain orientation for pathologic margin assessment.

FULL-THICKNESS EXCISION OF THE MASS

- Using electrocautery, a full-thickness excision of the mass is performed down to the deep perirectal tissue. A long needle-tip electrocautery device can often be helpful in providing access without obstructing visualization. It is easier to begin the dissection distally and work around the margins proximally; this allows for a more apparent identification of the perirectal tissue as it is encountered and helps to guide the rest of the proximal and deep extent of the excision (**FIGURE 5**).
- Special attention should be paid to create the electrocautery line of excision perpendicular to the rectal wall to avoid undermining the edges of the specimen and potentially compromising the resection margins.
- Once the perirectal fatty tissue is encountered, the mass is continually lifted away from this underlying fatty tissue and detached from it using the electrocautery. The goal is to remove a disc of tissue that contains the mass, adequate margins, and a portion of tissue deep to the mass to ensure adequate full-thickness excision and adequate pathologic evaluation. Special attention must be taken during the full-thickness excision of anteriorly located lesions because injury to the vagina or prostate can occur if the excision is carried too deeply.

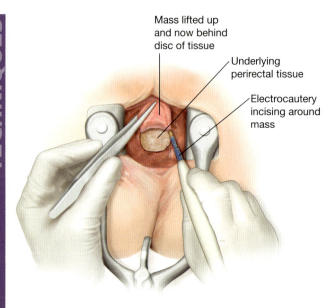

- As the excision proceeds, gentle traction of the orientation and stay sutures can provide additional tension to facilitate the excision or to bring the tissue closer to the operator.

FIGURE 5 • Full-thickness excision of the mass. Electrocautery is used to create a full-thickness defect through the rectal wall until the perirectal fat is identified. It is easier to begin at the most distal aspect of the lesion because visualization is better. Once the full-thickness defect is created, the free edge of tissue or a retraction suture is grasped to lift the mass and normal tissue away from the underlying perirectal fat as the excision proceeds proximally along the lateral aspects of the lesion, leaving the most proximal part of excision for last.

SUBMITTING THE SPECIMEN TO PATHOLOGY

- An important part of the TAE of a rectal mass is specimen orientation for the pathologist. After the mass has been excised, it should be fixed to a wax board with 22-gauge needles and hand delivered to the pathology suite so that the surgeon can speak directly to the pathologist for specimen orientation and margin assessment (**FIGURE 6**).
- The margins are inked and assessed. If tumor cells are present at any of the margins, additional tissue must be removed.

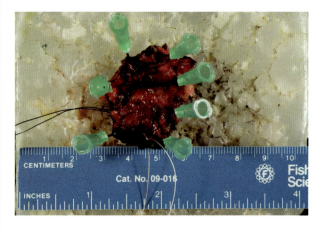

FIGURE 6 • Submitting the specimen to pathology. The resected specimen is then secured to a wax board with 22-gauge needles for proper orientation. Because orientation sutures were placed early in the case, there should be no confusion about the specimen orientation. The surgeon then brings the specimen to the pathology suite to confirm orientation with the pathologist and the margins are inked and assessed. If tumor cells are present at any of the margins, additional tissue must be removed.

CLOSURE OF THE RECTAL WALL DEFECT

- Once appropriate hemostasis is obtained and no additional margins need to be taken, attention is turned to the closure of the resultant rectal wall defect (**FIGURE 7**). Interrupted absorbable sutures are used to approximate the mucosa and submucosa. The sutures should be slightly spaced to allow for drainage to occur and to prevent hematoma formation (**FIGURE 8**). If there is difficulty obtaining adequate hemostasis, a running, locking suture starting at the apex of the surgical defect and moving toward the distal end of it can be used.
- The running suture is tied just before the end of the defect is reached, leaving a small opening for drainage to occur.
- Alternatively, the defect may be closed over a ¼" Penrose drain, secured into place with the final pass of the suture to allow fluid to drain. The patient will eventually pass the drain once the suture has dissolved.
- In the case of a large defect in which there is too much tension to reapproximate the mucosa, the defect may be left open to heal by secondary intention.
- After the defect has been closed, the retractors are removed, and a digital rectal examination is performed to confirm patency of the rectum.
- A rolled-up piece of hemostatic agent (Fibrillar, Gelfoam) may be placed into the rectum, overlying the suture line, to provide additional hemostasis.

Chapter 42 TRANSANAL EXCISION OF RECTAL TUMORS: OPEN TECHNIQUE 397

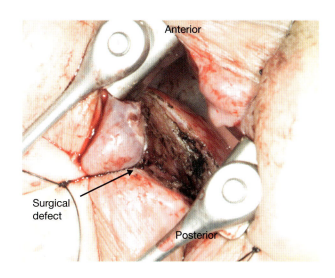

FIGURE 7 • Hemostasis of rectal defect. The resultant rectal defect is irrigated and hemostasis is obtained prior to closure.

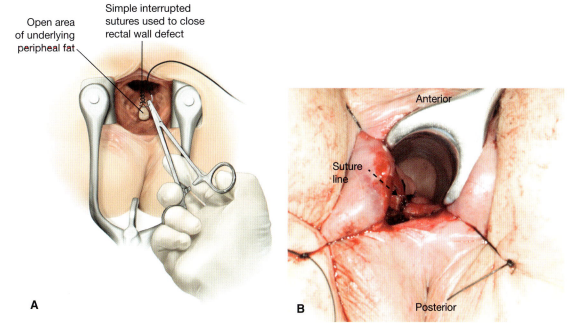

FIGURE 8 • Closure of the rectal wall defect. **A,** After appropriate hemostasis is obtained, the rectal wall defect is closed with a 2-0 Vicryl suture. **B,** Beginning at the most proximal aspect of the defect, the full-thickness rectal wall is reapproximated in a running fashion. The sutures are locked to provide better hemostasis, and the suture is tied just before the end of the defect is reached, leaving a small opening to allow drainage.

PEARLS AND PITFALLS

Preoperative	■ It is often more difficult to obtain adequate exposure in obese patients because of body habitus. Take extra time retracting the buttocks laterally with tape for prone cases, as well as using a Lone star retractor to help evert the anus and create better exposure. ■ High recurrence rates occur with lesions greater than T2 or other aggressive pathology (PNI, LVI). Re-review the pathology to ensure the lesion is appropriate for TAE.

Intraoperative	■ Avoid retractors that "push" the lesion away and use sutures if necessary to help bring the lesion more distal. ■ Avoid grasping the typically friable mass but instead use sutures to provide traction. ■ Place marking sutures early to avoid losing specimen orientation. ■ Full-thickness excision is confirmed by identification of perirectal fat. Pay special attention not to perform a partial-thickness excision. ■ Excision of anterior lesions run the risk of injury to the vagina or prostate. ■ Defects, especially when posterior, may be left open without reapproximating the rectal wall.
Postoperative	■ A consistent and aggressive bowel regimen is most important to prevent suture line disruption and keep the patient comfortable.

POSTOPERATIVE CARE

■ Patients usually have minimal, if any, pain immediately after a TAE. Patients may have spasms of the anal sphincter that can be treated symptomatically with muscle relaxants, but these are typically self-limited.

■ Patients, especially men, may have urinary retention postoperatively, which requires discharge home with a temporary urinary catheter.

■ Because of the fresh suture line, it is important that the patient be placed on an aggressive bowel regimen postoperatively to prevent suture line disruption. This should include a combination of stool softeners and fiber bulking agents, as well as mineral oil to lubricate the stool. Using such a bowel regimen will increase the postoperative comfort for the patient as well.

OUTCOMES

■ Five-year survival rates after TAE for patients with a T1 rectal cancer without nodal metastasis, LVI, and PNI are comparable with surgical resection and range from 70% to 87% for TAE compared with 80% to 93% for standard surgical resection. A retrospective study of 268 patients who underwent TAE or TME found that 10-year cancer-specific survival in the TAE and TME groups was not significantly different (98% vs 100%).[12]

■ Local recurrence rates have been shown to be statistically higher when TAE is performed vs standard surgical resection with local recurrence rates of 6% to 12.5% after TAE vs 2% to 7% after standard resection.

■ A prospective observational study across 282 hospitals found that, in comparison with radical resection, local resection was associated with lower postoperative complications but a significantly higher 5-year local tumor recurrence rate than did those who underwent radical resection. Tumor-free survival did not differ between the two groups.[13-15]

■ Salvage surgery in the form of a standard resection (low anterior or abdominoperineal resection) can be performed in cases of tumor recurrence after TAE, but R0 resection rates are typically low and survival is poor unless immediate salvage is performed at the time of recurrence diagnosis.[16]

■ Treatment of T2 lesions with TAE is still controversial. A recent multicenter, randomized trial to compare local excision with total mesorectal excision in downstaged low rectal cancer (GRECCAR 2), 148 patients 18 years and older with T2 low rectal cancer, of maximum size 4 cm, who were clinically good responders after chemoradiotherapy (residual tumor ≤2 cm) were randomly assigned before surgery to either local excision or total mesorectal excision. There was no difference between the local excision and total mesorectal excision groups in 5-year local recurrence (7% [95% confidence interval (CI) 3-16] vs 7% [3-16]; $p = .60$), metastatic disease (18% [CI 11-30] vs 19% [11-31]; $p = .73$), overall survival (84% [73-91] vs 82% [71-90]; $p = .85$), disease-free survival (70% [58-79] vs 72% [60-82]; $p = .68$), or cancer-specific mortality (7% [3-17] vs 10% [5-20]; $p = .53$). More data are still needed to support the local excision of T2 lesions but may be warranted in patients with multiple comorbidities who are unable to tolerate a larger surgical resection.[17-19]

■ TAE for the treatment of T3 lesions is not considered standard of care. There are case reports of successful outcomes using TAE for locally advanced tumors after downstaging with neoadjuvant chemoradiation therapy. Further prospective evaluation is needed to establish patient/pathologic criteria that will predict for successful outcome using TAE in more advanced tumors.

COMPLICATIONS

■ Bleeding
■ Infection/pelvic sepsis
■ Injury to the prostate or vagina for anteriorly located lesions
■ Pain (if resection involves the dentate line) or from postoperative scarring
■ Stenosis of the anus or rectum
■ Incontinence
■ Urinary retention

ALTERNATIVE SURGICAL STRATEGIES

■ TEM is a technique developed by Professor Gerhard Buess in the 1980s that allows for excision of rectal lesions with the use of instrumentation to maintain a stable pneumorectum. A retrospective study on patients with stage pT1 and pT2 rectal adenocarcinoma who underwent local excision from 1997 through mid-2006 compared TAE with TEM and found that, while the TEM patients less often had positive surgical margins, for patients with tumors ≥5 cm from the anal verge (AV), the estimated 5-year disease-free survival rate was similar between the TEM group (84.1%) and the TAE group (76.1%) ($p = .651$), and 40% of patients in the TAE group had lesions within 5 cm of the AV compared with only 2% in the TEM group ($p = .0001$), suggesting that TAE may be the preferred technique for lesions in the distal rectum likely secondary to difficulties maintaining pneumorectum.[20] Moreover, TEM has some disadvantages, such as the need for special equipment, expensive cost, and a steep learning curve that are not necessarily limitations in the TAE approach.[21]

- An alternative approach to proximal lesions is TAMIS, first described in 2010, useful for resection of proximal to mid-rectal lesions that are benign, early-stage malignancy, or with a noncurative intent in patients with advanced disease who are not candidates for radical surgery. Some of the advantages of TAMIS over TEM include rapid setup time, 360° vs 220° of visibility within the rectal lumen, the ability to universally adapt to any existing laparoscopic instrument, and the ease of lithotomy positioning within the operating theater (ie, better airway control).[22] In a recent retrospective study of patients with clinical T2 rectal cancer within 7 cm of the AV who received preoperative chemoradiotherapy followed by either TAE or TAMIS, 3-year local recurrence-free survival and disease free-survival were 100.0% and 97.1%, respectively.[23]

REFERENCES

1. National Comprehensive Cancer Network. Rectal Cancer (Version 1.2021). https://www.nccn.org/professionals/physician_gls/PDF/rectal.pdf
2. Christoforidis D, Cho HM, Dixon MR, Mellgren AF, Madoff RD, Finne CO. Transanal endoscopic microsurgery versus conventional transanal excision for patients with early rectal cancer. *Ann Surg.* 2009;249(5):776-782.
3. deBeche-Adams T, Nassif G. Transanal minimally invasive surgery. *Clin Colon Rectal Surg.* 2015;28(3):176-180.
4. Blumberg D, Paty PB, Guillem JG, et al. All patients with small intramural rectal cancers are at risk for lymph node metastasis. *Dis Colon Rectum.* 1999;42:881-885.
5. Endreseth BH, Myrvold HE, Romundstad P, et al. Transanal excision vs. major surgery for T1 rectal cancer. *Dis Colon Rectum.* 2005;48(7):1380-1388. Folkesson J, Johansson R, Pahlman L, et al. Population-based study of local surgery for rectal cancer. *Br J Surg.* 2007;94(11):1421-1426.
6. Hwang Y, Yoon YS, Bong JW, et al. Long-term transanal excision outcomes in patients with T1 rectal cancer: comparative analysis of radical resection. *Ann Coloproctol.* 2019;35(4):194-201.
7. Hahnloser D, Wolff BG, Larson DW, et al. Immediate radical resection after local excision of rectal cancer: an oncologic compromise? *Dis Colon Rectum.* 2005;48(3):429-437.
8. Ptok H, Marusch F, Meyer F, et al. Oncological outcome of local vs radical resection of low-risk pT1 rectal cancer. *Arch Surg.* 2007;142(7):649-655.
9. Kwok H, Bissett IP, Hill GL. Preoperative staging of rectal cancer. *Int J Colorectal Dis.* 2000;15:9-20.
10. Sitzler PJ, Seow-Choen F, Ho YH, et al. Lymph node involvement and tumor depth in rectal cancers: an analysis of 805 patients. *Dis Colon Rectum.* 1997;40:1472-1476.
11. Bipat S, Glas AS, Slors FJ, Zwinderman AH, Bossuyt PM, Stoker J. Rectal cancer: local staging and assessment of lymph node involvement with endoluminal US, CT, and MR imaging—a meta-analysis. *Radiology.* 2004;232(3):773-783.
12. Nash GM, Weiser MR, Guillem JG, et al. Long-term survival after transanal excision of T1 rectal cancer. *Dis Colon Rectum.* 2009;52(4):577-582.
13. Weiser MR, Landmann RG, Wong WD, et al. Surgical salvage of recurrent rectal cancer after transanal excision. *Dis Colon Rectum.* 2005;48(6):1169-1175.
14. Callender GG, Das P, Rodriguez-Bigas MA, et al. Local excision after preoperative chemoradiation results in an equivalent outcome to total mesorectal excision in selected patients with T3 rectal cancer. *Ann Surg Oncol.* 2010;17(2):441-447.
15. Garcia-Aguilar J, Shi Q, Thomas CR Jr, et al. A phase II trial of neoadjuvant chemoradiation and local excision for T2N0 rectal cancer: preliminary results of the ACOSOG Z6041 trial. *Ann Surg Oncol.* 2012;19(2):384-391.
16. Habr-Gama A, Perez RO, Nadalin W, et al. Operative versus nonoperative treatment for stage 0 distal rectal cancer following chemoradiation therapy: long-term results. *Ann Surg.* 2004;240(4):711-717.
17. You YN, Baxter NN, Stewar A, et al. Is the increasing rate of local excision for stage I rectal cancer in the United States justified? a nationwide cohort study from the National Cancer Database. *Ann Surg.* 2007;245(5):726-733.
18. Clancy C, Burke JP, Albert MR, O'Connell PR, Winter DC. Transanal endoscopic microsurgery versus standard transanal excision for the removal of rectal neoplasms: a systematic review and meta-analysis. *Dis Colon Rectum.* 2015;58(2):254-261.
19. Rullier E, Vendrely V, Asselineau J, et al. Organ preservation with chemoradiotherapy plus local excision for rectal cancer: 5-year results of the GRECCAR 2 randomised trial. *Lancet Gastroenterol Hepatol.* 2020;5(5):465-474.
20. Caycedo-Marulanda A, Jiang HY, Kohtakangas EL. Transanal minimally invasive surgery for benign large rectal polyps and early malignant rectal cancers: experience and outcomes from the first Canadian centre to adopt the technique. *Can J Surg.* 2017;60(6):416-423.
21. Lee TG, Lee SJ. Transanal single-port microsurgery for rectal tumors: minimal invasive surgery under spinal anesthesia. *Surg Endosc.* 2014;28:271-280.
22. Brodsky JT, Richard GK, Cohen AM, et al. Variables correlated with the risk of lymph node metastasis in early rectal cancer. *Cancer.* 1992;69:322-326.
23. Shin YS, Yoon YS, Lim SB, et al. Preoperative chemoradiotherapy followed by local excision in clinical T2N0 rectal cancer. *Radiat Oncol J.* 2016;34(3):177-185.

Chapter 43

Transanal Minimally Invasive Surgery for Rectal Lesions

Avo Artinyan and Daniel Albo

DEFINITION

- Transanal minimally invasive surgery (TAMIS) refers to a modification of transanal endoscopic microsurgery (TEM) which utilizes disposal multiport access devices in the place of a traditional nondisposable operating proctoscope. Other terms such as SILS-TEM have been used in the past, but have now been largely abandoned in favor of TAMIS.
- TEM refers to an approach for the local excision of lesions in the mid- to upper rectum described by Buess et al,[1] using a relatively large nondisposable operating proctoscope combined with either a stereoscopic telescope or a fiberoptic endoscope.
- TAMIS has largely replaced TEM due to the simplicity and low cost of multiport rectal access devices and the ability to incorporate widely available, traditional laparoscopic instrumentation.
- TAMIS and TEM both improve upon and complement the traditional Parks transanal excision (TAE) technique,[2] which describes the excision of low rectal lesions under direct vision with the aid of transanal retractors and standard surgical instruments. While TAE is appropriate for low rectal lesions, TAMIS is more suited for the excision of mid and upper rectal lesions.
- TAMIS is notably distinct from endoscopic mucosal resection (EMR) and other techniques that rely on flexible gastrointestinal endoscopes.
- The advantages associated with TAMIS and local excision in general vs radical surgery include lower morbidity, less pain, shorter operating times, shorter hospital stays, better functional outcomes, and avoidance of permanent colostomy.

DIFFERENTIAL DIAGNOSIS

- TAMIS can be used to treat a wide variety of both malignant and benign rectal conditions, including but not limited to large rectal adenomas, early rectal cancers, neuroendocrine tumors, gastrointestinal stromal tumors, endometriomas, and rectal strictures.
- These lesions encompass a wide variety of pathophysiologic entities with many common underlying complaints that alert the clinician to pathology within the distal large bowel and rectum.
- TAMIS can serve as both a diagnostic procedure and an effective therapeutic procedure in the appropriate setting.

PATIENT HISTORY AND PHYSICAL FINDINGS

- Patients with rectal lesions (for example, rectal polyps and rectal cancers) generally present with clinically evident or occasionally occult rectal bleeding. Those with early or small lesions may be completely asymptomatic with rectal pathology discovered on screening colonoscopy.

- A thorough history and physical examination should be performed, important components of which include the following:
  - Presence of *rectal pain and/or tenesmus*, which can often alert the surgeon to a more extensive lesion with sphincter/levator ani involvement
  - Presence of *obstructive symptoms*
  - Description of *anorectal function*, with any fecal incontinence or leakage documented preoperatively
  - *Urinary and erectile function*, with dysfunction documented preoperatively
  - A *detailed oncologic history* including both personal and family history of colorectal cancer, other malignancies, and hereditary cancer/polyposis syndromes
- Physical examination should include the following:
  - *Routine abdominal examination*, with particular attention to the presence of any surgical incisions, which may become pertinent should laparoscopy or laparotomy be necessary
  - *Digital rectal examination* with gross assessment of sphincter function and attention to palpable masses
  - *Bilateral inguinal nodal examination* for clinically evident nodal metastases
  - *Rigid proctoscopy by the surgeon* to define the anatomic parameters of the lesion
- Rigid proctoscopic examination is the most critical portion of the physical examination and is the key to proper selection of patients for TAMIS. Examination should be standardized and should document the following findings:
  - The distal and proximal extent of the lesion measured from the *anal verge*
  - Position of the lesion within the circumference of the rectum (anterior, posterior, or lateral)
  - Total circumference of the rectal wall involved by the lesion

IMAGING AND OTHER DIAGNOSTIC STUDIES

- A *complete colonoscopy* should be performed on all patients preoperatively. In the setting of possible colorectal neoplastic disease, the location of all polyps should be described, and all suspicious lesions should be endoscopically excised or biopsied if excision is not feasible. Lesions that are unresectable or are suspicious for invasive adenocarcinoma should be tattooed to facilitate resection if necessary in the future.
- For all suspicious rectal lesions (≤15 cm from anal verge on rigid proctoscopy), locoregional staging with *endorectal ultrasound* or *rectal protocol magnetic resonance imaging* should be performed to define the depth of the lesion (T stage) and possible nodal involvement (N stage).
- With all suspected or confirmed colorectal neoplastic disease, *complete staging computed tomography* (CT) *of the*

chest, abdomen, and pelvis should be performed to rule out metastatic disease.

- *Positron emission tomography/CT* should be used selectively for patients with suspected metastatic disease or those who are poor candidates for intravenous (IV) contrast secondary to renal insufficiency or contrast allergy.
- *Anal physiologic studies with manometry* should be strongly considered for patients with preoperative symptoms and signs of fecal incontinence to document preoperative sphincter function.

SURGICAL MANAGEMENT

Indications for Transanal Endoscopy Microsurgery

- *Large rectal polyps not amenable to colonoscopic resection* (usually sessile adenomatous polyps)
- *Rectal adenocarcinoma*: The indications for the local excision of rectal adenocarcinoma continue to evolve and have broadened with the completion of multidisciplinary trials such as the American College of Surgeons Oncology Group (ACOSOG) Z6041 trial. Because TAMIS is used to excise local disease and does not adequately address nodal disease, the degree to which the procedure is appropriate and successful is directly proportional to the likelihood of nodal metastases. In the combined literature, the risk of nodal disease is best predicted by T stage and is on the order of 5% to 10% for T1 lesions, 15% to 25% for T2 disease, and 35% to 75% for T3 disease. Other pathologic factors, such as lymphovascular invasion, are also useful in predicting risk of nodal disease and recurrence, and these are potentially applicable for patient selection (**TABLE 1**). *The desire to perform/undergo a minimally invasive procedure* should not supplant sound oncologic principles.
  - *Low-risk T1 disease*: Definitive therapy for rectal cancer should be reserved only for patients with low-risk T1 disease. This is also the current position of the National Comprehensive Cancer Network (NCCN).
  - *High-risk T1 or any T2 disease with combination therapy*: Multidisciplinary therapy with preoperative chemoradiation and TAMIS is a reasonable alternative for patients with high-risk T1 or T2 disease based on the results of the ACOSOG Z6041 trial. The risks and benefits of TAMIS vs radical resection need to be carefully discussed with the patient, particularly with respect to the higher risk of locoregional recurrence with local excision.
  - Lesions of any stage, technically amenable to TAMIS, in *patients who refuse radical resection*, appropriate discussion, and consent must be documented.
  - Lesions of any stage, technically amenable to TAMIS, for *palliative purposes*

- More recently we have used TAMIS as an alternative to "watch and wait" for locally advanced rectal cancers that have had a clinical complete or near complete response after preoperative therapy. We have termed this approach "excise, watch, and wait." The benefit of this approach is the ability to confirm pathologic complete response when present and decrease the risk of luminal cancer recurrence in patients with limited residual disease.
- Other *less common indications* for TAMIS include rectal carcinoids, endometriomas, angiodysplasia, rectal ulcers, rectal strictures, and other benign pathologies. We have also used TAMIS to excise anatomically favorable tailgut cysts. Just as with rectal adenocarcinoma, the decision to perform TAMIS in these settings should be based on sound clinical judgment and a thorough understanding of the anatomic limitations highlighted below.

Anatomic Considerations

- TAMIS is ideally suited for lesions whose *entire* extent falls within 5 to 15 cm from the anal verge.
  - The technical "sweet spot" for TAMIS is between 6 and 10 cm (midrectum), beyond which the surgeon has to contend with instrument limitations, diminished visualization and exposure, and the potential for peritoneal entry.
- TAMIS has been described for lesions proximal to 15 cm. However, peritoneal entry is much more likely with full-thickness excision in this setting, and appropriate expertise is required to perform an adequate and safe suture repair of the excision defect.
  - The likelihood of peritoneal entry is dependent on the circumferential location of the lesion (**TABLE 2**). For example, the mean distance to the peritoneal reflection anteriorly in men is at 9.7 cm, compared to 15.5 cm posteriorly. Dissection in the posterior midline above 15 cm is possible without frank peritoneal entry, as long as the visceral peritoneum of the rectosigmoid colon is not violated.[3]
- Lesions distal to 5 cm are usually covered in part or completely by the transanal access device. These lesions are more easily excised using conventional TAE.
- There is no absolute contraindication based on the total circumferential extent of the lesion, and complete circumferential excisions have been described. However, excision of lesions that occupy more than 40% of the circumference is technically much more challenging, may be associated with more advanced lesions, and can lead to compromised margins. Sound judgment, careful patient selection, and appropriate technical expertise are required.

Table 1: Additional Factors Associated With Increased/High Risk of Lymph Node Involvement/Local Recurrence

Poorly differentiated lesion
Lymphovascular invasion
Perineural invasion
Sm3 Kikuchi classification
Lesion diameter >4 cm

Table 2: Distance of Peritoneal Reflection From Anal Verge (Mean With Range, cm)

Location	Females	Males
Anterior	9 (5.5-13.5)	9.7 (7-16)
Lateral	12.2 (8.5-17)	12.8 (9-19)
Posterior	14.8 (11-19)	15.5 (12-20)

Adapted with permission from Najarian MM, Belzer GE, Cogbill TH, et al. Determination of the peritoneal reflection using intraoperative proctoscopy. Dis Colon Rectum. 2004;47(12):2080-2085.

Preoperative Preparation

- The key to the technical success of TAMIS is adequate visualization and exposure. As a result, preoperative mechanical bowel preparation is invaluable. We ask our patients to have a normal lunch and take a clear liquid diet with adequate hydration thereafter and nothing by mouth after midnight. We prefer a mechanical bowel preparation with two bottles of magnesium citrate in the afternoon the day before surgery, with a Fleet enema the night before and the morning of the procedure.
- In addition, we administered one dose of IV cefoxitin antibiotic within 1 hour of initiation of surgery.
- Appropriate informed consent should be obtained. In addition to the possibility of the more common complications, the consent process should address the following:
  - The potential need for reoperation based on pathologic findings (either repeat TAMIS or radical resection).
  - The likelihood of peritoneal entry for upper rectal lesions. For upper rectal lesions where peritoneal entry is a significant possibility, we routinely consent for possible laparoscopy and/or laparotomy with possible primary repair, radical resection, or ostomy.
  - Possible vaginal injury and subsequent rectovaginal fistula with anterior excisions in females.
  - Oncologic outcomes in comparison to radical resection, particularly the higher risk of locoregional recurrence with local excision.

Positioning

- Appropriate patient positioning is critical to the technical success of the procedure. Every effort should be made to position the patient such that the lesion is down at the 6 o'clock position.
- For posterior lesions, we prefer a high lithotomy position (**FIGURE 1A**).
- For anterior lesions, we prefer to place the patient in prone jackknife position on a split-leg table, with the surgeon positioned between the legs (**FIGURE 1B**).
- For lateral lesions, we place the patient in either one of the aforementioned positions and rotate the table to turn the lesion to 6 o'clock as much as possible. If the lesion cannot be placed completely down, then we have found that it is easier to perform the excision and repair when the lesion is oriented toward the dominant hand of the surgeon. The "circumferential sweet spot" for a right-handed surgeon in our experience is presented in **FIGURE 1C**.

Equipment

- Multiple transanal access platforms have been used and are appropriate for TAMIS. The standard procedure described by Parks[2] uses the operating transanal proctoscope by Wolf. Other transanal access platforms that have been used have incorporated equipment for single-incision laparoscopic surgery. These platforms have now gained US Food and Drug Administration (FDA) approval for transanal access. Although we have used a number of these systems, our preferred transanal access platform is the GelPOINT Path system manufactured by Applied Medical.
- We routinely use both standard and articulating laparoscopic instruments designed for single-incision laparoscopic surgery. In a typical case, we often use a 5-mm scope operated by the assistant, a standard Maryland grasper in the left surgeon's hand for grasping and retraction, and an articulating hook cautery or harmonic scalpel in the right surgeon's hand for excision. For repair, we use a standard laparoscopic needle driver.
- Our preferred energy sources are monopolar cautery and ultrasonic shears such as a harmonic scalpel for larger excisions.

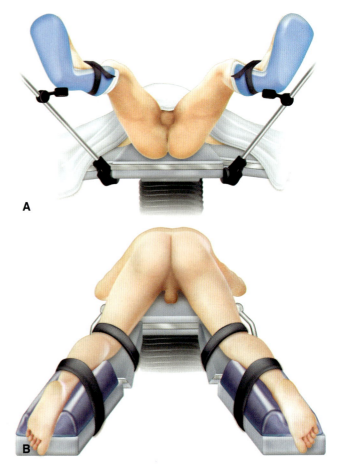

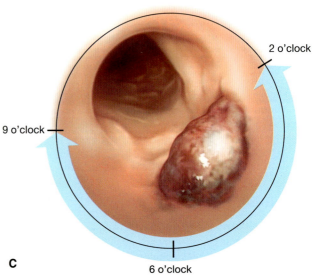

FIGURE 1 • **A,** High lithotomy position, perineal view (for posterior lesions). **B,** Modified prone jackknife on a split-leg table, posterior view, ideal for anterior lesions. **C,** Circumferential sweet spot for operative dexterity for a right-handed surgeon. Lesion, excision, and repair should ideally fall within 2 to 9 o'clock positions.

- The patient is placed under general endotracheal tube anesthesia, a Foley catheter is routinely inserted, and the patient is appropriately positioned.
- A minimal sterile preparation of the perineum is performed, and the patient is draped in standard fashion.
- We perform an intersphincteric block with 0.25% bupivacaine with epinephrine.
- The transanal access port is heavily lubricated, folded in and grasped from inside the port with a ring clamp (**FIGURE 2**), and then introduced gently into the rectum. Occasionally, gentle manual dilation of the sphincter is necessary to allow atraumatic placement of the port. We have found that the anal port naturally hugs the sphincters and stays in place and, therefore, does not routinely anchor the device with sutures.
- The instrument ports are first placed into the gel cap, and the gel cap is applied to the transanal port (**FIGURE 3**). Prior to applying the cap, we place one or two lightly lubricated Ray-Tec sponges into the rectum, which we then push into the proximal rectum in order to allow adequate insufflation of the distal rectum (**FIGURE 4**). The rectum is insufflated to 10 to 15 mm Hg as necessary.
- Placing one or more proximal Ray-Tec sponges limits the amount of insufflation to the remainder of the colon and helps maintain a clean working space free of any remnant fecal material (**FIGURE 4**).
- One of the difficulties we have found is periodic pneumorectum collapse. This can be limited by the following:
  - Inserting proximal Ray-Tecs as described earlier
  - Assuring an adequate prep, as we have noted that feculent material in the rectum and rectosigmoid will cause large bowel peristalsis
  - Avoiding excessive torque on the instruments to prevent loss of insufflation around the transanal access device
  - The use of an insufflation stabilization bag (Applied Medical)
  - Higher insufflation pressures to obtain adequate exposure
  - We do not like to use AirSeal, given the potential for distention of the proximal colon.
- The excision technique is divided into the four critical steps[4]:
  - Delineation of the excision margins (1 cm grossly in most instances) (**FIGURE 5**)
  - Full-thickness incision of the rectal wall into perirectal tissue (**FIGURE 6**)
  - Circumferential dissection and specimen removal (**FIGURE 7**)
  - Suture repair (**FIGURE 8**)
- We routinely mark 1-cm margins using a hook cautery device. These cautery marks can become extremely helpful later during the excision, particularly if visualization becomes compromised (**FIGURE 5**).
- A full-thickness incision is made 1 cm **distal** to the lesion using hook cautery, with the left hand lifting up the rectal wall to supply countertraction (**FIGURE 6**). The perirectal tissue is usually easily recognized by the presence of perirectal fat. Anteriorly the perirectal space may consist only of loose areolar tissue. This initial step must be performed with extreme caution with anterior and lateral lesions in order to prevent injury to genitourinary and vascular structures adjacent to the rectum. (Partial thickness resections can

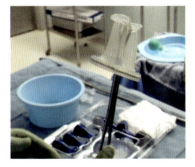

FIGURE 2 • The transanal port is folded in and grasped with ring clamps to facilitate insertion into anal canal.

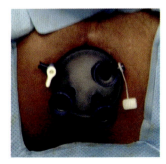

FIGURE 3 • Transanal access device with cap and ports inserted into anal canal.

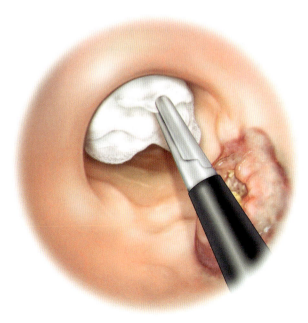

FIGURE 4 • Lightly lubricated Ray-Tec is inserted proximally to minimize proximal insufflation and limit soiling of operative field.

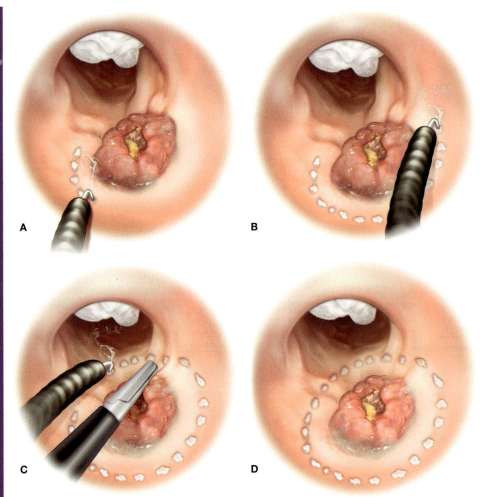

FIGURE 5 • Delineation of margins of excision, 1 cm in the majority of cases. (**A-D,** demonstrate progression of circumferential margin delineation).

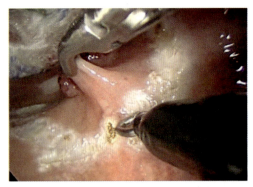

FIGURE 6 • Full-thickness incision of the rectal wall into perirectal fat.

be performed with incision and dissection in the submucosal space in a similar fashion but, in our institution, most partial thickness resections are performed endoscopically via EMR or endoscopic submucosal dissection by interventional gastroenterologists.)

- Once the perirectal space is entered, the perirectal fat is pushed away from the rectal wall with a combination of blunt and cautery dissection, and the rectal wall is progressively divided with hook cautery, hot scissors, or harmonic scalpel along the cautery line marked earlier in the case (**FIGURE 7**).
- This dissection is continued until the specimen is entirely free. Of note, the perirectal plane is *relatively* avascular, with occasional small mesorectal vessels to the rectal wall easily controlled with cautery. If the dissection does not proceed in a straightforward manner or is unusually bloody, the usual cause is dissection within an incorrect plane, or the lesion is more advanced than initially recognized.
- Once the specimen is free, the lesion is grasped, taking care to maintain appropriate orientation; the cap is lifted off the transanal access device; and the specimen is removed.
- The specimen is then properly oriented on a piece of Telfa dressing or preferably pinned to a foam needle counter with the pathologist in the room and sent for pathologic examination. Pinning the specimen allows proper assessment of the size of the margins given that there is significant contraction of the specimen after removal. Our pathologists will routinely ink and fix specimens with the pins in place. We perform frozen section examination selectively, only for suspicious margins on gross evaluation (**FIGURE 9**).

Chapter 43 TRANSANAL MINIMALLY INVASIVE SURGERY FOR RECTAL LESIONS 405

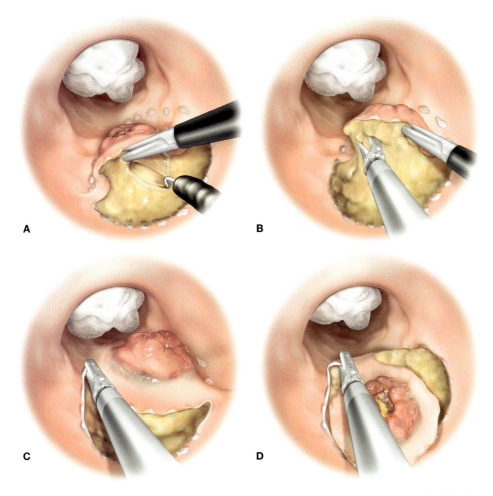

FIGURE 7 • Circumferential dissection of the lesion with 1-cm margins. The deep fat is taken with either hook cautery or harmonic scalpel. The rectal wall is then taken also with either cautery or harmonic scalpel. (**A-D,** demonstrate progression of circumferential dissection).

- Once the margins have been assessed and have been cleared, we proceed to perform a suture repair of the defect. The pneumorectum—which often exaggerates the size of the defect—can be decreased to facilitate closure. Even without this maneuver, very large defects can be reapproximated without significant difficulty.
- The defect can be repaired with a single running suture, or multiple interrupted sutures, transversely from right to left (**FIGURE 8**). Given that a single suture tends to be long and is somewhat tedious to handle in a small space, we prefer to place multiple shorter running sutures. We prefer a multifilament Vicryl suture, secured on one end with a Lapra-Ty. After running the suture for a number of throws, another Lapra-Ty is used to secure the remaining end, thus avoiding intracorporeal tying. Barbed suture (such as V-Loc™ or Quill™) can also be used. With this approach, we usually end up placing two to three running sutures to close a 180° defect.
- Once the repair is completed, the sponges are removed, the pneumorectum is released, and the transanal access device is gently pulled out. We place a rolled Gelfoam sponge soaked in lidocaine jelly into rectum. The sponge is resorbed and/or evacuated by the patient with the first postoperative bowel movement.

406 SECTION III RECTAL RESECTIONS

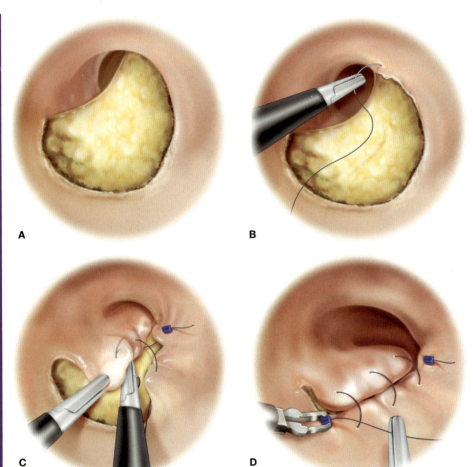

FIGURE 8 • Suture repair is completed transversely from right to left (surgeon's dominant to nondominant side). The sutures are secured on both ends with Lapra-Tys. A single running suture or two to three shorter running sutures may be used. (**A-D,** demonstrate progression of suture repair).

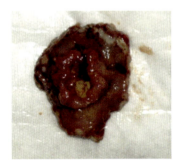

FIGURE 9 • Excised specimen is placed on Telfa, appropriately oriented and taken to pathology for gross and/or frozen examination.

PEARLS AND PITFALLS

Indications/patient selection	▪ Appropriate patient selection is critical both with respect to disease and size and location of lesion. ▪ Appropriate lesions are those 5-15 cm from anal verge, with sweet spot 6-10 cm (midrectum). ▪ Lesions >40% present a greater technical challenge, can lead to compromised margins, and may be associated with more advanced disease. ▪ Risk of peritoneal entry varies by circumferential position (anterior lesions carry the highest risk of peritoneal entry).
Positioning	▪ Always position the patient such that the lesion is down (6 o'clock). ▪ If 6 o'clock position is not completely possible, err toward surgeon's dominant hand.

Preoperative preparation	■ Adequate mechanical bowel preparation is required to facilitate visualization. ■ With poor prep, fecal material has tendency to migrate into the field.
Exposure	■ Ray-Tec sponge(s) placed proximally can limit insufflation of the proximal colon and keep the operative field clean.
Excision	■ Marking the margins with cautery and starting with a distal full-thickness incision facilitate the remainder of the dissection. ■ Harmonic scalpel is extremely useful but can cause a blanching artifact of the mucosa that can obscure the margins during dissection.
Repair	■ Defect is closed transversely from right to left using single running suture or two to three shorter running sutures. ■ Use of Lapra-Tys or barbed sutures obviates need for tying in a confined space.

POSTOPERATIVE CARE

■ For uncomplicated cases, we now routinely discharge patients home the same day after spontaneous urination.

■ If the excision is extensive or there is concern for peritoneal entry, the patient is admitted overnight for observation. In the absence of significant pain, fevers, bleeding, or urinary retention, the patient is discharged home on POD 1. If low-grade fevers are noted, CT scan examination with or without rectal contrast may be obtained to rule out inadvertent peritoneal entry or leak depending on clinical suspicion. With fevers in the absence of peritoneal leak, we have opted to use empiric antibiotics until resolution.

■ For the purposes of oncologic surveillance, given the concern for local recurrence, we survey the excision site with flexible sigmoidoscopy every 3 months for the first 6 months, then every 6 months for 2 years, followed by yearly and/or appropriate endoscopy and cancer screening, for a total of 5 years. In patients with invasive cancer, we perform CT scans of the abdomen and pelvis every 6 to 12 months for the first 3 years and then annually, for a total of 5 years, with the frequency determined by degree of suspicion.

OUTCOMES

Oncologic Outcomes

■ The oncologic success of TAMIS for rectal adenocarcinoma is dependent both on the *adequacy of technique* and on *appropriate patient selection*.
  ■ Local/locoregional recurrence is frequently the result of residual disease.
    - Luminal recurrences are likely related to residual disease at the excision site (suboptimal technique).
    - Nodal/regional recurrences are likely secondary to unrecognized nodal disease (suboptimal patient selection).
    - The risk of locoregional recurrence in low-risk T1 lesions excised with negative margins is comparable to radical resection (~5% *in most series*).
    - The risk of locoregional recurrence in unselected T1 and T2 patients is 10% or more and 30% or more, respectively, without additional therapy.[5]
    - Locoregional recurrences are usually salvageable with appropriate surveillance. Rarely salvage may entail multivisceral resection.
  ■ Overall survival with TAMIS should be comparable to radical resection in appropriately selected patients.

Complications

■ The TAMIS procedure, in large part, avoids the most severe complications of radical resection, including superficial and deep surgical site infections; anastomotic leaks; ventral hernia; postoperative bowel obstruction; and functional complications such as erectile dysfunction, urinary retention, and fecal incontinence.

■ The risk of operative mortality is significantly lower than that of radical surgery and is less than 1% in major series.

■ The risk of minor morbidity is less than 15% in most large series, with the risk of major morbidity of less than 5%.

■ Specific perioperative complications are as follows:
  ■ *Bleeding*: Postoperative bleeding is usually self-limited, with an infrequent need for transfusions. In a minority of cases, transanal or endoscopic ligation/cauterization may be necessary, with a very small likelihood of laparotomy and anterior resection.
  ■ *Functional complications*: Urinary retention and anal incontinence occur relatively infrequently and, in almost all cases, are transient. A brief period of anal leakage is often associated with traction injury from the transanal access device and usually resolves completely within a few months.
  ■ *Suture dehiscence*: Dehiscence can occur in approximately 15% of patients.
    - Most dehiscences of the extraperitoneal rectum are likely subclinical.
    - Suture dehiscences of the extraperitoneal rectum may present clinically with fevers or, in the case of large excisions, close to the anal sphincters, pain, and transient fecal incontinence.
    - Nonoperative management is the norm with antibiotics and expectant management. Attempts at closure almost always result in repeat dehiscence. We prefer to admit these patients initially for workup and to rule out progression of pelvic infection and discharge them on antibiotics when stable. Signs of progressive sepsis should prompt workup for abscess or peritoneal leak.
    - Most symptoms will resolve in approximately 4 to 6 weeks. In rare instances, laparoscopic or open abdominal exploration with fecal diversion may be necessary.

- **Peritoneal entry**: Unintended peritoneal entry is more common with anterior and lateral lesions and more common with upper rectal lesions. In most instances, this is recognized intraoperatively and can be managed with transanal suture repair. With high upper rectal lesions, peritoneal entry may be planned and, in this setting, should not be considered a complication. Significant expertise is required to perform an airtight repair, as suture dehiscence in this location will almost always lead to peritoneal soiling and peritonitis, necessitating abdominal exploration with repair, resection, or fecal diversion.
- **Rectal stricture**: The risk of stricture long term is less than 5% for primary excisions.
- Relatively rare complications include intraoperative injury to genitourinary structures; rectovaginal, rectourethral, and rectovesical fistulae; complications related to positioning; and medical complications not related to the technical portion of the procedure, such as *Clostridium difficile infection* and anesthetic complications.

REFERENCES

1. Buess G, Hutterer F, Theiss J, et al. A system for a transanal endoscopic rectum operation [in German]. *Chirurg.* 1984;55(10):677-680.
2. Parks AG. A technique for the removal of large villous tumours in the rectum. *Proc R Soc Med.* 1970;63:89-91.
3. Najarian MM, Belzer GE, Cogbill TH, et al. Determination of the peritoneal reflection using intraoperative proctoscopy. *Dis Colon Rectum.* 2004;47(12):2080-2085.
4. Smith RA, Anaya DA, Albo D, et al. A stepwise approach to transanal endoscopic microsurgery for rectal cancer using a single-incision laparoscopic port. *Ann Surg Oncol.* 2012;19(9):2859.
5. Garcia-Aguilar J, Mellgren A, Sirivongs P, et al. Local excision of rectal cancer without adjuvant therapy: a word of caution. *Ann Surg.* 2000;231(3):345-351.

Chapter 44

Laparoscopic Diverting Colostomies: Formation and Reversal

Jayson Moloney, David Graham Taylor, and Andrew RL Stevenson

DEFINITION

A colostomy is a surgically created communication through the body wall between the colon and the skin. There are several different kinds of colostomies, including the following:

- End colostomy: a colostomy in which a divided end of colon passes through the stomal trephine to open externally with a circumferential colocutaneous anastomosis (**FIGURE 1A**). A stomal trephine is a surgically created defect through layers of abdominal wall through which the colon passes to the external opening.
- Double-barreled colostomy: a colostomy in which two divided ends of colon pass through the stomal trephine to open externally, each via a circumferential anastomosis (**FIGURE 1B**).
- Loop colostomy: a colostomy in which a loop of colon passes through the stomal trephine to open externally via a colocutaneous anastomosis. A variable portion (usually 50%-75% of the circumference) of the antimesenteric colonic wall is opened for colocutaneous anastomosis, and the remainder of the colonic wall remains in continuity (**FIGURE 1C**).
- Tube colostomy: a colostomy in which a prosthetic tube passes from the colonic lumen through the abdominal wall to open externally.

PATIENT HISTORY AND PHYSICAL FINDINGS

General

- Diverting colostomies may be temporary or permanent. The possibility and likelihood of a stoma reversal must be taken into consideration prior to its formation.
- Whether creating or reversing a colostomy, detailed knowledge of the indication for colostomy is paramount. Diverting colostomies may be indicated by any combination of distally located pathology (ie, malignancy, obstruction, sepsis, fistula, inflammatory bowel disease), functional disorders (ie, pelvic floor or anal sphincter dysfunction), or recent or concurrent surgical procedure.

Formation

- Patient factors such as age, gender, body habitus, current medical comorbidities, and previous medical and surgical conditions along with psychological, social, and cultural issues must be elicited and taken into consideration.
- Physical examination primarily focused on the patient's body habitus, abdominal contour, and presence of abdominal scars is important in the consideration of the type and site of the stoma to be formed.

Closure

- Prior to embarking on reversal of colostomies, detailed knowledge is needed of the stoma creation and other operative procedures. Details such as type of stoma, resection of colon, peritoneal contamination, mobilization of splenic flexure, and marking of distal colon or rectum with a nonabsorbable suture are helpful in the operative planning process. In addition, up-to-date knowledge of the original pathology or indication necessitating formation of the stoma in the first instance is essential.

IMAGING AND OTHER DIAGNOSTIC STUDIES

- Whether creating or reversing a colostomy, preoperative investigation will be directed toward the underlying condition necessitating fecal diversion to exclude pathology proximal and/or distal to the actual or intended colostomy site.
- Unrecognized Crohn colitis, ileocolonic strictures, synchronous tumors, or other pathology may result in stomal complications or failure.

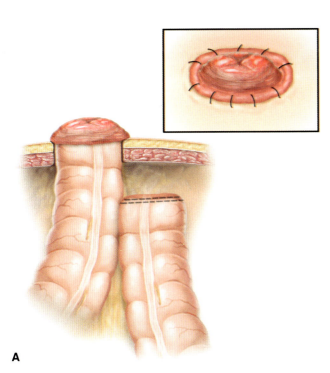

A

FIGURE 1 • **A,** End colostomy. **B,** Double-barreled colostomy. **C,** Loop colostomy.

409

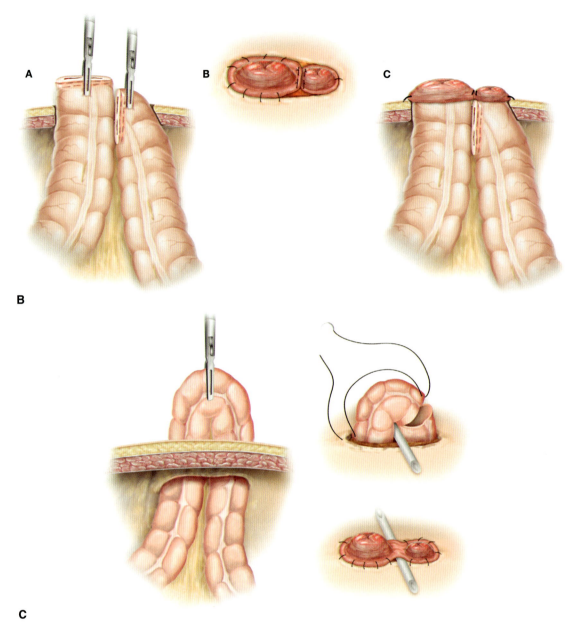

FIGURE 1 • Continued

- Colonoscopy, computed tomography (CT) scan, and/or colonic transit studies may help plan the type and site of stoma formation.

SURGICAL MANAGEMENT
Preoperative Planning

- It is critical to determine preoperatively which section of colon is to be used and if an end, double-barreled, or loop colostomy is to be formed.
- In the setting of proximal diversion for distal pathology, we prefer to use the sigmoid colon. Should this not be possible, we often opt for a diverting loop ileostomy. Alternatively, a transverse colostomy is an adequate option.

- The decision-making process regarding formation of an end, double-barreled, or loop colostomy is more complex and is illustrated in **TABLE 1**.
- Preoperative assessment and education, as well as preoperative stoma marking by an experienced stomal practitioner in conjunction with the surgeon, is highly recommended.
- Identifying the optimal stomal site should involve assessment of the patient standing, sitting, and supine. Factors involved in stomal site assessment are also listed in **TABLE 1**.

Perioperative Care

- Deep vein thrombosis (DVT) prophylaxis is recommended in the form of antithromboembolic compression stockings, sequential compression devices, and/or prophylactic heparin or low-molecular-weight heparin.

- A single 2-g dose of Cefoxitin is administered prior to incision unless contraindicated.

Patient Positioning

- For creation of sigmoid colostomy and reversal of end colostomy, the patient is positioned in a modified Lloyd–Davies position (**FIGURE 2A**) on a nonslip pressure area care mat. The right upper limb is secured in the neutral position by the patient's side padded to protect potential pressure points. Patients are prepped with an aseptic solution and draped with legging drapes and an under-buttock drape followed by square draping to expose the entire anterior and lateral abdominal wall.
- For creation of a transverse colostomy, and for the reversal of loop or double-barreled sigmoid colostomies, the patient is positioned supine, with the arms secured in the neutral position by the patient's side padded to protect potential pressure points (**FIGURE 2B**). For patients in the supine position, standard square draping is adequate.
- Bladder decompression with a urinary catheter is not necessary except for closure of end sigmoid colostomy.
- Gastric decompression with an orogastric tube, which is to be removed prior to completion of the general anesthetic, is used.
- The laparoscopic equipment is assembled with all cords and tubes exiting/entering the sterile field over the right side of the patient's chest.

Laparoscopic Equipment

- We prefer 5-mm balloon-tipped clear ports, except for a 12-mm balloon-tipped port used through the stomal site, and a nonballoon port for optical entry.
- We use a 5-mm 0° camera for insufflation-assisted optical entry into the peritoneal cavity and a 5-mm 30° camera at all other times.
- Monopolar diathermy attached to laparoscopic scissors is adequate in almost all laparoscopic techniques described in this chapter. Advanced energy devices are reserved for difficult dissections and for the closure of end colostomies. For intracorporeal stapling and dividing, we use 60-mm reticulating linear endostaplers with 1.8 mm closed staple height for division of colon and 1.2-mm cartridge for division of mesentery.
- For extracorporeal stapling and dividing, we use 75- to 80-mm linear staplers with 1.8 mm closed staple height for colonic division, 1.5 mm closed staple height for the longitudinal staple line of double-stapled side-to-side anastomosis, and 1.8 mm closed staple height for the transverse staple line of double-stapled side-to-side anastomosis.

Table 1: Decision Making Regarding Stoma Site and Type

Stoma position	Preferable: readily visible, accessible, and transrectus Avoid: skin creases, belt lines, scars/incisions, hernia, and bony prominences; lateral ostomies may interfere with arm motion while walking.
Sigmoid colostomy	Ideal site: LLQ, transrectus at a point one-third the distance between the umbilicus and the ASIS.
Transverse colostomy	Ideal site: RUQ, transrectus at a point one-third from the distance between the umbilicus and the junction of the costal margin and midclavicular line.
Stoma type	End colostomy: preferable for permanent stomas. Technically easier to construct and associated with a reduced complication rate. Advantageous in the difficult-to-construct stoma (eg, the obese abdomen). Double-barreled colostomy: usually reserved for stomas constructed during an operation in which a segment of colon has been resected and an anastomosis was not undertaken, but subsequent reversal is likely. Loop colostomy: preferable for temporary stomas and/or when there is distal obstruction
Obese patients	Consider an end colostomy. Division of the colon and part of the mesentery will give more length and allow easier passage of the stoma through the ST. Consider siting the stoma in the upper abdomen where there is thinner abdominal wall. (The lower abdomen adiposity is most pendulous.) Visualization and therefore appliance manipulation is compromised if the stoma is situated on the underside of an adipose roll or pendulous abdomen.

ASIS, anterosuperior iliac spine.

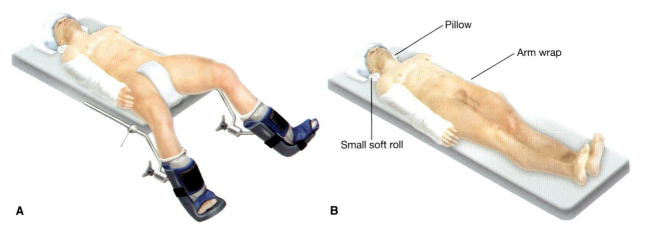

FIGURE 2 • **A**, Patient positioning: laparoscopic formation of sigmoid colostomy and laparoscopic reversal of end sigmoid colostomy. The patient is placed on a modified Lloyd-Davies position, with the legs on stirrups and the arms tucked to the side. All pressure points are padded to prevent neurovascular injuries. **B**, Patient positioning (lap formation of transverse colostomy).

Surgical Team Positioning

- Five surgical team configurations are described in this chapter (**FIGURE 3**).
- Configuration 1. The operating surgeon stands to the patient's left side, with the surgical assistant to the patient's right side and the instrument nurse adjacent to the patient's right knee.
- Configuration 2. The operating surgeon stands adjacent to the patient's right side with their right hand dissecting with the dissecting instrument via the right lower quadrant (RLQ) or suprapubic (SP) port and with their left hand using a bowel grasper via right upper quadrant (RUQ) port. The assistant stands to the surgeon's left side, with the camera in their right hand via the midline (ML) port and the bowel grasper via the stomal trephine (ST) or left lateral (LL) port site. The instrument nurse is adjacent to the patient's right knee. The monitor is placed adjacent to patient's left hip.
- Configuration 3. The operating surgeon stands to the patient's right side, with the dissecting energy device in their right hand via the ST or LL port and a bowel grasper in their left hand via the RUQ port. The assistant stands to the surgeon's left side, with the camera in their right hand via ML port site. The instrument nurse or a second assistant stands between the patient's lower limbs with a bowel grasper on their right or left hand via the RLQ port site. The monitor is placed adjacent to left side of the patient's chest.
- Configuration 4. The operating surgeon stands to the patient's right side with the assistant to the patient's left side and the instrument nurse adjacent to the patient's right knee.
- Configuration 5. The operating surgeon stands to the patient's left side, with the dissecting energy device in their right hand via the LUQ port and the bowel grasper in their left hand via ST port (three-port transverse colostomy formation technique) or via the left lower quadrant (LLQ) port (four-port transverse colostomy formation technique). The assistant stands to the surgeon's left side with the camera in their right hand via the ML port and bowel grasper in their left hand via the ST port. The instrument nurse stands adjacent to the patient's right knee. The monitor is placed adjacent to the right side of the patient's chest.

Port Placement

- Port placement planning and marking is important. The key to port placement is the RLQ port. The RLQ, RUQ, and ML ports should be placed a hand's breadth distance from each other.

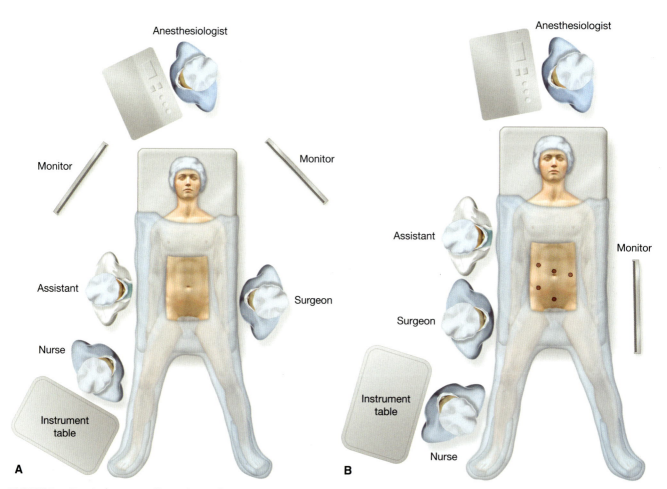

FIGURE 3 • Surgical team configuration and port placement. **A**, Configuration 1. **B**, Configuration 2. **C**, Configuration 3. **D**, Configuration 4. **E**, Configuration 5.

Chapter 44 **LAPAROSCOPIC DIVERTING COLOSTOMIES: FORMATION AND REVERSAL** 413

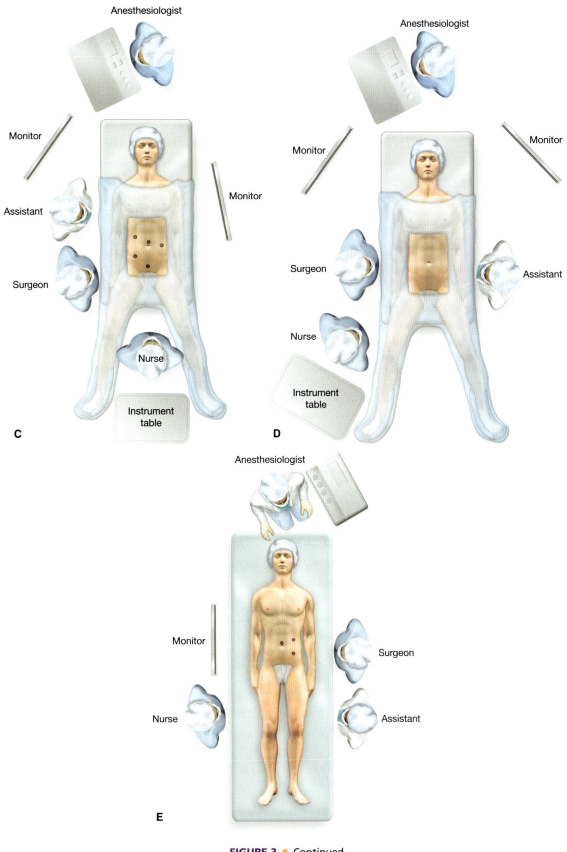

FIGURE 3 • Continued

414 SECTION III **RECTAL RESECTIONS**

- The RLQ port (5 mm) is inserted medial to, and at or just cranial to the level of the anterior superior iliac spine, just lateral to the path of the inferior epigastric vessels.
- The RUQ port (5 mm) is inserted a hand's breadth cranially along a craniocaudal line from the RLQ port.
- The ML port (5 mm) is placed via a small incision in the umbilicus or supraumbilically in obese patients with pendulous abdomens.

- The LL port (5 mm) is placed as laterally as possible at the level of the ML port. This port is optional, especially when the ST is created as the first step.
- The ST port (5 or 12 mm) is placed at the preoperatively marked stoma site. If an endoscopic linear stapler is to be used, a 12-mm port is mandatory.

LAPAROSCOPIC FORMATION OF SIGMOID COLOSTOMY

Creation of the Stomal Trephine and Port Insertion

- When sure about the need of a colostomy, we prefer to create the ST as the first step before the contour and layers of the abdominal wall have been altered by a pneumoperitoneum or surgical incisions.
- Using surgical team configuration 1 as previously described, a disc of skin at the preoperatively marked site is excised. Dissection through the subcutaneous adipose tissue proceeds to the anterior rectus sheath.
- The anterior rectus sheath is incised longitudinally enough to safely allow subsequent passage of the sigmoid colon but not excessive such that the patient is subjected to an unacceptably high risk of development of a parastomal hernia. The rectus muscle fibers are separated longitudinally.
- A small (<1 cm) incision is made in the posterior rectus sheath. The peritoneum is grasped and incised. A 5- or 12-mm balloon port is inserted via the peritoneal defect. A 12-mm Hg pneumoperitoneum is insufflated.
- A 5-mm 30° high-definition laparoscope is inserted.
- If unsure about the need of a colostomy, we delay formation of the ST until a later stage of the procedure. In these cases, we insufflate the pneumoperitoneum using a 5-mm insufflation-assisted optical entry port via the RUQ.

Lateral to Medial Colon Mobilization

- Configuration 2 is used. The operating table is placed in a Trendelenburg position rotated with the right side down.
- The bowel grasper in the surgeon's left hand retracts the rectosigmoid junction medially and cranially. The assistant's left-hand grasper may retract the proximal sigmoid colon or provide countertraction to the lateral wall of the pelvic brim.
- Dissection begins at the pelvic brim. The sigmoid is mobilized from lateral attachments (**FIGURE 4A**). The dissection proceeds in a lateral-to-medial direction toward the apex of the sigmoid mesentery.
- At this stage, the left ureter and gonadal vessels should be identified and preserved intact in the retroperitoneum (**FIGURE 4B**). As the mobilization of the sigmoid and descending colon mesentery continues proximally, anterior to the ureter and gonadal vessels, it is often advantageous to use configuration 3. The grasper held by the instrument nurse/second assistant retracts the colon distal to that retracted surgeon's left-hand grasper. The sigmoid and descending mesentery should be mobilized to the midline.

- When retracting the left colon during mobilization, it is useful to initially retract anteriorly and then medially. This ensures the colon acts as a "drape," eliminating the small bowel from the field of view.
- The extent of descending colon mobilization should be tailored to the patient. It is not usually necessary to fully mobilize the splenic flexure from its attachments, although a limited mobilization is sometimes helpful to avoid a retracted stoma, especially in the acute setting where a degree of edema, bowel dilatation, or mesocolic foreshortening exists. Generally, we recommend "overmobilization" to avoid undue tension. Inadequate mobilization at this stage will result in subsequent difficulty and frustration during passage of the colon through the ST and stomal maturation, resulting in a traumatized and often retracted stoma.

Sigmoid Colon Delivery Through Stomal Trephine

- Surgical team configuration 2 is used. The sigmoid colon is assessed to select the optimal segment for stomal formation (most often it is the sigmoid apex). Maximum mobility from proximal and distal colon and the mesentery and proximity to the intended stomal site are the most significant factors in this selection.
- If an end colostomy is planned, intracorporeal division of the colon with a stapler may be performed now (see "Colostomy Creation—End Colostomy").
- A stoma may become obstructed or ischemic unless correct orientation is ensured, without twisting. Correct orientation is confirmed, and the intended segment is grasped with a locking bowel grasper via the ST port. While marking of the bowel intracorporeally (using diathermy, sutures or clips) is useful, care must still be taken when delivering the bowel through the ST, as relying on markers alone is insufficient to avoid a 360° twist during this step. The assistant is instructed to ensure orientation is maintained by holding the shaft of the bowel grasper. Once exteriorized, the correct orientation must be strictly maintained during all subsequent steps until the stoma is finally matured.
- With the assistant holding the ST grasper, the surgeon moves to the left side of the patient to use configuration 1. The camera is withdrawn. The surgeon places two handheld retractors along the ST, retracting the rectus muscle fibers medially and laterally. The medial retractor is transferred to the assistant's right hand with the surgeon's right hand maintaining the lateral retractor. The surgeon's left hand takes control of the ST grasper, and subsequently the assistant's left hand takes control of the lateral retractor.
- The pneumoperitoneum is released. The surgeon's right hand extends the posterior sheath and peritoneal vertical incision

Chapter 44 LAPAROSCOPIC DIVERTING COLOSTOMIES: FORMATION AND REVERSAL

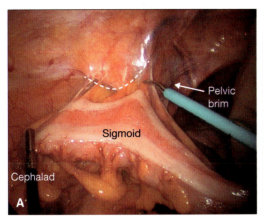
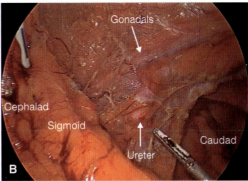

FIGURE 4 • Laparoscopic sigmoid colostomy: medial-to-lateral mobilization of the sigmoid colon. **A,** The sigmoid is mobilized by transecting the lateral peritoneal attachments *(dotted line)*, starting at the level of the pelvic brim. **B,** After transecting the lateral peritoneal attachments and mobilizing the sigmoid to the ML, the left ureter and gonadal vessels can be identified in the retroperitoneum as they cross the common iliac artery.

to an adequate length. The balloon of the port is deflated. The port is externalized along the shaft of the grasper. The colonic loop is then carefully externalized through the ST by extracting the ST grasper aided if required by nontraumatic bowel grasping (Rampley) forceps (**FIGURE 5**).

- Port closure precedes opening of the bowel and maturation of the stoma to maintain sterility. Port site incisions are closed with a 4-0 absorbable suture, and occlusive dressings are applied.

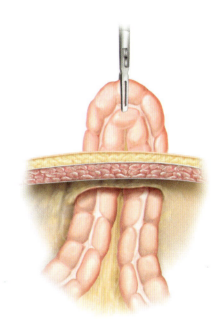

FIGURE 5 • Laparoscopic sigmoid colostomy: extraction of the sigmoid loop with a laparoscopic grasper inserted through the ST port site (the port has been removed).

COLOSTOMY CREATION

Loop Colostomy

- A supporting "rod" (optional) may be passed through a 5-mm defect in the mesentery adjacent to the apex of the externalized loop and sutured to the skin edge of the ST in the 3- and 9-o'clock positions (**FIGURE 6A**). Confirmation of correct colonic loop orientation is possible laparoscopically if deemed necessary.
- After port site closure, the apex of the colonic loop is opened by means of a transverse antimesenteric colotomy extending for 50% to 75% of the colonic circumference. The resulting proximal and distal limbs of the stoma are subsequently matured using between 8 and 12 seromuscular to subcuticular interrupted 3-0 absorbable sutures (**FIGURE 6B**). The stomal appliance is applied.

Double-Barreled Colostomy

- With an adequate length of sigmoid colonic loop (or both proximal and distal divided ends where a resection has been performed) externalized, a defect is created in the mesentery adjacent to the apex of the loop. The colon is then divided at this level with a linear stapler; the ends of the colon are grasped with nontraumatic bowel (eg, Rampley) forceps (**FIGURE 1B**).
- After port site closure, the staple line of the proximal limb is excised. Three seromuscular–subcuticular interrupted 3-0 absorbable sutures are placed (but not tied) in the 3-, 9-, and 12-o'clock positions of the skin edge of the ST and the cut edges of the opened proximal colon.

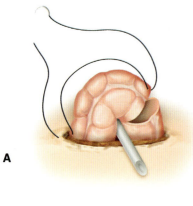

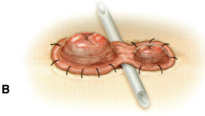

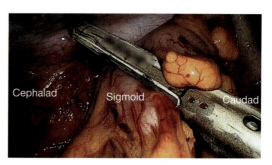

FIGURE 7 • Laparoscopic end sigmoid colostomy. The distal sigmoid colon is transected intracorporeally.

FIGURE 6 • Creation of a loop sigmoid colostomy. The apex of the colonic loop is opened transversely for 50% to 75% of the colonic circumference. The resulting proximal and distal limbs of the stoma are subsequently matured flush to the skin with interrupted absorbable sutures.

- A 10 mm length of one corner of the distal colonic staple line is excised. Three seromuscular–subcuticular interrupted 3-0 absorbable sutures are placed (and tied) in the 5-, 6-, and 7-o'clock positions of the ST and the small opening of the distal limb.
- The proximal sutures are tied. Additional seromuscular to subcuticular interrupted 3-0 absorbable sutures are placed at intervals between already placed sutures as necessary. A stomal appliance is applied.

End Colostomy

- For an end colostomy formation, instead of delivering the intact loop of sigmoid colon through the ST, the mobilized colon is transected intracorporeally.
- After identifying the optimal site for colonic division, a defect is created in the adjacent colonic mesentery with the energy device. The colon is then transected intracorporeally at this level with a 60-mm endoscopic linear stapler (**FIGURE 7**) inserted via the ST 12-mm port. Depending on the thickness of the adjacent mesentery and abdominal wall, a variable distance of mesentery is divided radially using an energy device, a linear cutting stapler with a vascular cartridge, or between ligation clips.
- The proximal colonic end is grasped with a locking bowel grasper via the ST port. Correct orientation is confirmed, and the assistant is instructed to ensure orientation is maintained by holding the shaft of the bowel grasper.
- The proximal colonic end is brought out through the ST port site as discussed previously.
- After port sit closure, the stoma is then matured with 8 to 12 seromuscular to subcuticular interrupted 3-0 absorbable sutures and a stomal appliance applied.

LAPAROSCOPIC FORMATION OF END TRANSVERSE COLOSTOMY

Creation of the Stomal Trephine and Port Placement and Mobilization

- Using surgical team configuration 4, the ST is created at the preoperatively marked site (if sure about the need of the colostomy). A 12- or 5-mm balloon port is inserted, and the pneumoperitoneum is insufflated.
- If unsure about the need of a colostomy, we delay formation of the ST until a later stage of the procedure. In these cases, we insufflate the pneumoperitoneum using a 5-mm insufflation-assisted optical entry port via the left upper quadrant.
- We use 5-mm ports in the LUQ and periumbilical locations and a 12-mm ST port (three-port technique) as described in the "Port Placement" section. An accessory LLQ port (four-port technique) is required in difficult omental mobilization cases.
- Configuration 5 is used, and the omentum is dissected from proximal transverse colon to prevent its passage into the ST (**FIGURE 8**).
- After identifying the optimal site for colonic division, formation of the colostomy can proceed as described earlier (see "Colostomy creation—End colostomy").

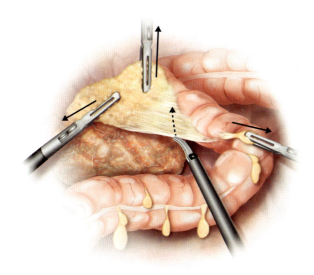

FIGURE 8 • Laparoscopic transverse colostomy. The omentum is separated from the transverse colon with an energy device.

CLOSURE OF A LOOP OR DOUBLE-BARRELED COLOSTOMY

Mobilization and Closure of Stoma

- In patients with a thin abdominal wall, we incise the mucocutaneous border circumferentially. In a patient with a thicker abdominal wall due to obesity or muscle bulk, we use an elliptical skin incision inclusive of the stoma with the long axis of the ellipse oriented transversely.
- The stoma is mobilized to the peritoneal cavity by means of sharp dissection. The colonic loop or ends should be adequately mobile to comfortably externalize beyond the skin.
- Closure of the colonic loop defect or anastomosis of the colonic ends can be achieved using either a hand-sewn single-layer seromuscular technique with 3-0 absorbable suture or a side-to-side double-stapled anastomotic technique with a linear stapling device (FIGURE 9A and B).
- The reanastomosed colon is returned to the peritoneal cavity. The fascial defect is closed craniocaudally with interrupted 0 absorbable sutures. The wound is lavaged with saline. Long-acting local anesthetic is infiltrated into the fascia and subcutaneous tissues.
- If a circumferential incision was used initially, the skin defect is reduced to a 5- to 10-mm-diameter defect by means of a subcuticular purse-string 3-0 absorbable suture. If an elliptical incision was used, the skin is closed with interrupted 3-0 absorbable subcuticular sutures. An occlusive dressing is applied.

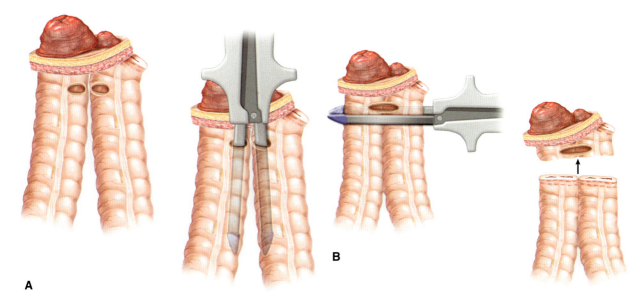

FIGURE 9 • Reversal of loop colostomy. A, The colostomy is resected with a linear stapler. B, A side-to-side stapled colocolonic anastomosis is performed with a linear stapler.

LAPAROSCOPIC CLOSURE OF END SIGMOID COLOSTOMY

Team Setup and Port Placement

- Surgical team configuration 2 is used. While it is appropriate to mobilize the stoma as the initial step to gain access to the peritoneal cavity and create pneumoperitoneum, we prefer to use a 5-mm insufflation-assisted optical entry port via the RUQ. This facilitates adhesiolysis in the region of the colostomy, which is made more difficult if the bowel has already been mobilized. Five-millimeter ports are inserted in the RLQ, RUQ, ML, and LL locations. The LL port is useful during mobilization of the descending colon and splenic flexure but may be omitted if this extent of mobilization is not required.
- A 12-mm ST port may be inserted after the stoma site after the stoma has been mobilized into the abdominal cavity. A 12-mm SP (optional) is inserted if the rectum and/or the inferior mesenteric artery (IMA) require transection using an endoscopic linear stapler and it is not ergonomically feasible to do so via the 12-mm ST port.

Mobilization (±Resection)

- With adequate Trendelenburg and right side rotated down positioning, further adhesiolysis proceeds as required to mobilize small bowel and omentum from the pelvis and remainder of the operative field.
- With no Trendelenburg but ongoing right side down positioning (using configurations 2 and then 3), the descending colon and splenic flexure (**FIGURE 10**) are mobilized medially as required, ensuring protection of the left ureter and gonadal vessels. The need for further mobilization of the proximal colon is dictated by its quality and the required length. Further mobilization (with or without resection) should be undertaken if there is insufficient length for a tension-free anastomosis or if the bowel is of inadequate quality for anastomosis (eg, excessive diverticulosis or inflammatory bowel disease). If necessary, additional mobilization or high division of the IMA (if not previously transected) may be performed using surgical team configuration 3. It is better to "overmobilize" rather than "undermobilize" the colon to achieve a tension-free anastomosis.
- When proximal mobilization has been performed and attention turns to the pelvis, there are generally two scenarios that the surgeon may encounter: (1) there is a distal sigmoid stump, with an intact IMA or (2) there is a distal rectal stump; the IMA may be intact or transected.
    - When there is a distal sigmoid with an intact IMA from the previous surgery:
        - Using configuration 2, the distal sigmoid stump is identified and mobilized from adhesions along with its mesentery along the lateral border ("lateral mobilization") toward the ML, ensuring protection of the left ureter and gonadal vessels (**FIGURE 4B**). Our preference is to resect any residual sigmoid colon, with eventual anastomosis occurring at the level of the upper rectum. As such, dissection continues distally to mobilize the left aspect of the upper mesorectum.

- With the assistant retracting the rectosigmoid junction anteriorly and cranially, the peritoneum is incised deep to the arch of the IMA/superior rectal vessels (SRVs) (**FIGURE 11**).
- Dissection of the avascular window deep to the IMA/SRV arch continues from medial to lateral until it becomes confluent with the previously performed LL mesocolon mobilization.

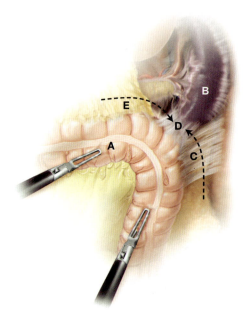

FIGURE 10 • Mobilization of the splenic flexure. The surgeon retracts the splenic flexure of the colon *(A)* downward and medially, exposing the attachments of the splenic flexure to the spleen *(B)*. The phrenocolic *(C)* and splenocolic *(D)* ligaments are transected in an inferior-to-superior and lateral-to-medial direction. The gastrocolic ligament *(E)* is then transected in a medial-to-lateral direction until both planes of dissection meet and the splenic flexure is fully mobilized.

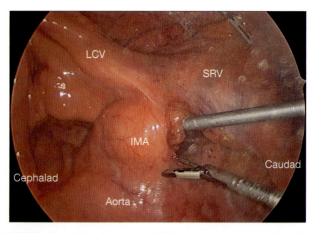

FIGURE 11 • IMA dissection. With the assistant retracting the rectosigmoid junction anteriorly and cranially, the peritoneum is incised deep to the arch of the superior rectal vessels (SRV). At this point, the IMA, taking off the aorta, can be seen with its terminal branches, the SRV and the LCV.

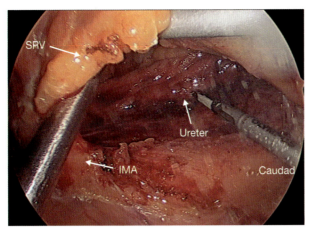

FIGURE 12 • Identification of the left ureter. After dissection of the IMA/SRV off the retroperitoneum, the left ureter is visualized and preserved intact prior to IMA transection.

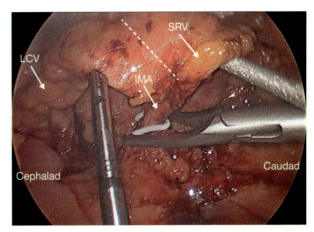

FIGURE 13 • IMA transection. The IMA is transected between endovascular clips at its origin off the aorta ("high" IMA ligation). If a high IMA ligation is not needed to achieve a tension-free anastomosis, a "low" transection can be performed across the LCV *(dotted line)*, preserving the IMA/SRV intact.

- The camera is rotated 90° clockwise to allow better visualization through the created window to the left pelvic sidewall and brim. The ureter should be visualized through this window (**FIGURE 12**).
- The second assistant or scrub nurse helps expose the retroperitoneal structures in this window by retracting the rectosigmoid junction and mesentery toward the anterior abdominal wall using the passing the suction/irrigator via the SP port under the IMA/SRV (**FIGURE 12**). The assistant's left hand grasper can then be repositioned proximally on the sigmoid stump to facilitate superior exposure for further dissection. Dissection continues cranially to identify and isolate the origin of the IMA off the aorta.
- If a "high" IMA division, proximal to the origin of the left colic vessels (LCVs), is mandated for the purposes of a tension-free anastomosis, the IMA can be divided with an endoscopic linear stapler or between clips (**FIGURE 13**), ensuring preservation of the left ureter and gonadal vessels.
- If adequate mobility and colonic length will permit subsequent colorectal anastomosis without high division of the IMA, the IMA is divided distal to the origin of the left colic artery (termed a "low" IMA division; **FIGURE 13**).
- The rectosigmoid junction and mesentery are further mobilized. The upper mesorectum is divided with the energy device, and the upper rectum is divided with an endoscopic linear stapler via the 12-mm SP port. The specimen is placed in an endoscopic pouch and can subsequently be removed via the ST at a later stage.
- When there is a rectal stump from the previous surgery:
  - If the IMA and upper rectum were divided at the time of the initial procedure, the rectal stump is identified and its end is mobilized. Rectal stump mobilization can be aided by per anal insertion of lubricated rectal "sizers" (by a second assistant or the scrub nurse). This maneuver also allows assessment of the degree of stricturing of the proximal end of the rectal stump, which is relatively common following a Hartmann procedure for acute indications such as complicated diverticulitis. When present, this inhibits passage of the circular endoluminal stapler and requires transection of the rectal stump in a more distal, favorable location for anastomosis.

Mobilization of the Colostomy

- This has been described previously (see "Closure of a Loop or Double-Barreled Colostomy—Mobilization and Closure of Stoma").

Colorectal Anastomosis

- Once mobilized, the bowel from the abdominal wall can be resected if desired, and if the bowel is of adequate quality for anastomosis the anvil of the circular stapler can be placed at this stage.
- The anvil of a circular endoscopic stapler is secured in the proximal colon using a purse-string suture. A purse-string applicator clamp is placed across the colon at the resection site; a purse-string suture is placed using a polypropylene suture on a straight needle. The colon is cut distal to but flush with the purse-string clamp. The clamp is released, and the cut edges are gently grasped with two Babcock forceps. The anvil of a 28 to 31 mm end-to-end anastomosis circular stapling device is inserted into the colonic end and the purse string tied to ensure closure of the colonic end around the stem of the anvil. The colonic end and anvil are returned to the peritoneal cavity.
- If a resection of distal sigmoid/rectal stump has occurred, the specimen can be removed in a bag via the ST defect after insertion of an appropriate wound protection device.
- Using surgical team configuration 2 with Trendelenburg positioning and after reinstigation of the pneumoperitoneum, an end-to-end the stapler colorectal anastomosis is fashioned (**FIGURE 14**).
- The stapler is inserted per anally, either by the surgeon or an experienced assistant, to the proximal limit of the rectal stump under laparoscopic visualization.

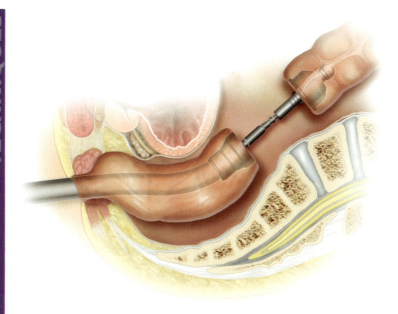

FIGURE 14 • Stapled end-to-end colorectal anastomosis.

- The stylet of the stapler is advanced through the proximal end of the rectal wall. The anvil and colonic end are grasped and the shaft of the anvil is "docked" onto the stylet. Colonic and mesenteric orientation is checked. The stylet, with anvil attached, is retracted into the head of the stapling device until appropriate tissue compression is achieved, ensuring no adjacent structures (eg, vagina) are incorporated.
- The stapling device is deployed. The stapling device is partially opened and removed per anally. Proximal and distal "donuts" are assessed for completeness.
- The colonic mesentery is inspected to ensure no small bowel is herniated deep to it.

- The integrity of the anastomosis is tested by air insufflation under water. The presence of air bubbles would indicate an anastomotic leak, necessitating a revision of the anastomosis. A pelvic drain is not used unless the anastomosis is extraperitoneal.
- Ports are removed. Port site closure is then performed, including fascial defect of any 12-mm ports. ST site closure has been described previously (see "Closure of a Loop Or Double-Barreled Colostomy—Mobilization and Closure of Stoma").

PEARLS AND PITFALLS

Important principles	■ Adequate preoperative preparation and planning ■ Adequate mobilization ■ Good blood supply ■ Appropriate aperture diameter
Permanent stomas	■ End colostomies are preferable over loop or double-barreled colostomies. ■ Consider prophylactic mesh placement, especially in patients at risk of parastomal hernias. We use the laparoscopic "buttonhole" or Sugarbaker technique.
Transverse colostomies	■ Avoid compromise to the left branch of the middle colic vessels, especially in situations in which the IMA may have been divided or compromised.
Tips in the obese patient	■ Aggressive preoperative weight loss is advisable: It reduces the thickness of the abdominal wall and the mesenteric bulk. ■ More extensive mobilization is required due to thicker abdominal wall. ■ Site the stoma further cranially than the standard position: The abdominal wall adipose tissue will be displaced caudally when the patient sits or stands. The abdominal wall is thinner in the upper abdomen, and lower sites may be out of view to the patient. ■ End colostomies are easier to construct and associated with fewer complications. The length available is superior, the mesenteric bulk is less, and the trephine aperture required is less. ■ A small Alexis wound protector/retractor placed through the ST often aids passage of the stoma. Cutting the inner ring aids removal of the device.

POSTOPERATIVE CARE

- Routine postoperative DVT prophylaxis is standard. An enhanced recovery style progression is routine with early mobilization and return to full diet.
- If a stoma has been created, stomal education should commence as early as possible (on the first postoperative day), as competency of stomal care is often the determining factor delaying patient discharge.
- When a colorectal anastomosis has been performed, our practice is to leave a rectal catheter in situ for 3 to 5 days. The rectal catheter is flushed with 20 mL of saline three times per day and remains in situ until the patient is passing flatus via or past the rectal catheter.

COMPLICATIONS

- Bleeding
- Anastomotic leak
- Wound infection
- Parastomal abscess
- Fistula
- Stomal retraction/stenosis
- Skin irritation/ulceration
- Stomal prolapse
- Parastomal or incisional hernia

SUGGESTED READINGS

1. Oliveira L. Laparoscopic stoma creation and closure. *Semin Laparosc Surg.* 2003;10(4):191-196.
2. Siddiqui MR, Sajid MS, Baig MK. Open vs laparoscopic approach for reversal of Hartmann's procedure: a systematic review. *Colorectal Dis.* 2010;12(8):733-741.
3. van de Wall BJ, Draaisma WA, Schouten ES, et al. Conventional and laparoscopic reversal of the Hartmann procedure: a review of literature. *J Gastrointest Surg.* 2010;14(4):743-752.

Chapter **45**

Surgical Management of Hemorrhoids

Bidhan Das

DEFINITION

- Hemorrhoids are a normal constituent of normal anorectal anatomy. The terms "hemorrhoid" or "hemorrhoidal disease" effectively refer to conditions related to the vascular cushions of the anal canal. The goal of any hemorrhoid treatment plan is the control of symptoms, rather the removal of these vascular cushions as a rule.
- Hemorrhoids, by their definition classically by Thomson in 1975, are specialized structures that act as vascular cushions contained within the submucosal space of the anal canal. It is thought that they serve to maintain closure of the anal canal and contribute to fecal continence.
- Hemorrhoidal tissue is not necessarily limited to the three cardinal "quadrants," and commonly, additional hemorrhoids in between these quadrants are found. Interestingly, hemorrhoidal tissue is neither artery nor vein, noting that histologically, they have no muscular wall and are, in fact, sinusoids.
- Hemorrhoid pathology is classified as either internal or external (**FIGURE 1**), relative to its position at the dentate line, and internal hemorrhoids are graded according to the severity of symptoms. It is exceedingly important to understand this functional anatomy before choosing the type of operative therapy.
- Operative hemorrhoidectomy classically describes the removal of both internal (proximal to the dentate line) and external hemorrhoidal tissue (distal to the dentate line).

However, new advances and procedures such as Doppler-guided hemorrhoidal ligation or transanal hemorrhoidal dearterialization (THD) can be performed with less pain and enhanced recovery times, as there is no cutting of the anoderm, and the operative field is proximal to the dentate line.
- Excisional hemorrhoidectomy remains the gold standard operation to which all treatments are compared, as its safety as well as durability has withstood the test of time. However, it remains a painful operation, and other measures may be weighed against a possibly higher recurrence rate with substantially reduced postoperative pain.
- Furthermore, with the rising population of patients on full anticoagulation because of the growing ability to treat severe cardiovascular diseases as chronic illnesses, older techniques such as sclerosant therapy become handy operative tools for the acutely bleeding patient, in whom further suturing runs the risk of further bleeding.

DIFFERENTIAL DIAGNOSIS

- Anal cancer, particularly melanoma
- Rectal prolapse (**FIGURE 2A** and **B**)
- Anorectal varices
- Perianal cyst disease
- Anal condyloma
- Pedunculated polyps
- Protruding anal papillae
- Anal skin tags, particularly sentinel tags associated with anal fissures
- Crohn's disease

PATIENT HISTORY AND PHYSICAL FINDINGS

- In order to treat hemorrhoids effectively, the other items in the differential diagnosis must be ruled out. Additionally, when considering surgical options, the pain of a traditional hemorrhoidectomy may be avoided by other methods that treat internal hemorrhoidal disease. Accurate diagnosis and determination of internal vs external hemorrhoidal disease must be ascertained to decide on the best operation for the patient.
- A thorough history and physical examination should be performed prior to treatment, including a detailed past medical history, present medications and allergies, and particularly conditions such as cirrhosis or previous treatment with radiation.
- Toileting behaviors, alteration in bowel function, and dietary changes must also be noted.
- Conditions that impair venous drainage and that push vascular cushions outward, behavioral/toileting abnormalities, and changes in sphincter function are all commonly believed to contribute toward worsening hemorrhoidal symptoms. Ultimately, venous congestion with subsequent hypertrophy of internal hemorrhoidal cushions leads to symptomatic hemorrhoids.

FIGURE 1 • Internal vs external hemorrhoids. Position of the hemorrhoids relative to the dentate line *(dotted arrow)* classifies them as internal (proximal to the dentate line) or external (distal to the dentate line).

Internal hemorrhoid   External hemorrhoid

422

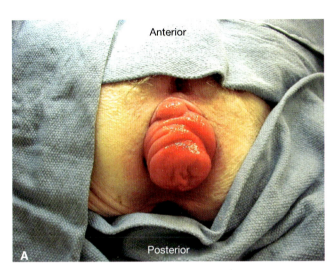
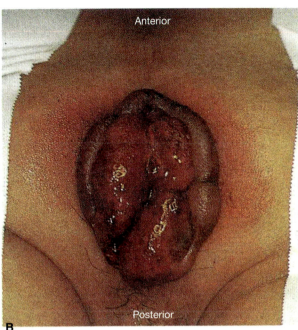

FIGURE 2 • Rectal prolapse. It is important to differentiate **(A)** rectal prolapse from **(B)** prolapsing internal hemorrhoids.

- Prolonged straining increases abdominal pressure, which then impairs venous return, thus making the hemorrhoidal cushions unable to decompress transient congestion. Supportive tissues of the cushions then become gradually more and more attenuated, leading to prolapse of the cushion. Further prolapse then increases the possibility of trapping blood in the cushions with less abdominal pressure, thus causing progressive enlarging. Continued prolonged straining is an important preoperative history point because the behavior will need to be modified in the postoperative period to reduce pain and can worsen the efficacy of suture ligation operations.
- Dietary factors and toileting behavior are also critical issues because they not only impair postoperative recovery, but they can also promote postsurgical anal fissures, compounding a difficult postoperative recovery.
- Cirrhotic patients are at high risk for having anorectal varices, which are often mistaken for hemorrhoidal cushions. Elective hemorrhoidectomy for anorectal varices is fraught with excessive bleeding even to the point of hemodynamic instability in the stable patient once dissection for a misdiagnosis has started.
- A complete rectal examination, which includes not just a digital rectal examination (DRE) but anoscopy and proctoscopy, is essential to the diagnosis. It is important to distinguish between rectal prolapse vs mucohemorrhoidal protrusion. Proctoscopy aids in the diagnosis of inflammatory bowel disease while allowing control of bleeding and biopsy. The number, location, grade designation, and relative size of hemorrhoids should be noted.

IMAGING AND OTHER DIAGNOSTIC STUDIES

- Given a thorough physical examination, imaging or other diagnostic modalities are rarely indicated.

SURGICAL MANAGEMENT

Preoperative Planning

- Patients do not require bowel preparation for hemorrhoidectomy of any kind. Often, a simple enema before operation is sufficient for evacuation of the rectum. A rigid proctoscopy in the operating room before starting the procedure not only completes the preparation but also reviews the rectal mucosa for any signs of inflammation that may alter the surgical therapy or alert the surgeon to a heretofore unknown cause of straining.
- The operation can be performed using a number of anesthetic choices and options, including general anesthesia, local anesthesia with intravenous sedation, or even regional anesthesia.
- Sequential compression devices (SCDs) are placed on the patient prior to the induction of general anesthesia.
- When performing a THD procedure, a patient should be examined for the presence of external hemorrhoidal disease. The operating surgeon may feel that there is more benefit in performing a traditional hemorrhoidectomy when there is a substantial external component that could be worsened by an internal ligation procedure, which could cause subsequent levator spasm and tenesmus postoperatively.
- When performing rubber band ligation of internal hemorrhoids, an office setting is most often well tolerated.

Positioning

- Multiple positions are excellent for hemorrhoidectomy operations, including lateral Sims position (**FIGURE 3**), prone jackknife (**FIGURE 4**), or high lithotomy (**FIGURE 5**) using C-type "candy cane" footholders. Anesthesia concerns and surgical needs often are satisfied with the use of high lithotomy position. It is important to note that for prone jackknife, the folding mechanism of the operating table should be at the patient's hip for maximal exposure, whereas in

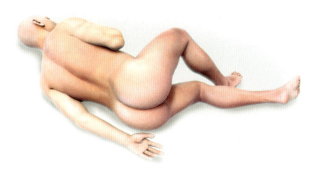

FIGURE 3 • Sims position.

lithotomy the sacrum should be at the very edge of the bed. In smaller patients, a flattened and folded blanket or bedroll can be placed under the sacrum to provide some elevation of the perineum and forward projection.

- Lithotomy patients using the C-type footholders often benefit from 45° angling of the footholder base toward the patient's head, whereas the "C" should be orthogonal to the patient's body. SCD/Venodyne boot cords can be tucked behind the adjustment flanges of the footholders.

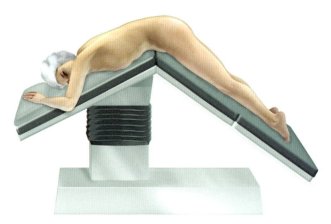

FIGURE 4 • Prone jackknife position.

Such a position pushes the patient's knees cephalad and feet medially.

- For lithotomy patients undergoing either traditional hemorrhoidectomy or THD, an under-the-buttocks drape with a plastic drain pocket can be used to store the Doppler device or to clip instruments while suture ligating or sewing for ready access.

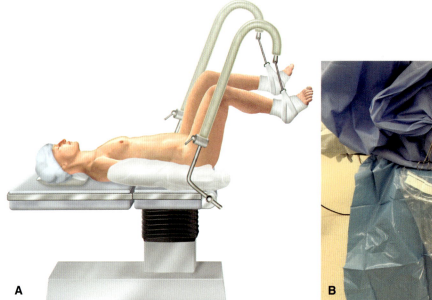

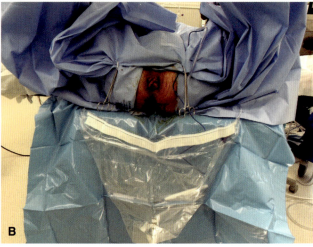

FIGURE 5 • **A,** Lithotomy position with C-type (candy canes) footholders. **B,** Final Setup for High Lithotomy with under-the-Buttocks drape with plastic pouch; white band can be used to hold instruments.

TRADITIONAL EXCISIONAL HEMORRHOIDECTOMY (CLOSED FERGUSON TECHNIQUE)

Delineation of Hemorrhoidal Cushions and Skin Incisions

- After performing a proper anoscopy using serial dilation of graded Hill-Ferguson retractors, a hemorrhoidal bundle can be readily exposed. Using a forceps or hemostatic clamp, the hemorrhoidal cushions can be gathered to facilitate the skin incision, which should spare the anoderm but include the hemorrhoidal bundle. This incision can be minimized by undermining directly underneath the hemorrhoidal bundle at the distal aspect and cutting inward directly into the anal canal to start the dissection (**FIGURE 6**).

Dissection of the Hemorrhoidal Vascular Tissue From the Internal Sphincter

- After cutting directly under the hemorrhoid bundle distally and through the dermis, a Metzenbaum scissor carefully and sharply separates the vascular submucosal tissues from the

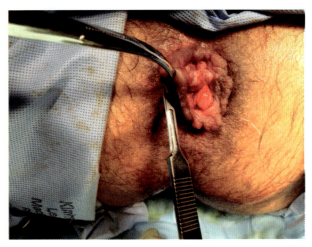

FIGURE 6 • Delineation of hemorrhoidal cushions and skin incision. Elevation of the anoderm with a clamp distal to the hemorrhoidal cushion allows for a precise incision.

adherent, often fibrous internal sphincter and intersphincteric groove (**FIGURE 7**).
- A rule of thumb: Dissect the sphincter from the hemorrhoid rather than hemorrhoidal tissue from the sphincter.

Continued Skin Excision and Pedicle Isolation

- As the surgeon dissects the sphincter off the hemorrhoid, a substantial "tunnel" is created; to save anoderm, the edges of the "tunnel" are simply cut directly toward the proximal aspect of the hemorrhoid, which can help make the operation progress by better easily delineating the hemorrhoidal bundle.
- As the incision reaches a point proximally, the hemorrhoid bundle is delineated completely and isolated cephalad, and in such a manner the vascular pedicle of the hemorrhoid is effectively isolated.

Pedicle Clamp, Specimen Removal, and Suture Ligation

- With the hemorrhoidal tissue narrowed down to a pedicle, this vascular structure can be clamped with a hemostat, the specimen cut and removed, and a suture ligature of absorbable suture can be applied, leaving the tail long (**FIGURE 8**).

Closure

- Using the same suture and the pedicle suture ligation as an elevated anchor, continuous (**FIGURE 9**) or running, locking bites can be taken to close the incision, grabbing small fibers of the internal sphincter as one works distally to anchor the cut edges and promote hemostasis.
- Upon leaving the limits of the anal sphincter and thus the mucosa, no further deeper tissue anchoring is used. One variant of the closure is to tie the suture to itself, every two bites, which can effectively act as a mucosal proctopexy until the end of the mucosal opening is reached. The suture is tied to itself at the distal aspect of the anoderm.
- The same process is repeated in the other two quadrants and can be modified for areas that are not in the traditional quadrants.

Hemostasis Assessment and Packing

- After completion of hemorrhoidectomy, a repeat examination using Hill-Ferguson retractors is performed to ensure continued hemostasis. After verification of hemostasis, a Surgicel is tucked into the anal canal, which can be removed at any time or with first flatus or defecation. Should bleeding be encountered, an interrupted suture or figure-of-8 suture can be applied liberally.

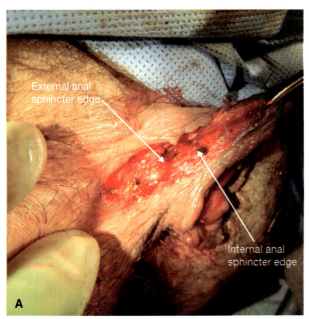
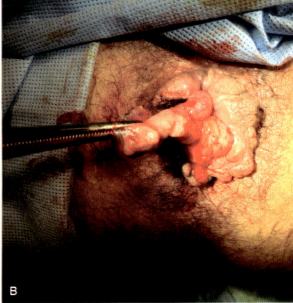

FIGURE 7 • **A,** Dissection of the hemorrhoidal vascular tissue from the internal sphincter. Using scissors, dissect the sphincter from the hemorrhoid rather than hemorrhoidal tissue from the sphincter. **B,** The pedicle is isolated.

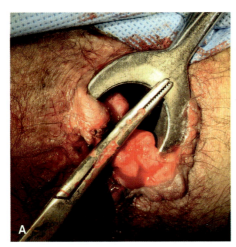
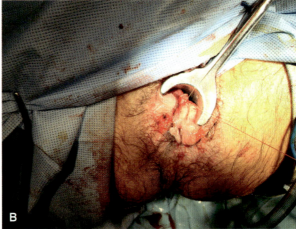

FIGURE 8 • **A,** Suture ligation of hemorrhoidal vascular pedicle. After the hemorrhoidal pedicle has been transected at its origin and the hemorrhoidal tissue has been removed, the pedicle is suture ligated for hemostasis. **B,** Suture is kept long, as an anchoring stitch.

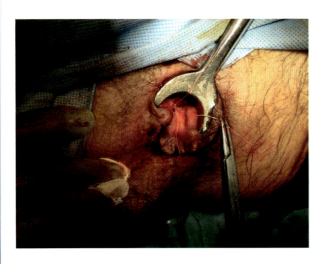

FIGURE 9 • Closure. Using the same suture and the pedicle suture ligation as an elevated anchor, continuous or running, locking bites can be taken to close the incision, grabbing small fibers of the internal sphincter as one works distally to anchor the cut edges and promote hemostasis.

RUBBER BAND LIGATION OF HEMORRHOIDS

Isolation of the Hemorrhoidal Cushion

- Anoscopy is performed using serial dilation of either graded Hill-Ferguson retractors or office anoscopy (Buie, Hirschman, lighted Welch Allyn) to demonstrate that there is an internal hemorrhoid of grade II or III classification.
- Pressure can then be placed against the anoscope, which will make the already protruding hemorrhoid even more prominent (**FIGURE 10**).

Rubber Band Application

- With the anoscope pressure being maintained, a Barron ligator is used to ligate the hemorrhoid (**FIGURE 11**) by first passing the hemorrhoid-seizing forceps through the window of the ligator after the ligator has been loaded.
- The forceps then grab the protruding internal hemorrhoid as broadly as possible (**FIGURE 11A** and **B**) and the ligator is pushed directly down onto the hemorrhoid until the base of the hemorrhoid is reached while seizing forceps has the hemorrhoid still elevated.
- The ligator fires the rubber band around the base of the hemorrhoid (**FIGURE 11C**). It is of the *utmost* importance that the ligation is performed definitively proximally to the dentate line (**FIGURE 11D**).

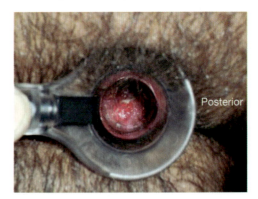

FIGURE 10 • Hemorrhoidal banding: isolation of the hemorrhoidal pedicle with an anoscope.

Chapter 45 SURGICAL MANAGEMENT OF HEMORRHOIDS   427

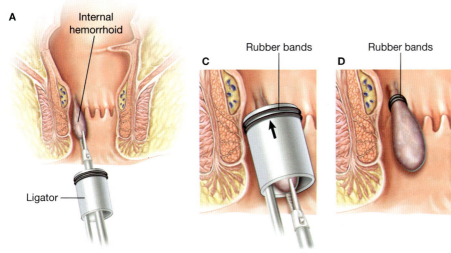

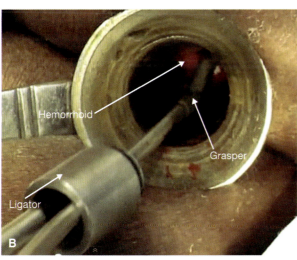

FIGURE 11 • Rubber band application. **A** and **B,** The forceps grab the protruding internal hemorrhoid as broadly as possible. **C,** The ligator is pushed directly down onto the hemorrhoid until the base of the hemorrhoid is reached. **D,** The ligator fires the rubber band around the base of the hemorrhoid. It is of the *utmost* importance that the ligation is performed definitively proximally to the dentate line *(dotted arrow)*.

Maintenance of Band Ligation

- To complete the procedure, a fine gauge short needle (25 gauge) is used to instill 2 to 3 mL of local anesthetic submucosally on the "cap" of the ligated hemorrhoid to create a large "mushroom" that will prevent slippage of the rubber band.

SUTURE LIGATION OF INTERNAL HEMORRHOIDS

Suture Ligation

- After anoscopy demonstrates the internal hemorrhoid, a figure-of-eight suture of absorbable suture material is placed to completely encompass the hemorrhoidal bundle without passing the needle through the cryptoglandular interface and thus reducing the chance of abscess.
- The suture is tied in such a way that the knot lies toward the most cephalad portion of the internal hemorrhoid. Such a placement can sometimes gather and fixate the internal hemorrhoid proximally in addition to the vascular ligation.

DOPPLER-GUIDED LIGATION OF THE HEMORRHOIDAL TERMINAL ARTERY BRANCHES AND MUCOSAL PROCTOPEXY USING TRANSANAL HEMORRHOIDAL DEARTERIALIZATION DEVICE

Isolation of Distal Branches of the Hemorrhoidal Arteries

- The THD device is a specifically designed anoscope/proctoscope equipped with a Doppler probe that faces outward and a light source attached to a pivot cage for a specifically designed suture and needle driver set (**FIGURE 12A**). Continuous Doppler audio waveform is provided with a double crystal that is made to focus and capture the larger diameter arteries located in the superficial layers of the rectal wall.
- Following lubrication and a thorough anoscopy using serial dilation with graded Hill-Ferguson retractors, the proctoscope is inserted through the anal canal reaching the distal rectum (roughly 6-7 cm from the anal verge).
- By moving the proctoscope with the Doppler ultrasound activated, one can hear the waveforms generated and isolate the six strongest waveforms that correlate to six equidistant positions around the anal canal (**FIGURE 12B**).

Transfixion With Suture Ligature

- Once a hemorrhoidal artery is located, the rectal mucosa and submucosal wall are transfixed with a figure-of-eight/"Z-stitch" to ligate the artery (**FIGURE 12C**). This transfixion suture is performed with the provided 2-0 absorbable polyglycolic acid with a 5/8-in needle at the prefabricated notch, inserting the needle driver tip into the provided pivot cage (**FIGURE 12D**), which is in the center of the proctoscope's lumen. The pivot cage is used twice to perform an appropriate figure-of-8/Z-stitch to ligate the artery.
- The suture is then tied after the Doppler probe is removed. This removal allows the operating surgeon's finger to slide deep into the anal canal to set the knot. The tail is left long, as this suture will act as an anchor for the upcoming mucosal proctopexy.

Mucosal Proctopexy

- Holding the THD proctoscope as a continued retractor and holding the long anchor tail against the scope, mucosal and submucosal bites can be taken to eliminate the prolapse of the hemorrhoid or mucosa. These bites are taken distal to the transfixion site at a step size of half a centimeter and can be tied back to the anchor stitch to create the "mucopexy" (**FIGURE 13**).
- Note that this mucopexy terminates at least 5 mm proximally to the dentate line and is tied to the first anchor stitch for a substantial mucosal proctopexy and to avoid potential abscess formation.
- This procedure is repeated five more times for a completed procedure.
- At the conclusion, an anoscopic examination of each suture site is performed to verify no undue bleeding which can be treated with suture ligation. A Surgicel light packing is placed in the anal canal and can be removed any time or by first flatus or defecation.

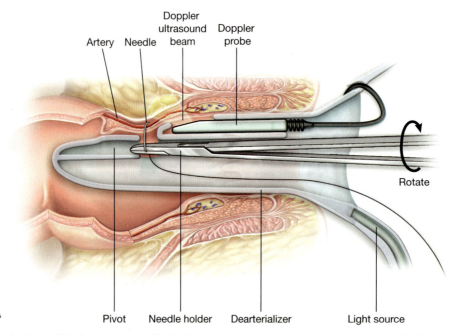

FIGURE 12 • The THD device. **A,** This device is a specifically designed anoscope/proctoscope equipped with a Doppler probe that faces outward and a light source attached to a pivot cage for a specifically designed suture and needle driver set. **B,** Using the Doppler ultrasound, one can hear the waveforms generated and isolate the six strongest waveforms that correlate to six equidistant positions around the anal canal. **C,** Once a hemorrhoidal pedicle is located, the rectal mucosa and submucosal wall are transfixed with a figure-of-8/Z-stitch to ligate the pedicle. **D,** Detailed view of needle holder with the provided 2-0 polydioxanone (PDS) suture on a 5/8-in needle inserted into the pivot.

Chapter 45 SURGICAL MANAGEMENT OF HEMORRHOIDS 429

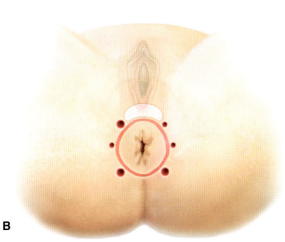

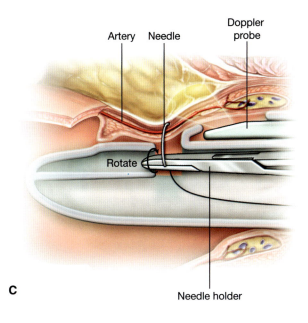

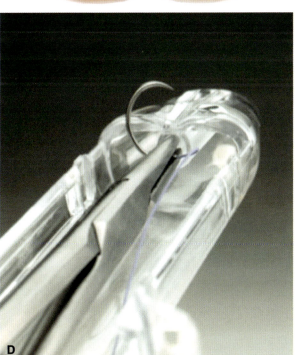

FIGURE 12 • Continued

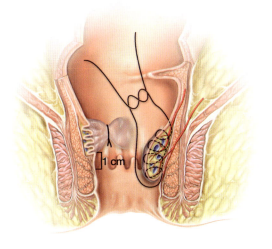

FIGURE 13 • Mucosal proctopexy. Holding the THD proctoscope as a *continued* retractor and holding the long anchor tail against the scope, mucosal and submucosal bites can be taken to eliminate the prolapse of the hemorrhoid or mucosa. These bites are taken distal to the transfixion site at a step size of half a centimeter and can be tied back to the anchor stitch to create the mucopexy. This mucopexy terminates at least 5 mm proximally to the dentate line and is tied to the first anchor stitch for a substantial mucosal proctopexy and to avoid potential abscess formation.

SCLEROSANT INJECTION OF HEMORRHOIDS

Delineation of Hemorrhoidal Cushions and Verification of Anatomy

- After performing a proper anoscopy using serial dilation of graded Hill-Ferguson retractors, a hemorrhoidal bundle can be readily exposed using a Hill-Ferguson retractor with countertraction provided by the opposite hand holding a gauze. At this point, it is essential to note that there should be no external component and that the internal hemorrhoids to be targeted are grades I and II.
- Using an angled spinal needle (18- to 22-gauge with a bend of 30° an inch from the tip), the proximal aspect of the hemorrhoidal bundle is found and a submucosal injection of a sclerosant solution of the surgeon's choice, usually between 3 and 5 mL in volume, is performed (**FIGURE 14**).
- Accurate injection reveals swelling of the mucosa without blanching of the mucosa, with a "striation sign" indicative of bridging hemorrhoidal veins.

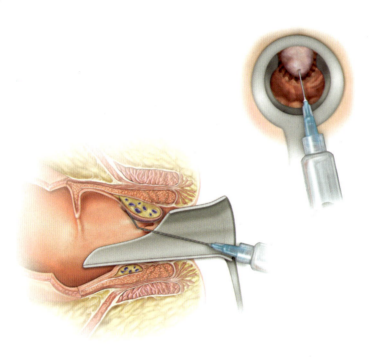

FIGURE 14 • Sclerosant injection of hemorrhoids. Using an angled spinal needle (18- to 22-gauge with a bend of 30° an inch from the tip), the proximal aspect of the hemorrhoidal bundle is found and a submucosal injection of a sclerosant solution of the surgeon's choice, usually between 3 and 5 mL in volume, is performed.

PEARLS AND PITFALLS

Indications	■ A thorough evaluation of the anorectum with classification of the hemorrhoidal cushions is essential in picking the optimal procedure. ■ Ruling out inflammation or prior radiation can help prevent wound complications. ■ Operative hemorrhoidal treatment requires a failure of conservative therapy. ■ Sclerotherapy has limited indications but is invaluable in the anticoagulated patients, as it creates no bleeding. ■ Doppler-guided techniques are for those with internal hemorrhoidal disease without external components.
Incisions	■ Sparing the anoderm reduces postoperative pain and anal stenosis. ■ In traditional hemorrhoidectomy, isolation of the hemorrhoidal pedicle can be done as soon as the hemorrhoidal bundle narrows. Never "chase the hemorrhoid" proximally into the rectum—it can be very difficult to ligate a lost "bleeder" appropriately if it retracts and such a proximal dissection will not improve the patient's symptoms of bleeding, irritation, or prolapse.
Dissection and suturing	■ Including fibers of the underlying sphincter during running closure of the mucosal gap may prevent a dissection-based hematoma. ■ When performing a mucosal proctopexy or a suture ligation, it is important that the stitch remains proximal to the dentate line to prevent cryptoglandular interface abscess formation. ■ Using a long initial anchor stitch for the hemorrhoidal pedicles can always provide a mucosal proctopexy by gathering the mucosa and tying back to the anchor while closing. ■ In order to reduce the risk of anal stenosis, minimize the amount of normal tissue resected/incorporated between hemorrhoidectomy sites. A small anodermal incision with submucosal dissection of the vascular tissue may also help.

Hemostasis	▪ Surgical hemostasis is paramount. ▪ Up to 5-8 postoperative days, the hemorrhoidal pedicle can slough or suffer from infection and cause pronounced bleeding. ▪ Most postoperative bleeding occurs as a result of poor ligation and requires urgent suture ligation.
Proctopexy	▪ Although the anchor stitch is often well affixed, the mobility of mucohemorrhoidal prolapse makes for an insufficient proctopexy if the knot that is made between the anchor and the running suture is not set proximally by the operating surgeon. The proctopexy is meant to gather the mucosal tissues and slide them cephalad; as such, the knot must lie near the anchoring suture, not toward the anal verge.
Rubber band ligation	▪ It is imperative that the band is placed 1-2 cm proximal to the dentate line to minimize postbanding pain. ▪ Many surgeons only band one hemorrhoid at each visit to minimize discomfort; multiple ligations are associated with greater pain, vasovagal syncope, and urinary retention. ▪ Should vasovagal symptoms or substantial discomfort occur, injection of a local anesthetic with epinephrine can be performed to help alleviate symptoms; perhaps, the best treatment is to remove the band. ▪ Although banding seems trivial, there are several reported cases of necrotizing pelvic infections leading to sepsis and even death after elective band ligation. It is also advised that the surgeon be mindful of treating the immunocompromised patient.
Sclerotherapy	▪ Some surgeons are concerned about intravenous injection of sclerosant, so withdrawal with the injecting needle is helpful before injecting. ▪ Intramucosal injection (induces mucosal blanching) must be avoided because it can lead to sloughing and ulcerations. ▪ No mucosal swelling, however, may mean the injection is too deep and can result in prostatic abscess, pyelophlebitis, and small soft tissue/rectal ulceration.

POSTOPERATIVE CARE

▪ These operations can all be safely performed in the outpatient setting.

▪ A bare minimum of intravenous fluids should be administered to reduce the risk of postoperative urinary retention. We limit our intraoperative fluid use to less than 200 mL.

▪ Routine use of diluted liposomal bupivacaine (Exparel) has dramatically reduced postoperative pain, shortened recovery, and reduced postoperative narcotic use.

▪ Postoperatively, warm water tub soaks are used to relax the levators, reduce levator spasm, and alleviate urinary retention.

▪ Postoperatively, we prescribe a low-dose narcotic (hydrocodone-acetaminophen), an oral nonsteroidal anti-inflammatory drug (NSAID) (ketorolac 10 mg three times a day for 5 days), and a low-dose muscle relaxant (diazepam 2 mg orally three times a day to assist with pelvic floor spasm). Prescription narcotic medications are unnecessary after in-office rubber band ligation.

▪ The patient is given instructions to consume a high-fiber diet (25 g/d), slowly increase water intake to match fiber intake, refrain from straining, and consume a daily or twice-daily dose of a stool softener such as polyethylene glycol.

▪ Signs and symptoms of vasovagal episodes or pelvic sepsis are explained to the patient.

OUTCOMES

▪ Operative excisional hemorrhoidectomy has, by far, the lowest recurrence rate but results in increased patient pain postoperatively. Recurrence rates are quoted at 1.4%.

▪ Doppler-guided ligation is a newer modality of treating hemorrhoids that still has yet to attain long-term follow-up data to accurately assess recurrence rates. In a study of 170 patients with a majority having grade III disease (82.7%), control of bleeding was obtained in 159 patients (93.5%) and control of prolapse in 152 (89.5%), with mean follow-up 11.5 ± 12 (range, 1-41) months.

▪ Eighty percent of patients with grade I or II hemorrhoids will note improvement in symptoms after rubber band ligation and up to 70% will remain completely symptom-free. The recurrence rate, though, is higher with banding than with surgical excision.

▪ The results of sclerotherapy in resolving internal hemorrhoids have been evaluated in small trials and retrospective reviews. Many researchers have found the benefits of injection therapy to be short-lived and somewhat comparable to diet control. However, in the actively bleeding/oozing anticoagulated patient, a modality that does not promote further bleeding may be invaluable. Khoury et al prospectively randomized 120 patients with grades I and II disease to single vs multiple injections, with nearly 90% reporting resolution or improvement in symptoms 1 year after injection and no difference with regard to the number of treatment sessions required.

COMPLICATIONS

▪ Bleeding with severe hemorrhage (occurring less than 5% of all cases)

▪ Urinary retention

▪ Infection of closed hemorrhoidectomy sites

▪ Fecal impaction

▪ Anal stenosis

▪ Skin necrosis

▪ Intramucosal or suture abscess from ligation techniques

▪ Cryptoglandular abscess

▪ Tenesmus

- Persistent or excessive levator spasm
- Pelvic sepsis, necrotizing soft tissue infections, anorectal necrosis
- Systemic absorption of sclerosant solution leading to acute respiratory distress syndrome (ARDS)

SUGGESTED READINGS

1. Bailey HR, Ferguson JA. Prevention of urinary retention by fluid restriction following anorectal operations. *Dis Colon Rectum*. 1976;19:250-252.
2. Barron J. Office ligation treatment of hemorrhoids. *Dis Colon Rectum*. 1963;6:109.
3. Jayaranam S, Colquhoun PH, Malthaner RA. Stapled versus conventional surgery for hemorrhoids. *Cochrane Database Syst Rev*. 2006;18:CD005393.
4. Khoury GA, Lake SP, Lewis MC, et al. A randomized trial to compare single with multiple phenol injection treatment for haemorrhoids. *Br J Surg*. 1985;72:741-742.
5. Ratto C, Donisi L, Parello A, et al. Evaluation of transanal hemorrhoidal dearterialization as a minimally invasive therapeutic approach to hemorrhoids. *Dis Colon Rectum*. 2010;53:803-811.
6. Thomson WH. The nature of haemorrhoids. *Br J Surg*. 1975;62(7):542-552.
7. Wrobleski DE, Corman ML, Veidenheimer MC, et al. Long-term evaluation of rubber ring ligation in hemorrhoidal disease. *Dis Colon Rectum*. 1980;23:478-482.

Chapter 46 Surgical Management of Anal Fissures

Daniel Albo

DEFINITION
- An anal fissure is an acute longitudinal tear or a chronic ovoid ulcer in the squamous epithelium of the anal canal.
- They are also often referred to as fissure in ano.
- The exact etiology of anal fissures is debated. Risk factors that increase the likelihood of developing an anal fissure include the following:
  - Increased sphincter tone
  - Chronic constipation
  - Straining to have a bowel movement, especially if the stool is large, hard, and/or dry
  - Sedentary lifestyle
  - Sexual practices: anal intercourse, insertion of anal/rectal foreign bodies
  - Overly tight or spastic anal sphincter muscles: failure of relaxation of the anal sphincter during bowel movements
  - Decreased blood flow to the perianal skin
  - Scarring in the anorectal area
  - Inflammatory bowel disease, such as Crohn disease and ulcerative colitis
  - Anal cancer, especially after radiation therapy
  - Tuberculosis
  - Sexually transmitted diseases (such as syphilis, gonorrhea, chlamydia, chancroid, HIV)
  - Leukemic infiltrates
  - Decreased blood flow to the anorectal area
  - Anal fissures are also common in women after childbirth and in young infants
  - Women are more commonly affected than men (58% vs 42%)

DIFFERENTIAL DIAGNOSIS
- Hemorrhoids (specially thrombosed hemorrhoids)
- Anal canal cancer
- Anal trauma

PATIENT HISTORY AND PHYSICAL FINDINGS
- Patients typically present with intense anal pain during and especially after defecation. The pain can last for several minutes to a few hours after having a bowel movement.
- Although patients are often asymptomatic between bowel movements, they often develop a "fear of defecation" and may try to avoid defecation secondary to the pain.
- Chronic constipation is common.
- Some bright red anal bleeding, especially on the toilet paper, is common.
- On physical examination, the anus appears tight and spastic. The pain is usually severe enough that the patient will not tolerate a digital rectal examination in the office.
- On anoscopy, which oftentimes is done under conscious sedation due to severe anal pain, the fissure is usually linear, although ovoid-shaped fissures are oftentimes seen as well.
- Anal fissures are almost universally present along the posterior midline in men and they are often associated with a sentinel skin tag at the squamous-columnar epithelial junction (anal verge). In women, they can also be seen on an anterior location (**FIGURE 1**).
- Anal fissures seen in Crohn disease and tuberculosis are frequently painless.

IMAGING AND OTHER DIAGNOSTIC STUDIES
- Diagnosis is made by visual inspection. Unless findings suggest a specific cause or the appearance and/or location is unusual, further studies are not required.
- In selected cases, flexible sigmoidoscopy or colonoscopy may be indicated.

SURGICAL MANAGEMENT
- The majority of anal fissures will resolve with medical management and will not require surgery.
- Medical management includes the following:
  - Aggressive prevention of constipation
    - Increase fiber and decrease fat in the diet
    - Fiber supplementation

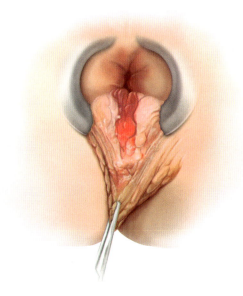

FIGURE 1 • Anal fissure. With an anoscope inserted in the anal canal, an anal fissure can be seen in the posterior midline of the squamous epithelium of the anal canal. A sentinel skin tag can be seen on the distal end of the fissure on the anal verge.

- Increase water intake
- Use of moist pads (flushable baby wipes) for wiping and anal hygiene
- Avoiding straining or prolonged sitting on the toilet
- Soaking in a warm bath (also called a sitz bath), 10 to 20 minutes several times a day, to promote the relaxation of the anal muscles
■ These conservative measures lead to healing of the anal fissure in a few weeks to a few months in 80% to 90% of patients. However, when these conservative measures alone are not successful, pharmacologic intervention can also be instituted. This includes the following:
- Topical nitrates ointment: Examples include nitroglycerin ointment 0.4% (Rectiv) and glyceryl trinitrate ointment (Rectogesic). Although effective, they are dose dependent. Disabling headaches are common at higher doses, making patient compliance with the treatment unreliable.
- Topical calcium channel blockers, including nifedipine or diltiazem ointment, are as effective as nitrate ointments but with significantly less side effects. Examples include topical nifedipine 0.3% with lidocaine 1.5% ointment and diltiazem 2% ointment.
■ Combination of medical therapies may offer up to 98% cure rates.
■ A combined surgical and pharmacologic treatment, administered by colorectal surgeons, is periodic direct injection of botulinum toxin (Botox) into the anal sphincter to relax it. Oftentimes, these injections prove less and less potent with each application. With patients spending thousands of dollars and not achieving a permanent cure, they oftentimes elect to have surgery.
■ When conservative medical therapy fails, surgery is considered.

Preoperative Planning

■ Mechanical bowel preparation is not necessary.
■ Fleet enemas are prescribed for the night before and the morning of surgery to clear the rectal vault.
■ Intravenous cefoxitin is administered within 1 hour of skin incision.
■ A preoperative time-out and briefing is conducted with the entire surgical team in attendance.
■ An anal block with bupivacaine extended-release liposome injection is associated with both pain relief for 72 hours and a 45% reduction in total opioid consumption at 72 hours.

Positioning

■ The patient is placed supine on a modified lithotomy position with the legs on padded stirrups to prevent neurovascular injuries to the calves (**FIGURE 2**).

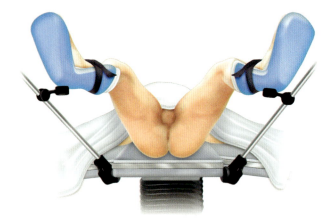

FIGURE 2 • Modified lithotomy position. The legs are placed on stirrups with padding to help prevent neurovascular injuries.

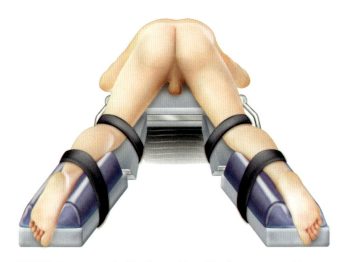

FIGURE 3 • Prone jackknife position. The lower extremities are placed on a split-leg table position to allow the surgeon to operate from in between the patient's legs.

■ Alternatively, the patient can be placed in a prone jackknife position on a split-leg table, with the surgeon positioned between the legs (**FIGURE 3**). The buttocks are spread apart with tape.
■ The author prefers to perform these procedures under general anesthesia.
■ Using headlights is critical for good visualization.

CLOSED LATERAL INTERNAL SPHINCTEROTOMY (TRANSCUTANEOUS)

- Using lubrication, perform a gentle anal dilation with two fingers.
- An anoscope is used to confirm the presence of the anal fissure.
- With the patient on a modified lithotomy position and palpating with the tip of your right index finger, identify the anal intersphincteric groove (**FIGURE 4**). The intersphincteric groove is a distinct groove in the anal canal, forming the lower border of the pecten analis, marking the change between the subcutaneous part of the external anal sphincter and the border of the internal anal sphincter.
- For the closed internal lateral sphincterotomy, the author prefers to use a cataract scalpel due to the vertical plane of the cutting edge of the blade (**FIGURE 5**), as opposed to the oblique plane of the cutting edge of a no. 11 blade. This makes it easier to cut the internal sphincter more evenly as the scalpel is withdrawn from the intersphincteric groove.

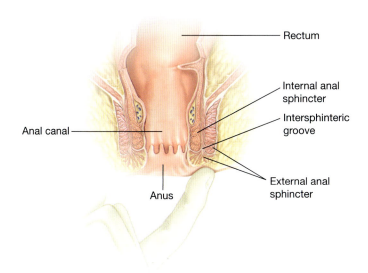

FIGURE 4 • The intersphincteric groove. The intersphincteric groove can be easily palpated by the surgeon's right index finger between the external and internal anal sphincters.

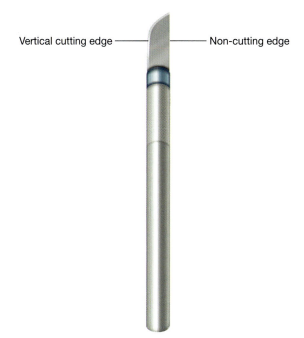

FIGURE 5 • A cataract scalpel. This scalpel's blade has a vertical cutting edge and a blunt edge on the opposite side, making its shape and size ideal to insert in the intersphincteric groove.

- Place your left index finger in the anal canal. In cases of HIV or hepatitis B/C infection, insert an anal speculum instead of inserting your own finger as a precaution to avoid potential transmission of communicable disease in case of inadvertent injury to your index finger during the sphincterotomy.
- Using a no. 11 blade scalpel on your right hand, create a small opening on the skin overlying the intersphincteric groove on the patient's left lateral side. Performing the closed lateral internal sphincterotomy on the anal canal's left lateral side is easier for a right-handed surgeon to perform (scalpel in your dominant hand).
- Introduce a cataract blade scalpel through this skin opening and into the intersphincteric groove, with the blade of the knife in between the internal and external anal sphincter muscles and until the tip of the blade is located just distal to the level of the dentate line (**FIGURE 6**). The blade should be inserted parallel to the sphincter muscles, so that it is oriented on an anterior/posterior direction, therefore preventing accidental cutting of the external sphincter on the way in.
- Alternatively, you can use a no. 11 blade scalpel if a cataract scalpel is not available.
- Now, turn the blade of the cataract scalpel 90° so that the left lateral cutting edge is facing inward, toward the internal anal sphincter.
- Press the cutting edge of the blade toward your index finger (placed in the anal canal), cutting the internal sphincter in the process (**FIGURE 7**). As you withdraw the scalpel outward, finish cutting the internal sphincter evenly in one sweeping motion. Repeat this maneuver if necessary.
- If you transected the internal sphincter appropriately, you should feel the anus relax immediately.
- Avoid cutting the mucosa of the anal canal because this could lead to troublesome anal fistulae postoperatively. In

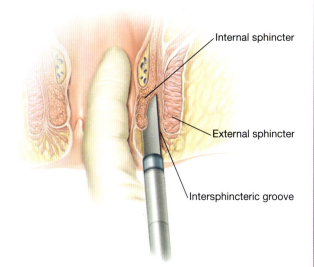

FIGURE 6 • Closed internal lateral sphincterotomy: insertion of the cataract scalpel into the intersphincteric groove. The blade of the cataract scalpel is inserted into the groove, parallel to the plane of the sphincters, in order to avoid inadvertent injury to the external sphincter upon insertion.

the event that the anal canal mucosa is cut, reapproximate it with running fast-absorbable 3-0 suture. The presence of your index finger in the anal canal allows you to feel the blade as it cuts through the internal sphincter and helps prevent cutting the mucosa of the anal canal.

- Minor bleeding from the skin opening at the end of the procedure is not uncommon; holding pressure from inside

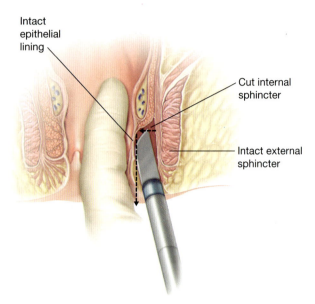

FIGURE 7 • Closed internal lateral sphincterotomy. The cataract scalpel blade is first pushed internally toward the anal canal and is then withdrawn (*dotted arrows*), cutting the internal sphincter in the process. The index finger inside the anal canal allows the surgeon to gauge the proper depth of transection through the sphincter without violating the epithelial lining of the anal canal.

Intact epithelial lining
Cut internal sphincter
Intact external sphincter

and outside the anal canal is usually all that is necessary to achieve hemostasis. If more troublesome bleeding occurs from the transected internal sphincter muscle bed, you can inject thrombin glue into the area and hold pressure. In the rare cases where the bleeding does not stop, you may have to open the overlaying mucosa of the anal canal to expose the bleeder and control it surgically.

- Place a tampon in the anal canal at the completion of the procedure for hemostasis; the patient can remove it postoperatively.
- In patients with large left lateral hemorrhoids, the closed lateral internal sphincterotomy can be performed on the patient's right lateral side, in between the right anterior and right posterior hemorrhoidal pedicles. This helps reduce the risk of bleeding from a transected hemorrhoidal pedicle. The technique used is the same as the one described here, but using your right index finger in the anal canal and cutting with the scalpel in your left hand.

OPEN LATERAL INTERNAL SPHINCTEROTOMY

- Using lubrication, perform a gentle anal dilation with two fingers.
- An anal speculum is inserted to confirm the presence of the anal fissure and to expose the anal canal.
- With the patient on a modified lithotomy position and palpating with the tip of your right index finger, identify the anal intersphincteric groove (**FIGURE 4**). The intersphincteric groove is a distinct groove in the anal canal, forming the lower border of the pecten analis, marking the change between the subcutaneous part of the external anal sphincter and the border of the internal anal sphincter.
- Make a radial incision with a no. 15 blade scalpel over the intersphincteric groove on the patient's left lateral side and extend it toward the anal canal for a distance of 1 to 1.5 cm (**FIGURE 8A**).
- Performing the open lateral internal sphincterotomy on the anal canal's left lateral side is easier for a right-handed surgeon to perform. In patients with large left lateral hemorrhoids, the closed lateral internal sphincterotomy can be performed on the patient's right lateral side, in between the right anterior and right posterior hemorrhoidal pedicles. This helps reduce the risk of bleeding from a transected hemorrhoidal pedicle.
- Using Metzenbaum scissors to develop a submucosal plane, separate the anal mucosa from the underlying internal sphincter (**FIGURE 8B**).
- The distal aspect of the internal anal sphincter and the medial aspect of the external anal sphincter are exposed.

- The intersphincteric groove is dissected gently with Metzenbaum scissors, completely separating the internal sphincter from the external sphincter.
- The internal sphincter is then transected full thickness (**FIGURE 8C**) under direct visualization with Metzenbaum scissors to the level of the dentate line (typically about 2 cm in length).
- If you transected the internal sphincter appropriately, you should feel the anus relax immediately.
- Hemostasis is carefully achieved with electrocautery.
- The incision is closed with a running, rapidly absorbable 3-0 suture (**FIGURE 8D**).
- Place a tampon in the anal canal at the completion of the procedure for hemostasis.

Other Procedures

- The Lord procedure: Dilation of the anus is performed initially with two fingers and then slowly stretching the anal canal (over 2-3 minutes) until it accommodates four fingers. The dilation, performed by moving the two fingers around in a circular fashion, accomplishes what was originally described as a "controlled" disruption of the internal sphincter. The problem is that there is really no way of controlling the disruption of the sphincter in this way and it is easy to disrupt the external sphincter as well. This procedure has largely been abandoned due to an unacceptably high incidence of anal incontinence associated with it.
- Excision of the fissure with posterior open sphincterotomy: This procedure has also been largely abandoned due to the deformity that it produces in the anal canal and unacceptably high incidence of anal incontinence associated with it.

Chapter 46 SURGICAL MANAGEMENT OF ANAL FISSURES   437

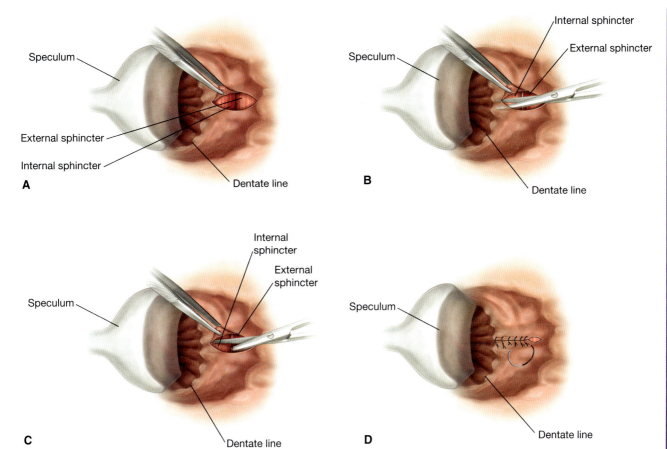

FIGURE 8 • Open internal lateral sphincterotomy. **A**, A radial skin incision is made. **B**, A submucosal dissection is performed exposing the internal and external anal sphincters. **C**, The internal sphincter is cut to the level of the dentate line. **D**, The skin incision is closed with running absorbable suture.

PEARLS AND PITFALLS

Patient positioning	▪ The author prefers the modified lithotomy position with the legs elevated.
Visualization	▪ Using headlights is critical for good visualization.
Intersphincteric groove	▪ It is critically important to properly identify the intersphincteric groove. ▪ Gentle palpation with the tip of the right index finger allows for easier localization of this groove.
Closed internal lateral sphincterotomy	▪ A left lateral internal sphincterotomy is easier to perform for a right-handed surgeon. ▪ A right lateral internal sphincterotomy may be preferred in patients with large left lateral hemorrhoids. ▪ Using a cataract blade greatly facilitates a more uniform transection of the internal sphincter. ▪ Cut the internal sphincter as you withdraw the blade out. ▪ Having your left index finger inside the anal canal helps prevent accidently cutting the anal mucosa.
Open internal lateral sphincterotomy	▪ Separate the internal and external sphincters. ▪ Cut the internal sphincter to the level of the dentate line. ▪ This results in higher incidence of anal sphincter dysfunction postoperatively when compared to the closed technique.
Postoperative care	▪ Aggressive prevention of constipation with a bowel regimen is mandatory.

POSTOPERATIVE CARE

- This procedure is typically performed on an outpatient basis.
- The patient removes the anal tampon the day after surgery or during the first bowel movement.
- Aggressive prevention of constipation with a bowel regimen is mandatory.
- The patient is placed on a high-fiber, low-fat diet.
- The author recommends over-the-counter fiber supplementation (totaling 25-35 g of fiber per day). Stool softeners and increasing water intake are also necessary to promote soft bowel movements and to aid in the healing process.
- Judicious use of laxatives.
- Nonsteroidal anti-inflammatory agents are prescribed. Narcotic use is used sparingly due to their tendency to induce constipation.
- Warm sitz baths for comfort purposes are used.
- Wiping after bowel movements is only allowed with flushable baby wipes (no toilet paper) to prevent irritation.
- Use of zinc oxide ointments may help accelerate the healing of deep anal fissures.

OUTCOMES AND POSTOPERATIVE COMPLICATIONS

- Garcia-Aguilar and colleagues have published perhaps the most comprehensive analysis of outcomes after open internal sphincterotomy (OIS) and closed internal sphincterotomy (CIS).
- Overall, both techniques accomplish excellent results in terms of resolution of pain and healing of the fissure.
- Differences in persistence of symptoms (3.4% OIS vs 5.3% CIS), recurrence of the fissure (10.9% vs 11.7% CIS), and need for reoperation (3.4% OIS vs 4% CIS) were statistically not significant.
- However, statistically significant differences were seen in the percentage of patients with permanent postoperative difficulty controlling gas (30.3% vs 23.6%; $P < .062$), soiling underclothing (26.7% vs 16.1%; $P < .001$), and accidental bowel movements (11.8% vs 3.1%; $P < .001$) between those who underwent OIS and those who had CIS.
- Although 90% of patients reported general overall satisfaction, more patients undergoing CIS (64.4%) than OIS (49.7%) were very satisfied with the results of the procedure.
- The author concluded that lateral internal sphincterotomy is highly effective in treatment of chronic anal fissure but is associated with significant permanent alterations in continence. CIS is preferable to OIS because it effects a similar rate of cure with less impairment of control.

SUGGESTED READINGS

1. Cross KL, Massey EJ, Fowler AL. The management of anal fissure: ACPGBI position statement. *Colorectal Dis*. 2008;10(suppl 3):1-7.
2. Garcia-Aguilar J, Belmonte C, Wong WD, et al. Open vs. closed sphincterotomy for chronic anal fissure: long-term results. *Dis Colon Rectum*. 1996;39(4):440-443.
3. Garg P, Garg M, Menon GR. Long-term continence disturbance after lateral internal sphincterotomy for chronic anal fissure: a systematic review and meta-analysis. *Colorectal Dis*. 2013;15(3):e104-e117.
4. Herzig DO, Lu KC. Anal fissure. *Surg Clin North Am*. 2010;90(1):33-44.
5. Nelson RL, Chattopadhyay A, Brooks W, et al. Operative procedures for fissure in ano. *Cochrane Database Syst Rev*. 2011;11:CD002199.
6. Nelson RL, Thomas K, Morgan J, et al. Non surgical therapy for anal fissure. *Cochrane Database Syst Rev*. 2012;2:CD003431.

Chapter 47

Operative Treatment of Rectal Prolapse: Perineal Approach (Altemeier and Modified Delorme Procedures)

Valerie P. Bauer

DEFINITION

- Rectal prolapse is a "falling down" of the rectum caused by weakness in surrounding supportive tissues. Straining during constipation secondary to functional disorders of elimination (anismus) and anatomic causes of outlet obstruction such as middle and anterior pelvic organ prolapse (enterocele, sigmoidocele, rectocele, hysterocele, and cystocele) are major risks factors. Other risk factors include low anterior cul-de-sac, multiparity, anal sphincter muscle weakness, levator diastasis, redundant rectosigmoid, and neurologic disease.[1] Recognition of the type of prolapse determines operative approach. Internal intussusception includes all layers of the rectum and rectosigmoid through the rectum and into the anal canal but not beyond. Partial-thickness prolapse involves protrusion of the redundant **mucosal** layer of the rectum for a distance of 1 to 3 cm from the anal margin (**FIGURE 1A**). True prolapse consists of a full-thickness protrusion of all layers of the rectum through a sliding hernia of the cul-de-sac so that the rectum is out of the body (**FIGURE 1B**).[2]

DIFFERENTIAL DIAGNOSIS

- Prolapsed and incarcerated internal hemorrhoids may appear similar to rectal prolapse. The appearance of concentric folds differentiate rectal prolapse from hemorrhoidal prolapse, which appears as radial invaginations relative to anatomic location of the internal hemorrhoidal cushions.
- Enterocele and sigmoidocele is the combined prolapse of posterior vaginal wall and herniation of the respective segments of bowel through the anterior cul-de-sac, which may cause anterior rectal prolapse and bleeding.
- Hysterocele and cystocele involve vaginal prolapse, which can also contribute to the "pulling down" of the fascial support of the rectum.
- Rectal cancer or polyps may act as a lead point from which colorectal prolapse occurs, hence underscoring the importance of diagnostic colonoscopy to rule out proximal mucosal pathology as a cause of intussusception.
- Inflammatory colitides should be considered for findings of isolated rectal ulceration, seen in the anterior rectum at the point of retroperitoneal fixation, where repeated internal prolapse forms. A discrete anterior solitary rectal ulcer is approximately 4 to 10 cm from the anal verge.

PATIENT HISTORY AND PHYSICAL FINDINGS

- Successful perineal proctosigmoidectomy for full-thickness prolapse (Altemeier) and mucosectomy for partial mucosal prolapse (modified Delorme) depends on proper determination of type of prolapse. Therefore, accurate history and recognition of physical examination findings is of paramount importance.
- Surgery for isolated internal prolapse is currently not performed in lieu of conservative management to include dietary and behavioral modifications, such as pelvic muscle rehabilitation for treatment of functional elimination disorders. However, future understanding of the relationship between posterior internal pelvic organ prolapse and middle/anterior pelvic organ prolapse may redefine guidelines for surgical indication using a multidisciplinary approach to multiorgan repair to include colorectal, urogynecology, and urology subspecialists.
- A thorough history must identify causes of constipation (and excessive straining) such as dietary and social behaviors (inadequate fiber intake, sedentary lifestyle), medications, and medical conditions (hypothyroidism, electrolyte disturbances, interstitial cystitis, pelvic organ prolapse, anxiety, or psychiatric disturbances).
- Past surgical history of multiple prior pelvic operations (hysterectomy, sacrocolpopexy, coloproctostomy) increases

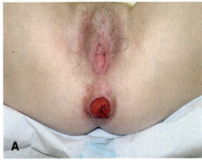

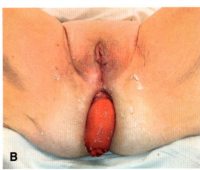

FIGURE 1 • Presentation of full-thickness rectal prolapse. **A,** Mucosal prolapse showing concentric circles of mucosal folds in association with hysterocele. **B,** Large prolapse in recurrent disease after a failed Altemeier procedure showing engorged mucosa and loss of concentric folds.

operative risk for complication. Prior abdominal repair of rectal prolapse with rectosigmoid resection is a contraindication to perineal proctectomy due to altered mesenteric blood flow and risk for distal ischemia.

- Risk factors for colorectal cancer and polyps is determined through family history and personal history of changes in bowel habits, bleeding, and results of most recent colonoscopy.

- Obstetric and urogynecologic history aims to determine risk factors for anal muscle weakness and pelvic organ prolapse, such as number of intrauterine pregnancies, term vaginal deliveries, large-birth-weight baby, prolonged labor, use of forceps, high-grade vaginal tear, absence of controlled episiotomy, and urinary incontinence. In addition, nulliparity has been associated with higher incidence of rectal prolapse as well.[3,4]

- Initial presentation is commonly described as "something falling out that has to be pushed back in." Other possible initial complaints include a feeling of fullness in the pelvis, severe pain (levator muscle spasm), bleeding, incomplete evacuation with splinting or positional maneuvers to eliminate, excessive straining, mucus or fecal staining, perineal discomfort and burning (due to chronic moisture), improved pain on lying down, and fecal urgency with "nothing there."

- Initial anorectal examination is done in prone jackknife or lateral Sims position. It begins with inspection of the perianal skin. In the absence of grossly visible prolapse at the anal margin, a patulous anus, fecal smearing, and thickening (lichenification) of anoderm due to chronic perineal moisture suggests rectal or mucosal prolapse. The appearance of the anus may be flat due to loss of compliance and function of the pelvic floor musculature (perineal descent syndrome). Visible scars due to episiotomy or prior anorectal surgery should be noted.

- Vaginal examination may reveal anterior vaginal prolapse (cystocele) or posterior vaginal wall prolapse (rectocele, enterocele).

- Digital rectal examination determines anal sphincter tone and function. Patients with full-thickness prolapse often have little to no resting or squeeze tone due to levator muscle separation and pudendal nerve damage. Patients are asked to squeeze to give some indication of sphincter strength (diagnostic of fecal incontinence). Digital palpation of the perineal body may also reveal anterior thinning and sphincteric defect due to prior obstetric injury or other mechanisms of levator separation.

- Digital compression in the anterior rectum may reveal rectocele. The patient should be asked to strain during digital palpation to evaluate for paradoxical contraction or lack of anal sphincter relaxation (indicative of functional elimination disorder, anismus). Similarly, exaggerated strain may reproduce internal prolapse and/or rectocele, which is appreciated by luminal protrusion into the posterior wall of the vagina.

- Anorectal examination uses a side-viewing anoscope (Hirschman) to evaluate the anal canal. Internal hemorrhoids may or may not prolapse with rectal prolapse. However, they may be inflamed, bleeding, or thrombosed due to excessive straining from outlet obstruction caused by the prolapse. Patients with rectal prolapse complain more of hemorrhoidal disease due to a lack of awareness of rectal prolapse. Rigid proctosigmoidoscopy allows for evaluation of the rectum and sigmoid up to 25 cm from the anal verge for evidence of prolapse or other mucosal disease. Anterior solitary rectal ulcer is classically seen between the first and second valve of Houston and represents the point of recurrent internal prolapse. Release of air insufflation and having the patient bear down as the scope is withdrawn will prolapse redundant tissue into the aperture of the proctosigmoidoscope, which is diagnostic of rectal prolapse in the office.

IMAGING AND OTHER DIAGNOSTIC STUDIES

- Having the patient squat or strain, especially after administration of fleet enema, will help protrude the prolapsed rectum. This test is performed in the clinic and is diagnostic of rectal prolapse (toilet test).

- Defecography uses fluoroscopic imaging to evaluate the structure and function of posterior, middle, and anterior pelvic floor during the three phases of elimination—rest, squeeze, and strain. It may be used to diagnose rectal prolapse if it is not clinically evident. Pelvic floor structures are visualized using thick barium paste instilled into the rectum, a barium-impregnated tampon in the vagina, oral contrast for small bowel, and intravenous contrast for visualization of the bladder. Internal rectal prolapse is demonstrated during strain in image (**FIGURE 2A** and **B**).

- Pelvic floor physiology testing determines preoperative functional baseline of the anal sphincter, especially when there is associated fecal incontinence. These tests include anal manometry, rectal sensation, and anal electromyography (EMG).

- Pudendal nerve terminal motor latency determines neurogenic impediment to anal sphincter muscle function. Although pudendal neuropathy is not a contraindication for repair of rectal prolapse, its presence may predict poor outcome in improvement of fecal incontinence associated with rectal prolapse after surgery and should be discussed with the patient preoperatively.[5]

SURGICAL MANAGEMENT

Preoperative Planning

- Perineal repair of rectal prolapse is favored for patients with high-risk surgical comorbidities. Therefore, medical and cardiac risk stratification should be obtained prior to surgery and discussed with every patient, including the possibility of complication due to comorbid condition.

- Surgery is done under general anesthesia; however, in the high-risk population, the procedure can be performed under spinal or even local anesthesia.

- Patients undergo preoperative bowel preparation and fleet enemas before the procedure.

- Previous intra-abdominal resection for repair of rectal prolapse increases ischemic complications from subsequent perineal resections, and it is considered a relative contraindication to perineal repair.

Positioning

- The patient may be placed in lithotomy position using candy cane or Allen stirrups or in prone jackknife position.

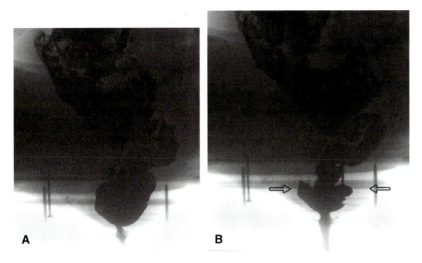

FIGURE 2 • **A,** Cine defecography during the initial strain phase of elimination shows foreshortening of rectum with early internal intussusception. **B,** The prolapse progresses with strain, but not beyond the anal canal, illustrating internal rectorectal intussusception *(arrows)* without mucosal or full-thickness prolapse.

PERINEAL PROCTECTOMY (ALTEMEIER PROCEDURE)

Preparation After Anesthesia Induction

- Rigid proctosigmoidoscopy is performed to ensure there is clean preparation. Residual stool may be suctioned and the rectum irrigated with saline or diluted Betadine solution until clean.
- A full perineal and vaginal preparation is performed using Betadine solution.
- A Foley catheter is inserted.
- Local anesthesia, using a total of 30 mL 0.25% Marcaine with 1:200,000 epinephrine, is infiltrated through a 22-gauge spinal needle in the intersphincteric groove circumferentially.
- A Lone Star retractor system (CooperSurgical Inc, Trumbull, CT) is positioned using small hooked retractors placed at the dentate line circumferentially (**FIGURE 3**).

Incision

- The prolapsed segment is grasped with Babcock clamps.
- Electrocautery is used to score a circumferential incision 1 to 1.5 cm proximal to the dentate line. This is deepened through all the layers of the rectal wall circumferentially (**FIGURE 4**).
- Clamps are applied to the distal edge of the rectum.

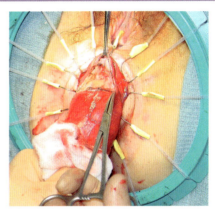

FIGURE 4 • A full-thickness incision is placed 1 to 1.5 cm from the anal verge using electrocautery around the rectum.

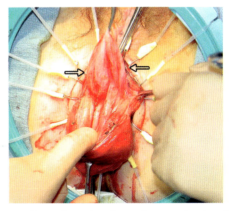

FIGURE 5 • Sharp dissection frees the anterior hernia sac (as noted by the *arrows*) from the prolapsed rectal tissue.

Anterior Dissection of the Hernia Sac

- A deep pouch of Douglas is often encountered and dissected free from the anterior segment of the rectum (**FIGURE 5**).
- The hernia sac is resected, allowing access to the intraabdominal cavity and delivery of excess redundant bowel.

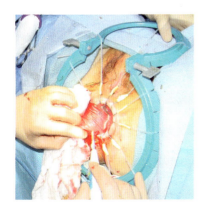

FIGURE 3 • Placement of the Lone Star retractor using hooked elastic bands attached to the dentate line in a circumferential fashion.

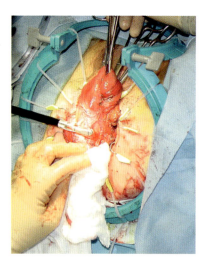

FIGURE 6 • An energy device that enables sealing of mesorectal vasculature may be used to safely and rapidly divide the mesorectum in the process of mobilizing the redundant rectal prolapse.

- The peritoneal edges are reapproximated using absorbable suture, thus excluding the abdominal cavity.

Posterior Dissection

- An energy device, such as Enseal (Ethicon Endo-Surgery Inc, Cincinnati, OH), may be used to seal and divide the mesorectum (**FIGURE 6**).
- Redundant bowel is freely delivered (**FIGURE 7A**). The extent of delivery may vary according to the degree of prolapse and extent of surgical dissection (**FIGURE 7B**).

Posterior Levatorplasty

- A modification of the Altemeier operation involves the addition of a levatorplasty, which is the plication of either the anterior or the posterior levator ani muscles with long-term absorbable sutures such as polydioxanone (PDS). Placation of either the anterior or posterior levator muscles decreases pelvic outlet aperture and decreases recurrence while improving continence.[6] Anterior levatorplasty is associated with a higher incidence of dyspareunia than posterior levatorplasty.
- The levator ani muscle is grasped on each side with a Babcock clamp and reapproximated using two to three interrupted sutures (**FIGURE 8**). Care should be taken to ensure that two fingerbreadths pass through the remaining aperture to avoid excessive compression of the rectum and subsequent constipation.
- If the peritoneal cavity is entered, the peritoneum is closed with absorbable sutures. The bowel is fastened to the peritoneum and anterior tissue using interrupted absorbable sutures.

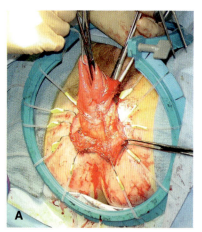
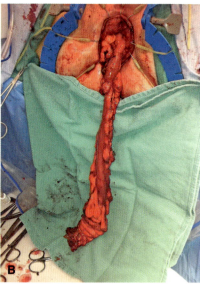

FIGURE 7 • **A** and **B**, Variable degrees of redundant prolapse may be observed in the mobilization and delivery of bowel.

Resection of Redundant Rectosigmoid

- The level of transection is determined by the viability of the bowel and approximation to the proximal free edge of the distal resected cuff. Division begins anteriorly. In order to prevent retraction of the rectum into the pelvis, four corner sutures are placed and left tagged prior to completely transecting the rectum.
- Absorbable 2-0 Vicryl sutures are placed full thickness in interrupted fashion, reapproximating the bowel.
- Upon completion, rigid proctoscopy is performed to ensure the viability of the bowel proximal to the anastomosis and also to assess the integrity of the bowel, ruling out a possible perforation that might have been incurred during the dissection.
- The Lone Star retractor is removed and the anastomosis is interiorized.

Chapter 47 OPERATIVE TREATMENT OF RECTAL PROLAPSE   443

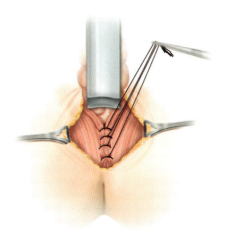
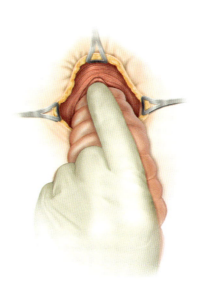

FIGURE 8 • Plication technique of the posterior levator ani muscles. Note that two fingerbreadths pass through the remaining aperture in the reapproximated levator ani muscle to avoid excessive compression of the rectum and subsequent constipation.

DELORME PROCEDURE

- This procedure was described by Delorme in 1900, for repair of mucosal prolapse, and involves stripping of the mucosa from the prolapsed bowel, placating the denuded muscular wall, and reanastomosing the mucosal rings.[7]

Preparation After Anesthesia Induction

- The patient is positioned and prepared in a manner similar to that of an Altemeier procedure.

- The submucosa is infiltrated using a local anesthetic such as 0.25% bupivacaine with 1:200,000 epinephrine in order to reduce bleeding and facilitate the plane of dissection.

Incision

- A circular incision is made through the mucosa approximately 1 cm proximal to the dentate line (**FIGURE 9A**).
- A sleeve of mucosa and submucosa is sharply dissected from the underlying muscle to the apex of the protruding bowel and the point at which there is some tension (**FIGURE 9B**).

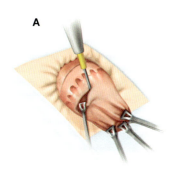
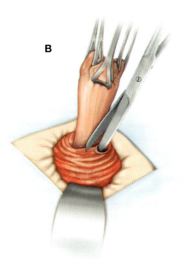

FIGURE 9 • **A**, The mucosa is dissected 1.0 to 1.5 cm proximal to the dentate line, and **(B)** it is then stripped off of the muscularis propria.

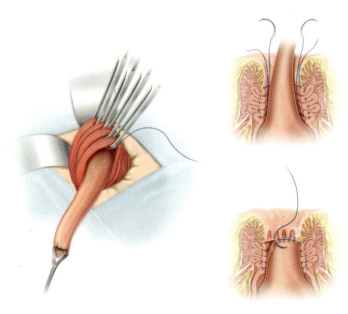

FIGURE 10 • The muscularis propria is plicated in all four quadrants.

Plication of muscularis propria

- The denuded muscle (muscularis propria) is prepared for longitudinal plication by placing serial Allis clamps in each quadrant. Vicryl sutures are placed in all four quadrants, beginning from proximal to the incised mucosa and ending at the level to where the mucosa is dissected (**FIGURE 10**).

- The placating sutures are tied after confirmation of absolute hemostasis.

Resection and anastomosis

- The stripped mucosa is then excised and anastomosed to the distal mucosa with interrupted absorbable sutures.

PEARLS AND PITFALLS

Indications	▪ A thorough history and physical examination should be obtained, including in-office administration of enema to reproduce and confirm full-thickness or partial rectal prolapse. ▪ Clinical suspicion for internal prolapse may be diagnosed with symptoms of incomplete defecation and defecogram showing rectorectal intussusception with or without obstruction. ▪ Prior history of rectal prolapse repair increases risk for ischemia on subsequent perineal repair if the initial procedure involved division of mesenteric blood flow. ▪ Complete colonoscopic evaluation should be performed to rule out proximal cause of obstructed defecation or prolapse.
Dissection	▪ Identification, resection, and closure of the anterior hernia are important for obliterating the hernia sac contributing to the anterior prolapse. ▪ Care should be taken to prevent division of the mesentery proximal to the bowel edge in order to minimize anastomotic ischemia and tension.
Levatorplasty	▪ Placation of either the anterior or posterior levator muscles decreases pelvic outlet aperture and decreases recurrence while improving continence. ▪ Anterior levatorplasty is associated with higher incidence of dyspareunia. ▪ Posterior levatorplasty should allow two fingerbreadths between the bowel and muscle approximation to minimize constipation postoperatively.
Rigid proctosigmoidoscopy	▪ Evaluates for potential unrecognized rectal perforation that may have been undetected during the dissection.

POSTOPERATIVE CARE

- Regular diet is usually resumed on postoperative day 1.
- The Foley catheter is removed the day after surgery. The patient can be discharged on postoperative day 1.
- A bowel regimen should be implemented to minimize constipation and excessive straining postoperatively. The patient should be educated to take adequate fiber intake and gentle cathartics, such as milk of magnesia, each day for 2 weeks until the anastomosis has healed. Avoidance of excess straining should be stressed, along with orders for nothing per rectum.

OUTCOMES

- Perineal proctosigmoidectomy has variable reported recurrence rates ranging from 10% to 25% in large clinical studies. The addition of posterior levatorplasty improves recurrence rates down to 7.7% and also increases time to recurrence from 13.3 to 45.5 months.[6]
- The Delorme procedure has similarly high recurrence rates but has been favored to perineal proctosigmoidectomy in cases of extreme comorbid conditions or failed surgery for prolapse.[8]

COMPLICATIONS

- Anastomotic dehiscence (intrapelvic leakage is uncommon) is usually due to tension and/or poor blood supply. Therefore, extreme care must be taken to mobilize the bowel adequately and to avoid transecting the mesentery too far proximally.
- Bleeding occurs in 5% of patients, with resulting pelvic hematoma.
- Anastomotic stricture: Most patients will develop some degree of stricture, but it rarely requires dilatation.

REFERENCES

1. Nigro ND. An evaluation of the cause and mechanism of complete rectal prolapse. *Dis Colon Rectum.* 1966;9(6):391-398.
2. Altemeier WA, Culbertson WR, Schowengerdt C, et al. Nineteen years' experience with the one-stage perineal repair of rectal prolapse. *Ann Surg.* 1971;173(6):993-1006.
3. Menees SB, Smith TM, Xu X, et al. Factors associated with symptom severity in women presenting with fecal incontinence. *Dis Colon Rectum.* 2013;56(1):97-102.
4. Kahn MA, Stanton SL. Posterior colporrhaphy: its effects on bowel and sexual function. *Br J Obstet Gynaecol.* 1997;104:82-86.
5. Birnbaum EH, Stamm L, Rafferty JF, et al. Pudendal nerve terminal motor latency influences surgical outcome in rectal prolapse. *Dis Colon Rectum.* 1996;39(11):1215-1221.
6. Chun SW, Pilarski AJ, You SY, et al. Perineal rectosigmoidectomy for rectal prolapse: role of levatorplasty. *Tech Coloproctol.* 2004;8(1):3-8.
7. Tsunoda A, Yasuda N, Noboru Y, et al. Delorme's procedure of rectal prolapse: clinical and physiological analysis. *Dis Colon Rectum.* 2003;46:1260-1265.
8. Senapati A, Nicholls RJ, Thomson JP, et al. Results of Delorme's procedure for rectal prolapse. *Dis Colon Rectum.* 1994;37:456-460.

Chapter 48

Operative Treatment of Rectal Prolapse: Transabdominal Approach

Karin M. Hardiman

DEFINITION
- Rectal prolapse is the full-thickness protrusion of the rectum through the anus. The rectum intussuscepts and then progresses outward to come out of the anus.

DIFFERENTIAL DIAGNOSIS
- It is important to differentiate rectal prolapse from prolapsing hemorrhoids (**FIGURE 1**), as the treatment paradigms are completely different. Rectal prolapse is prolapsing rectal tissue that has full concentric rings. Prolapsing internal hemorrhoids is a mucosal prolapse in three separate bundles.

PATIENT HISTORY AND PHYSICAL FINDINGS
- Rectal prolapse is most common in multiparous elderly women with long-standing constipation. A small percentage is also seen in young male patients. Scleroderma and psychiatric disorders are also more common in patients with rectal prolapse.
- Patients describe having tissue extrude from their anus that usually retracts on its own or with manual pressure. Prolapse is most often associated with episodes of straining but it can occur even with ambulation, especially in elderly female patients. It is important to elicit how much they are prolapsing, how often, and how much it is bothering them in order to decide whether to operate. Prolapse is often associated with mild bleeding and mucus discharge.
- It is important to elicit any bowel habits dysfunction that has to be addressed. Recurrence rates of prolapse are higher after surgery when severe constipation or obstructed defecation due to pelvic floor dysfunction is not addressed.
- The patient should be asked about their continence as the surgeries for prolapse described here do not immediately improve continence. After prolapse surgery, about half of patients have some improvement in continence over time, but if their incontinence is severe and they cannot squeeze on examination, they may be better served with an ostomy. Intense preoperative counseling is critical.
- Associated gynecologic and/or urologic pelvic floor dysfunction issues (including difficulty with urination and uterine prolapse) commonly seen in rectal prolapse patients should be addressed in a multidisciplinary fashion together with a urogynecologist.
- Patients often come with digital photographs of their prolapse that allow for confirmation of the diagnosis. Otherwise, it is important to elicit the prolapse in the clinic to be able to differentiate it from prolapsing hemorrhoids.
- The best way to confirm the rectal prolapse is to give the patient 5 minutes on the toilet to elicit the prolapse and then examine them. Rectal prolapse looks like a single long tube sticking out with concentric ring; prolapsing hemorrhoids look like multiple individual quadrants of tissue (**FIGURE 1**).
- Physical examination should include digital rectal examination to assess for masses. Having the patient push during the examination allows the examiner to feel for enterocele,

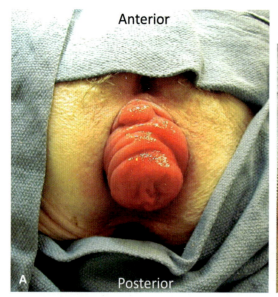
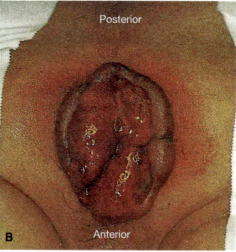

FIGURE 1 • It is important to differentiate **(A)** rectal prolapse from **(B)** prolapsing internal hemorrhoids. Rectal prolapse is prolapsing tissue that has full concentric rings (patient is in supine position, in candy canes). Prolapsing internal hemorrhoids is a mucosal prolapse in three separate bundles (patient is in a prone jackknife position).

rectocele, and cystocele. In addition, the patient should be asked to squeeze to assess the sphincter muscles.
- Patients with an incarcerated rectal prolapse may on occasion present to the emergency room. In these cases, the treatment depends on the appearance of the bowel. If viable, gentle reduction with sedation, reassurance, and education are usually all that is needed and the patient can follow up electively; if not viable, a perineal proctectomy is needed.

IMAGING AND OTHER DIAGNOSTIC STUDIES

- Any patient being evaluated for rectal prolapse should have a colonoscopy to rule out either a malignancy acting as the lead point of the prolapse or a synchronous tumor.
- In patients that are unable to elicit prolapse or bring you a picture, a defecography can be very helpful. During this procedure, the patient's small bowel, rectum, and vagina are all filled with contrast and the patient is asked to have a barium bowel movement while the radiologist takes a video. This often demonstrates the prolapse along with other types of pelvic floor dysfunction. The prolapse may not be seen on defecography, as evacuation of barium requires less straining than evacuation of hard stool in constipated patients.

SURGICAL MANAGEMENT

Operative Planning and Strategy

- The choice of operation is dependent on many factors including patient health, prior surgeries, the operating surgeon's comfort with laparoscopy, and whether the patient has a history of constipation.
- If the patient is healthy enough, then an abdominal rather than a perineal approach should be offered due to the lower risk of recurrence. Otherwise, they may be better served with a lower risk perineal operation or no operation at all.
- Rectal prolapse is not dangerous unless incarcerated, so not all patients are offered operation.
- Abdominal surgery for rectal prolapse should include dissection posterior to the mesorectum with fixation of the mobilized rectum just below the sacral promontory, as this fixation decreases the risk of recurrence. The fixation can be performed with sutures or with mesh.
- In constipated patients, resection of the sigmoid colon is recommended. In these cases, although not proven beneficial by Cochrane review of available evidence, either a full bowel preparation or just enemas can be performed preoperatively at the surgeon's discretion.
- The surgery can be performed open or laparoscopically. Laparoscopic surgery is associated with significant short-term advantages over open surgery.
- Preoperative antibiotics are given within 1 hour of incision to decrease the risk of postoperative wound infection and are stopped within 24 hours of surgery.
- Heparin prophylaxis is given perioperatively to lower the risk of deep vein thrombosis.

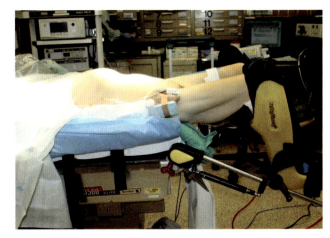

FIGURE 2 • Patient positioning for laparoscopic rectal prolapse repair. The patient is placed in a lithotomy position with the thighs parallel to the ground to avoid conflict with the surgeon's arms. The patient is placed on a beanbag with both arms tucked and taped to the table over a towel.

Positioning

- Any rectal prolapse should be reduced manually prior to starting the operation.
- For laparoscopic operations, the patient is placed on a lithotomy position with the legs on Yellofin stirrups and with the thighs parallel to the ground to avoid conflict with the surgeon's arms and instruments (FIGURE 2). Avoid pressure on the calves (to prevent deep vein thrombosis) and on the lateral peroneal nerves (to prevent foot drop).
- Both arms are tucked and padded to avoid neurovascular injuries (for open cases, the arms are placed on arm boards laterally). All lines and cords are kept out of the tucking.
- Tape the patient across the chest over a towel to secure them to the operating room (OR) table.

LAPAROSCOPIC SUTURE RECTOPEXY

Insufflation, Port, and Team Setup

- The abdomen is accessed with either a Veress needle or a Hassan port at the inferior portion of the umbilicus and carbon dioxide (CO_2) pneumoperitoneum is established.
- Port placement (FIGURE 3): A 5-mm infraumbilical camera port is inserted for the 30° camera. Three 5-mm working ports are inserted in the right lower quadrant, the right upper quadrant, and the left lower quadrant.
- The surgeon stands on the patient's right side, with the scrub nurse next to them. The assistant stands on the left side of the table (FIGURE 4).

Posterior Dissection

- The patient is placed in a steep Trendelenburg position with the left side up. The bowel is placed in the upper abdomen. The sigmoid colon and rectum are often very redundant and can be hard to manipulate. At times, this may require additional port placement.

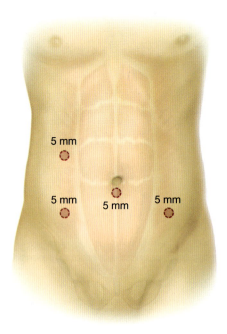

FIGURE 3 • Laparoscopic rectopexy port placement. A 5-mm infraumbilical camera port is inserted for the 30° camera. Three 5-mm working ports are inserted in the right lower quadrant, the right upper quadrant, and the left lower quadrant.

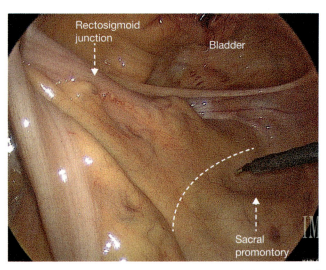

FIGURE 5 • The rectosigmoid is pulled toward the abdominal wall, tenting out the base of its mesentery peritoneum at the sacral promontory. The peritoneum is incised along the root of the mesocolon (dotted line) across the promontory toward the right posterolateral cul-de-sac.

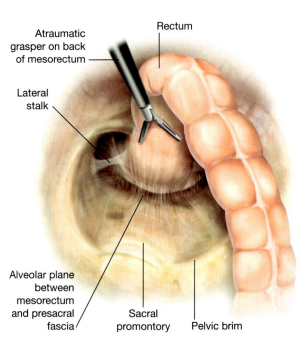

FIGURE 6 • The rectum is lifted anteriorly toward the abdominal wall in order to reveal the alveolar plane between the mesorectum and the presacral fascia.

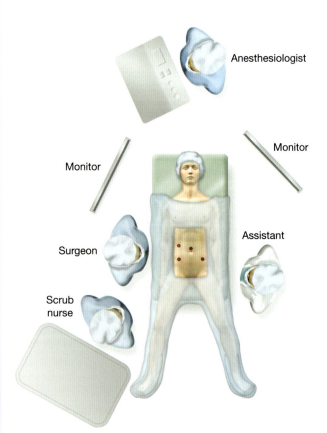

FIGURE 4 • Operating room team setup. The surgeon stands on the patient's right side with the scrub nurse next to them. The assistant stands on the left side of the table.

- The rectosigmoid is pulled toward the abdominal wall, tenting upward the base of its mesentery at the sacral promontory (**FIGURE 5**). The peritoneum is incised along the root of the mesocolon with cautery across the promontory and toward the right and left posterolateral aspect of the cul-de-sac.
- The rectum is then lifted anteriorly toward the abdominal wall in order to reveal the alveolar plane in the presacral space located between the mesorectum and the presacral fascia (**FIGURE 6**). Dissect the presacral space distally with

Chapter 48 OPERATIVE TREATMENT OF RECTAL PROLAPSE: TRANSABDOMINAL APPROACH

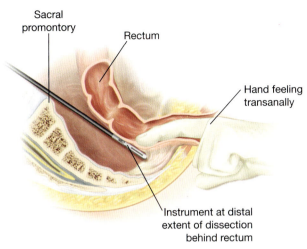

FIGURE 7 • Digital rectal examination allows palpating an instrument placed at the distal end of dissection, confirming that the posterior dissection has reached the top of the anal canal.

an energy device until reaching just above the levator ani muscles and the anal canal. Digital rectal examination may be needed to confirm the distal extent of dissection is appropriate (FIGURE 7).

- Avoid penetration into the endopelvic fascia along the lateral pelvic wall, because this can lead to serious bleeding from the hypogastric vein and its branches. Also, dissecting into the presacral fascia could result in catastrophic bleeding from the presacral venous plexus.
- The sympathetic nerves should be identified and preserved intact in the retroperitoneum.
- Minimize unnecessary dissection of the lateral rectal stalks.

Rectopexy

- Completely reduce the prolapse by retracting the rectosigmoid junction in a cephalad direction.
- The rectopexy sutures (braided nonabsorbable or absorbable sutures) are placed starting just below the top of the promontory. While retracting the rectum anteriorly, three sutures are placed along the midline, from the presacral fascia to the back of the mesorectum, placing the most distal stitch first (FIGURE 8). SH needles will fit through 5-mm ports if the curve of the needle is slightly flattened.
- When placing these stitches, it is important to have the needle enter at a right angle to the bone and then turn the

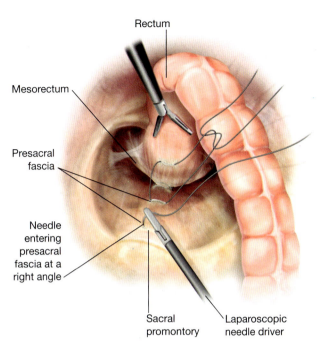

FIGURE 8 • Stitch placement for rectopexy. The stitches are placed along the midline, starting with the first one a few centimeters distal to the promontory and moving upward. The needle should enter the presacral fascia at a right angle. When bone is felt, turn the needle to encircle a wide swath of presacral fascia. Pull up on the mesorectum and place the stitch through the back of the mesorectum to pull the rectum upward when tying the knots.

needle after the bone is felt so that a wide swath of presacral fascia is incorporated in the stitch (FIGURE 8). Pull up on the mesorectum and place the stitch through the back of the mesorectum to pull the rectum upward when tying the knots. It is helpful to use a knot pusher or an automatic tying device to tie the knots in the narrow confines of the presacral space.
- Another important tip is not to remove any misplaced stitches but instead to just tie them, as removal can result in significant bleeding from the presacral veins.

Closure

- Assess the abdomen for hemostasis; remove all ports, and close skin incisions with absorbable suture.

HAND-ASSISTED LAPAROSCOPIC SURGERY RESECTION RECTOPEXY

- Hand-assisted laparoscopic surgery (HALS) in colorectal surgery has the same short-term outcome advantages of conventional laparoscopic-assisted (LA) surgery over open surgery, including less pain, faster recovery, lower incidence of wound complications, and reduction of cardiopulmonary complications, especially in the obese and in the elderly.
- Advantages of HALS over conventional LA colorectal surgery include the following:

- Reintroduces tactile feedback into the field
- Shorter learning curves; easier to teach
- Shorter operative times and lower conversion to open rates
- Higher usage rates of minimally invasive surgery

Port Placement, Team, and Operating Room Setup

- Start by placing a hand access port through a 5- to 6-cm Pfannenstiel incision. Care is taken to avoid bladder injury (FIGURES 9 and 13).
- Insufflate the CO_2 pneumoperitoneum; a 5-mm port is placed through the hand port.

- Insert a 5-mm supraumbilical camera port.
- Insert two 5-mm working ports in the right and left lower quadrants, respectively.
- The operating team and OR setup is otherwise identical as previously described (**FIGURE 4**).

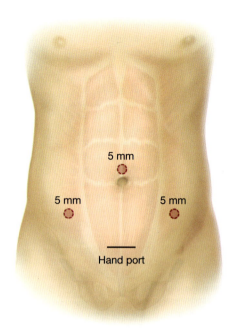

FIGURE 9 • Hand-assisted laparoscopic surgery (HALS) rectopexy port placement. A 5-mm supraumbilical camera port is inserted for the 30° camera. Two 5-mm working ports are inserted in the right lower quadrant and the left lower quadrant. The hand port (GelPort) is inserted through a 5- to 6-cm Pfannenstiel incision.

POSTERIOR DISSECTION

- The patient is placed in a steep Trendelenburg position with the left side up. Using your right hand, gently pull the small bowel out of the pelvis and place it in the upper abdomen. A laparotomy sponge, inserted via the hand port, can be used to hold the small bowel out of the pelvis and also to clean the camera tip intracorporeally.
- The sigmoid colon and rectum are often very redundant and can be hard to manipulate. HALS greatly facilitates this maneuver. If necessary, insert an additional port for this purpose.
- Using the hand, the rectosigmoid junction is pulled toward the anterior abdominal wall and pubis, tenting out the peritoneum at the sacral promontory. This peritoneum is incised with cautery across the promontory and toward the posterolateral cul-de-sac on the right and left sides.
- The rectum is then lifted anteriorly toward the abdominal wall in order to reveal the alveolar plane in the presacral space located between the mesorectum and the presacral fascia (**FIGURE 6**). Dissect the presacral space distally with an energy device until reaching just above the anal canal. Digital rectal examination may be needed to confirm the distal extent of dissection is appropriate.
- Avoid penetration into the endopelvic fascia along the lateral pelvic wall, because this can lead to serious bleeding from the hypogastric vein and its branches. Also, dissecting into the presacral fascia could result in catastrophic bleeding from the presacral venous plexus.
- The sympathetic nerves should be identified and preserved intact in the retroperitoneum.
- Minimal dissection of the lateral rectal stalks should be performed.

Sigmoid Resection

- This step should only be performed if the patient has a redundant colon and severe constipation.
- The mesentery of the sigmoid colon is separated from the retroperitoneum bluntly by medial to lateral dissection starting at the original opening made in the peritoneum at the sacral. The inferior mesenteric artery is lifted up and the left ureter and gonadal vessel are identified and left intact in the retroperitoneum (**FIGURE 10**).
- Once this dissection reaches the abdominal sidewall, the attachments between the sigmoid colon and the lateral peritoneum are divided.
- The mesentery to the bowel to be resected is divided with the LigaSure or Harmonic, staying close to the bowel until the top of the rectum is reached distally and the point appropriate for anastomosis is reached proximally. This proximal point is where the proximal colon reaches the rectum in the position it will be in after the rectopexy.
- The bowel is divided distally at the top of the rectum as defined by the splaying of the teniae coli. This division can be done with a laparoscopic gastrointestinal anastomosis (GIA), Contour, or thoracoabdominal (TA) stapler placed through the hand port. This position is estimated by pulling the top of the rectum up to the top of the sacral promontory. The proximal bowel is then pulled through the hand port and is divided extracorporeally. A 31-mm end-to-end anastomosis (EEA) anvil is then placed in the open end of the descending colon.
- The end-to-end colorectal anastomosis with a 31-mm EEA (**FIGURE 11**) is performed after the rectopexy sutures are placed but before they are tied.
- An underwater air test is performed to check for anastomotic leak (**FIGURE 12**). Perform after tying the rectopexy sutures. Perform this test with a colonoscope so that the anastomosis can be viewed at the same time. An air leak would indicate a disruption in the anastomotic line and may necessitate revision of the anastomosis.
- If there is undue tension on the anastomosis, the lateral and retroperitoneal attachments to the descending colon should be divided.

Chapter 48 OPERATIVE TREATMENT OF RECTAL PROLAPSE: TRANSABDOMINAL APPROACH 451

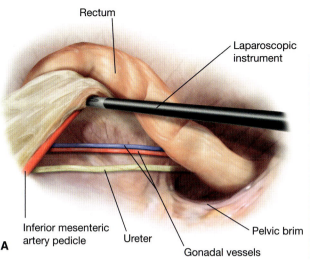
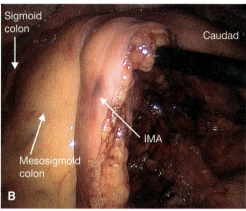

FIGURE 10 • Schematic **(A)** and operative **(B)** pictures. Medial to lateral mobilization of the mesosigmoid colon. The mesentery of the sigmoid colon is separated from the retroperitoneum bluntly by medial to lateral dissection starting at the original opening made in the peritoneum at the sacral promontory. The inferior mesenteric artery (IMA) is lifted up and the left ureter and gonadal vessel are identified and left intact in the retroperitoneum.

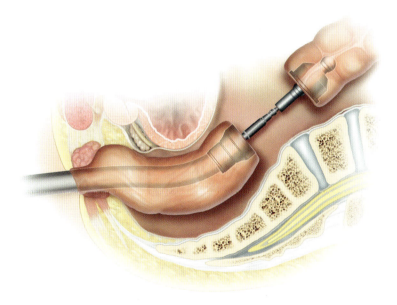

FIGURE 11 • The end-to-end colorectal anastomosis is performed with a 31-mm end-to-end anastomosis (EEA).

Rectopexy

- The lid of the hand port can be left on or off for placement of the rectopexy sutures depending on surgeon preference.
- The rectopexy sutures are to be placed starting just below the top of the promontory. Along, braided nonabsorbable suture on an SH needle is used to perform suture rectopexy. Alternatively, absorbable suture or mesh can be used.
- The rectum is held out of the way with a retractor, and three sutures are placed in the midline from the presacral fascia to the back of the mesorectum, placing the most distal stitch first (**FIGURE 8**).

- When placing these stitches, it is important to have the needle enter the tissue at a right angle to the bone and then turn the needle after the bone is felt so that a wide swath of presacral fascia is encircled. Another tip is not to remove any misplaced stitches but instead to just tie them, as removal can result in significant bleeding from the presacral veins.
- The rectum should be pulled up (with any prolapse reduced) and the stitch should then be placed through the back of the mesorectum such that the rectum is hitched up higher on the sacrum than it was previously. This should be repeated for each of the three stitches.
- If a resection is being performed, place the sutures, tag them, and then tie them after performing the anastomosis.

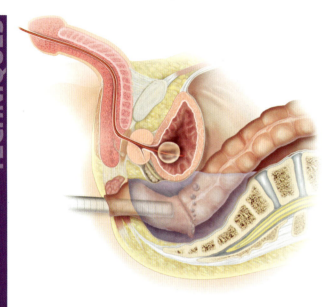

Closure

- The rectus muscles and peritoneum can be approximated with absorbable suture or not.
- The anterior fascia is closed with running polydioxanone (PDS) sutures.
- The wound is irrigated and the skin is closed with running absorbable subcuticular sutures.
- The 5-mm port sites are closed with absorbable subcuticular sutures.

FIGURE 12 • An underwater air test is performed to check for anastomotic leak. An air leak would indicate a disruption in the anastomotic line and may necessitate revision of the anastomosis.

OPEN RECTOPEXY WITH OR WITHOUT SIGMOID RESECTION

Pfannenstiel Incision

- Make a 10-cm Pfannenstiel incision two fingerbreadths above the pubis. Divide the anterior fascia with cautery, taking care to leave the rectus muscles intact. This division should curve superiorly at the lateral edges so as not to divide the oblique muscles.
- Create a plane between the anterior fascia and the anterior surface of the rectus muscle using cautery and finger dissection while lifting up on the fascia with Kocher clamps (**FIGURE 13**). This plane should extend down to the pubis inferiorly and superiorly up about 6 cm.
- Find the midline between the rectus muscles and sharply enter the abdomen several centimeters from the pubis in order to avoid entering the bladder.
- With the bladder retracted medially, the posterior rectus sheet/peritoneum is incised inferolaterally in order to avoid injuring the bladder (**FIGURE 14**). This can be done bilaterally or on one side or the other.
- Place a wound protector (**FIGURE 15**).

Posterior Dissection

- Place the patient in Trendelenburg position. Place a Bookwalter (or similar) retractor for exposure.
- Pull the rectosigmoid forward and incise the peritoneum at the sacral promontory. At the top of the promontory, the sympathetic hypogastric nerves should be identified and preserved. They form a wishbone here and extend forward

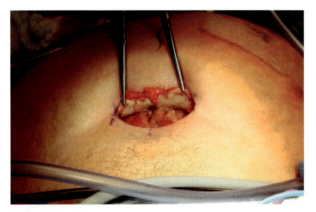

FIGURE 13 • Pfannenstiel incision. The plane between the anterior fascia and the anterior surface of the rectus muscle has been created while lifting up on the rectus fascia with Kocher clamps. This plane should extend down to the pubis inferiorly and superiorly up about 6 cm.

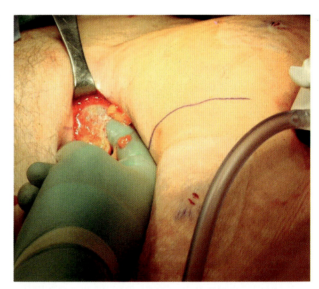

FIGURE 14 • Pfannenstiel incision. The posterior rectus sheet/peritoneum is incised inferolaterally with the bladder retracted medially to avoid injuring the bladder.

Chapter 48 OPERATIVE TREATMENT OF RECTAL PROLAPSE: TRANSABDOMINAL APPROACH   453

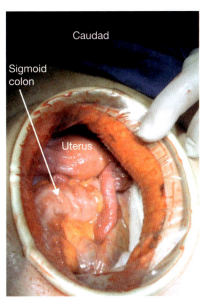

FIGURE 15 • Placement of the wound protector.

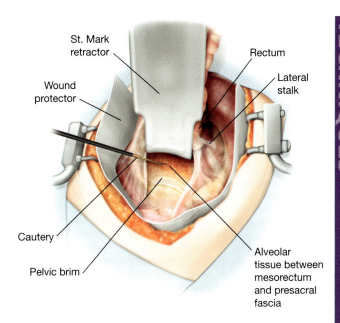

FIGURE 17 • Exposure of the presacral space using the St. Mark retractor. Place the retractor behind the mesorectum and pull forward and upward to reveal the alveolar plane of the presacral space. The dissection is carried down to the level of the pelvic floor; reposition the retractor frequently to maintain the proper tension to reveal the correct tissue plane.

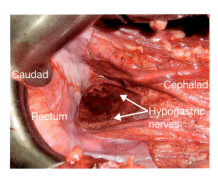

FIGURE 16 • Identification of the hypogastric nerves. At the top of the promontory, the sympathetic hypogastric nerves should be identified and preserved. They form a wishbone here and extend forward around the rectum.

around the rectum (**FIGURE 16**). If these are divided in a male patient, the consequence is retrograde ejaculation.
- Place a St. Mark retractor in this peritoneal opening, pull forward and superiorly on the rectum, and divide the alveolar plane between the mesorectum and the presacral fascia with the Bovie cautery, taking care to stay out of the presacral venous plexus (**FIGURE 17**).
- As the dissection proceeds, the St. Mark retractor should be placed more distally so that appropriate tension is always maintained. This dissection should be carried out posterior to the rectum down to the level of the pelvic floor.
- The lateral stalks should be left intact as much as possible during this dissection. Useful tools for this dissection include the long tip for the Bovie as well as the extender that can be placed between the long tip and the handpiece and bariatric St. Mark retractors.
- Check the extent of the distal dissection by placing one hand or surgical instrument in the abdomen at the most distal extent of the dissection and then reach under the drapes to place a finger in the anus to feel the other hand through the posterior rectal wall. The dissection should extend to the top of the anal canal.
- Any prolapse should again be reduced at this time.

Sigmoid Resection

- This step should only be performed if the patient has a very redundant sigmoid colon and severe constipation. The technique for open sigmoidectomy has been described elsewhere in this book.
- The bowel is divided distally at the top of the rectum as defined by the splaying of the teniae.
- The proximal point of transection is where the proximal colon reaches the proximal rectum in the position it will be in after the rectopexy. This position is estimated by pulling the top of the rectum up to the top of the sacral promontory.
- The colorectal anastomosis with 31-mm EEA stapler is performed after the rectopexy sutures are placed but before they are tied.

Rectopexy

- The rectopexy sutures are to be placed starting just below the top of the sacral promontory. Use a long, braided nonabsorbable suture on an SH needle to perform the suture rectopexy, or absorbable suture or even mesh that is attached to the promontory and then sutured to the rectum or mesorectum can also be used.
- The rectum is held out of the way with a retractor and three sutures are placed in the midline from the presacral fascia to the back of the mesorectum, placing the most distal stitch first.
- When placing these stitches, it is important to have the needle enter the presacral tissue at a right angle to the bone and then turn the needle after the bone is felt so that a wide swath of presacral fascia is encircled (**FIGURE 8**). Another tip

SECTION III RECTAL RESECTIONS

is not to remove any misplaced stitches but instead to just tie them as removal can result in significant bleeding from the presacral veins.

- The rectum should be pulled up (with any prolapse reduced) and the stitch should then be placed through the back of the mesorectum such that the rectum is hitched up higher on the sacrum than it was previously. This should be repeated for each of the three stitches.
- Alternatively, the stitches can be attached to the lateral stalk on one side or the other.

- If a resection is being performed, place the sutures, tag them with hemostats, and then tie them after performing the anastomosis with a 31-mm EEA stapler.

Closure

- The rectus muscles and peritoneum can be approximated with absorbable suture or not.
- The anterior fascia is then closed with running PDS sutures.
- The wound is irrigated and the skin closed with running absorbable subcuticular sutures.

PEARLS AND PITFALLS

Diagnosis	• Must differentiate rectal prolapse from prolapsing internal hemorrhoids.
Posterior dissection	• Must stay in the correct plane and in the midline; otherwise, severe bleeding may occur.
Sigmoid resection	• Perform resection only in patient's very redundant sigmoid colons and with severe underlying constipation. • The anastomosis should be tension-free and without redundancy.
Rectopexy	• Always check and be sure that the rectal prolapse is reduced before performing the rectopexy. • Place sutures through presacral fascia below the top of promontory. • Tie, rather than remove, misplaced presacral stitches to avoid bleeding.

POSTOPERATIVE CARE

- The orogastric tube is removed at the completion of the case.
- Patients are offered liquids the day of surgery and their diets are advanced to a general diet as tolerated. Reasons not to advance the diet include nausea, vomiting, and abdominal distention. Flatus is not needed for diet advancement but is preferred prior to discharge home.
- Length of stay varies, with laparoscopic and HALS suture rectopexy often being as short as 2 days and open resection rectopexy as long as 7 days.
- Chemical and mechanical prophylaxis for deep vein thrombosis should be started in the operating room and should be continued postoperatively.
- Early ambulation is important.
- Pain is managed with a combination of narcotic and nonnarcotic medications, starting with mostly intravenous medications and quickly converting over to oral medications.
- The Foley catheter is left in place for 2 days due to the low pelvic dissection. Upon removal, the patient should attempt to void frequently and intermittent straight catheterization should be performed as needed for retention. Some patients will continue to need this at home.
- Patients should be placed on fiber and/or an osmotic laxative such as MiraLAX as soon as they are able to tolerate oral intake. The goal is one or two soft bowel movements a day such that straining is avoided. The medication can be titrated at home to reach this goal as not all patients have a bowel movement prior to discharge.

OUTCOMES

- Recurrence rates are very low, with most series reporting less than 5% recurrence.

- If recurrence occurs in the case of rectopexy alone, rectopexy can be performed again with or without resection.
- If recurrence occurs after resection and rectopexy, further attempts at repair must be chosen carefully so as not to devascularize any bowel.

COMPLICATIONS

- Pelvic bleeding in the postoperative period is avoided by meticulous technique and hemostasis. If it occurs and is not profuse, it will usually stop by withholding all anticoagulants.
- Wound infection is the most common complication and should be treated by opening the skin and packing the wound until healing occurs.
- The risk of anastomotic leak is 2% to 5%.

SUGGESTED READINGS

1. Fleming FJ, Kim MJ, Gunzler D, et al. It's the procedure not the patient: the operative approach is independently associated with an increased risk of complications after rectal prolapse repair. *Colorectal Dis.* 2012;14(3):362-368.
2. Kairaluoma MV, Kellokumpu IH. Epidemiologic aspects of complete rectal prolapse. *Scand J Surg.* 2005;94(3):207-210.
3. Karas JR, Uranues S, Altomare DF, et al. No rectopexy versus rectopexy following rectal mobilization for full-thickness rectal prolapse: a randomized controlled trial. *Dis Colon Rectum.* 2011;54(1):29-34.
4. Luukkonen P, Mikkonen U, Jarvinen H. Abdominal rectopexy with sigmoidectomy vs. rectopexy alone for rectal prolapse: a prospective, randomized study. *Int J Colorectal Dis.* 1992;7(4):219-222.
5. Marderstein EL, Delaney CP. Surgical management of rectal prolapse. *Nat Clin Pract Gastroenterol Hepatol.* 2007;4(10):552-561.
6. McKee RF, Lauder JC, Poon FW, et al. A prospective randomized study of abdominal rectopexy with and without sigmoidectomy in rectal prolapse. *Surg Gynecol Obstet.* 1992;174(2):145-148.
7. Varma M, Rafferty J, Buie WD. Practice parameters for the management of rectal prolapse. *Dis Colon Rectum.* 2011;54(11):1339-1346.

Chapter 49 Perirectal Abscess and Perianal Fistula

Vijian Dhevan, Roger M. Galindo, and Henry A. Reinhart

DEFINITION

- The principle underlying cause for most inflammatory anorectal diseases, such as perirectal abscess and perianal fistula, is often an anorectal infection. Anorectal infections originate in anal crypts, ducts, and glands, which can also involve nearby blood vessels and lymphatics.
- Fistulas and abscesses can present similarly with pain, inflammation, and drainage.
- Abscesses and fistulas are not treated as separate entities. The development of one can lead to the other. A fistula is a tract of inflammatory origin that has its primary opening in an anal crypt in the anal canal and has a secondary opening in the anus, perianal area, or perianal skin.
- An anal sinus is like a fistula; however, it ends blindly in the perianal or perirectal space.
- The three stages of an anorectal infection progress from the acute phase to the chronic phase via three methods. The first method is spontaneous drainage of the abscess through the anus. The second method is by spontaneous rupture of the abscess into the surrounding tissue or perianal tissue. The third method is by an incision and drainage procedure. While the first method results in the formation of a sinus, the second and third methods result in the formation of a perianal fistula.
- Anorectal infections can be divided into three stages. Stage one is where infectious material invades one or more of the crypts and/or glands. Stage two is where the infection is carried into the surrounding spaces, which includes the perianal and perirectal spaces. Stage three is the resulting effects of this infection/inflammation, which includes abscess, sinus, and fistula.
- The areas that perirectal abscesses occupy are potential anatomical spaces. In total, there are five possible anatomical spaces that must be considered (**FIGURE 1**).
- These five anatomical spaces include the left and right pelvirectal space, the retrorectal space, and the left and right ischiorectal space. The two pelvirectal spaces and the retrorectal space lie above the pelvic diaphragm (supralevator compartment), while the ischiorectal spaces lie below the pelvic diaphragm (infralevator compartment). The proximity and the location of the rectum with these spaces is of importance for diagnosis as well as for planning of surgical procedures.
- Of the sites for these potential perirectal abscesses, the general make up is perianal 60%, ischiorectal 20%, intersphincteric 5%, above the pelvic floor (supralevator) 4%, and submucosal 1%.

DIFFERENTIAL DIAGNOSIS

- Prostatitis with or without abscess must be ruled out in males via radiography or physical examination.
- Infected pilonidal cysts can present in a similar fashion and can usually be ruled out with physical examination.
- Thrombosed hemorrhoids cause pain and swelling and can also be ruled out on physical examination.

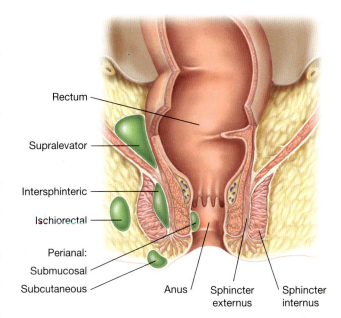

FIGURE 1 • Five potential anatomical locations of perirectal abscesses.

PATIENT HISTORY AND PHYSICAL FINDINGS

- A detailed history and physical examination are important to help distinguish other etiologies of pain. A history of repeated perirectal abscesses or spontaneous periodic perianal drainage may indicate untreated fistula disease. A detailed rectal examination can help distinguish the various causes of pain, although anoscopy is usually avoided in the awake patient. Careful attention must be paid to the patient presenting with sepsis as they may have Fournier's gangrene. Questions concerning past medical history such as immunocompromise, Crohn disease, malignancy, and previous anorectal surgery are important to ask.
- Throbbing anal/perianal pain is the usual complaint of a patient with an abscess. This is secondary to the perianal and perineal rich tissue somatic nerve supply. Deep abscesses involving the suprapelvic spaces generally manifest without discomfort due to the lack of somatic nerve supply. However, a deep abscess can cause acute septic symptoms such as chills, fevers, generalized malaise, and leukocytosis.
- A patient with a fistula can have periodic spontaneous drainage at a site away from the anal opening. Any draining opening noted near the anal, perianal, or perineal skin should be considered a secondary opening of a fistula. The opening may have nearby granulation tissue or discolored skin, be housed within an old scar, or have an appearance of an opening that has healed.
- Careful digital examination may reveal a cord-like structure. An examination under anesthesia would generally show purulent

material oozing from the abscess cavity or fistula. However, if no internal opening is noted one cannot rule out the existence of a fistula or a sinus as the pliable tissue within the anorectal canal could be collapsed at the time of examination.

- Abscesses with resulting sinus tracts and/or fistulas usually arise from organisms originating from the gastrointestinal tract such as *Escherichia coli* or other gram-negative aerobic bacteria or anaerobe bacteria from the colon like *Bacteroides splanchnicus*. There are some perianal abscesses that arise from boils, carbuncles, or furuncles that are usually caused by *Staphylococcal* organisms. Thus, getting a culture form the abscess drainage can be helpful in determining the origin of the abscess.

IMAGING AND OTHER DIAGNOSTIC STUDIES

- While imaging is not required it may be useful to gauge the extent and severity of the abscess. Imaging such as contrast-enhanced computed tomography (and/or MRI) can also be useful in the diagnosis of supralevator abscesses when physical examination is not diagnostic. Owing to the ubiquitous use of computed tomography at the authors' institution it is usually available at the time of surgical consult.

SURGICAL MANAGEMENT

Positioning

- Different patient positions on the operating room table can be utilized, including a lithotomy position with Yellofin or Allen stirrups (**FIGURE 2**) and lithotomy position with C-type (candy canes) footholders (**FIGURE 3**). In most cases, a lithotomy position is adequate. However, this author (VD) feels the best visualization is achieved with the patient in a prone jack knife position (**FIGURE 4**).

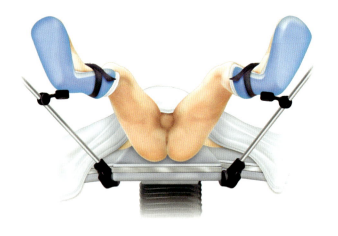

FIGURE 2 • Modified lithotomy position. The legs are placed on Yellofin or Allen stirrups. The patient is firmly secured to the table to allow table position changes during the procedure. The arms are tucked and all pressure points are padded to prevent nerve and/or vascular injuries.

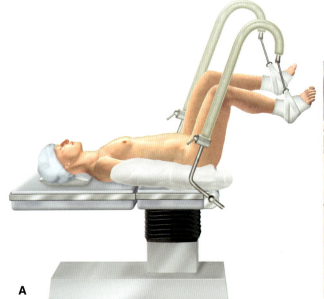

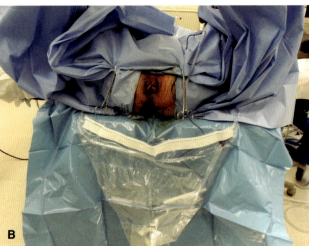

FIGURE 3 • **A,** Lithotomy position with C-type (candy canes) footholders. **B,** Final setup for high lithotomy with under-the-buttocks drape with plastic pouch; white band can be used to hold instruments.

Chapter 49 PERIRECTAL ABSCESS AND PERIANAL FISTULA 457

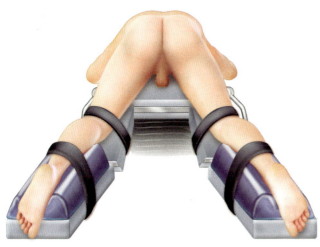

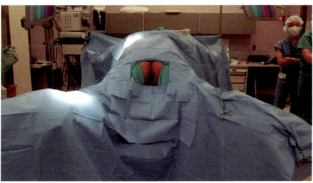

FIGURE 4 • Prone position. The arms are resting without straining on arm boards. The lower extremities are resting on a splittable configuration. The patient is firmly secured to the table for position changes during the procedure. All pressure points are padded to prevent nerve and/or vascular injuries.

ABSCESSES

- The treatment of choice for any abscess is incision and drainage. Conservative management is never advised as a delay in drainage can lead to chronic problems, complicated fibrosis, and potential anal dysfunction and chronic pain. Drainage requires accurate localization. Careful examination and imaging can assist in this regard. Often, an examination under anesthesia is required due to the extreme pain the patient may have and the need to properly drain the entire cavity.
- Perianal abscess: Incision and drainage can be performed in the emergency room or in the clinic. Drainage is usually achieved with a cruciate incision. Careful attention should be taken to ensure all purulent material is drained and any loculations are broken. The cavity should be copiously irrigated. An appropriately sized opening will allow the cavity to be irrigated without risk of formation of a second collection. This should also allow for quick healing.
- Ischiorectal abscesses: Incision and drainage is usually accomplished in the operating room. It can be achieved with a cruciate incision or an oval incision at the point of maximum fluctuation. Careful attention should be taken to ensure all purulent material is drained and any loculations are broken. The cavity can be irrigated to verify all purulent material is removed. One must verify that there is not a bilateral component. The author's preference is to pack in the operating room and to remove the packing within hours and irrigate the wound at least three times a day and with every bowel movement. This will keep the cavity clean and allow for closure from the inside out.
- Intersphincteric and Supralevator abscesses: These can be difficult to identify. Preoperative imaging is required. The patient should be taken to the operating room where an examination under anesthesia can be conducted. An incision is made within the anal canal below the dentate line and dissection with scissors is conducted upward. Once the cavity is incised, a drainage catheter should be left in place (ie, a Penrose drain) to avoid the levator muscle contracting and preventing adequate drainage of remaining material.
- Submucosal abscesses: These are usually tackled in the operating room with an examination under anesthesia. An anal retractor (ie, a Hill-Ferguson or a bivalve self-retaining retractor) is used and the mucosa overlying the abscess is opened and copiously irrigated.

TECHNIQUES

PERIANAL FISTULA

- Depending on the original location of the perirectal abscess that originated it, Dr. Parks classification described five main types of perianal fistula (**FIGURE 5**).
- The main methods of treatment for perianal fistula are fistulotomy, seton placement, mucosal flaps, fibrin glue, and fistula plugs. The guiding principle is to identify the external and internal openings. This sometimes cannot be performed at the time of abscess drainage as there is significant inflammation and the chance of creating a false passage is high. In the operating room an examination under anesthesia is conducted. In most cases a lithotomy position is adequate; however, this author feels best visualization is achieved with the patient in a prone jack knife position. An anal speculum is used and the internal opening can be found with rigid probes, or gentle injection of peroxide with visualization of bubbling from the internal opening. If the internal opening is distal to the sphincteric mechanism, the overlying tissue can be opened and the fistulae tract can be marsupialized. If only a very small amount of striated muscle is encountered this can also be divided. However, if a moderate or significant amount of anal sphincteric muscle is encountered then a soft seton should be placed. The path of the fistula usually follows the Goodsall rule (**FIGURE 6**) except in cases of inflammatory bowel disease.
- The Goodsall rule states that a fistula with the external opening anterior to an imaginary transverse line across the anus has its internal opening at the same radial position and for an external opening posterior to this line, the internal opening is in the midline posteriorly with a horseshoe track.
- Seton placement is usually reserved for fistula tracts that are within the sphincter mechanism or tracking above the mechanism. The same method of identifying the internal opening is used. The author prefers to use a Hewson suture passer placed through the fistula tract. Then a vessel loop is pulled through the tract and tied in place. Ample pressure on the vessel loop will not only allow for adequate drainage of the tract but will also draw the fistula out from the sphincter mechanism. In refractory cases, a soft seton should be replaced with a cutting seton (ie, a 0-silk tie). Weekly tightening of the seton will allow for adequate advancement of the seton to draw the fistula out of the sphincter mechanism.
- Fistula plugs and fibrin glue
    - These are two newer methods used for closure of fistulas. Fibrin glue is used when both the internal and external openings are clearly identifiable and the tract can be easily accessed. The tip of the applicator is placed in the tract after it has been mechanically deepithelialized. The

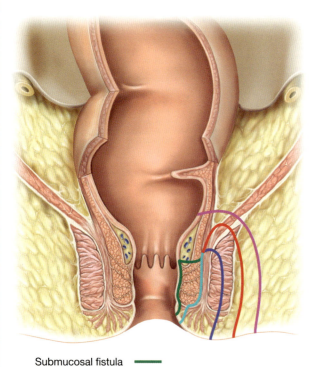

Submucosal fistula
Intersphincteric fistula

FIGURE 5 • Parks perianal Fistula classification. There are five different potential perianal fistula tracts depending on the perirectal abscess location that originated the fistula.

FIGURE 6 • The Goodsall rule.

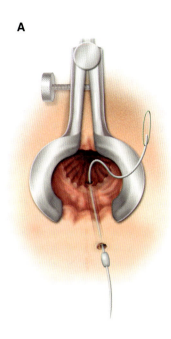 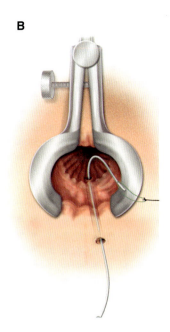

FIGURE 7 • Fistula plug technique.

glue is injected as the applicator is retracted leaving the fistula tract occluded with the glue. This method may have to be repeated for complete closure of the tract.
- Similar methods are used for the fistula plug, but instead of placing glue, a commercially available plug is pulled through the tract. The inner and outer cuffs are then sutured in place (FIGURE 7).

- Mucosal advancement is a technique usually used for extrasphincteric or suprasphincteric fistulas. The external fistula tract is excised and left open to allow for adequate drainage and the internal opening is then covered with an anal mucosa advancement flap. For this procedure to be successful any existing infection needs to be adequately drained and adequate exposure is mandatory.

PEARLS AND PITFALLS

Preoperative planning	■ A bowel prep is useful but not mandatory.
Technique	■ A dilute mixture of blue dye and hydrogen peroxide injected into the abscess cavity can sometimes help locate an internal fistula opening. ■ A small incision may not allow for adequate drainage and lead to a recurrence.

POSTOPERATIVE CARE

- If an adequate incision is made there is usually adequate drainage and the wound does not require repeat packing.
- Postoperative antibiotics are usually not required in straightforward cases in patients who are not immunocompromised.

COMPLICATIONS

- Aggressive fistulotomy involving a significant portion of the sphincter complex may result in anal incontinence.
- Inadequate incision size in abscess drainage may result in recurrence.
- Anal problems are pervasive, embarrassing, and vexing to patients. Primary care providers should be well versed in addressing these concerns, which uncommonly require referral for specialty care. In addition, anal symptoms and findings may herald previously undiagnosed underlying illness.[1]

REFERENCE

1. Klein JW. Common anal problems. *Med Clin North Am.* 2014;98(3):609-623. doi:10.1016/j.mcna.2014.01.011

Chapter 50

Surgical Management of Pilonidal Disease

Vijian Dhevan and Henry A. Reinhart

DEFINITION

- Pilonidal comes from the term "pilus" which means hair, and nidus, which means nest. Pilonidal disease (PD) is the manifestation of an inflammatory reaction to the pilonidal cyst in the sacrococcygeal region.
- The embryologic origin is thought to include the hair follicle being lost in the ectodermal layer in the subcutaneous tissue at or near the midline in the sacrococcygeal region. The cavity of the cyst communicates with the exterior via pores, and this is the reason that pilonidal cysts usually are associated with hair.
- This is more prevalent in hirsute individuals, obese individuals, males, poor hygiene, and sedentary lifestyle. Organisms can enter via the pores and fester in the cavity.
- Mostly PD appears to be caused by loose hairs that penetrate the skin. Friction and pressure, skin rubbing against skin, tight clothing, bicycling, long periods of sitting, or similar factors force the hair down into skin. Three elements are instrumental in this process: (1) the invader, hair; (2) the force, causing hair penetration; and (3) the vulnerability of the skin.
- Incidence of PD is about 26 per 100,000 population. Pilonidal disease occurs predominantly in males, at a ratio of about 3 to 4:1. It occurs predominantly in white patients, typically in the late teens to early twenties, decreasing after age 25, and rarely occurs after age 45.
- Local irritation to the subcutaneous (SC) site, positive family history of PD, sedentary life style, and obesity are common in patients with PD (all factors between 34% and 50% occurrence in PD).

DIFFERENTIAL DIAGNOSIS

- Perirectal abscess
- Anorectal fistula
- Simple abscess, carbuncle, furuncle
- Hidradenitis suppurativa
- Pyoderma gangrenosum
- Syphilitic granuloma
- Tuberculous granuloma
- Inflammatory bowel disease
- Epidural abscess
- Congenital abnormalities
- Inclusion dermoid/teratoma
- Skin malignancy (ie, squamous cell carcinoma)

PATIENT HISTORY AND PHYSICAL FINDINGS

- The most prominent clinical presentation of PD is pain and swelling at the sacrococcygeal region about 4 to 5 cm posterior to the anal orifice associated with midline pits that may have tracts traveling laterally.

- Irritation and inflammation can lead to abscess formation that can either spontaneously drain to the exterior via one of the many pores or can cause an expanding area of fluctuance.
- Chronic pilonidal disease often manifests as recurrent or persistent drainage and pain.
- On physical exam, the patient is usually afebrile and nontoxic. Commonly, the patient has typical findings of an abscess, including redness, warmth, local tenderness, and fluctuance with or without induration. A tender mass with sinus drainage may be present. Loose hair may be seen projecting from the site.

IMAGING AND DIAGNOSTIC STUDIES

- Diagnosing pilonidal disease is usually clinical and should not require imaging.
- Ultrasound (US) has been shown to help diagnose extent of disease although the findings usually corroborate physical exam findings.
- Magnetic resonance imaging (MRI) can be used in more complicated cases such as fistulas, inflammatory bowel disease, and other causes besides pilonidal cyst.

SURGICAL MANAGEMENT

- The authors prefer patients to undergo hair removal prior to any surgical intervention, if possible.
- Hair removal can be achieved by shaving, which is not the recommended technique due to the hair regrowing quickly, by waxing, which is more economical, or by laser hair removal, which is the preferred method.
- Hair removal surrounding the pilonidal cyst will allow for better chances of primary closure of the wound at the time of surgery.
- Adequate time should be given to allow for the skin to heal prior to surgery.
- Removal of the hair within the cyst is optimal to eliminate the occurrence of abscesses while the surrounding permanent hair removal is being conducted.
- When the patient presents to the emergency department with an infected pilonidal cyst, the initial management should be incision and drainage:
  - It can be performed under local anesthesia or conscious sedation.
  - The patient is placed in a prone position.
  - The incision should be placed longitudinally and should be made off the midline, through the skin and subcutaneous tissues, entering the cyst cavity.
  - Pus and debris is evacuated and all ingrown hair is removed.
  - The wound is irrigated and packed lightly and a cover dressing with 4 × 4 gauze and an ABD pad is secured with surgical tape.
  - The patient can then be followed up in the surgery clinic.

- For patients that recur after incision and drainage, three options for surgical treatment of the pilonidal cyst include:
  1. Exteriorization of the cyst complex
  2. En Bloc excision and primary closure with or without flaps
  3. En Bloc excision and closure by secondary intention

EXTERIORIZATION OF THE CYST COMPLEX

- The authors do not routinely utilize this procedure.
- In the exteriorization procedure, the patient is positioned in the prone jack knife position.
- The extent of the cyst cavity is gauged with probes. All hair is removed.
- Then, the cavity is opened, and all of the channels are connected. The overlapping skin is excised. This should provide a divot or a saucer-shaped wound that can form the base of the healed incision.
- See **FIGURE 1**.

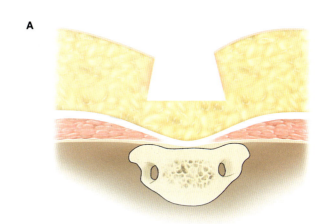
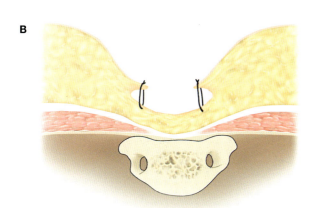
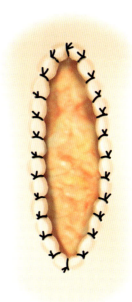

FIGURE 1 • Evagination. **A,** Pilonidal complex is excised. **B** and **C,** Edges are sutured to the underlying tissue to create a new base that will eventually form the new skin.

EN BLOC EXCISION AND PRIMARY CLOSURE

- The en bloc excision and primary closure utilizes a prone jack knife position.
- An elliptical incision is made and dissection to the base of the cyst cavity is undertaken.
- Once all the affected tissue is removed, then closure can be attempted via a primary nontissue mobilization closure, which should utilize an incision that is not in the midline.
- A Z-plasty or variation of the z-plasty (rhomboid flap, advancement flap, v-y plasty, cleft lift) may be used to minimize wound tension (see **FIGURES 2** and **3**).
- A technique that is being popularized currently is the Bascom flap, which is an excision of the pits with an extension including the most diseased side to excise pits and tracts en bloc.
- The opposite side is then undermined to create a flap, which is then closed primarily.
- This appears to have promising outcomes since the closure is then off of the midline and the depth of the

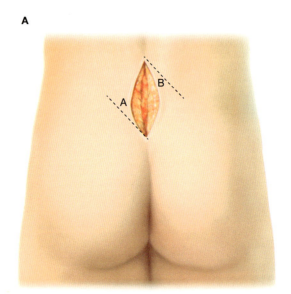

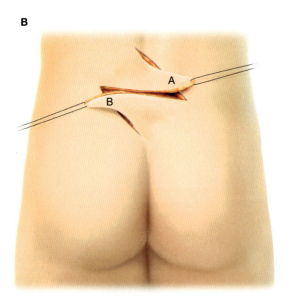

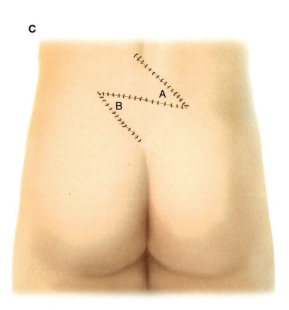

FIGURE 2 • Z-plasty. Initial resection in an elliptical format, then mobilization of tissue flaps by initial incision from apex of the eclipse in a 45° cut to establish a triangular flap. The top flap **(B)** is mobilized to the lower tangential cut apex and the lower flap **(A)** is mobilized to the top tangential cut apex. Flaps sutured in place.

Chapter 50 SURGICAL MANAGEMENT OF PILONIDAL DISEASE   463

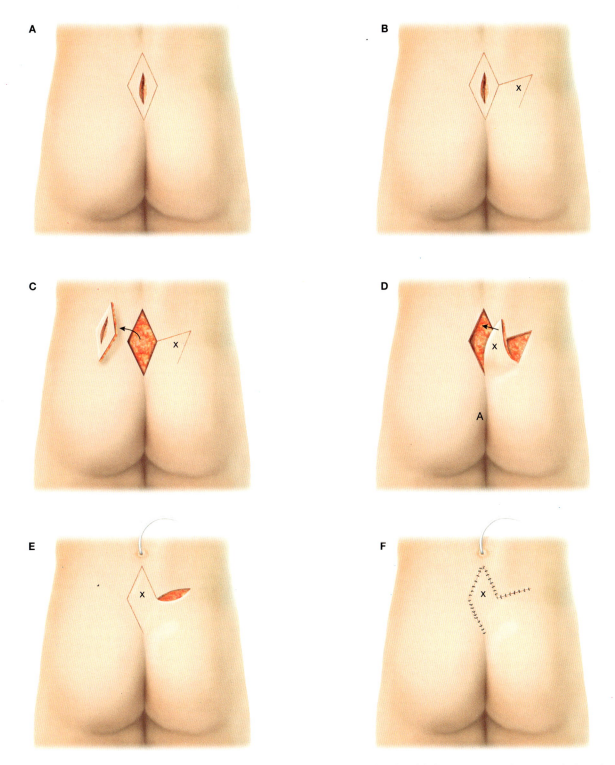

FIGURE 3 • Rhomboid reconstruction. **A** and **C**, Pilonidal complex excised in a rhomboid fashion. **B**, Triangular cut made from lateral edge. **D-F**, Triangular flap mobilized to cover the resected area and sutured in place with the approximation of the triangular cut in a linear fashion.

gluteal cleft is no longer profound. A drain can be left postoperatively.
- Other types of closure include the Karydakis flap, which is an elliptical excision of diseased tissue with closure off of midline.
- There are other types of flaps also used, although more evidence is needed prior to evaluate these types. The locations and extent of diseased tissue usually dictates what type of closure is needed (1) (see **FIGURE 4**).

SECTION III RECTAL RESECTIONS

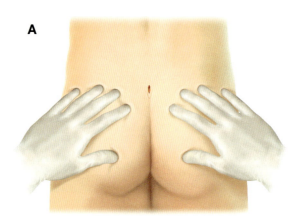

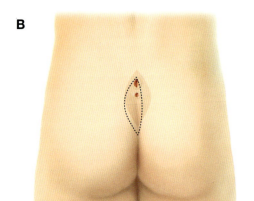

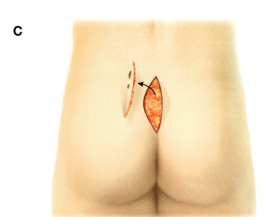

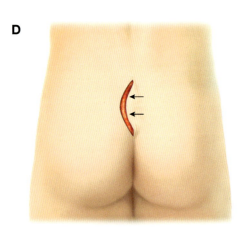

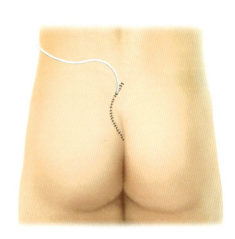

FIGURE 4 • Bascom lift. **A,** Working are made to adequately measure the distance of resection and mobilization. **B** and **C,** Pilonidal complex is excised with an elliptical incision favoring one side. **D** and **E,** Contralateral flap is lifted from the midline cleft and mobilized to the ipsilateral cut edge and sutured in place.

EN BLOC EXCISION AND CLOSURE BY SECONDARY INTENTION

- The patient is positioned in the prone jack knife position.
- An elliptical incision is made and dissection to the base of the cyst cavity is undertaken. Then, the incision is either packed with routine dressing changes or preferably a negative pressure dressing, which can expedite closure. This type of treatment may be required in wounds that have a significant amount of infection in which the surrounding tissue does not lend itself to primary closure.

Chapter 50 **SURGICAL MANAGEMENT OF PILONIDAL DISEASE** **465**

PEARLS AND PITFALLS

Initial presentation	▪ Incision and drainage is sufficient in the majority of cases. Pack the wound and send the patient home on oral antibiotics that cover skin flora. ▪ Removal of ingrown hair within the cyst is optimal to eliminate the occurrence of abscesses.
Preoperative management	▪ Hair removal allows for better chances of primary closure of the wound at the time of surgery. Laser is most effective. ▪ Adequate time should be given to allow for the skin to heal prior to surgery.
Surgical management	▪ Prone jack knife position provides best exposure. ▪ Blue dye may be injected into the pits to ensure complete excision during surgery using an angiocatheter without the needle. ▪ Avoid closure in the midline. ▪ Encourage good hygiene to avoid recurrences. ▪ Recurrences are best managed by more complex flap reconstructions.

POSTOPERATIVE CARE

▪ After surgical care is dependent on the type of surgery performed, which includes drain removal if a flap was utilized, routine dressing changes if a wound was left open, and pain control.

COMPLICATIONS

▪ If an inadequate resection is performed, there is a high likelihood of recurrence. Recurrence of the abscess is by far the most common complication, reported to be between 40% and 50%, although 58% will heal primarily by 5 weeks.

▪ If the initial intervention was minimally invasive such as an incision and drainage or pit picking, then a flap may be the best follow-up intervention.

▪ A *Cochrane Database of Systematic Reviews* article published in 2007 showed no significant difference in outcomes between techniques involving primary closure vs healing by secondary intention, though the review did recommend off-line closure when primary closure is performed. A series of

treatments of the local region with phenol have also been described, with a low incidence of recurrence reported.

▪ Other complications include wound infection, wound dehiscence, and poor cosmesis among others.

▪ Squamous cell carcinoma after recurrence of pilonidal disease is rare. When diagnosed, it requires en bloc surgical resection and appropriate oncologic care with local radiation and possibly chemotherapy.

SUGGESTED READINGS

1. Grabowski J, Oyetunji TA, Goldin AB, et al. The management of pilonidal disease: a systematic review. *J Pediatr Surg.* 2019;54(11):2210-2221.
2. Keighley MRB. Anorectal disorders. In: Baker RJ, Fisher JE, eds. *Mastery of Surgery.* Vol. II. 4th ed. Lippincott Williams & Wilkins publisher; 2002:1638.
3. Nesselrod JP. The anal canal and rectum. In: Davis L, ed. *Christopher's Textbook of Surgery.* 7th ed. W.B Saunders Company Publication; 1960:714.
4. Nixon AT, Garza RF. *Pilonidal Cyst and Sinus.* Stat Pearls; 2022.

Chapter **51** | # Surgical Management of Peritoneal Carcinomatosis

Cristian D. Valenzuela, Perry Shen, Edward A. Levine, and Konstantinos I. Votanopoulos

DEFINITION

- The term peritoneal surface disease (PSD) describes the intra-abdominal dissemination of neoplasms to peritoneal surfaces, and is a term complementary, but not identical to peritoneal carcinomatosis.
- Cytoreductive surgery (CRS) and hyperthermic intraperitoneal chemotherapy (HIPEC) have been shown to be effective treatment options for a variety of epithelial malignancy primaries. The scope of this chapter is to analyze the role of CRS/HIPEC in the management of selected colon cancer patients with peritoneal dissemination.
- Colon cancer carcinomatosis rarely presents solely with PSD distribution without nodal or parenchymal lesions.
- The operation is a two-step process:
  - Surgical resection (CRS) of involved organs and peritoneal surfaces, followed by
  - Delivery of heated chemotherapy (HIPEC) to the peritoneal cavity.
- During HIPEC, a heated chemotherapy solution is circulated in the abdominal cavity to treat any cancer cells that may remain after CRS. Delivering chemotherapy at the time of cytoreduction allows for targeted distribution in the peritoneal cavity, with tumor to drug concentrations higher than that achieved with systemic chemotherapy.
- Thus, the theoretical advantage of CRS/HIPEC, which is now routinely performed at specialized centers, is that it treats macroscopic disease surgically and microscopic disease pharmacologically.
- The goal for CRS/HIPEC applied to PSD from colon cancer is the complete cytoreduction of all macroscopic disease prior to perfusion with HIPEC. Therefore, appropriate candidates are identified based not only on their ability to tolerate CRS but also on the likelihood of obtaining a complete cytoreduction.
- Currently, it is not clinically possible to categorize colon cancer patients based on propensity to spread on peritoneal surfaces vs metastasis to distant parenchymal organs. This weakness must be taken into consideration in the design of any clinical trial inclusive of HIPEC, which by itself has locoregional and not systemic effects.
- Careful selection of patients can help ensure that only those who can expect to have the greatest benefits are subjected to the inherent risks of this treatment paradigm.

PATIENT SELECTION

- Patient selection is based predominantly on the extent of disease and the functional reserves of the patient.
- Preoperative evaluation includes complete history and physical examination, review of previously obtained pathology, and infused computed tomography (CT) of the chest, abdomen, and pelvis or dedicated abdominal magnetic resonance imaging (MRI).

- Preoperative lab work includes complete blood counts, a comprehensive metabolic pannel, liver function panel, hemoglobin A1c level, and carcinoembryonic antigen (CEA) levels.
- Our selection criteria include the following:
  - The patient is medically fit to undergo CRS/HIPEC without signs of the kidney, liver, or bone marrow dysfunction preoperatively.
  - The patient's Eastern Cooperative Oncology Group (ECOG) functional status is less than or equal to 2.
  - There is no extra-abdominal disease or retroperitoneal disease.
  - There is low-volume peritoneal disease (preferably a peritoneal carcinomatosis index [PCI] less than 14) that is potentially completely resectable.
  - Any parenchymal hepatic metastasis should be limited and should not require major anatomic liver resection.
  - Malignant ascites and bowel obstructions are predictors of incomplete resection and worse overall survival.

IMAGING AND OTHER DIAGNOSTIC STUDIES

- MRI may detect PSD with up to 100% sensitivity, yet has a significantly high false-positive rate, especially after prior operations. This is because MRI is incapable of recognizing a difference between scar tissue and recurrent PSD.
- Positron emission tomography is rarely used given that sensitivity and specificity are prohibitively low, especially in patients with limited disease.
- Endoscopy can allow clinicians to tattoo second colonic primaries in less than 5% of the patients. Endoscopic ultrasonography is unlikely to change the management of these patients.
- Diagnostic laparoscopy can assist in determining the extent and stage of PSD prior to CRS/HIPEC.
- The PCI is the most used staging system for PSD. It provides a way to standardize the extent of disease. It has been shown to have prognostic value and certain scores have been used as a cutoff in deciding when CRS/HIPEC is appropriate. Calculating the PCI involves dividing the abdomen into nine regions and the small bowel into four regions. For each region, a score of 0 (no tumor), 1 (tumor up to 0.5 cm), 2 (tumor up to 5 cm), or 3 (tumor > 5 cm) is applied to assist in understanding tumor burden. Scores for each of the 12 regions are tabulated to derive the PCI score.
- We calculate ascites score in patients with voluminous ascites (**FIGURES 1** and **2**) based on preoperative imaging. Patients with colorectal primaries and ascites score greater than 3 (or three out of nine abdominal areas containing ascitic fluid while on supine position on the CT table) have minimal chances to achieve a complete CRS. In these patients, after upfront systemic chemotherapy, we start the operation with diagnostic laparoscopy to establish resectability.

Chapter 51 SURGICAL MANAGEMENT OF PERITONEAL CARCINOMATOSIS   **467**

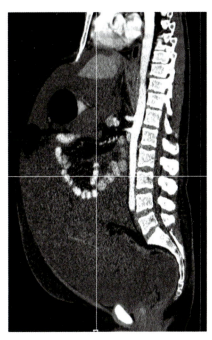

FIGURE 1 • Contrast-enhanced computed tomography of a patient with large volume of malignant ascites. The peritoneal carcinomatosis index (PCI) is calculated based on the size of solid disease components but it is not possible to distinguish solid components from ascitic fluid in patients with a large volume of malignant ascites. In these cases, we use the ascites score to evaluate patients for the operation.

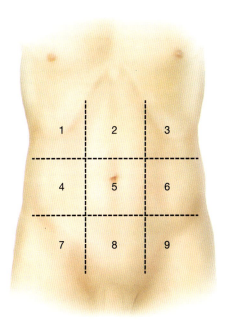

FIGURE 2 • Schematic for calculating the ascites score. One point is assigned for the presence of malignant ascites in each of nine abdominal regions on supine computed tomography. The nine regions correlate with those used to calculate the peritoneal carcinomatosis index.

SURGICAL MANAGEMENT
Preoperative Planning
- Preoperative assessment includes a complete history and physical examination, laboratory evaluation consisting of complete blood counts, comprehensive metabolic panel, hemoglobin A1C level, CEA level, and a blood type with cross-match of four units of packed red blood cells.
- Postsplenectomy vaccines are routinely administered at least 2 weeks prior to operations in which splenectomy is anticipated, based on imaging findings.
- At the surgeon's discretion, ureteral stents may be placed prior to incision. This is generally appropriate for patients with a high probability of ureteral involvement, prior retroperitoneal surgical exploration, or large volume of disease.
- We use mechanical and antibiotic bowel preparation preoperatively routinely. Patients with a bowel obstruction may benefit from the use of enemas. Bowel obstruction is a poor prognostic sign for achieving a compete cytoreduction.
- Prophylactic antibiotics are administered prior to induction of anesthesia.
- Both mechanical and pharmacologic deep vein thrombosis (DVT) prophylaxis is instituted unless contraindicated.

Positioning and Team Setup
- The majority of patients are positioned in a supine position. In rectal cancers or other cases for which a low anterior resection (LAR) is anticipated, a modified lithotomy position is preferred (**FIGURE 3**).

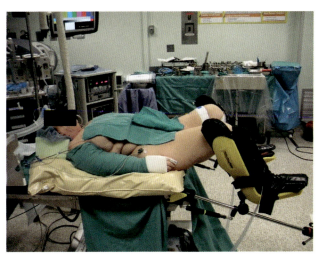

FIGURE 3 • Patient positioning. If a low anterior resection is anticipated, the patient is placed in a modified lithotomy position. The thighs are positioned level with the abdomen, allowing placement of a self-retaining retractor, avoiding excessive pressure between the retractor and the patient's thighs. The arms are tucked. All pressure points are padded to prevent neurovascular and muscular injuries.

- In the modified lithotomy position, the legs are placed in Allen or Yellofin stirrups. All pressure points are padded to prevent neurovascular injuries and/or calf myonecrosis.
- The thighs are positioned level with the abdomen, as this allows placement of a self-retaining retractor without creating excessive pressure between the retractor and the patient's thighs.

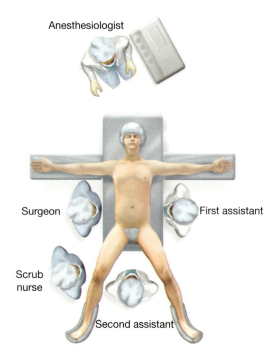

- The perineum is positioned flush with the edge of the operating room table.
- The arms are placed in a neutral position and supported with suitable armrests.
- The surgeon starts at the patient's right side, with the assistant standing to the patient's left side and with the scrub nurse standing to the surgeon's right side (**FIGURE 4**). If the patient is in a modified lithotomy position, a second assistant would be standing in between the patient's legs.

FIGURE 4 • Team setup. The surgeon starts on the patient's right side, with the assistant standing on the patient's left side, and with the scrub nurse standing on the surgeon's right side. A second assistant, if available, stands between the patient's legs.

CYTOREDUCTIVE SURGERY

- After prepping and draping the abdomen, an incision is made from the xiphoid to the pubis to facilitate complete exposure of the peritoneal cavity.
- If the falciform ligament is present, it is resected in continuity with the round ligament prior to placing a fixed retractor (Bookwalter or bilateral Thompson).
- All adhesions from previous operations are lysed to allow all areas of the peritoneal cavity to be exposed to HIPEC.
- It is important at this point to proceed with a detailed mapping of the distribution of disease prior to commencing with any organ resection. Invasion of major vascular retroperitoneal structure or disease at the porta hepatis should not be undertaken for colon cancer–induced PSD.
- CRS is then undertaken to remove all visible tumor deposits, if possible. Only peritoneal surfaces involved by tumor deposits are stripped from the abdominal wall, using electrocautery and blunt dissection.
- The greater omentum is routinely removed, as it is nearly always a site of tumor deposits in patients with carcinomatosis (**FIGURE 5**). Any other involved tissue or organ not vital to survival is also removed. During resection of the lesser omentum (if there is no gross involvement), effort should be made to attempt to preserve the vagal branches innervating the stomach. This will spare the patient long-term gastroparesis and will significantly improve postoperative quality of life.
- Splenectomy is performed in cases of direct involvement or any identified involvement of the left hemidiaphragm, to facilitate a complete diaphragmatic stripping. Attention should be taken to avoid injury to the tail of the pancreas. If a distal pancreatectomy is performed, a drain should be

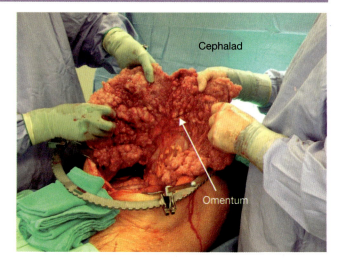

FIGURE 5 • Intraoperative photograph of a patient with peritoneal carcinomatosis. Thickening of the omentum from tumor implants is referred to as "omental cake."

left in place in the left upper quadrant of the abdomen. The incidence of pancreatic leak is not higher in CRS/HIPEC compared to other indications, but associated mortality is significantly higher in this context and should be taken into consideration.

- Intraoperatively, if the surgeon believes complete macroscopic cytoreduction (defined as R01/R1 or CC-0) is not possible or carries undue risk for the patient, the operation is aborted or tailored to delay bowel obstruction without, if possible, any visceral resections, as incomplete CRS offers no survival advantage in colon cancer–induced PSD.

Chapter 51 **SURGICAL MANAGEMENT OF PERITONEAL CARCINOMATOSIS** **469**

- If bowel resection is required, no data exist regarding the timing of creating an anastomosis; thus, any anastomosis required could be made prior to or following HIPEC. Required ostomies are created following HIPEC.

- We encourage the use of diverting loop ileostomies when LAR with primary anastomosis is performed.

GRADING THE RESECTION

- The grade of resection is judged by the surgeon at the conclusion of the cytoreduction.
- Residual disease is evaluated by measuring the diameter of the largest remaining tumor deposits.
- The two classification systems in use are the R level of resection and the completeness of cytoreduction (CC) score (**TABLE 1**). Complete cytoreduction of all gross disease is designated R0 or R1 or CC-0.
- We define complete CRS as no macroscopic evidence of disease at completion of CRS and we group R0/R1 resections together. We rarely claim R0 resection in peritoneal carcinomatosis, except in oligometastatic (ie, low PCI) peritoneal disease. In addition, the pathologist cannot practically evaluate the margins, due to the plethora of specimens that CRS typically produces.

Table 1: Grade of Resection

R Status	Diameter of Largest Remaining Tumor Deposits	Completeness of Cytoreduction Score
—	0 mm	CC-0N—no visible disease following neoadjuvant chemotherapy
R0—clear margins		CC-0S—no visible disease remains
R1—involved margins		
R2a	2.5 mm	CC-1
	5 mm	CC-2
R2b	>5-20 mm	
R2c	>20-25 mm	CC-3
	>25 mm	

The two classification systems in use are the R status of resection and the completeness of cytoreduction (CC) score. Complete cytoreduction of all gross disease is designated R0 or R1 or CC-0.

HYPERTHERMIC INTRAPERITONEAL CHEMOTHERAPY

- The decision of whether to proceed with HIPEC is based on the degree of cytoreduction achieved and is also influenced by institutional protocols. Although HIPEC has a role in patients following a complete cytoreduction, it is unlikely to prolong survival following incomplete cytoreduction. However, we do perfuse patients with massive malignant ascites identified at exploration, even if a complete cytoreduction is not achieved, to palliate the severity of ascites production and improve tolerance of systemic chemotherapy.
- Several factors that influence the efficacy of the intraperitoneal chemotherapy include dose, timing, distribution, temperature, tumor responsiveness, tumor size, systemic chemotherapy, and prior surgery.
- The ratios of peritoneal drug concentrations to plasma drug concentrations are dependent both on the molecular weight and water solubility of the chemotherapy (**TABLE 2**). The most used chemotherapeutic agents for colon cancer are mitomycin C (MMC) and oxaliplatin.

- Heating the chemotherapy increases the penetration of agents into tumor deposits and enhances their cytotoxic effects. The desired temperature of the perfusate in the abdomen ranges from 40 to 42 °C. To compensate, the patient is cooled during HIPEC to prevent systemic hyperthermia. Lowering room temperature and using room temperature intravenous fluids accomplish this through passive cooling.
- Perfusion for colon primaries at our institution is generally maintained for 120 minutes with MMC (30 mg at induction followed by 10 mg an hour later) or oxaliplatin (200 mg/m²). Perfusion times may be decreased to avoid systemic absorption in patients deemed to be particularly susceptible to adverse effects of chemotherapy. Factors that may make a patient more susceptible to drug toxicity include extensive peritonectomy, poor performance status, or advanced age.
- The perfusate is drained following the designated time period for perfusion. The abdomen is explored once again, and anastomoses or ostomies are created as necessary. We do not routinely place drains, except for patients undergoing distal pancreatectomy. The abdomen is closed, and the procedure is concluded.
- Several techniques for perfusing with HIPEC have evolved. All consist of a closed circuit to maintain consistent hyperthermia and temperature monitoring (**FIGURE 6A** and **B**). There is insufficient evidence to support one technique over another.

Hyperthermic Intraperitoneal Chemotherapy Delivery Modalities: The Closed Abdominal Technique

- The closed technique is one of the two most commonly used HIPEC techniques.
- This technique involves the placement of inflow and outflow catheters through the skin prior to suturing the skin closed in a temporary, yet watertight manner (**FIGURE 7**).

Table 2: Chemotherapeutic Agents Used in Hyperthermic Intraperitoneal Chemotherapy for Colorectal Cancer

Agent	Molecular Weight	Peritoneal Fluid Concentration to Plasma Concentration Ratio
Floxuridine	246 Da	2000:1
Mitomycin C	334 Da	75:1
Oxaliplatin	397 Da	25:1

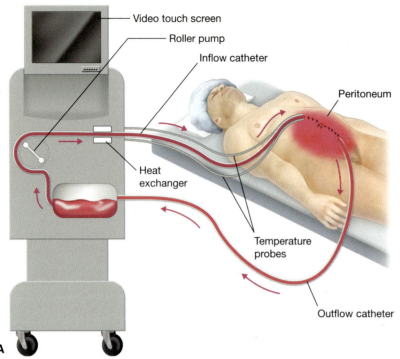

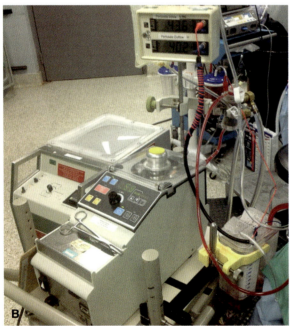

FIGURE 6 • **A,** Schematic of a hyperthermic intraperitoneal chemotherapy perfusion circuit. **B,** Photograph of the perfusion circuit. Flow of isotonic fluid is established into the patient. Inflow and outflow temperatures are monitored and the perfusate is titrated to an outflow temperature of 40-42 °C. The chemotherapeutic agent is added at this point. The perfusate exits the patient, is filtered, and is cycled back through the heat pump and into the patient for the set period of time.

- Temporarily closing at the level of the skin while leaving the fascia open allows contact of the perfusate to the likely contaminated subcutaneous tissue on either side of the incision.
- The operating room personnel massage the abdomen (gently shaking it in a back-and-forth rocking fashion) to help distribute the perfusate throughout the abdomen (**FIGURE 8**).
- The increased pressure in the closed technique theoretically provides deeper penetration of the chemotherapy into tissues.
- For these reasons, the closed technique is our preferred approach to delivering HIPEC.

Hyperthermic Intraperitoneal Chemotherapy Delivery Modalities: The Open or Coliseum Technique

- The open technique is also a commonly used HIPEC method.
- This HIPEC technique involves suturing plastic sheeting circumferentially around the patient's skin incision and securing it to the fixed retractor (**FIGURE 9**). This expands the potential space with a "coliseum-like" device, which allows the bowel to float freely in a larger volume of perfusate.
- This technique theoretically increases exposure of all surfaces to the chemotherapy.

Chapter 51 SURGICAL MANAGEMENT OF PERITONEAL CARCINOMATOSIS   471

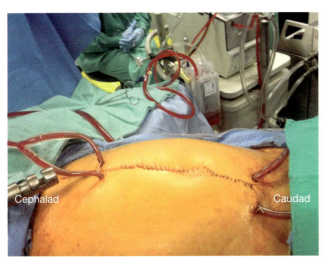

FIGURE 7 • A photograph depicting the closed abdominal technique. There are two inflow and two outflow cannulas that allow the abdomen to be in continuity with the perfusion circuit. The abdomen has been closed temporarily with a running suture at the skin level.

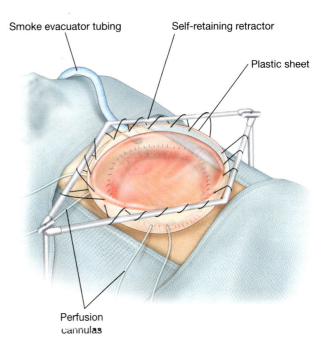

FIGURE 9 • The open or "coliseum" hyperthermic intraperitoneal chemotherapy technique involves suturing plastic sheeting circumferentially around the patient's skin incision and securing it to the fixed retractor. This expands the potential space with a "coliseum-like" device, which allows the bowel to float freely in a larger volume of perfusate.

- The open technique allows the surgeon to manipulate the intra-abdominal contents and may facilitate a more even distribution of heat and agent throughout the abdomen.
- Due to concern regarding exposure of operating room personnel to the chemotherapeutic agent with the open technique, specialized education and training of involved personnel is mandatory. Other safety efforts include restriction of operating room traffic, smoke evacuators, filtration masks, and waterproof gowns.

Hyperthermic Intraperitoneal Chemotherapy Delivery Modalities: Other Techniques

- Other modalities of perfusion have been developed to combine the advantages of both the open and closed techniques but are not widely used.
- These techniques may provide more even drug and temperature distribution; however, they are generally complex and do not eliminate all safety risks to operating room personnel.

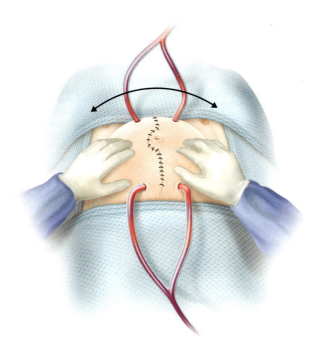

FIGURE 8 • Distribution of the perfusate in the closed hyperthermic intraperitoneal chemotherapy technique. The operating room personnel massage the abdomen (gently rocking back and forth) to help distribute perfusate throughout the abdomen.

472 SECTION III **RECTAL RESECTIONS**

PEARLS AND PITFALLS

CRS/HIPEC goal	▪ Complete cytoreduction prior to HIPEC infusion.

Patient selection	▪ It is critical to select appropriate candidates. Important elements to assess include the following:
	  ▪ Patient's performance status
	  ▪ Extent and distribution of disease
	▪ Consider use of laparoscopy for staging.

CRS	▪ Remove everything with tumor deposits: nonvital organs and peritoneum. ▪ If a bowel resection is required, an anastomosis may be created prior to or following HIPEC. Required ostomies are created following HIPEC. ▪ The two predominating classification systems are used: R status of resection and the CC score.
HIPEC	▪ Perfuse for 120 minutes at 40-42 °C. ▪ Temperature >42 °C greatly increases morbidity/mortality. ▪ The closed abdomen and open (coliseum) techniques are most frequently used.
Postoperative care	▪ ICU monitoring is required in about 30% of patients. ▪ Postoperative grade III/IV morbidity is around 27%: A high index of clinical suspicion is required.

POSTOPERATIVE CARE

- The goal is for endotracheal extubation in the operating room, followed by hemodynamic support and close fluid monitoring, possibly in the intensive care unit (ICU).
- Thirty percent of our patients require ICU monitoring for a median stay of 1 day, whereas 70% are admitted directly to the floor.
- An enhanced recovery after surgery (ERAS) protocol is followed postoperatively modified to the personalized extent of visceral resections.
- Patients are kept nil per os (NPO) until exhibiting return of bowel function. Nasogastric tubes are used as necessary.
- The Foley catheter is removed within 48 hours; however, it is kept for 5 days in cases where an LAR was performed and for 10 days in cases of a cystectomy or bladder repair.
- Intravenous patient-controlled analgesia or thoracic epidural analgesia is used postoperatively at the discretion of the surgeon.
- Mechanical and pharmacologic DVT prophylaxis is started on the day of the operation.
- Aggressive chest physical therapy is instituted. Early ambulation is encouraged.
- The median hospital stay for our first 1000 CRS/HIPEC patients is 8 days.
- Postdischarge follow-up: Patients are discharged home with 2 to 4 weeks of prophylactic enoxaparin, and are initially seen for a postoperative checkup 2 weeks following discharge from the hospital. Follow-up thereafter includes a history and physical examination, tumor markers, and contrast-enhanced CT imaging of the chest, abdomen, and pelvis every 3 months.

COMPLICATIONS

- Given the extent of the surgical resection required to achieve adequate cytoreduction, postoperative morbidity is significant. Major perioperative morbidity over the last 5 years for our institution is 27%, with 3.8% perioperative mortality.
- Complications are frequently divided into two groups: secondary to the operation itself, or to toxicity from the chemotherapeutic agents.
- The complications of CRS essentially depend on the combination of organs resected and are similar with that described in the general surgery literature. The severity of complications may be significantly variable and depends on the physiologic reserves of the patient (which are commonly depleted), the extent of CRS, ECOG status, and the impact of chemotherapy.
- Twenty-three percent of patients are likely to require a blood transfusion at some point during their operation or postoperative hospitalization.
- Predictors of postoperative morbidity include older age, higher PCI, greater number of visceral resections, poorer performance status, and higher chemotherapy drug dose.
- Morbidity and mortality rates are related to the experience of the center performing CRS/HIPEC.
- Common causes of death are bowel perforation, respiratory failure, bone marrow suppression, thromboembolic events, and sepsis.
- Preoperative baseline factors such as diabetes, presence of ascites, bowel obstruction, and poor performance status are the predictors of increased perioperative mortality.
- Despite significant risk of morbidity and mortality, CRS/HIPEC often remains the last hope that many of these patients have for improved long-term survival. Therefore, balanced evaluation of complication risk following CRS/HIPEC must be compared to inherent complications of PSD and its natural history without such treatment.

OUTCOMES

- The completeness of cytoreduction has been shown to be an important independent predictor of survival. The average rate of complete cytoreduction among high-volume centers is about 60% to 75%.
- Predictors of incomplete cytoreduction include poor performance status, disease outside of the peritoneal cavity, more than three hepatic metastases, biliary or ureteral obstruction,

multifocal bowel obstructions, presence of malignant ascites, and extensive disease within the gastrohepatic ligament.

- A consensus statement on the locoregional treatment of colorectal PSD recommends CRS/HIPEC as the treatment of choice for patients without distant metastatic disease and in whom complete cytoreduction is deemed feasible.
- CRS/HIPEC in our institution has a median survival of 33.6 months in colorectal cancer patients who achieved a complete CRS and 21.2 months if CRS/HIPEC is performed with synchronous hepatic resection of limited liver disease in patients pretreated with more than one line of systemic chemotherapy. This must be compared with the 10 to 14 months median survival obtained with second-line chemotherapy and the 3 months median survival obtained with third-line chemotherapy for stage IV colorectal cancer patients.
- The PRODIGE 7 randomized controlled trial, a recently published European study on colorectal cancers with PSD, found an absence of overall survival benefit of CRS/HIPEC over CRS alone. Although adequately powered, a methodological criticism of this study is that HIPEC was applied with a shorter perfusion time (30 minutes) compared to the commonly used protocols in the United States (120 minutes). Additional prospective studies are needed to define the true benefit in colorectal cancer with peritoneal disease.
- It is important to note that systemic chemotherapy and CRS/HIPEC are complementary treatments and are not mutually exclusive.
- These patients should be treated in a multidisciplinary fashion. Multiple lines of chemotherapy will likely result in decreased ECOG functional status, which is a well-documented predictor of increased postoperative morbidity and mortality. Conversely, upfront CRS/HIPEC resulting in major morbidity will deprive the patient from timely administration of systemic chemotherapy.
- Patient quality of life is another key outcome following CRS/HIPEC. Our quality-of-life data indicate that patients return to their baseline between 3 and 6 months postoperatively. The expected decrease in quality of life immediately following such therapy and its duration should be communicated to patients considering CRS/HIPEC.
- Future directions will include the use of personalized ex vivo organoid platforms to define efficacy of both HIPEC and systemic chemotherapy options for each patient separately.

MAIN POINTS OF CYTOREDUCTIVE SURGERY/HYPERTHERMIC INTRAPERITONEAL CHEMOTHERAPY FOR PATIENTS WITH PERITONEAL SURFACE DISEASE FROM COLON CANCER

- CRS/HIPEC involves surgical resection of all seeded organs and peritoneal surfaces followed by heated chemotherapy within the abdomen, with the goal of complete cytoreduction.
- When planning CRS/HIPEC for patients with PSD from colonic primary lesions, appropriate patient selection hinges on the feasibility of obtaining a complete CC-0 cytoreduction and the patient's ability to undergo the procedure. Results of the PRODIGE 7 trial suggest that CRS combined with systemic chemotherapy results is a meaningful survival benefit in colorectal cancer patients with peritoneal disease.
- The sensitivity of preoperative CT in determining distribution of disease is small.

- The goal of CRS/HIPEC is the removal of all visible disease prior to perfusion with HIPEC. Incomplete cytoreduction offers no survival benefit in patients with peritoneal disease from colonic primary lesions.
- Many factors influence the efficacy of HIPEC. There are also many ways to perform HIPEC, each with their own advantages and disadvantages.
- Close monitoring is required postoperatively, as complication rates are high. Clinicians should maintain a high index of suspicion for complications.
- CRS/HIPEC may offer a survival benefit in low-volume patients with colon cancer–induced PSD when a complete cytoreduction is obtained. This treatment modality should be offered in addition to systemic chemotherapy.
- CRS/HIPEC may potentially be repeated in appropriately selected patients with recurrence limited to the peritoneal cavity, and may be associated with prolonged survival.

SUGGESTED READINGS

1. Elias D, Lefevre JH, Chevalier J, et al. Complete cytoreductive surgery plus intraperitoneal chemohyperthermia with oxaliplatin for peritoneal carcinomatosis of colorectal origin. *J Clin Oncol.* 2009;27(5):681-685

2. Esquivel J, Elias D, Baratti D, et al. Consensus statement on the loco regional treatment of colorectal cancer with peritoneal dissemination. *J Surg Oncol.* 2008;98(4):263-267.

3. Forsythe SD, Sasikumar S, Moaven O, et al. Personalized identification of optimal HIPEC perfusion protocol in patient-derived tumor organoid platform. *Ann Surg Oncol.* 2020;27(13):4950-4960.

4. Glehen O, Kwiatkowski F, Sugarbaker PH, et al. Cytoreductive surgery combined with perioperative intraperitoneal chemotherapy for the management of peritoneal carcinomatosis from colorectal cancer: a multi-institutional study. *J Clin Oncol.* 2004;22(16):3284-3292.

5. Hill AR, McQuellon RP, Russell GB, et al. Survival and quality of life following cytoreductive surgery plus hyperthermic intraperitoneal chemotherapy for peritoneal carcinomatosis of colonic origin. *Ann Surg Oncol.* 2011;18(13):3673-3679.

6. Levine EA, Stewart JH, Shen P, et al. Intraperitoneal chemotherapy for peritoneal surface malignancy: experience with 1000 patients. *J Am Coll Surg.* 2014;218(4):573-585.

7. Newman NA, Votanopoulos KL, Stewart JH, et al. Cytoreductive surgery and hyperthermic intraperitoneal chemotherapy for colorectal cancer. *Minerva Chir.* 2012;67(4):309-318.

8. Quenet F, Elias D, Roca L, et al. Cytoreductive surgery plus hyperthermic intraperitoneal chemotherapy versus cytoreductive surgery alone for colorectal peritoneal metastases (PRODIGE 7): a multicentre, randomised, open-label, phase 3 trial. *Lancet Oncol.* 2021;22(2):256-266.

9. Randle RW, Swett KR, Swords DS, et al. Efficacy of cytoreductive surgery with hyperthermic intraperitoneal chemotherapy in the management of malignant ascites. *Ann Surg Oncol.* 2014;21(5):1474-1479.

10. Sarnaik AA, Sussman JJ, Ahmad SA, et al. Technology of intraperitoneal chemotherapy administration: a survey of techniques with a review of morbidity and mortality. *Surg Oncol Clin N Am.* 2003;12(3):849-863.

11. Stewart JH, Shen P, Levine EA. Intraperitoneal hyperthermic chemotherapy for peritoneal surface malignancy: current status and future directions. *Ann Surg Oncol.* 2005;12(10):765-777.

12. Verwaal VJ, Bruin S, Boot H, et al. 8-year follow-up of randomized trial: cytoreduction and hyperthermic intraperitoneal chemotherapy versus systemic chemotherapy in patients with peritoneal carcinomatosis of colorectal cancer. *Ann Surg Oncol.* 2008;15(9):2426-2432.

13. Verwaal VJ, van Ruth S, de Bree E, et al. Randomized trial of cytoreduction and hyperthermic intraperitoneal chemotherapy versus systemic chemotherapy and palliative surgery in patients with peritoneal carcinomatosis of colorectal cancer. *J Clin Oncol.* 2003;21(20):3737-3743.

14. Valenzuela CD, Levine EA, Mangieri CW, et al. Repeat cytoreductive surgery with hyperthermic intraperitoneal chemotherapy for cancers with peritoneal metastasis: A 30-year institutional experience. *Ann Surg Oncol.* 2022. doi:10.1245/s10434-022-11441-3. PMID: 35286531.

Chapter 52

Enhanced Recovery After Surgery

Dhruvesh M. Ramson and Andrew G. Hill

DEFINITION

- Enhanced recovery after surgery (ERAS) refers to evidence-based, patient-focused multidisciplinary perioperative care clinical pathways/protocols that aim to reduce the surgical stress response, optimize physiological function, and improve recovery following surgery.
- The 2012 "Guidelines for Perioperative Care in Elective Colonic Surgery: Enhanced Recovery After Surgery (ERAS) Society Recommendations" was the first ERAS clinical pathway published. There are now other validated similar clinical pathways published by the ERAS Society in several different general surgery subspecialties.
- The ERAS Society is composed of an international consortium of surgeons constituted in April 2011. They performed a comprehensive review of all available evidence for every aspect of colorectal surgery perioperative care using MEDLINE, Embase, and Cochrane databases from 1996 to 2012.
- Data analyzed included review articles, case series, nonrandomized studies, randomized control studies, meta-analyses, and systematic reviews.
- ERAS uses a Cochrane checklist for methodological quality. Quality of evidence and recommendations are based on the Grading of Recommendations, Assessment, Development, and Evaluation (GRADE) system.
- These protocols have been shown to reduce morbidity, enhance recovery, and shorten the length of stay following major colorectal surgery.
- There are several key evidence-based elements to an ERAS protocol. Keys to a successful ERAS protocol are:
  - Multidisciplinary team approach
  - Longitudinal care integration encompassing the entire perioperative period (pre, intra, and postoperative care)

- Strict adherence to the clinical pathway
- Detailed ongoing compliance and audit monitoring by a dedicated ERAS advance practice provider
- Careful attention paid to patients who are unable to achieve care goals or milestones
- ERAS clinical pathways require no new technology and have been proven to be greatly cost-effective, to maximally improve quality of care, and to significantly reduce the cost of care in colorectal surgery. And, yet, their adoption, especially in the United States has been slow.

PERIOPERATIVE MANAGEMENT

Preadmission Management

- Key preadmission ERAS components are summarized in **TABLE 1**.
- Preoperative prehabilitation and optimization of medical comorbidities including cardiovascular, respiratory, and renal disease is very important. This is achieved through clinical evaluation, risk assessment, medication optimization, and the creation of a plan for anesthesia.
- Conditions associated with increased perioperative risk requiring for extensive evaluation and optimization include:
  - Advanced age and frailty
  - Cardiovascular disease
  - Cerebrovascular disease
  - Neurologic disease
  - Pulmonary disease
  - Obstructive sleep apnoea
  - Renal disease
  - Liver disease
  - Endocrine disease

Table 1: Preadmission Management ERAS Recommendations

Item	Recommendation	Evidence level	Recommendation grade
Preoperative information, education, and counseling	Patients should routinely receive dedicated preoperative counseling.	Moderate	Strong
Preoperative optimization	Preoperative medical optimization is necessary before surgery. Smoking and alcohol consumption (alcohol abusers) should be stopped 4 wk before surgery.	*Alcohol*: Low *Smoking*: High	Strong
Management of anemia	Attempts to correct should be made prior to surgery. Blood transfusions should be avoided.	High	Strong
Preoperative nutrition	Preoperative routine nutritional assessment should be performed. Perioperative fasting should be minimized. Oral nutritional support may be used to supplement total intake for a period of at least 7-10 days.	Moderate	Strong
Preoperative bowel preparation	Mechanical bowel preparation should not be used routinely in colonic surgery.	High	Strong
Preoperative fasting and carbohydrate treatment	Clear fluids should be allowed up to 2 h and solids up to 6 h prior to induction of anesthesia. Preoperative oral carbohydrate treatment should be used routinely. In diabetic patients carbohydrate treatment can be given along with the diabetic medication.	Solids and fluids: Moderate Carbohydrate loading, overall: Low	Fasting guidelines: Strong Preoperative carbohydrate drinks: Strong

Chapter 52 **ENHANCED RECOVERY AFTER SURGERY** **475**

- Anaemia
- Malnutrition and obesity
- Thromboembolic disease
- Social and behavioral factors such as cigarette smoking, excessive alcohol consumption, and illicit drug use should be addressed.
- Malnutrition is a modifiable risk factor which places patients at risk of decreased immune function, delayed wound healing, and organ dysfunction. Preoperative nutrition goals are to assess the patient for preexisting malnutrition, optimize surgical readiness by managing malnutrition, and support anabolism for recovery.
- Preoperative exercise programs are incorporated into some ERAS protocols; however, at present there is limited evidence to suggest that they impact upon clinically important outcomes.

Patient Education and Counseling

- ERAS guidelines recommend preadmission counseling and education.
- A variety of approaches are acceptable, including personal counseling, printed materials, and electronic media, alone or in combination. Whatever approach is used, patient education should include discussions regarding the surgical procedure, anesthesia, routine postoperative care, expected course of recovery, recovery milestones, expected date of discharge, and "warning signs" that warrant a surgical review following discharge.
- These efforts may reduce anxiety, improve recovery, enhance would healing, and decrease hospital length of stay.
- Preoperative education by a stoma nurse specialist improves postoperative quality of life by facilitating early patient psychological adaptation to the significant lifestyle changes associated with having a stoma. In addition, preoperative stoma site selection is critical for minimization of postoperative complications. The site should be selected through collaboration of the surgeon, stoma nurse specialist, and patient.
- The evidence level for preoperative patient education is: Moderate. The recommendation grade is: Strong.

Preoperative Optimization

Smoking Cessation and Abstinence From Alcohol

- Active smokers are at increased risk for perioperative complications.
- To reduce this risk, at least 4 weeks of abstinence from smoking is required. Surgery is associated with an increased incidence of spontaneous smoking cessation and may represent the best time for patients to stop smoking permanently. A variety of approaches are effective.
- Alcohol abuse is also associated with an increased risk of postoperative complications.
- ERAS guidelines strongly recommend 4 weeks of preoperative abstinence for alcohol abusers.
- The evidence level for smoking and alcohol cessation preoperatively is: High for smoking, and Low for alcohol. The recommendation grade is: Strong for both smoking and alcohol cessation preoperatively.

Preoperative Nutrition

- The risk of complications is increased in patients with unintentional weight loss of 5% to 10% or more.

- Patients with higher nutritional risk benefit from preoperative nutritional treatment.
- For malnourished patients, oral nutritional supplementation (or additional parenteral nutrition when indicated) has the best effect if started 7 to 10 days preoperatively and is associated with a reduction in the prevalence of infectious complications and anastomotic leaks.
- ERAS recommendation:
  - Preoperative routine nutritional assessment offers the opportunity to correct malnutrition and should be offered. Preoperatively, patients at risk of malnutrition should receive nutritional treatment preferably using the oral route for a period of at least 7 to 10 days.
  - The quality of evidence for this recommendation is: Moderate. The recommendation grade is: Strong.

Management of Anemia

- Anemia is common in patients presenting for colorectal surgery and increases all-cause morbidity. Attempts to correct it should be made prior to surgery.
- Newer preparations of intravenous iron have a low risk of adverse reactions and are more effective than oral iron at restoring hemoglobin concentrations in both iron deficiency anemia and anemia of chronic disease.
- Ideal hemoglobin targets remain somewhat controversial, but it is recommended a minimum hemoglobin concentration of 60 to 100 g/L. Patients cardiac, pulmonary, and renal comorbidities are at higher risk and a target hemoglobin >80 g/L is desirable.
- Blood transfusion has long-term effects and should be avoided if possible.
- The quality of evidence for these recommendations is: High. The recommendation grade is: Strong.

Fasting Guidelines

- NPO after midnight prior to surgery is one of the most widely prescribed orders in all of surgery. It works on the assumption that it increases gastric pH, reduces gastric volume, and that it reduces aspiration of gastric contents into the lungs during induction of anesthesia. It has been orally transmitted from generation to generation of surgeons. Problem is, it is NOT supported by ANY evidence. On the contrary, fasting induces dehydration and electrolyte imbalances at a time when the body will be under significant surgical stress.
- Using a Cochrane review of more than 22 randomized clinical trials, ERAS concluded that preoperative fasting DOES NOT reduce gastric content, does not increase gastric pH, and, importantly, does not reduce the incidence of regurgitation and/or aspiration perioperatively.
- ERAS recommendation:
  - Avoid prolonged preoperative fasting and, instead, ERAS endorses electrolyte and carbo-loading preoperatively. The following fasting intervals prior to the induction of anesthesia for surgery are recommended:
    - No oral intake within 2 to 3 hours of surgery.
    - Clear liquids are encouraged up to 2 to 3 hours prior to surgery. Some protocols include the administration of a carbohydrate and electrolyte-rich drink (400 mL drink with 12.5% maltodextrins) 2 hours prior to the onset of anesthesia.

476 SECTION III **RECTAL RESECTIONS**

- Solid intake is encouraged up to 6 hours prior to surgery.
  - This practice leads to less preoperative thirst, hunger and anxiety, reduces postoperative insulin resistance, and minimizes postoperative losses of nitrogen and protein, better maintaining lean body mass and muscle strength perioperatively. In essence, it converts the patient from the "fasted" to a "metabolically fed" state.
  - The evidence level for this recommendation is: Moderate. The recommendation grade is: Strong.

Bowel Preparation

- The routine use of preoperative mechanical bowel preparation (MBP) remains a controversial topic in colorectal surgery
- In 2011, ERAS performed Cochrane review with 18 RCTs of MBP including 5805 patients. Overall, they found no differences in anastomotic leaks, wound infections, overall complications, or perioperative mortality. In fact, 2 studies showed increased anastomotic leaks and 1 study showed increased infectious complications in patients receiving MBP preoperatively
- ERAS recommendation:
  - MBP should not be used routinely in colonic surgery
  - The evidence level for this recommendation is: High. The recommendation grade is: Strong
  - However, recent evidence conflicts with this recommendation. In a study utilizing the NSQIP database and including 8442 patients receiving MBP with antibiotics, MBP without antibiotics, or no preparation, MBP with antibiotics was independently associated with reduced incidences of surgical site infection (SSI) [odds ratio (OR) = 0.40; 95% confidence interval (CI), 0.31-0.53], anastomotic leak (OR = 0.57; 95% CI, 0.35-0.94), and postoperative ileus (OR = 0.71; 95% CI, 0.56-0.90) compared with no MBP at all. MBP without antibiotics was not associated with decreased rates of SSI, anastomotic leak, or ileus.
  - A recent meta-analysis of seven randomized controlled trials with a total of 1769 patients undergoing elective colorectal surgery found that oral systemic antibiotics plus MBP reduced the incidence of total and incisional surgical site infection compared with systemic antibiotics alone or

MBP alone (total: 7.2% vs 16.0%, $P < .00001$; incisional: 4.6% vs 12.1%, $P < .00001$).
- Thus, ERAS guidelines regarding the use of MBP may need to be revisited in the future.

Preoperative Management

Preoperative management recommendations are summarized in **TABLE 2**.

Thromboprophylaxis

- Patients undergoing colorectal resection are at high risk of developing deep vein thrombosis (DVT) due to age, existence of malignancy, in addition to the nature and length of surgery. Patients identified as being at moderate to highrisk of DVT or pulmonary embolism (PE) should be given chemical and mechanical thromboprophylaxis perioperatively.
- Chemical prophylaxis is typically achieved by subcutaneous administration of unfractionated or low-molecular-weight heparin. This may be given immediately before surgery or shortly after. Evidence for the timing of the first dose of chemical prophylaxis remains unclear and may be dictated by surgeon and local institute preference.
- Mechanical methods of thromboprophylaxis include intermittent pneumatic compression (IPC), graduated compression stockings (GCS), and the venous foot pump. IPC is superior to no prophylaxis and GCS and may offer benefit when used in addition to low-molecular-weight heparin.
- Extended postoperative prophylaxis should be continued for 28 days after surgery for patients with colorectal cancer.
- The evidence level for this recommendation is: High. The recommendation grade is: Strong.

Preanesthetic Medication

- Psychological distress (pre- and postoperative anxiety) may increase perioperative analgesic requirements and postoperative complication rates.
- The adverse side effects of drugs, such as benzodiazepines, opioids, or beta-blockers, can limit their use as anxiolytic preanesthetic medications.

Table 2: Intraoperative Management ERAS Recommendations

Item	Recommendation	Evidence level	Recommendation grade
Prophylaxis against thromboembolism	Patients should wear well-fitting compression stockings, have intermittent pneumatic compression, and receive pharmacological prophylaxis with LMWH. Extended prophylaxis for 28 d should be given to patients with colorectal cancer.	High	Strong
Preanesthetic medication	Avoid routine use of long- or short-acting sedative medication before surgery because it delays immediate postoperative recovery.	Moderate	Strong
PONV	A multimodal approach to PONV prophylaxis should be adopted in all patients undergoing major colorectal surgery. If breakthrough NV occurs, it should be treated using a multimodal approach.	High	Strong
Preoperative fluid management	Patients should reach the anesthetic room in as close a state to euvolemia as possible and any preoperative fluid and electrolyte excesses or deficits should be corrected.	Moderate	Strong
Antimicrobial prophylaxis and skin preparation	Routine prophylaxis using intravenous antibiotics should be given 30-60 min before initiating surgery. Additional doses should be given during prolonged operations according to half-life of the drug used. Preparation with chlorhexidine-alcohol should be used.	High	Strong

Chapter 52 **ENHANCED RECOVERY AFTER SURGERY** **477**

- Effective communication strategies, including attending a preoperative educational session with information for patients on the intent of ERAS pathways, can successfully reduce patient anxiety and improve their perioperative experience.
- ERAS recommendation:
  - Preoperative education can reduce patient anxiety to an acceptable level without the need for anxiolytic medication. Pharmacologic anxiolysis with long- or short-acting sedative medication (especially benzodiazepines and especially in the elderly) should be avoided if possible before surgery.
  - Opioid-sparing multimodal preanesthetic medication can be used with a combination of acetaminophen, nonsteroidal anti-inflammatory drug (NSAIDs), and gabapentinoids. All should be dose adjusted according to age and renal function.
  - Gabapentinoids should preferably be limited to a single lowest dose to avoid sedative side effects.
  - The evidence level for this recommendation is: Moderate. The recommendation grade is: Strong.

Prevention of Nausea and Vomiting

- Prevention of nausea and vomiting (PONV) is fundamental for patients undergoing colorectal surgery.
- Nausea and vomiting affect up to 50% to 80% of patients postoperatively. When severe, it may result in dehydration and delayed return of adequate nutrition intake or may require the placement of a nasogastric tube, increase intravenous fluid administration postoperatively, prolong hospital stay, and increase healthcare costs.
- ERAS recommendation:
  - A multimodal approach to PONV prophylaxis should be considered in all patients.
  - Patients with 1 to 2 risk factors should ideally receive a two-drug combination prophylaxis using first-line antiemetics. Patients with >2 risk factors should receive 2 to 3 antiemetics.
  - If nausea and/or vomiting still occur, despite prophylaxis, salvage therapy should be provided using a multimodal approach using different classes of drugs from those used for prophylaxis.
  - The evidence level for this recommendation is: High. The recommendation grade is: Strong.

Preoperative Fluid and Electrolyte Therapy

- It is imperative that the patient should reach the anesthetic room in as close a state to euvolemia as possible.
- Avoidance of prolonged preoperative fasting, provision of clear liquids (including carbohydrate drinks) for up to 2 hours prior to the induction of anesthesia, and avoidance of mechanical bowel preparation help reduce the incidence of preoperative fluid and electrolyte deficits and substantially reduced intraoperative fluid requirements.
- Any preoperative fluid and electrolyte excesses or deficits must be corrected.
- ERAS recommendation:
  - Patients should reach the anesthetic room in as close a state to euvolemia as possible and any preoperative fluid and electrolyte excesses or deficits should be corrected.
  - The evidence level for this recommendation is: Moderate. The recommendation grade is: Strong.

Preoperative Antimicrobial Prophylaxis

- A Cochrane review of 206 RCTs including 43,451 patients showed that:
  - Chlorhexidine vs betadine preoperative skin preparation reduced postoperative wound infections by 40%.
  - Intravenous (IV) antibiotics covering enteric flora administered 30 to 60 min preoperatively decrease postoperative wound infections by 76%.
- ERAS recommendation:
  - Prophylaxis with IV antibiotics should be given within 60 minutes before incision as a single-dose administration to all patients undergoing colorectal surgery.
  - In patients receiving oral mechanical bowel preparation, oral antibiotics should be given.
  - Skin disinfection should be performed using chlorhexidine–alcohol-based preparations. Evidence is insufficient to support advanced measures such as antiseptic showering, routine shaving, and adhesive incise sheets.
  - The evidence level for this recommendation is: High. The recommendation grade is: Strong.

Intraoperative Management

Intraoperative management ERAS recommendations are summarized in **TABLE 3**.

Table 3: Intraoperative Management ERAS Recommendations

Item	Recommendation	Evidence level	Recommendation grade
MIS vs open surgery	MIS for colonic resections has clear advantages vs open surgery and is recommended if the expertise is available. MIS is an enabler for successful administration of several ERAS components.	High	Strong
Standard anesthetic protocol	A standard anesthetic protocol allowing rapid awakening should be given. The anesthetist should control fluid therapy, analgesia, and hemodynamic changes to reduce the metabolic stress response.	Rapid awakening: Low Cerebral monitoring: High	Strong
Intraoperative fluid therapy	The goal of perioperative fluid therapy is to maintain euvolemia. A perioperative near-zero fluid balance approach should be preferred. Goal-directed fluid therapy should be adopted especially in high-risk patients and in patients undergoing surgery with large intravascular fluid loss.	High	Strong
Preventing intraoperative hypothermia	Intraoperative maintenance of normothermia to keep body temperature >36 °C should be observed routinely. Preoperative warming is encouraged.	High	Strong
Drainage of peritoneal cavity after colonic anastomosis	Routine drainage should not be routinely used.	High	Strong

478 SECTION III **RECTAL RESECTIONS**

Surgical Access: Minimally Invasive Surgery (MIS) vs Open Surgery

- MIS leads to significant improvements in short-term outcomes without compromising oncological outcomes when compared to open surgery. Outcome advantages include less pain, faster recovery, more complete recovery, lower incidence of wound infections and incisional hernias, and shorter length of hospital stay.
- MIS is both an important enabling technology for many of the elements of ERAS and an independent predictor of good outcome. It independently has the capacity to reduce complications, which is the goal of an ERAS program. MIS enables reduced pain and opiate requirement, early mobilization, less impact on fluid shifts, and reduced ileus.
- The relative influences of laparoscopy and enhanced recovery protocols have been compared in several trials. The LAFA study was a multicenter RCT, which randomized patients to laparoscopic and open segmental colectomy and "fast track" and "standard care" within nine Dutch centers. The median hospital stay was 2 days shorter after laparoscopic resection and the best outcomes with the least impact on the immune system was in the group receiving both minimally invasive surgery and ERAS protocol. Regression analysis showed that laparoscopic surgery was the only predictive factor to reduce hospital stay and morbidity.
- The EnROL trial randomized between laparoscopic and open colorectal resection within an enhanced recovery protocol and measured physical fatigue at 1 month as its primary outcome. Median hospital stay was 2 days shorter after laparoscopic surgery. A meta-analysis of protocol-driven care and laparoscopic surgery for colorectal cancer concluded that the combination reduced colorectal cancer surgery complications, but not mortality.
- ERAS recommendation:
  - A minimally invasive approach to colon and rectal cancer has clear advantages for improved and more rapid recovery, reduced general complications, reduced wound-related complications including incisional hernia and fewer adhesions. It is also an enabler for successful administration of many of the major components of ERAS such as opiate-sparing analgesia and optimized fluid therapy.
  - Quality of evidence: High.
  - Recommendation grade: Strong.

Standard Anesthetic Protocol

- ERAS protocols favor strategies involving multimodal analgesic agents and avoidance of long-acting anesthetic agents.
- Typical anesthetic regimes include:
  - Lowest possible dosing and typically include a short-acting anesthetic agent such as propofol and inhaled anesthetics such as sevoflurane.
  - Avoidance of premedications such as benzodiazepines, which are associated with an increased risk of respiratory depression and postoperative sedation.
  - Avoidance of long-acting opioids.
  - Avoidance of long-acting paralytic agents.
  - Use of a peripheral nerve stimulator to prevent profound muscle paralysis.

- Reversal of paralytic agents at the conclusion of surgery to prevent ongoing paralysis, which may be associated with postoperative respiratory complications.
- ERAS recommendation:
  - The use of short-acting anesthetics, cerebral monitoring to improve recovery and reduce the risk for postoperative delirium, monitoring of the level, and complete reversal of neuromuscular block are recommended.
    - Quality of evidence: Short-acting anesthetics: Low.
    - Recommendation grade: High.
    - Quality of evidence: Use of Cerebral Monitoring: High.
    - Recommendation grade: Strong.
    - Quality of evidence: Reducing intra-abdominal pressure during laparoscopic surgery facilitated by neuromuscular block: Low.
    - Recommendation grade: Weak.
    - Quality of evidence: Monitoring (objective) the level and complete reversal of neuromuscular block: High.
    - Recommendation grade: Strong.

Intraoperative Fluid Management

- Fluid management is centered on the maintenance of euvolemia and avoidance of hypovolemia or disproportionate fluid administration that may result in pulmonary complications.
- There are various strategies that may be implemented:
  - Restrictive fluid therapy aims to prevent fluid overload by replacing only fluid that is lost during surgery. It is the optimal strategy for minimization of fluid administration.
  - Goal-directed fluid therapy centers on the administration of fluids in order to achieve physiological goals such as stroke volume variation, systolic pressure variation, or pulse pressure variation. Such a strategy may be unnecessary if avoidance of preoperative dehydration and early preoperative nutrition are achieved.
- ERAS recommendation:
  - The goal of perioperative fluid therapy is to maintain fluid homoeostasis avoiding fluid excess and organ hypoperfusion. A perioperative near-zero fluid balance approach should be preferred. Goal-directed fluid therapy should be adopted especially in high-risk patients and in patients undergoing surgery with large intravascular fluid loss.
  - Inotropes should be considered in patients with poor contractility (CI < 2.5 L/min).
  - Quality of evidence: High.
  - Recommendation grade: Strong.

Preventing Intraoperative Hypothermia

- Monitoring body temperature intraoperatively and the standardized use of body warmers are important as body temperature changes can occur due to exposure during surgery and the impairment of body temperature regulation mechanism as a consequence of anesthesia.
- Changes in body temperature are associated with morbidity including coagulopathy, adverse cardiac events, and increased surgical site infections.
- Risk factors for intraoperative hypothermia include prolonged procedures (>2 hours), older patients, and patients with minimal adipose tissue.
- Methods to conserve body temperature include warming and humidification of anesthetic gases, warming IV

and irrigation fluids, and forced air warming blankets and devices. In addition, the ambient temperature should be at least 21 °C.
- Another area to minimize hypothermia is the use of pre-warming prior to the OR.
- Laparoscopic surgery reduces heat loss vs open surgery.
- ERAS recommendation:
  - Reliable temperature monitoring should be undertaken in all colorectal surgical patients and methods to actively warm patients to avoid inadvertent perioperative hypothermia should be employed.
  - Inotropes should be considered in patients with poor contractility (CI < 2.5 L/min).
  - Quality of evidence:
    - Maintenance of normothermia: High

- Monitoring of temperature: High
- Prewarming: Moderate
- Recommendation grade: Strong

Avoidance of Drains

- ERAS protocols advocate for the avoidance of peritoneal drains. Evidence suggests that when used in an elective setting, drains are not associated with reduced morbidity or mortality and do not decrease the rate of, nor negate the deleterious effects of, anastomotic leakage.
- ERAS recommendation:
  - Pelvic and peritoneal drains show no effect on clinical outcome and should not be used routinely.
  - Evidence level: High.
  - Recommendation grade: Strong.

PEARLS AND PITFALLS

Preadmission	- Patient education (including stoma site selection)
	- Pre-operative optimisation of medical comorbidities
	- Correct anaemia
	- Preoperative Nutrition. Use immunonutrition in malnourished patients
	- Selective bowel preparation
	- Avoid NPO
	- Carbohydrate drink 2 hours prior to surgery
Preoperative	- Chemical and mechanical thromboprophylaxis
	- No premedication
	- Multimodal prevention of nausea and vomiting
	- Routine use of prophylactic antibiotics prior to induction of anaesthesia
	- Maintain euvolemic state
Intraoperative	- Laparoscopic surgery is one of the most important ERAS elements enabler and should be used whenever expertise is available
	- Use a standard anesthetic protocol to reduce metabolic impact and allow for rapid reawakening
	- Maintain a euvolemic state. Goal-directed fluid therapy should be used
	- Prevent perioperative hypothermia
	- Use multimodal analgesia including TEA for open surgery and TAP blocks for laparoscopic surgery
	- Avoidance of drains and nasogastric tubes
Postoperative	- Use multimodal analgesia including the use of paracetamol, NSAIDs, lidocaine drips, and gabapentin
	- Early mobilization is key as it prevents postoperative complications
	- Maintain a euvolemic state
	- Early urinary catheter removal
	- Multimodal Prevention of postoperative ileus. Early oral nutrition
	- Early discharge

POSTOPERATIVE CARE

See **TABLE 4**.

Avoidance of Nasogastric Tubes

- Routine placement of nasogastric tubes is contraindicated. A Cochrane meta-analysis of 33 trials with >5000 patients undergoing abdominal surgery confirmed significant differences by an earlier return of bowel function. And a decrease in pulmonary complications in a nasogastric tube was avoided. Another recent meta-analysis of RCTs including 1416 patients undergoing colorectal surgery showed that pharyngolaryngitis and respiratory infections were less frequent if postoperative nasogastric decompression was avoided.
- There are no data to support the use of prophylactic nasogastric decompression in reducing postoperative anastomotic leakage.

- ERAS recommendation:
  - Nasogastric tubes should not be used routinely. If inserted during surgery, they should be removed before reversal of anesthesia.
  - Quality of evidence: High
  - Recommendation grade: Strong

Postoperative Analgesia

- Postoperative analgesia resulting in adequate pain control is essential in ERAS pathways in colorectal surgery.
- Goals of pain management are to improve the comfort of the patient, facilitate early postoperative mobilization, and subsequent rehabilitation.
- Multimodal analgesia strategies center on minimization of opioid use. The benefit of using a multimodal approach to

480 SECTION III RECTAL RESECTIONS

Table 4: Postoperative Management ERAS Recommendations

Item	Recommendation	Evidence level	Recommendation grade
Nasogastric intubation	Postoperative nasogastric tubes should not be used routinely. Nasogastric tubes inserted during surgery should be removed before reversal of anesthesia.	High	Strong
Postoperative analgesia	Use multimodal analgesia. Avoid use of opioids. Goals: Improve comfort, facilitate early mobilization, and rehabilitation.	Moderate	Strong
Thoracic epidural analgesia	Gold-standard after open surgery for minimizing metabolic stress response and providing analgesia postoperatively in open surgery. Not recommended after laparoscopic surgery.	High	Strong
Lidocaine infusion	The analgesia benefit is in both open surgery and laparoscopic colorectal surgery.	High	Strong
Transversus abdominis plane (TAP) block	TAP blocks reduce opioid consumption and improve recovery in minimally invasive surgery.	Moderate	Strong
Postoperative fluid therapy	Net "near-zero" fluid and electrolyte balance should be maintained. For maintenance needs, hypotonic crystalloids should be used. For replacement of losses, balanced solutions are preferred. Hypotension during epidural analgesia should be treated with vasopressors after ensuring the patient is euvolemic.	Neutral fluid balance: High Hypotonic crystalloids for maintenance needs: Low Balanced salt solutions instead of 0.9% saline: Low	Strong
Urinary drainage	Routine transurethral bladder drainage for 1 (low risk of urinary retention patients) to 3 d (high risk of urinary retention) is recommended.	High	Strong
Prevention of postoperative ileus	A multimodal approach is recommended: multimodal analgesia, avoid nasogastric tube, use of goal-directed fluid therapy. Chewing gum, coffee, bisacodyl, magnesium oxide, and alvimopan may be included.	Multimodal prevention: High. Alvimopan: Moderate. Bisacodyl, magnesium oxide, and coffee: Low	Thoracic epidural, fluid overload, nasogastric decompression, chewing gum, and alvimopan: Strong Oral magnesium: Weak
Postoperative glucose control	Hyperglycemia should be avoided to avoid complications. ERAS protocol reduces insulin resistance and improves glycemic control. Insulin should be used judiciously to maintain blood glucose as low as feasible with the available resources.	Moderate	Strong
Early mobilization	Prolonged immobilization increases the risk of pneumonia, insulin resistance, and muscle weakness. Patients should therefore be mobilized early.	Moderate	Strong

pain management is based on the concept that several multiple pain-reducing mechanisms will improve pain control while avoiding the side effects of each drug.

- General principals of pain management include:
  - Use of nonopioid analgesics such as paracetamol and NSAIDs.
  - Management of somatic pain by infiltration of long-acting local anesthetic agents at port sites, local anesthetic delivery techniques such as rectus sheath catheters, and regional anesthesia such as epidural blockade, or transversus abdominis plane (TAP) blockade.
- ERAS recommendation:
  - Avoid opioids and apply multimodal analgesia in combination with spinal/epidural analgesia or TAP blocks when indicated
  - Quality of evidence for multimodal opioid-sparing analgesia: Moderate
  - Recommendation grade: Strong

Postoperative Analgesia: Epidural Blockade

- The use of lidocaine infusions to reduce opioid use and nausea in colorectal surgery is now well established.
- Published dosing ranges from 1.5 to 3 mg/kg/h depending on the bolus given (0-1.5 mg/kg). Continuous ECG monitoring is advised. Nurses should be aware of potential toxicity symptoms (tinnitus, circumoral tingling, blurred vision, tongue paresthesia).

- The analgesia benefit is in both open surgery and laparoscopic colorectal surgery.
- This beneficial effect appears to last longer than the infusion itself. Studies have been inconsistent in the duration of use of the infusion with some stopping at the end of surgery while others continue between 12 and 24 hours postoperatively
- ERAS recommendation:
  - Lidocaine infusions can reduce opiate consumption after surgery
  - Quality of evidence: High
  - Recommendation: Strong

Postoperative Analgesia: Abdominal Wall Blocks

- The role of epidural analgesia within the setting of an ERAS program has been questioned, especially with regard to laparoscopic operations. Interest in local anesthetic abdominal walls blocks, as a component of multimodal analgesia, has thus increased.
- TAP blocks are the most widely studied. TAP blocks provide analgesic coverage to the anterior abdominal wall from T10 to L1 and have been demonstrated to provide an opioid-sparing approach in colorectal surgery
- ERAS recommendation:
  - TAP blocks reduce opioid consumption and improve recovery. Both ultrasound-guided and laparoscopic approaches have been described.
  - Quality of evidence: Moderate

- Recommendation: TAP blocks in minimally invasive surgery: Strong

Postoperative Fluid Therapy

- The main goal of postoperative fluid therapy is to maintain a euvolemic state, avoiding excessive intravenous fluid administration.
- Principles for postoperative fluid administration include:
  - Discontinuation of intravenous fluid therapy as soon as oral fluids can be tolerated
  - Infusion of balanced salt solutions prior to oral intake commencing
  - Limited boluses of balanced salt solution to manage hemodynamic instability/inadequate urine output
- There are limited data to support the commonly goal directed therapy outcome of 0.5 mL/kg/h of urine output.
- Routine use of postoperative diuretics without specific clinical indication is contraindicated due to the risk of depletion of intravascular volume.
- ERAS recommendation:
  - Net "near-zero" fluid and electrolyte balance should be maintained. To cover pure maintenance needs, hypotonic crystalloids should be used (rather than isotonic crystalloids, which contain high concentrations of sodium and cations).
  - For replacement of losses, saline 0.9% and saline-based solutions should be avoided, with balanced solutions being preferred.
  - In patients receiving epidural analgesia, arterial hypotension should be treated with vasopressors after ensuring the patient is euvolemic.
  - Quality of evidence:
    - Neutral fluid balance: High
    - Hypotonic crystalloids for maintenance needs: Low
    - Balanced salt solutions instead of 0.9% saline: Low
- Recommendation grade: Strong

Early Urinary Catheter Removal

- Early removal of urinary catheters is important as they are associated with risk of urinary tract infection and may delay efforts in early ambulation.
- Early removal is not associated with an increased risk of urinary retention and may decrease hospital length of stay.
- ERAS recommendation:
  - Routine transurethral catheterization is recommended for 1 to 3 days after colorectal surgery. The duration should be individualized based on known risk factors for retention: male gender, epidural analgesia, and pelvic surgery.
  - Patients at low risk should have routine removal of catheter on the first day after surgery, while patients with moderate or high risk require catheterization for up to 3 days.
  - Quality of evidence: High
  - Recommendation grade: Strong

Prevention of Postoperative Ileus

- Prolonged postoperative ileus is a major cause of patient discomfort, impaired nutrition, delayed discharge, and increased costs.

- Core elements for decreasing ileus include:
  - Minimization of opioid analgesia
  - Use of minimal access surgery
  - Eliminating prophylactic nasogastric tube placement
  - Maintenance of euvolemia

There is some evidence to suggest that peripherally acting mu-opioid receptor antagonists may reduce postoperative ileus and are used in some ERAS protocols.

Postoperative Glycaemic Control

- ERAS recommendation:
  - Hyperglycemia is a risk factor for complications and should therefore be avoided.
  - Several interventions in the ERAS protocol prevent insulin resistance and improve glycemic control with no risk of causing hypoglycemia.
  - For inpatients, insulin should be used judiciously to maintain blood glucose as low as feasible with the available resources.
  - Quality of evidence: Moderate
  - Recommendation grade: Strong

Early Oral Nutrition

- The traditional practice of withholding oral nutrition until return of bowel function should be avoided.
- Early resumption of oral intake is important to maintain a well-fed metabolic state.
- Diet can be safely resumed within a few hours postsurgery when the patient is fully conscious.
- Early nutrition is associated with a reduced risk of infectious complications.
- Postoperative nutritional support can be achieved with the use of high-calorie drinks which decrease the post-operative protein deficit
- The recent ESPEN guideline on perioperative nutrition presented an extensive review of multiple RCTs and meta-analysis and concluded that perioperative use of immuno-nutrition with enteral feeds rich with immunomodulators (such as L-arginine, L-glutamine, omega-3 fatty acids, and nucleotides) reduces postoperative infectious complications and should be given to malnourished patients undergoing major cancer surgery.
- ERAS recommendation:
  - Most patients can and should be offered food and oral nutrition supplementationfrom the day of surgery. Perioperative immunonutrition in malnourished patients is beneficial in colorectal cancer surgery.
  - Quality of evidence: Moderate.
  - Recommendation grade: Strong.

Early Mobilization

- Early postoperative mobilization is a crucial component of all ERAS protocols. This is typically achieved through a multidisciplinary approach including physiotherapy and occupational therapy.
- Early mobilization has a role in the prevention of:
  - Postoperative pneumonia
  - Venous thromboembolism
  - Postoperative ileus

- ERAS recommendation:
  - Early mobilization through patient education and encouragement is an important component of ERAS programs.
  - Prolonged immobilization is associated with a variety of adverse effects and patients should therefore be mobilized as early as possible.
  - Quality of evidence: Moderate
  - Recommendation grade: Strong

COMPLICATIONS

Prediction of Infective Complication

- C-reactive protein (CRP) has been demonstrated to be a useful negative predictor of postoperative infective complications and is commonly used to guide discharge.
- Studies suggest that a postoperative day 3 CRP <150 mg/L is highly predictive of an uncomplicated recovery.

OUTCOMES

Early Discharge

- The ultimate goal of ERAS programs is to facilitate enhanced recovery and accelerated return to normal activities.
- Many protocols do not require the resumption of bowel function prior to discharge.

Colonic vs Rectal Resections

- It is essential that ERAS protocols distinguish between colectomy and proctectomy, as each of these are distinct operations requiring some differences in perioperative care protocols with differing endpoints.
- Patients undergoing proctectomy are likely to have undergone neoadjuvant chemotherapy and typically have undergone full bowel preparation, which introduces issues of fluid and electrolyte balance. Extensive pelvic dissection may require urinary catheter drainage for longer periods than colon resection patients do. Furthermore, proctectomy is associated with a higher prevalence of stomas which require further preoperative planning (**FIGURE 1**).

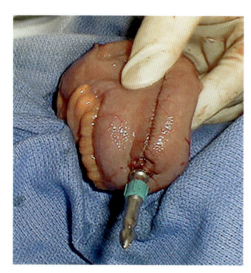

FIGURE 1 • Intraoperative picture demonstrating fashioning of ileal pouch during laparoscopic surgery. (Reprinted with permission from Delaney CP. *Operative Techniques in Laparoscopic Colorectal Surgery*. 2nd ed. Wolters Kluwer; 2014. Figure 18.10.1.)

Setting Up and Maintaining an ERAS Protocol

- A team-based approach is imperative in the successful implementation of an ERAS program. A team-based approach incorporates all members of the multidisciplinary team including surgeon, anesthetist, nurse, pharmacist, physiotherapist, occupational therapist, and dietician.
- Separation of elective and acute cases is imperative due to the fundamental differences in the underlying pathophysiology and hence needs of these two groups. Elective colorectal surgery patients typically have shorter length of stays and separating these two groups of patients on the ward can help to achieve this outcome.
- Simplicity in an ERAS protocol is imperative in its implementation and success. Modern protocols must be evidence based, cost effective, and easy to implement. Too many unnecessary elements result in a protocol that is cumbersome and difficult to implement and maintain.
- Discharge planning should commence prior to admission. Successful early discharge is achieved when discharge is discussed with patients and families prior to the day of discharge. Patients and families benefit from early warnings and preparation time. Discharge discussions should start at the first clinic appointment.
- Regular audit of outcomes with scheduled appraisal of success and failures must be engineered into the program. This is crucial in ensuring the long-term success and sustainability of any ERAS program. Audit is an essential part of clinical governance and helps to maintain compliance with the ERAS protocol.

Audit of Compliance

- Recording of outcomes and measurement of compliance with the elements of an ERAS protocol are vital and should be audited regularly.
- There are a variety of tools for measuring compliance such as smart order sets or electronic systems.

SUGGESTED READINGS

1. Delaney CP, Fazio VW, Senagore AJ, Robinson B, Halverson AL, Remzi FH. "Fast track" postoperative management protocol for patients with high co-morbidity undergoing complex abdominal and pelvic colorectal surgery. *Br J Surg*. 2001;88(11):1533-1538. doi:10.1046/j.0007-1323.2001.01905.x
2. Gustafsson UO, Scott MJ, Hubner M, et al. Guidelines for perioperative care in elective colorectal surgery—enhanced recovery after surgery (ERAS®) society recommendations: 2018. *World J Surg*. 2019;43(3):659-695. doi:10.1007/s00268-018-4844-y
3. Hill AG. Enhanced recovery after surgery: tips and tricks for success. *ANZ J Surg*. 2021;91(3):228-229. doi:10.1111/ans.16533
4. Kehlet H, Wilmore DW. Evidence-based surgical care and the evolution of fast-track surgery. *Ann Surg*. 2008;248(2):189-198. doi:10.1097/SLA.0b013e31817f2c1a
5. Ljungqvist O, Scott M, Fearon KC. Enhanced recovery after surgery: a review. *JAMA Surg*. 2017;152(3):292-298. doi:10.1001/jamasurg.2016.4952
6. Scott MJ, Baldini G, Fearon KC, et al. Enhanced Recovery After Surgery (ERAS) for gastrointestinal surgery, part 1: pathophysiological considerations. *Acta Anaesthesiol Scand*. 2015;59(10):1212-1231. doi:10.1111/aas.12601
7. Wick EC, Galante DJ, Hobson DB, et al. Organizational culture changes result in improvement in patient-centered outcomes: implementation of an integrated recovery pathway for surgical patients. *J Am Coll Surg*. 2015;221(3):669-677.

Index

Note: Page numbers followed by "*f*" indicate figures and "*t*" indicate tables.

A

Abdominal cavity, laparoscopic small bowel resection, 2–3, 2*f*

Abdominal laparoscopic proctosigmoidectomy, 291–294, 291*f*–294*f*

Abdominoperineal resection (APR), 244
  hand-assisted laparoscopic surgery (HALS)
    complications, 334
    descending colon mobilization, 328
    descending colostomy creation, 332–333
    descending mesocolon, medial to lateral dissection of, 327–328, 327*f*
    differential diagnosis, 322
    equipment and instrumentation, 323
    imaging and diagnostic studies, 322–323
    inferior mesenteric artery (IMA), 326–327, 326*f*–327*f*
    inferior mesenteric vein (IMV), 325–326
    intracorporeal proximal transection, 328
    levator ani muscle, transection of, 330–331, 330*f*–331*f*
    open transperineal approach, 331–332, 331*f*–332*f*
    outcomes, 334
    patient history, 322
    patient positioning, 323
    pearls and pitfalls, 333
    pelvic dissection, 328–330, 329*f*–330*f*
    pelvic inlet, sigmoid colon mobilization off, 328, 328*f*
    perineal wound closure, 332
    physical findings, 322
    port placement, 324
    postoperative care, 333
    preoperative preparation, 323
    surgical team setup, 323
    team positioning and draping, 323–324, 324*f*
  laparoscopic technique
    bottom-up technique, 310–311, 311*f*
    colostomy completion, 319, 319*f*–320*f*
    complications, 321
    equipment and instrumentation, 308
    exploration and exposure, 310, 310*f*
    extraperitoneal colostomy technique, 316, 317*f*
    imaging and diagnostic studies, 307
    indications for, 307
    outcomes, 320–321
    patient history, 307
    pearls and pitfalls, 320
    perineal closure, 319, 319*f*–320*f*
    perineal dissection, 317, 318*f*
    perineal rectum and specimen extraction, dissection of, 318–319
    port placement, 308–310, 309*f*
    positioning, 308, 308*f*
    postoperative care, 320

    preoperative planning, 308
    sigmoid colon, mobilization and division of, 312–313, 313*f*
    top-down technique, 311, 311*f*–312*f*
    total mesorectal excision (TME), 314–316, 314*f*–316*f*
  open technique
    complications, 305
    descending colostomy, 304–305
    differential diagnosis, 298
    exposure, 299–300, 299*f* 300*f*
    imaging and diagnostic studies, 298
    inferior mesenteric artery, 300, 300*f*–301*f*
    outcomes, 305
    patient history, 298
    pearls and pitfalls, 305
    perineal wound, closure of, 304
    perineum dissection, 303, 303*f*–304*f*
    physical findings, 298
    positioning, 298–299, 299*f*
    postoperative care, 305
    preoperative planning, 298
    rectum mobilization, 301–303, 301*f*–302*f*
    sigmoid colon mobilization, 300, 300*f*–301*f*
  robotic-assisted laparoscopic surgery technique
    colostomy and closure, 343
    complications, 344
    descending and sigmoid mesocolon, lateral mobilization of, 338
    descending and sigmoid mesocolon, medial to lateral dissection of, 338
    exploration and robotic docking, 337
    imaging and diagnostic studies, 335–336
    incision, 337, 337*f*
    intracorporeal proximal transection, 339
    mesorectal dissection, 339–341, 339*f*–342*f*
    outcomes, 344
    patient history, 335
    pearls and pitfalls, 344
    perineal procedure, 342–343, 343*f*
    physical findings, 335
    port placement and instruments, 337, 337*f*
    positioning, 336, 336*f*
    postoperative care, 344
    preoperative planning, 336
    presacral plane, 337, 338*f*
    vascular division, 338, 338*f*

Acute colitis, 203

Adenocarcinoma, 63

Adhesiolysis, 11

AIRSEAL-CONMED 8-mm laparoscopic insufflation port, 80

Alexis® retractor, 119, 119*f*

Alvarado score, 48

Alvimopan, 128, 229

American Joint Committee on Cancer (AJCC) stage, 77

Anal fissure
  closed lateral internal sphincterotomy, 434–436, 435*f*–436*f*
  complications, 438
  differential diagnosis, 433
  imaging and diagnostic studies, 433
  open lateral internal sphincterotomy, 436, 437*f*
  outcomes, 438
  patient history, 433
  pearls and pitfalls, 437
  physical findings, 433
  positioning, 434
  postoperative care, 438
  preoperative planning, 434
  surgical management, 433–434

Anastomosis, low anterior rectal resection
  creation of, 283
  division of rectum, 283
  ileostomy, creation of, 283
  specimen extraction, 283

Anastomotic leak
  colon/rectal injuries, 243
  hand-assisted laparoscopic surgery (HALS), 117
  laparoscopic transverse colectomy, 109
  left hemicolectomy, robotic-assisted technique, 147

Anesthesia
  induction, preparation after, 441
  for right hemicolectomy, 55

Anterior compartment dissection, 383–386, 384*f*–385*f*

Antibiotic prophylaxis, 29, 55

Appendectomy. *See* Laparoscopic appendectomy

Appendicitis Inflammatory Response (AIR) score, 48

Appendix
  exposure of, 50
  transection of, 51–52, 51*f*–52*f*

Ascending colon
  hand-assisted laparoscopic surgery (HALS), 74, 74*f*–75*f*
  mobilization, 55, 56*f*
  single-incision laparoscopic technique, 83, 83*f*

B

Bleeding
  laparoscopic transverse colectomy, 108
  left hemicolectomy, robotic-assisted technique, 147

Bookwalter retractor, 119

I-1

I-2 **INDEX**

Bottom-up technique, 310–311, 311*f*
Bowel necrosis, colon/rectal injuries, 243
Bowel resection
   hand-assisted laparoscopic surgery (HALS), 75, 76*f*
   transverse colectomy, 97, 98*f*
Bowel transection, 58, 58*f*

C
Carbohydrate loading, 128
Carcinoembryonic antigen (CEA), 323
   hand-assisted laparoscopic surgery (HALS), 71
   left hemicolectomy, 118
   low anterior rectal resection (LAR), 245
      laparoscopic technique, 254
   sigmoid colectomy
      hand-assisted laparoscopic surgery (HALS), 166
      open technique, 148
   total abdominal colectomy (TAC)
      hand-assisted laparoscopic surgery (HALS), 216
Carter–Thomason suture-passer device, 7, 7*f*
Cecum
   hand-assisted laparoscopic surgery (HALS), 72
   tattooed lesion in, 54, 54*f*
Cefoxitin, 55
Ceftriaxone, 55
Chlorhexidine, 128
Circulating tumor DNA (ct-DNA), 79
Closed lateral internal sphincterotomy, 434–436, 435*f*–436*f*
Colectomy
   abdominal. *See* Total abdominal colectomy (TAC)
   laparoscopic. *See* Laparoscopic transverse colectomy
   robotic. *See* Robotic total abdominal colectomy
   sigmoid. *See* Sigmoid colectomy
   transverse. *See* Transverse colectomy
Colitis, 203
Coloanal anastomosis, 244
   total mesorectal excision with, 295, 295*f*–296*f*
      abdominal laparoscopic proctosigmoidectomy, 291–294, 291*f*–294*f*
      complications, 297
      differential diagnosis, 287
      imaging and diagnostic studies, 287, 288*f*
      outcomes, 297
      patient history, 287
      pearls and pitfalls, 296–297
      physical findings, 287
      positioning, 288, 289*f*
      postoperative care, 297
      preoperative planning, 287–288, 288*f*
      stoma creation, 296, 296*f*
      transanal, intersphincteric resection of rectum, 289–291, 289*f*–290*f*
Colon cancer, 203
Colonic inertia, 204
Colonoscopy
   complicated diverticulitis, 185, 186*f*
   laparoscopic transverse colectomy, 101
   left hemicolectomy
      hand-assisted laparoscopic surgery (HALS), 135
      laparoscopic technique, 128
      open technique, 118

low anterior rectal resection (LAR), 244
right hemicolectomy
   hand-assisted laparoscopic surgery (HALS), 71
   robotic-assisted technique, 89
   single-incision laparoscopic technique, 79
robotic total abdominal colectomy, 229
sigmoid colectomy
   hand-assisted laparoscopic surgery (HALS), 165
   laparoscopic technique, 157, 158*f*
   open technique, 148
total abdominal colectomy (TAC)
   hand-assisted laparoscopic surgery (HALS), 216
   open technique, 195
Colon/rectal injuries, 237
   colorectal resection with anastomosis, 239
   colostomy creation, 241, 242*f*
   complications, 243
   creating anastomosis, 239–240, 240*f*–241*f*
   differential diagnosis, 237
   full-thickness injuries, 238
   imaging and diagnostic studies, 237
   mesenteric injuries, 238
   operative exposure and assessment for, 238
   outcomes, 243
   patient history and physical findings, 237
   pearls and pitfalls, 242
   postoperative care, 243
   primary repair, 238, 238*f*
   serosal (partial-thickness) injuries, 238
   surgical management, 237
Colostomy
   colorectal anastomosis, 419–420, 420*f*
   completion, 319, 319*f*–320*f*
   complications, 421
   end sigmoid colostomy, laparoscopic closure of, 418–420
   end transverse colostomy, laparoscopic formation of, 416, 417*f*
   laparoscopic diverting colostomies
      double-barreled colostomy, 415–416
      end colostomy, 416
      imaging and diagnostic studies, 409–410
      laparoscopic equipment, 411–412
      loop colostomy, 415
      patient history, 409
      patient positioning, 411
      perioperative care, 410–411
      physical findings, 409
      port placement, 412–414
      preoperative planning, 410, 411*t*
      sigmoid colostomy, laparoscopic formation of, 414–415, 415*f*
      surgical team positioning, 412
   loop/double-barreled colostomy, closure of, 417, 417*f*
   mobilization, 418–419, 418*f*, 419
   pearls and pitfalls, 420
   postoperative care, 421
   team setup and port placement, 418
Complicated diverticulitis
   differential diagnosis, 185
   Hartmann procedure/emergency sigmoid colectomy
      abdominal closure, 193
      abdominal entry, containing contamination, 192
      colon mobilization and resection, 192–193
      complications with, 194
      outcomes with, 194
      pearls and pitfalls, 193

postoperative care, 193–194
stoma creation, 193
imaging and diagnostic studies, 185, 186*f*
laparoscopic elective sigmoid colectomy, bladder repair
   abdominal access and port placement, 187, 188*f*
   closure, 191
   colon division, 191
   colorectal anastomosis, 191, 192*f*
   descending colon and splenic flexure, 188, 190*f*
   extraction incision, 191
   inferior mesenteric/superior hemorrhoidal artery pedicle, 187–188, 188*f*–189*f*
   rectosigmoid, separation, and fistula repair, 191, 191*f*
patient history and physical findings, 185
surgical management
   patient positioning, 187, 187*f*
   preoperative planning, 186–187
Computed tomography (CT)
   abdominoperineal resection (APR), 322
   coloanal anastomosis, 287
   colon/rectal injuries, 237
   complicated diverticulitis, 185, 186*f*
   enterocutaneous fistula (ECF) with, 19, 19*f*
   hand-assisted laparoscopic surgery (HALS), 322
   inflammatory bowel disease, 9
   laparoscopic appendectomy, 49, 49*f*
   laparoscopic right hemicolectomy, 64
   laparoscopic small bowel resection, 1
   laparoscopic transverse colectomy, 101
   left hemicolectomy
      laparoscopic technique, 128
      open technique, 118
      robotic-assisted technique, 143
   low anterior rectal resection (LAR)
      hand-assisted laparoscopic surgery (HALS), 265
      laparoscopic technique, 253
   right hemicolectomy, 54
      hand-assisted laparoscopic surgery (HALS), 71
      robotic-assisted technique, 89
      single-incision laparoscopic technique, 79
   robotic total abdominal colectomy, 229
   sigmoid colectomy
      hand-assisted laparoscopic surgery (HALS), 165–166
      laparoscopic technique, 157, 157*f*
      single-incision laparoscopic surgery technique, 176
   total abdominal colectomy (TAC)
      hand-assisted laparoscopic surgery (HALS), 216
      laparoscopic technique, 203
      open technique, 195
   transverse colectomy, 93*f*, 94
      hand-assisted laparoscopic surgery (HALS), 110, 110*f*
Contrast-enhanced abdominal computed axial tomography, 148
COVID-19, 80
Crohn disease
   duodenal, 16
   enterocutaneous fistula (ECF) with, 19
   laparoscopic right hemicolectomy, 63
   nonstricturing, nonpenetrating, 9
   penetrating, 9
   stricturing, 9
CT. *See* Computed tomography (CT)
Cytoreductive surgery, 468–469

INDEX **I-3**

D

Deep vein thrombosis (DVT), 116, 323
  left hemicolectomy, laparoscopic technique, 134
  sigmoid colectomy
    hand-assisted laparoscopic surgery (HALS), 166
    open technique, 155
  total abdominal colectomy, hand-assisted laparoscopic surgery, 216
Delorme procedure, 443–444, 443f–444f
Descending colon
  complicated diverticulitis, 188
  hand-assisted laparoscopic surgery (HALS), 113
  mobilization, 348, 348f
  total abdominal colectomy (TAC), 221–222
Descending mesocolon
  hand-assisted laparoscopic surgery (HALS), 112, 112f
  left hemicolectomy, laparoscopic technique, 131–132
  sigmoid colectomy, hand-assisted laparoscopic surgery (HALS), 170, 170f
  total abdominal colectomy (TAC), 221, 222f
Diarrhea, 46
Digital rectal examination (DRE), 276
Diverticulitis, 185
Divided loop ileostomy, creation of, 33
  abdominal wall aperture creation, 33
  ileal limb preparation and placement, 34, 34f
  stoma maturation, 34, 34f
  stoma site skin incision, 33
Drop test, laparoscopic small bowel resection, 2, 2f
Duodenal Crohn disease, 16
Duodenal perforation, 1
Duodenojejunal bypass, 13–14, 14f–15f

E

EAF. *See* Enteroatmospheric fistula (EAF)
ECF. *See* Enterocutaneous fistula (ECF)
End ileostomy
  creation of
    abdominal wall aperture creation, for stoma, 30, 30f–31f
    abdominal wall skin incision for, 30
    ileal limb preparation and placement, 31
    ileal mobilization, 30
    stoma maturation, 32
    stoma site skin incision, 30
  reversal of
    anastomosis after takedown of, 38, 38f
    distal bowel segment, preparation of, 37–38
    fascial closure, 38
    mobilization and resection, 37, 37f
    stoma closure, 37
    stoma site skin closure, 38
End-loop ileostomy
  creation of
    abdominal wall aperture creation, 35
    ileal limb preparation and placement, 35, 35f
    stoma maturation, 35
    stoma site skin incision, 35
  imaging and diagnostic studies, 37
  patient history and physical findings, 36–37
  reversal, 36
  surgical management, 37
Endorectal ultrasound (ERUS)
  laparoscopic technique, 253

low anterior rectal resection (LAR), 244
Endoscopic tissue biopsy, 93
Enhanced recovery after surgery (ERAS), 285
  anemia management, 475
  bowel preparation, 476
  complications, 482
  fasting guidelines, 475–476
  intraoperative management, 476t, 477–479
  left hemicolectomy, robotic-assisted technique, 143
  outcomes, 482
  pearls and pitfalls, 479
  perioperative management
    preadmission management, 474–475, 474t
  postoperative care, 479–482
  preoperative management, 476–477, 476t
  preoperative nutrition, 475
  robotic total abdominal colectomy, 229
  sigmoid colectomy, hand-assisted laparoscopic surgery (HALS), 174
  total abdominal colectomy (TAC), 195
Enhanced recovery protocols, 285
Enteroatmospheric fistula (EAF), 18
  nonsurgical closure of
    abdominal wound and fistula control, 25, 26f
    fibrin glue, closure of, 25, 26f
    newborn with, 25, 25f
    peritoneal contamination control, 25, 26f
  surgical closure of, 23
    abdominal wound and fistula version, 23, 24f
    en bloc resection, 24, 24f
    intestinal transit and abdominal wall, reconstruction of, 24, 24f–25f
    peritoneal contamination control, 23, 24f
Enterocolonic anastomosis, 68, 69f
Enterocutaneous fistula (ECF). *See also* Enteroatmospheric fistula (EAF)
  classifications of, 18
  complications with, 27
  imaging and diagnostic studies, 19–20, 19f
  open abdomen and multiple enteroatmospheric fistulas, 18, 18f
  pearls and pitfalls, 26–27, 26f
  prognostic factors, 18–19, 18f, 19t
  surgical management
    preoperative planning, 20–21
    surgical tips, 21–22, 21f–23f
Epidural pain, 55
Euglycemia, 128
Extracorporeal anastomosis, 85, 85f
Extraperitoneal colostomy technique, 316, 317f

F

Familial adenomatous polyposis (FAP), 203
Female pelvis, sagittal section of, 378, 379f
Finney strictureplasty, 12, 12f
Fistulograms, 19
Fluoroquinolones, 55
Foley catheter, 2
  duodenojejunal bypass, 13
  hand-assisted laparoscopic surgery (HALS), 71
  single-incision laparoscopic technique, 86

G

Gastrocolic ligament, 121, 122f, 132
Gastrografin, 19
Gastrojejunal bypass
  hand-sewn technique, 13, 14f

stapled technique, 13, 14f
GelPort hand-assisted device, 111
Glucagon-like peptic-2 (GLP-2) therapy, 20

H

HALS. *See* Hand-assisted laparoscopic surgery (HALS)
Hand access device, open proctectomy through, 374, 374f–375f
Hand-assisted laparoscopic surgery (HALS)
  abdominoperineal resection (APR)
    complications, 334
    descending colon mobilization, 328
    descending colostomy creation, 332–333
    descending mesocolon, medial to lateral dissection of, 327–328, 327f
    differential diagnosis, 322
    equipment and instrumentation, 323
    imaging and diagnostic studies, 322–323
    inferior mesenteric artery (IMA), 326–327, 326f–327f
    inferior mesenteric vein (IMV), 325–326
    intracorporeal proximal transection, 328
    levator ani muscle, transection of, 330–331, 330f–331f
    open transperineal approach, 331–332, 331f–332f
    outcomes, 334
    patient history, 322
    patient positioning, 323
    pearls and pitfalls, 333
    pelvic dissection, 328–330, 329f–330f
    pelvic inlet, sigmoid colon mobilization off, 328, 328f
    perineal wound closure, 332
    physical findings, 322
    port placement, 324
    postoperative care, 333
    preoperative preparation, 323
    surgical team setup, 323
    team positioning and draping, 323–324, 324f
  left hemicolectomy, 135
    anastomosis, 140, 141f
    assessment of reach, 140
    complications with, 142
    entering abdomen and initial exposure, 136–137, 136f–137f
    imaging and diagnostic studies, 135
    lateral to medial dissection, 140, 140f
    mesenteric dissection, medial to lateral, 137–139, 137f–139f
    outcomes with, 142
    patient history and physical findings, 135
    pearls and pitfalls, 141–142
    postoperative care, 142
    splenic flexure mobilization, 139, 139f
    surgical management, 135–136, 136f
    transverse colon mesentery, 140, 140f
  low anterior rectal resection (LAR), 265
    abdomen closure, 273
    anastomosis, 272–273, 273f
    complications, 275
    differential diagnosis, 265
    extracorporeal proximal transection, 272
    imaging and diagnostic studies, 265
    inferior mesenteric artery (IMA), 267–268, 268f
    inferior mesenteric vein (IMV), 269, 269f
    left colon mobilization, 269, 270f
    operative team setup, 266–267, 267f
    outcomes, 274–275
    patient history and physical findings, 265

I-4   INDEX

Hand-assisted laparoscopic surgery (HALS)
(*continued*)
  pearls and pitfalls, 274
  pelvic dissection and distal rectal
    transection, 271, 272*f*
  port placement, 266–267, 266*f*
  postoperative care, 274
  splenic flexure mobilization, 270–271,
    270*f*–271*f*
  surgical management, 265–266, 266*f*
  rectal prolapse, 449–450, 450*f*
  right hemicolectomy
    ascending colon, lateral mobilization, 74,
      74*f*–75*f*
    bowel resection and anastomosis, 75, 76*f*
    closure, 76
    complications with, 77
    exposure, 72, 72*f*
    hepatic flexure and proximal transverse
      colon, 75, 75*f*
    ileocolic pedicle division, 73, 73*f*
    imaging and diagnostic studies, 71
    indications for, 71
    outcomes with, 77
    patient history and physical findings, 71
    pearls and pitfalls, 77
    postoperative care, 77
    right mesocolon mobilization, 73, 73*f*–74*f*
    surgical management, 71, 72*f*
  sigmoid colectomy, 165
    complications with, 174
    descending mesocolon, 170, 170*f*
    differential diagnosis, 165
    extracorporeal proximal transection, 172
    imaging and diagnostic studies, 165–166
    inferior mesenteric artery (IMA),
      169–170, 170*f*
    inferior mesenteric vein (IMV), 168–169,
      169*f*
    intracorporeal colorectal anastomosis,
      172, 173*f*
    intracorporeal distal transection,
      171–172, 172*f*
    lateral descending colon mobilization,
      170, 171*f*
    outcomes with, 174
    patient history and physical findings, 165
    pearls and pitfalls, 174
    port placement, 167, 168*f*
    postoperative care, 174
    sigmoid colon mobilization, 170, 171*f*
    splenic flexure mobilization, 170–171,
      171*f*–172*f*
    surgical management, 166–167,
      166*f*–167*f*
    wound closure, 173
  total abdominal colectomy (TAC), 216
    ascending colon, lateral mobilization of,
      224–225, 226*f*
    ascending colon, medial to lateral
      mobilization of, 224, 225*f*
    complications with, 228
    descending mesocolon, 221, 222*f*
    differential diagnosis, 216
    extracorporeal mobilization and proximal
      transection, 225–226, 226*f*
    hepatic flexure, 222–223, 223*f*
    ileocolic pedicle, 224, 225*f*
    imaging and diagnostic studies, 216
    inferior mesenteric artery (IMA),
      220–221, 220*f*–221*f*
    inferior mesenteric vein (IMV), 219–220,
      220*f*

intracorporeal distal transection, 225, 226*f*
intracorporeal ileorectal anastomosis,
  226–227, 226*f*
middle colic vessels (supramesocolic
  approach), 223–224, 224*f*
operative field setup, 218, 219*f*
outcomes with, 228
patient history and physical findings, 216
pearls and pitfalls, 227
port placement, 218
postoperative care, 227–228
sigmoid and descending colon, 221–222,
  222*f*
splenic flexure, 222, 223*f*
surgical management, 216–218,
  217*f*–218*f*
wound closure, 227
transverse colectomy, 110
  complications with, 117
  descending colon, 113
  descending mesocolon, 112, 112*f*
  differential diagnosis, 110
  extracorporeal transection and
    anastomosis, 115–116, 116*f*
  imaging and diagnostic studies, 110, 110*f*
  inferior mesenteric vein (IMV), 111–112,
    112*f*
  left colic artery, 112–113, 113*f*
  middle colic vessels (supramesocolic
    approach), 115, 115*f*
  operative field setup, 111
  outcomes with, 117
  patient history and physical findings, 110
  pearls and pitfalls, 116
  pelvic inlet, sigmoid off, 113, 114*f*
  port placement, 111
  postoperative care, 116
  right colon, 115
  splenic flexure, 113, 114*f*
  surgical management, 110–111, 111*f*
Hand-sewn anastomosis, 353, 353*f*–354*f*
Hasson technique, 102
Hasson trocar, 50
Heineke–Mikulicz strictureplasty, 11, 11*f*
Hemogram, 48
Hem-O-Lock clips, appendiceal base with, 51,
  51*f*
Hemorrhoids, 422
  complications, 431–432
  differential diagnosis, 422
  doppler-guided ligation of the hemorrhoidal
    terminal artery branches, 428–429,
    428*f*–429*f*
  imaging and diagnostic studies, 424
  internal hemorrhoids, suture ligation of, 427
  mucosal proctopexy, 428, 429*f*
  outcomes, 431
  patient history, 422–423
  pearls and pitfalls, 430–431
  physical findings, 422–423
  positioning, 423–424, 424*f*
  postoperative care, 431
  preoperative planning, 423
  rubber band ligation, 426–427, 426*f*–427*f*
  sclerosant injection of, 430, 430*f*
  traditional excisional hemorrhoidectomy,
    424–425, 424*f*–426*f*
  transanal hemorrhoidal dearterialization
    device, mucosal proctopexy using,
    428–429, 428*f*–429*f*
Hepatic flexure, 75, 75*f*
  hand-assisted laparoscopic surgery (HALS),
    222–223, 223*f*

robotic-assisted technique, 91
transverse colectomy, 95, 96*f*
Hepatic flexure and right colon mobilization,
  373–374, 373*f*–374F
Hepatic flexure mobilization, 55, 56*f*, 196,
  197*f*
Hereditary nonpolyposis colorectal cancer
  (HNPCC), 214
Hernia sac, anterior dissection of, 441–442
Hyperthermic intraperitoneal chemotherapy,
  469, 469*t*
  delivery modalities, 469–471, 470*f*
  open/coliseum technique, 470, 471*f*

I

Ileal transection, 58, 58*f*
Ileocolic pedicle, 197, 198*f*
Ileocolic pedicle (ICP), 56, 57*f*, 72, 72*f*, 73, 73*f*
Ileocolic vessels, 89, 90*f*
Ileocolonic anastomosis, 59, 59*f*–61*f*
Ileorectal anastomosis, total abdominal
  colectomy (TAC), 201, 201*f*
Ileostomy
  appliance, placement of, 36, 36*f*
  laparoscopic creation of, 35, 41
    ileal limb preparation and placement, 36
    stoma maturation, 36
    stoma orientation, 36
    stoma site skin incision and port
      placement, 36
  reversal, 41
  surgical management
    antibiotic prophylaxis, 29
    intraoperative positioning, 29
    preoperative planning, 28–29
    stoma education, 29
    stoma site marking, 29, 29*f*
Ileotransverse bypass, 15, 15*f*
Inadvertent extracolonic India ink injection, 79
Incision and trocar placement, 371, 371*f*
Incision placement, 346
Inferior mesenteric artery (IMA), 279,
  279*f*–280*f*, 300, 300*f*–301*f*, 348, 349*f*
  complicated diverticulitis, 187, 189*f*
  left hemicolectomy
    hand-assisted laparoscopic surgery
      (HALS), 136, 137*f*
    laparoscopic technique, 131, 131*f*
  low anterior rectal resection (LAR)
    hand-assisted laparoscopic surgery
      (HALS), 267–268, 268*f*
  sigmoid colectomy
    hand-assisted laparoscopic surgery
      (HALS), 169–170, 170*f*
    laparoscopic technique, 160–161,
      160*f*–161*f*
    open technique, 152, 152*f*
    single-incision laparoscopic surgery
      technique, 180, 180*f*
  total abdominal colectomy (TAC), 200, 200*f*
    hand-assisted laparoscopic surgery
      (HALS), 220–221, 220*f*–221*f*
    laparoscopic technique, 209, 209*f*–210*f*
Inferior mesenteric vein (IMV), 279, 279*f*
  hand-assisted laparoscopic surgery (HALS),
    111–112, 112*f*
  left hemicolectomy
    hand-assisted laparoscopic surgery
      (HALS), 138, 139*f*
    laparoscopic technique, 130–131, 130*f*
    robotic-assisted technique, 145–146, 145*f*
  low anterior rectal resection (LAR)

INDEX I-5

hand-assisted laparoscopic surgery (HALS), 269, 269f
sigmoid colectomy
hand-assisted laparoscopic surgery (HALS), 168–169, 169f
total abdominal colectomy (TAC)
hand-assisted laparoscopic surgery (HALS), 219–220, 220f
laparoscopic technique, 210–211, 211f
Inflammatory bowel disease (IBD), 195
bowel evaluation, 11
complications with, 16
differential diagnosis, 9
duodenal strictures, 16
Finney strictureplasty, 12, 12f
Heineke–Mikulicz strictureplasty, 11, 11f
ileotransverse bypass, 15, 15f
imaging and diagnostic studies, 9–10
incision placement, 11
outcomes with, 16
patient history and physical findings, 9
pearls and pitfalls, 16
postoperative care, 16
side-to-side isoperistaltic strictureplasty, 12, 13f
small bowel bypass
duodenojejunal bypass, 13–14, 14f–15f
gastrojejunal bypass, 13, 14f
surgical management
patient positioning, 10
preoperative planning, 10
preparation, 10
Intestinal fistulas, 18
Intestinal reconstruction, 388
Intra-abdominal abscess, 243

J
J-pouch construction, 375, 375f–376f
J-pouch ileoanal anastomosis, 364, 364f–365f

L
Laparoscopic appendectomy
appendiceal base, 50, 50f
appendix
exposure of, 50
transection of, 51–52, 51f–52f
closure, 52
complications with, 53
differential diagnosis, 48
imaging and diagnostic studies, 48–49, 48f–49f
mesoappendix division, 51, 51f
outcomes with, 53
patient history and physical findings, 48
pearls and pitfalls, 53
postoperative care, 53
specimen retrieval, 52, 52f
surgical management
indications for, 49
patient and team positioning, 49, 49f
port placement, 49–50, 49f–50f
preoperative planning for, 49
Laparoscopic-assisted (L) ports, 278f, 279
Laparoscopic elective sigmoid colectomy, bladder repair
abdominal access and port placement, 187, 188f
closure, 191
colon division, 191
colorectal anastomosis, 191, 192f

descending colon and splenic flexure, 188, 190f
extraction incision, 191
inferior mesenteric/superior hemorrhoidal artery pedicle, 187–188, 188f–189f
rectosigmoid, separation, and fistula repair, 191, 191f
Laparoscopic jejunostomy feeding tube placement, 44–45, 44f–45f
Laparoscopic right hemicolectomy, 63
closure, 69
complications with, 70
diagnostic studies, 64, 64f
enterocolonic anastomosis, 68
closure of, 68, 69f
extracorporeal transection, 68, 69f
ileocolic mesentery, medial to lateral mobilization, 65–66, 66f–67f
indications for
adenocarcinoma, 63
benign pathology, 63
carcinoid, 63
neoplastic pathology, 63
lateral colon mobilization, 67, 67f–68f
outcomes with, 70
patient history and physical findings, 63–64, 63t
pearls and pitfalls, 69
port placement, 65, 65f
postoperative care, 70
surgical management, 64, 65f
vascular transection, 65–66
Laparoscopic small bowel resection
abdominal cavity, access to, 2–3, 2f
closure, 7, 7f
complications with, 8
differential diagnosis, 1
disease identification, 4, 4f
imaging and diagnostic studies, 1
mesenteric window, 4, 4f–5f
outcomes with, 8
patient history and physical findings, 1
pearls and pitfalls, 7–8
port placement, 3, 3f–4f
postoperative care, 8
small bowel anastomosis, 5–6, 5f–6f
specimen
placement, 5, 5f
removal, 7
surgical management
patient positioning, 2
preoperative planning, 1–2
Laparoscopic suture rectopexy, 447–449, 447f–449f
Laparoscopic transverse colectomy, 101
complications with, 108–109
exploration, 103, 103f
imaging and diagnostic studies, 101
lateral attachments and omentum, 106, 106f
outcomes with, 108
patient history and physical findings, 101
pearls and pitfalls, 108
pedicle ligation, 103, 103f–104f
postoperative care, 108
retromesenteric dissection, 104, 105f–106f
skin incisions, 102, 102f
specimen exteriorization and anastomosis, 107, 107f
surgical management, 101, 102f
Laparotomy
left hemicolectomy
hand-assisted laparoscopic surgery (HALS), 137

open technique, 119
sigmoid colectomy, open technique, 150
Lateral colon mobilization, 67, 67f–68f
Lateral compartment dissection, 381–383, 381f–382f
Lateral descending colon mobilization, 170, 171f
Left colic artery, 112–113, 113f
Left colon
mobilization, 371–372, 371f
splenic flexure, mobilization of, 279–280, 279f–280f
Left hemicolectomy
hand-assisted laparoscopic surgery (HALS), 135
anastomosis, 140, 141f
assessment of reach, 140
complications with, 142
entering abdomen and initial exposure, 136–137, 136f–137f
imaging and diagnostic studies, 135
lateral to medial dissection, 140, 140f
mesenteric dissection, medial to lateral, 137–139, 137f–139f
outcomes with, 142
patient history and physical findings, 135
pearls and pitfalls, 141–142
postoperative care, 142
splenic flexure mobilization, 139, 139f
surgical management, 135–136, 136f
transverse colon mesentery, 140, 140f
laparoscopic technique
abdominal wound closure, 132
complications with, 134
descending mesocolon, 131–132
differential diagnosis, 127
extracorporeal resection and anastomosis, 132, 133f
gastrocolic ligament and lesser sac, 132
imaging and diagnostic studies, 128
inferior mesenteric artery (IMA), 131, 131f
inferior mesenteric vein (IMV), 130–131, 130f
left colic artery, 131
lymphovascular pedicle resection, 127, 127f
omentum placement, 129, 130f
operative field setup, 129, 129f
outcomes with, 134
patient history and physical findings, 127–128
pearls and pitfalls, 133–134
port placement, 129, 129f
postoperative care, 134
splenic flexure mobilization, 132, 132f
surgical management, 128, 129f
white line of Toldt, 132
open technique, 118
colon extraction and anastomosis, 124, 124f–125f
complications with, 126
differential diagnosis, 118
dual (medial and lateral) approach, 121, 122f–123f
imaging and diagnostic studies, 118
laparotomy, 119
lateral to medial dissection, 123, 123f
left colon mesentery, 120, 121f
outcomes with, 126
patient history and physical findings, 118
pearls and pitfalls, 126
peritoneal cavity, 119, 125

I-6 INDEX

Left hemicolectomy (*continued*)
    peritoneal sectioning, 120, 120*f*
    peritoneum, 120, 121*f*
    postoperative care, 126
    sigmoid colon, 120, 120*f*
    surgical field preparation, 119, 119*f*–120*f*
    surgical management, 118, 119*f*
    vascular isolation, 123–124, 124*f*
  robotic-assisted technique, 143
    colorectal anastomosis, 146–147, 146*f*–147*f*
    complications with, 147
    differential diagnosis, 143
    dissection, 144–145, 145*f*
    docking, 144
    imaging and diagnostic studies, 143
    inferior mesenteric artery (IMA), 145–146, 145*f*
    inferior mesenteric vein (IMV), 145–146, 145*f*
    patient history and physical findings, 143
    pearls and pitfalls, 147
    postoperative care, 147
    proximal transection point and mesentery, 146
    rectosigmoid colon, 146, 146*f*
    small bowel positioning, 144, 144*f*
    surgical management, 143
    trocar placement, 144, 144*f*
Lesser sac
  left hemicolectomy, laparoscopic technique, 132
  transverse colectomy, 94–95, 95*f*
Leukocyte scintigraphy, 10
Ligament of Treitz, 43, 43*f*
  hand-assisted laparoscopic surgery (HALS), 111, 112*f*
  left hemicolectomy, 138, 139*f*
Loop ileostomy, 28
  abdominal wall aperture creation, 32
  ileal limb preparation and placement, 32, 33*f*
  imaging and diagnostic studies, 28, 37
  patient history and physical findings, 28, 36–37
  reversal, 36, 38, 39*f*
  stoma maturation, 32, 33*f*
  stoma site skin incision, 32
  surgical management, 37
Low anterior rectal resection (LAR)
  anastomosis, 283, 284*f*
  coloanal anastomosis, 248, 248*f*–249*f*
  complications, 251, 285
  differential diagnosis, 244
  enhanced recovery protocols, 285
  hand-assisted laparoscopic surgery (HALS), 265
    abdomen closure, 273
    anastomosis, 272–273, 273*f*
    complications, 275
    differential diagnosis, 265
    extracorporeal proximal transection, 272
    imaging and diagnostic studies, 265
    inferior mesenteric artery (IMA), 267–268, 268*f*
    inferior mesenteric vein (IMV), 269, 269*f*
    left colon mobilization, 269, 270*f*
    operative team setup, 266–267, 267*f*
    outcomes, 274–275
    patient history and physical findings, 265
    pearls and pitfalls, 274
    pelvic dissection and distal rectal transection, 271, 272*f*
    port placement, 266–267, 266*f*

    postoperative care, 274
    splenic flexure mobilization, 270–271, 270*f*–271*f*
    surgical management, 265–266, 266*f*
  imaging and diagnostic studies, 244–245, 276–277, 277*f*, 277*t*
  inferior mesenteric artery, transection of, 279, 279*f*–280*f*
  inferior mesenteric vein, transection of, 279, 279*f*
  laparoscopic technique, 253
    anastomosis techniques, 262–263, 262*f*–263*f*
    anterior dissection of, 260, 260*f*
    complications with, 264
    differential diagnosis, 253
    hand-sewn anastomosis, 263, 263*f*
    imaging and diagnostic studies, 253–254
    lateral dissection of, 259–260
    low anterior resection, 255, 255*f*–256*f*
    omental dissection and splenic flexure mobilization, 256, 256*f*
    operative steps, 255
    outcomes with, 264
    patient history and physical findings, 253
    pearls and pitfalls, 263
    pelvic dissection of, 260
    posterior dissection of, 259, 259*f*
    postoperative care, 264
    proximal dissection of, 261, 261*f*–262*f*
    surgical management, 254–255, 254*f*–255*f*
    total mesorectal excision (TME), 258–259, 258*f*
    vascular oncologic approach, 256–258, 257*f*–258*f*
  left colon and splenic flexure, mobilization of, 279–280, 279*f*–280*f*
  outcomes, 251, 285
  patient history, 244, 276
  pearls and pitfalls, 251, 284
  physical examination, 276
  physical findings, 244
  positioning, 278–279
  postoperative care, 251, 285
  preoperative planning, 277–278
  rectal cancer, minimally invasive *vs.* open resection for, 276
  robotic-assisted laparoscopic technique, 276
  robotic total mesorectal excision, 281–282, 281*f*–282*f*
  surgical management, 245, 245*f*
  total mesorectal excision (TME)
    abdominal exploration, 245
    colonic mesentery and splenic flexure, 245–246, 246*f*
    incision, 245
    lateral rectal ligaments, 247, 248*f*
    left and sigmoid colon, 245
    rectum and hypogastric nerve identification, 247, 247*f*
    rectum and proximal colonic transection, 247, 248*f*
    small bowel retraction, 245
    vessel ligation and left ureter identification, 246, 246*f*
Low molecular weight heparin (LMWH), 214

M

Magnetic resonance enterography (MRE)
  inflammatory bowel disease, 9
  laparoscopic small bowel resection, 1
Magnetic resonance imaging (MRI)

abdominoperineal resection (APR), 322
enterocutaneous fistula (ECF) with, 20
hand-assisted laparoscopic surgery (HALS), 322
laparoscopic appendectomy, 49
laparoscopic small bowel resection, 1
low anterior rectal resection (LAR), 244
  hand-assisted laparoscopic surgery (HALS), 265
  laparoscopic technique, 253
  restorative proctocolectomy with ileal pouch-anal anastomosis (RP/IPAA), 354
right hemicolectomy
  single-incision laparoscopic technique, 79
  sigmoid colectomy, single-incision laparoscopic surgery technique, 177
  total abdominal colectomy (TAC), 195
  transverse colectomy, 94
MANTRELS score, 48
Medicaid insurance, 156
Mesoappendix, 51, 51*f*
Metronidazole, 55
Middle colic vessels (supramesocolic approach), 115, 115*f*, 223–224, 224*f*
Molecular residual disease (MRD), 79
Monopolar scissors, 281
MRE. *See* Magnetic resonance enteroclysis (MRE)
MRI. *See* Magnetic resonance imaging (MRI)
Mucosal proctopexy, 428, 429*f*

N

National Surgical Quality Improvement Program (NSQIP), 142
Neurogenic bowel, 204
Nonocclusive bowel necrosis, 46
Normothermia, 128
Nutritional assessment, 42

O

Obesity, 63
Omentum dissection, 94–95, 95*f*
Open jejunostomy feeding tube placement, 43–44, 43*f*
Open lateral internal sphincterotomy, 436, 437*f*

P

Patient induction/positioning, 369, 369*f*–370*f*
Pedicle ligation, laparoscopic transverse colectomy, 103, 103*f*–104*f*
Pelvic abscess, 155
Pelvic exenteration
  abdominal phase
    anterior compartment dissection, 383–386, 384*f*–385*f*
    intestinal reconstruction, 388
    lateral compartment dissection, 381–383, 381*f*–382*f*
    perineal closure and reconstruction, 388–389
    perineal phase, 388
    posterior compartment dissection, 385*f*–387*f*, 386–387
    urinary reconstruction, 388
  compartments, 378, 378*f*
  complications, 390, 391*t*
  female pelvis, sagittal section of, 378, 379*f*
  imaging and diagnostic studies, 379–380, 380*f*
  outcomes, 390

INDEX I-7

patient history, 378–379
pearls and pitfalls, 389–390
physical findings, 378–379
positioning, 380–381, 381f
postoperative care, 390
preoperative planning, 380
Perianal fistula, 458–459, 458f–459f
complications, 459
differential diagnosis, 455
imaging and diagnostic studies, 456
patient history, 455–456
pearls and pitfalls, 459
physical findings, 455–456
positioning, 456, 456f–457f
postoperative care, 459
potential anatomical locations, 455f
Perineal closure, 319, 319f–320f, 388–389
Perineal dissection, 317, 318f
Perineal phase, 388
Perineal proctectomy, 441, 441f–443f
Perineal rectum dissection, 318–319
Perineal wound, closure of, 304
Perineum dissection, 303, 303f–304f
Perirectal abscess, 457
complications, 459
differential diagnosis, 455
imaging and diagnostic studies, 456
patient history, 455–456
pearls and pitfalls, 459
physical findings, 455–456
positioning, 456, 456f–457f
postoperative care, 459
potential anatomical locations, 455f
Peritoneal carcinomatosis
complications, 472
cytoreductive surgery, 468–469
hyperthermic intraperitoneal chemotherapy,
469, 469t, 473
delivery modalities, 469–471, 470f
open/coliseum technique, 470, 471f
imaging and diagnostic studies,
466, 467f
outcomes, 472–473
patient selection, 466
pearls and pitfalls, 472
positioning and team setup, 467–468,
467f–468f
postoperative care, 472
preoperative planning, 467
resection, grading of, 469, 469t
Pfannenstiel incision, 173, 178, 178f
Pilonidal disease (PD)
complications, 465
cyst complex, exteriorization of, 461, 461f
differential diagnosis, 460
En bloc excision
primary closure, 462–463, 462f–464f
secondary closure, 464
imaging and diagnostic studies, 460
patient history, 460
pearls and pitfalls, 465
physical findings, 460
postoperative care, 465
surgical management, 460–461
Pneumoperitoneum, 72, 89
Positive FIT-DNA test, 79
Positron emission tomography (PET)
low anterior rectal resection (LAR)
laparoscopic technique, 254
sigmoid colectomy, single-incision
laparoscopic surgery technique, 177
single-incision laparoscopic technique, 79
Posterior compartment dissection, 385f–387f,
386–387

Posterior dissection, 442, 442f, 447–449,
448f–449f
Posterior levatorplasty, 442, 443f
Pouch-anal anastomosis, 375, 375f–376f
Presacral plane, single-incision laparoscopic
surgery technique, 179–180, 180f
Proximal transverse colon, 75, 75f, 91

R

Raja Isteri Pengiran Anak Saleha Appendicitis
(RIPASA) score, 48
Rectal cancer, 276
Rectal prolapse
perineal approach
anesthesia induction, preparation after,
441
complications, 445
Delorme procedure, 443–444, 443f–444f
differential diagnosis, 439
hernia sac, anterior dissection of, 441–442
imaging and diagnostic studies, 440, 441f
incision, 441
outcomes, 445
patient history, 439–440
pearls and pitfalls, 444
perineal proctectomy, 441, 441f–443f
positioning, 440
posterior dissection, 442, 442f
posterior levatorplasty, 442, 443f
postoperative care, 445
preoperative planning, 440
redundant rectosigmoid resection, 442
transabdominal approach
closure, 449
complications, 454
differential diagnosis, 446, 446f
hand-assisted laparoscopic surgery
(HALS), 449–450, 450f
imaging and diagnostic studies, 447
insufflation, port, and team setup, 447,
448f
laparoscopic suture rectopexy, 447–449,
447f–449f
operative planning and strategy, 447
outcomes, 454
patient history, 446–447, 446f
pearls and pitfalls, 454
positioning, 447, 447f
posterior dissection, 447–449, 448f–449f,
450–452, 451f–452f
postoperative care, 454
rectopexy, 449, 449f
sigmoid resection, open rectopexy with/
without, 452–454, 452f–453f
Rectal wall defect, closure of, 396, 397f
Rectopexy, 449, 449f
Rectosigmoid colon, left hemicolectomy, 146,
146f
Rectum mobilization, 301–303, 301f–302f
Redundant rectosigmoid resection, 442
Restorative proctocolectomy with ileal
pouch-anal anastomosis (RP/IPAA)
hand-assisted laparoscopic surgery (HALS)
complications, 377
differential diagnosis, 368
hand access device, open proctectomy
through, 374, 374f–375f
hepatic flexure and right colon
mobilization, 373–374, 373f–374F
imaging and diagnostic studies, 368, 368f
incision and trocar placement, 371, 371f
J-pouch construction, 375, 375f–376f
left colon mobilization, 371–372, 371f

outcomes, 377
patient history, 368
patient induction/positioning, 369,
369f–370f
patient preparation, 369
pearls and pitfalls, 376
physical findings, 368
postoperative care, 377
pouch-anal anastomosis, 375, 375f–376f
splenic flexure mobilization, 372–373,
372f–373F
surgical management, 369
temporary diverting loop ileostomy
construction, 376, 376f
open technique
complications, 355
descending colon mobilization, 348, 348f
differential diagnosis, 345
diverting stoma and closure creation, 354
hand-sewn anastomosis, 353, 353f–354f
imaging and diagnostic studies, 345
incision placement, 346
inferior mesenteric artery transection, 348,
349f
outcomes, 355
patient history, 345
pearls and pitfalls, 354
physical findings, 345
positioning, 345–346, 346f
postoperative care, 354
pouch creation, 350–351, 350f–351f
preoperative planning, 345
proctectomy, 349–350, 349f–350f
right colon, mobilization of, 346,
346f–347f
stapled anastomosis, 352
transverse colon mobilization, 347, 347f
single-incision laparoscopic technique
complications, 367
diagnostic laparoscopy, 358, 358f
diverting loop ileostomy, 365, 366f
ileoanal pouch anastomosis, 365
ileoanal pouch formation, 364,
364f–365f
imaging and diagnostic studies, 357
instrumentation, 357
J-pouch ileoanal anastomosis, 364,
364f–365f
outcomes, 367
patient history, 356
patient positioning, 357–358, 357f
pearls and pitfalls, 366
physical findings, 356
postoperative care, 366–367
proctectomy and total mesorectal
excision, 361–362, 361f–362f
right colon mobilization, 359, 359f
single multichannel port technique, 358,
358f
splenic flexure mobilization, 360–361,
360f–361f
transanal single-port total mesorectal
excision, 362–364, 363f–364f
transverse colon, mobilization of,
359–360, 359f–360f
Retraction placement and orientation sutures,
395, 395f
Retromesenteric dissection, laparoscopic
transverse colectomy, 104, 105f–106f
Retroperitoneal plane, single-incision
laparoscopic surgery technique, 180,
180f
Right colon mobilization, 55, 56f, 346,
346f–347f

I-8 INDEX

Right hemicolectomy
anesthesia, 55
bowel transection, 58, 58f
closure, 61
complications with, 62
differential diagnosis, 54
hand-assisted laparoscopic surgery (HALS)
ascending colon, lateral mobilization, 74, 74f–75f
bowel resection and anastomosis, 75, 76f
closure, 76
complications with, 77
exposure, 72, 72f
hepatic flexure and proximal transverse colon, 75, 75f
ileocolic pedicle division, 73, 73f
imaging and diagnostic studies, 71
indications for, 71
outcomes with, 77
patient history and physical findings, 71
pearls and pitfalls, 77
postoperative care, 77
right mesocolon mobilization, 73, 73f–74f
surgical management, 71, 72f
ileocolonic anastomosis, 59, 59f–61f
imaging and diagnostic studies, 54, 54f
incision, 55
laparoscopic, 63
closure, 69
complications with, 70
diagnostic studies, 64, 64f
enterocolonic anastomosis, 68, 69f
extracorporeal transection, 68, 69f
ileocolic mesentery, medial to lateral mobilization, 65–66, 66f–67f
indications for, 63
lateral colon mobilization, 67, 67f–68f
outcomes with, 70
patient history and physical findings, 63–64, 63t
pearls and pitfalls, 69
port placement, 65, 65f
postoperative care, 70
surgical management, 64, 65f
vascular transection, 65–66
patient history and physical findings, 54
patient positioning, 55
pearls and pitfalls, 61
postoperative care, 61
right colon mobilization, 55, 56f
robotic-assisted technique, 88
complications with, 92
contraindications, 88
hepatic flexure, 91
ileocolic vessels, identification and ligation of, 89, 90f
indications, 88
intracorporeal anastomosis, 91, 91f
middle colic vessel ligation, 91
patient history and physical findings, 88
pearls and pitfalls, 92
port placement and exploratory laparoscopy, 89, 90f
proximal transverse colon, 91
reinspection and closure, 91
retroperitoneal plane and duodenum identification, 90, 90f
right colon and terminal ileum, 91
surgical management, 89
trunk of Henle, 91
single-incision laparoscopic technique
ascending mesocolon, 82–83, 82f–83f
complications with, 86
diagnostic laparoscopy, 81–82, 81f

differential diagnosis, 78
extracorporeal anastomosis, 85, 85f
extracorporeal transection, 84, 84f
imaging and diagnostic studies, 79
intraoperative indocyanine bowel perfusion, 84, 84f
midtransverse colon, 84, 84f
midtransverse colon mesentery, 83, 84f
outcomes with, 86
patient history and physical findings, 78–79, 78t
pearls and pitfalls, 85–86
postoperative care, 86
surgical management, 79–80, 80f
terminal ileal mesentery, 83, 83f
wound closure, 85
surgical management, 55
vascular anatomy of, 54, 54f
vascular pedicle transection, 56–57, 58f
Right mesocolon mobilization, 73, 73f–74f
Robotic-assisted laparoscopic surgery technique, 276
abdominoperineal resection (APR)
colostomy and closure, 343
complications, 344
descending and sigmoid mesocolon, lateral mobilization of, 338
descending and sigmoid mesocolon, medial to lateral dissection of, 338
exploration and robotic docking, 337
imaging and diagnostic studies, 335–336
incision, 337, 337f
intracorporeal proximal transection, 339
mesorectal dissection, 339–341, 339f–342f
outcomes, 344
patient history, 335
pearls and pitfalls, 344
perineal procedure, 342–343, 343f
physical findings, 335
port placement and instruments, 337, 337f
positioning, 336, 336f
postoperative care, 344
preoperative planning, 336
presacral plane, 337, 338f
vascular division, 338, 338f
left hemicolectomy, 143
colorectal anastomosis, 146–147, 146f–147f
complications with, 147
differential diagnosis, 143
dissection, 144–145, 145f
docking, 144
imaging and diagnostic studies, 143
inferior mesenteric artery (IMA), 145–146, 145f
inferior mesenteric vein (IMV), 145–146, 145f
patient history and physical findings, 143
pearls and pitfalls, 147
postoperative care, 147
proximal transection point and mesentery, 146
rectosigmoid colon, 146, 146f
small bowel positioning, 144, 144f
surgical management, 143
trocar placement, 144, 144f
right hemicolectomy, 88
complications with, 92
contraindications, 88
hepatic flexure, 91
ileocolic vessels, identification and ligation of, 89, 90f

indications, 88
intracorporeal anastomosis, 91, 91f
middle colic vessel ligation, 91
patient history and physical findings, 88
pearls and pitfalls, 92
port placement and exploratory laparoscopy, 89, 90f
proximal transverse colon, 91
reinspection and closure, 91
retroperitoneal plane and duodenum identification, 90, 90f
right colon and terminal ileum, 91
surgical management, 89
trunk of Henle, 91
Robotic colectomy, 88
Robotic total abdominal colectomy, 229
abdominal access, 231
bowel resection and anastomosis, 233–234, 234f
complications with, 235
differential diagnosis, 229
ileocolic mesentery and right colon, 231–232, 231f–232f
imaging and diagnostic studies, 229
inferior mesenteric artery, 233, 233f
inferior mesenteric vein and distal transverse colon, 232–233, 232f
middle colic vasculature, 231
outcomes with, 235
patient history and physical examination, 229, 229f
pearls and pitfalls, 234
postoperative care, 235
surgical management, 229–231, 230f–231f
Robotic total mesorectal excision, 281–282, 281f–282f

S
Sepsis, 20
Sequential compression devices (SCDs), 80
Side-to-side isoperistaltic strictureplasty, 12, 13f
Sigmoid colectomy
hand-assisted laparoscopic surgery (HALS), 165
complications with, 174
descending mesocolon, 170, 170f
differential diagnosis, 165
extracorporeal proximal transection, 172
imaging and diagnostic studies, 165–166
inferior mesenteric artery (IMA), 169–170, 170f
inferior mesenteric vein (IMV), 168–169, 169f
intracorporeal colorectal anastomosis, 172, 173f
intracorporeal distal transection, 171–172, 172f
lateral descending colon mobilization, 170, 171f
outcomes with, 174
patient history and physical findings, 165
pearls and pitfalls, 174
port placement, 167, 168f
postoperative care, 174
sigmoid colon mobilization, 170, 171f
splenic flexure mobilization, 170–171, 171f–172f
surgical management, 166–167, 166f–167f
wound closure, 173
laparoscopic technique, 157
anastomosis, 163, 163f

complications with, 164
differential diagnosis, 157
imaging and diagnostic studies, 157, 157f–158f
inferior mesenteric artery (IMA), 160–161, 160f–161f
lateral peritoneal attachments, 161–162
medial to lateral mobilization, 161, 161f
operating team setup, 159, 159f
outcomes with, 164
patient history and physical findings, 157
pearls and pitfalls, 164
port placement, 159, 160f
postoperative care, 164
sigmoid colon, 162–163, 162f
splenic flexure, 161–162, 162f
surgical management, 157–159, 159f
wound closure, 163
open technique, 148
anastomosis, 153–154, 153f–154f
closure, 155
colon transection, 152, 153f
complications with, 155
differential diagnosis, 148
disparities, 155–156
imaging and diagnostic studies, 148
inferior mesenteric artery (IMA), 152, 152f
inspection, 150
laparotomy, 150
left colon and left ureter, 150, 150f–151f
operating team setup, 149, 149f
outcomes with, 155
patient history and physical findings, 148
patient positioning, 149, 149f
pearls and pitfalls, 155
postoperative care, 155
splenic flexure, 151, 151f
surgical field preparation, 150
surgical management, 148–149
single-incision laparoscopic surgery technique, 176
bowel continuity, 182–183, 182f–183f
bowel diversion, 183
bowel division, 181, 181f
complications with, 184
exploration and adhesions, lysis of, 179
high vascular division, 180, 180f
imaging and diagnostic studies, 176–177, 176f
incision and port placement, 178, 178f
lateral attachments and splenic flexure takedown, 181, 181f
outcomes with, 184
patient history and physical findings, 176
pearls and pitfalls, 184
postoperative care, 184
presacral plane, 179–180, 180f
retroperitoneal plane, 180, 180f
surgical management, 177, 177f
technical alternatives, 183
Sigmoid colon mobilization, 300, 300f–301f, 312–313, 313f
Sigmoid mesocolon, 279
Sigmoid resection, open rectopexy with/without, 452–454, 452f–453f
Single-incision laparoscopic surgery technique restorative proctocolectomy with ileal pouch-anal anastomosis (RP/IPAA)
complications, 367
diagnostic laparoscopy, 358, 358f
diverting loop ileostomy, 365, 366f
ileoanal pouch anastomosis, 365
ileoanal pouch formation, 364, 364f–365f

imaging and diagnostic studies, 357
instrumentation, 357
J-pouch ileoanal anastomosis, 364, 364f–365f
outcomes, 367
patient history, 356
patient positioning, 357–358, 357f
pearls and pitfalls, 366
physical findings, 356
postoperative care, 366–367
proctectomy and total mesorectal excision, 361–362, 361f–362f
right colon mobilization, 359, 359f
single multichannel port technique, 358, 358f
splenic flexure mobilization, 360–361, 360f–361f
transanal single-port total mesorectal excision, 362–364, 363f–364f
transverse colon, mobilization of, 359–360, 359f–360f
right hemicolectomy
ascending mesocolon, 82–83, 82f–83f
complications with, 86
diagnostic laparoscopy, 81–82, 81f
differential diagnosis, 78
extracorporeal anastomosis, 85, 85f
extracorporeal transection, 84, 84f
imaging and diagnostic studies, 79
intraoperative indocyanine bowel perfusion, 84, 84f
midtransverse colon, 84, 84f
midtransverse colon mesentery, 83, 84f
outcomes with, 86
patient history and physical findings, 78–79, 78t
pearls and pitfalls, 85–86
postoperative care, 86
surgical management, 79–80, 80f
terminal ileal mesentery, 83, 83f
wound closure, 85
sigmoid colectomy, 176
bowel continuity, 182–183, 182f–183f
bowel diversion, 183
bowel division, 181, 181f
complications with, 184
exploration and adhesions, lysis of, 179
high vascular division, 180, 180f
imaging and diagnostic studies, 176–177, 176f
incision and port placement, 178, 178f
lateral attachments and splenic flexure takedown, 181, 181f
outcomes with, 184
patient history and physical findings, 176
pearls and pitfalls, 184
postoperative care, 184
presacral plane, 179–180, 180f
retroperitoneal plane, 180, 180f
surgical management, 177, 177f
technical alternatives, 183
Single plus one sigmoidectomy, 176
Small bowel bypass, 9. See also Inflammatory bowel disease
duodenojejunal bypass, 13–14, 14f–15f
gastrojejunal bypass, 13, 14f
Small bowel follow-through (SBFT), 19
Specimen extraction dissection, 318–319
Splenic flexure
complicated diverticulitis, 188, 190f
hand-assisted laparoscopic surgery (HALS), 113, 114f
left hemicolectomy

hand-assisted laparoscopic surgery (HALS), 139, 139f
laparoscopic technique, 132, 132f
left hemicolectomy, open technique, 121, 122f–123f
mobilization, 57, 58f, 372–373, 372f–373f
sigmoid colectomy
hand-assisted laparoscopic surgery (HALS), 170–171, 171f–172f
laparoscopic technique, 161–162, 162f
open technique, 151, 151f
single-incision laparoscopic surgery technique, 181, 181f
total abdominal colectomy (TAC), 196, 197f
hand-assisted laparoscopic surgery (HALS), 222, 223f
laparoscopic technique, 212, 212f
transverse colectomy, 95, 96f
Splenic injury, 108
Splenocolic ligament, 121, 122f–123f
Spontaneous fistula, probability of, 18, 19t
Stapled anastomosis, 352
Stapled ileocolonic anastomosis, 59, 59f–60f
Stricturing disease, 9
Strictureplasty, 9
contraindications to, 10
Finney strictureplasty, 12, 12f
Heineke–Mikulicz strictureplasty, 11, 11f
indications for, 10
recurrence following, 16
side-to-side isoperistaltic strictureplasty, 12, 13f
Subjective Global Assessment Score, 42
Suture line failure, 243
Systemic inflammatory response syndrome (SIRS), 19

T

TAC. See Total abdominal colectomy (TAC)
Temporary diverting loop ileostomy construction, 376, 376f
Terminal ileal mesentery, 83, 83f
Terminal ileum, 91
Top-down technique, 311, 311f–312f
Total abdominal colectomy (TAC)
hand-assisted laparoscopic surgery (HALS), 216
ascending colon, lateral mobilization of, 224–225, 226f
ascending colon, medial to lateral mobilization of, 224, 225f
complications with, 228
descending mesocolon, 221, 222f
differential diagnosis, 216
extracorporeal mobilization and proximal transection, 225–226, 226f
hepatic flexure, 222–223, 223f
ileocolic pedicle, 224, 225f
imaging and diagnostic studies, 216
inferior mesenteric artery (IMA), 220–221, 220f–221f
inferior mesenteric vein (IMV), 219–220, 220f
intracorporeal distal transection, 225, 226f
intracorporeal ileorectal anastomosis, 226–227, 226f
middle colic vessels (supramesocolic approach), 223–224, 224f
operative field setup, 218, 219f
outcomes with, 228
patient history and physical findings, 216
pearls and pitfalls, 227

I-10 INDEX

Total abdominal colectomy (TAC) (*continued*)
  port placement, 218
  postoperative care, 227–228
  sigmoid and descending colon, 221–222, 222*f*
  splenic flexure, 222, 223*f*
  surgical management, 216–218, 217*f*–218*f*
  wound closure, 227
  laparoscopic technique, 203
    complications with, 215
    ileorectal anastomosis/end ileostomy, 212–213, 213*f*
    imaging and diagnostic studies, 203–204
    inferior mesenteric artery (IMA), 209, 209*f*–210*f*
    inferior mesenteric vein (IMV), 210–211, 211*f*
    left colon mobilization, 209
    outcomes with, 214–215
    patient history and physical findings, 203
    pearls and pitfalls, 214
    port placement, 204–205, 205*f*
    postoperative care, 214
    rectal transection, 212, 212*f*
    right and middle mesenteric vasculature, 208, 208*f*
    right colon mobilization, 206–207, 206*f*–207*f*
    splenic flexure mobilization, 212, 212*f*
    surgical management, 204, 204*f*
    team setup, 204–205, 205*f*
    transverse colon mobilization, 207, 207*f*
  open technique, 195
    ascending colon mobilization, 196, 196*f*
    closure, 201
    complications with, 202
    descending colon mobilization, 199, 199*f*
    differential diagnosis, 195
    distal division, 200, 200*f*
    ileorectal anastomosis, 201, 201*f*
    imaging and diagnostic studies, 195
    incision and access, 196
    patient history and physical findings, 195
    pearls and pitfalls, 201–202
    postoperative care, 202
    proximal division, 197–198, 198*f*
    surgical management, 195
    transverse colon mobilization, 196, 197*f*
  robotic, 229
    abdominal access, 231
    bowel resection and anastomosis, 233–234, 234*f*
    complications with, 235
    differential diagnosis, 229
    ileocolic mesentery and right colon, 231–232, 231*f*–232*f*
    imaging and diagnostic studies, 229
    inferior mesenteric artery, 233, 233*f*
    inferior mesenteric vein and distal transverse colon, 232–233, 232*f*
    middle colic vasculature, 231
    outcomes with, 235
    patient history and physical examination, 229, 229*f*
    pearls and pitfalls, 234
    postoperative care, 235
    surgical management, 229–231, 230*f*–231*f*
Total mesorectal excision (TME), 314–316, 314*f*–316*f*
  low anterior rectal resection (LAR)
    abdominal exploration, 245
    colonic mesentery and splenic flexure, 245–246, 246*f*

incision, 245
    lateral rectal ligaments, 247, 248*f*
    left and sigmoid colon, 245
    rectum and hypogastric nerve identification, 247, 247*f*
    rectum and proximal colonic transection, 247, 248*f*
    small bowel retraction, 245
    vessel ligation and left ureter identification, 246, 246*f*
Transanal excision (TAE) of rectal tumors
  alternative surgical strategies, 398–399
  complications, 398
  full-thickness excision of the mass, 395–396, 396*f*
  imaging and diagnostic studies, 392–393
  lesion exposure, 394, 394*f*
  outcomes, 398
  patient history, 392
  patient positioning, 393, 393*f*, 393*t*
  pearls and pitfalls, 397–398
  physical findings, 392
  postoperative care, 398
  preoperative planning, 393, 393*t*
  rectal wall defect, closure of, 396, 397*f*
  retraction placement and orientation sutures, 395, 395*f*
  specimen to pathology, 396, 396*f*
  surgical margin, 394–395, 394*f*
Transanal, intersphincteric resection of rectum, 289–291, 289*f*–290*f*
Transanal minimally invasive surgery (TAMIS)
  anatomic considerations, 401
  complications, 407–408
  differential diagnosis, 400
  equipment, 402–405, 403*f*–406*f*
  imaging and diagnostic studies, 400–401
  indications for, 401
  outcomes, 407
  patient history, 400
  pearls and pitfalls, 406–407
  physical findings, 400
  positioning, 402, 402*f*
  postoperative care, 407
  preoperative preparation, 402
Transverse colectomy
  hand-assisted laparoscopic surgery (HALS), 110
    complications with, 117
    descending colon, 113
    descending mesocolon, 112, 112*f*
    differential diagnosis, 110
    extracorporeal transection and anastomosis, 115–116, 116*f*
    imaging and diagnostic studies, 110, 110*f*
    inferior mesenteric vein (IMV), 111–112, 112*f*
    left colic artery, 112–113, 113*f*
    middle colic vessels (supramesocolic approach), 115, 115*f*
    operative field setup, 111
    outcomes with, 117
    patient history and physical findings, 110
    pearls and pitfalls, 116
    pelvic inlet, sigmoid off, 113, 114*f*
    port placement, 111
    postoperative care, 116
    right colon, 115
    splenic flexure, 113, 114*f*
    surgical management, 110–111, 111*f*
  laparoscopic, 101
    complications with, 108–109
    exploration, 103, 103*f*
    imaging and diagnostic studies, 101

lateral attachments and omentum, 106, 106*f*
    outcomes with, 108
    patient history and physical findings, 101
    pearls and pitfalls, 108
    pedicle ligation, 103, 103*f*–104*f*
    postoperative care, 108
    retromesenteric dissection, 104, 105*f*–106*f*
    skin incisions, 102, 102*f*
    specimen exteriorization and anastomosis, 107, 107*f*
    surgical management, 101, 102*f*
  open technique, 93
    abdominal closure, 99
    bowel resection and anastomosis, 97, 98*f*
    complications with, 100
    differential diagnosis, 93
    hepatic flexure and splenic flexure, 95, 96*f*
    imaging and diagnostic studies, 93–94, 94*f*
    incision and abdominal exploration, 94
    middle colic vessels, isolation and division of, 96, 97*f*
    omentum dissection and lesser sac exposure, 94–95, 95*f*
    outcomes with, 99
    patient history and physical findings, 93, 93*f*
    pearls and pitfalls, 99
    postoperative care, 99
    surgical management, 94
Transverse colon
  mesentery, 140, 140*f*
  mobilization, 347, 347*f*
Tube jejunostomy
  complications with, 46–47
  imaging and diagnostic studies, 42
  laparoscopic jejunostomy feeding tube placement, 44–45, 44*f*–45*f*
  open jejunostomy feeding tube placement, 43–44, 43*f*
  outcomes with, 46
  patient history and physical findings, 42
  pearls and pitfalls, 46
  postoperative care, 46
  surgical management
    patient positioning, 42
    preoperative planning, 42

U

Ulcerative colitis, 9
Ultrasound (US)
  colon/rectal injuries, 237
  enterocutaneous fistula (ECF), 19
  inflammatory bowel disease, 9
  laparoscopic appendectomy, 48, 48*f*
  single-incision laparoscopic technique, 79
Ureteric injury, 147
Urinary reconstruction, 388

V

Vacuum-assisted closure (VAC) therapy, 21, 21*f*
Vascular pedicle transection, 56–57, 58*f*
Venous thromboembolic prophylaxis, 55
Venous thromboembolism (VTE), 214
Veress needle, laparoscopic small bowel resection, 2, 2*f*

W

Witzel technique, 43, 43*f*

QUADM 0523